For Anna, Giuseppe
and Paolo... again.
More than ever
G.A.S.

To my family
G. Di F.

Giulio Aniello Santoro • Giuseppe Di Falco

Benign Anorectal Diseases

Diagnosis with Endoanal and Endorectal Ultrasound and New Treatment Options

Foreword by

G.G. Delaini

Springer

Giulio Aniello Santoro, M.D., Ph.D.
Head, Section of Anal Physiology and Ultrasound
Coloproctology Service
Department of Surgery
Regional Hospital-Treviso
Italy
giulioasantoro@yahoo.com
www.endorect.com

Giuseppe Di Falco, M.D.
Chairman, Department of Surgery
Regional Hospital-Treviso
Italy

Anatomical drawings by Nadia Simeoni (Turin, Italy)

Library of congress control number: 2005933616

ISBN-10 88-470-0336-9 Springer Milan Berlin Heidelberg New York
ISBN-13 978-88-470-0336-1 Springer Milan Berlin Heidelberg New York

Springer is a part of Springer Science+Business Media
springer.com

Cover design: Estudio Calamar, Barcelona, Spain
Typesetting: ITG sas, Turin, Italy

Foreword

Pathology is the accomplished tragedy;
Physiology is the basis on which our treatment rests.

Samuel Butler

Benign anorectal diseases are quite common among the general population. Although the exact incidence is unknown, we estimate an overall prevalence of 3–7%. Most of these diseases significantly affect patients' quality of life. For example, fecal incontinence is a devastating condition, and it is the second leading cause of admission to long-term care facilities in the United States. Besides, more than US $400 million is spent each year for adult diapers necessitated by fecal incontinence.

During the last 10 years, the attention given by the media to these diseases has led to less embarrassment and fewer social stigmas associated with them, which in turn has led to a greater willingness for sufferers to talk openly about their conditions and seek medical care.

Fistula-in-ano, obstructed defecation, and fecal incontinence are still major surgical challenges. The high rate of surgical failure and the need for repeat surgery are common experiences of physicians dealing with these conditions. One reason for these poor results is the lack of comprehensive knowledge about the pathophysiology of these diseases, and therefore, surgery treats the symptoms and not the causes. In the last decade, funding opportunities for benign anorectal disease research has increased vastly. The turning point was a better comprehension of anatomic damage, determined by magnetic resonance imaging and endoanal–endorectal ultrasound. The latter is becoming the paramount diagnostic instrument for use by colorectal surgeons, as it allows a clear understanding of underlying anatomic defects. Paradoxically, even if the method most likely to alter management of these diseases is endoanal–endorectal ultrasound, there remains a lack of formal training programs in most countries. The investigation is usually carried out by interested clinicians. It is clear that endoanal-endorectal ultrasound is heavily operator dependent, and it is most important that accreditation be put in place to ensure quality assurance.

Benign anorectal diseases: Diagnosis with endoanal and endorectal ultrasound and new treatment options offers a balanced and clear overview on the approach to these conditions. Ranging from the endosonographic anatomy of the normal anal canal and the rectum, through the ultrasonographic assessment of the different benign anorectal diseases to state-of-the-art surgical therapy and new treatment options by expert authors, this book offers a major contribution to the effort of standardizing diagnostic and therapeutic approaches. High-quality and extensive illustrations along with practice-orientated guidelines make this book a fundamental reference for all specialists – from colorectal surgeons to gastroenterologists, radiologists and gynecologists.

Verona, January 2006

Professor Gian Gaetano Delaini, M.D.
Chairman, Clinica Chirurgica
University of Verona, Italy

Preface

Benign anorectal and perineal diseases occur very frequently and should be considered a social problem, constituting an important economic burden to health care resources.

Fecal incontinence has a major impact on quality of life. The true prevalence of this devastating condition is grossly underestimated due to embarrassment experienced by patients often reluctant to admit their symptoms. In the majority of cases, fecal incontinence occurs in women with an obstetric injury, and symptoms may develop even in an elderly population who experienced vaginal deliveries earlier in life.

Anorectal fistula is a common disorder. Understanding the anatomy and pathogenesis of fistulas is mandatory to identify the primary fistula tract and the internal opening; to ascertain whether there are secondary tracts, horseshoe configurations, or abscesses; and to tailor treatment accordingly. Recurrences are frequently a result of the surgeon's failure to expose the entire fistula tract out of fear of impairing anal continence.

Obstruction defecation syndrome is another common benign anorectal disease, which is characterized by an impaired expulsion of the bolus after calling to defecate. Patients complain of different symptoms that often lead to a poor quality of life. This condition may be due to a broad range of causes, and the precise pathophysiology should always be cleared to offer the appropriate management of these complex cases.

In the last two decades, different tests and procedures for evaluating benign anorectal and perineal diseases developed, improving our knowledge of the pathogenesis of these disorders. Within these techniques, endoanal and endorectal ultrasonography have become an important, integral part of the routine colorectal practice because of their accessibility, relative simplicity of performance, and low cost. Anal endosonography is used most often to detect anal sphincter defects in patients with fecal incontinence, to classify anal fistulas and perianal abscesses, and to evaluate patients with obstructed defecation, providing important diagnostic and prognostic information and directly altering management. A major advance has been the recent introduction of high-resolution, three-dimensional ultrasound with surface- and volume-rendered modes, which has resulted in a better understanding of normal and abnormal anorectal patterns.

For these reasons, 2 years after publishing the *Atlas of Endoanal and Endorectal Ultrasonography: Staging and Treatment Options for Anorectal Cancer*, we felt the necessity to present this second book, *Benign Anorectal Diseases: Diagnosis with Endoanal and Endorectal Ultrasound and New Treatment Options*. This book is the fruit of over 10 years of personal experience in this field and of a collaborative effort by radiologists, gastroenterologists, and colorectal surgeons. Sections I and II present a broad base of information on fundamental principles of ultrasound imaging and currently available equipment for endoanal and endorectal ultrasonography, with new technical developments in three-dimensional reconstruction. Section III provides the state of the art in pelvic floor imaging, with considerable detailed description of endosonographic anatomy of the normal anal canal and rectum. Magnetic resonance imaging of the anorectal region and pelvic structures is also described. Sections IV and V extensively evaluate the role of endoanal ultrasonography in the assessment of patients with fecal incontinence, perianal sepsis, and fistula-in-ano. Accuracy and reliability of ultrasonography is reported, along with a detailed review of recent ultrasound literature and a critical comparison between ultrasound and magnetic resonance imaging. Section VI focuses on updates in the evaluation of outlet obstruction. Here, the conventional defecographic study is discussed, along with the new procedures of endorectal ultrasound, dynamic anorectal endosonography, transvaginal ultrasonography, transperineal dynamic ultrasonography, and dynamic magnetic resonance defecography. Section VII focuses on the description of other physiologic procedures, such as manometry and electromyography, in an effort to show which testings are really necessary and should be recommended in evaluating benign anorectal disorders. Sections VIII–X assess the more practical aspects of treatment options for anal fistulas; traditional and innovative surgical techniques for fecal incontinence, including dynamic graciloplasty, artificial anal sphincter, sacral neuromodulation, radiofrequency delivery, bulking agent injection, biofeedback, and other nonoperative modalities; and for outlet obstruction. Indications, contraindications, risks, benefits, and limitations are accurately examined.

Considerable space has been dedicated to drawings illustrating anatomy and techniques and to two-dimensional and three-dimensional echographic images in order to help the reader to learn how to see and interpret ultrasound and to provide more experienced proctologists with an opportunity to review and reassess their techniques.

We wish to express our deep appreciation to all colleagues, among the foremost experts with outstanding qualifications in this complex field, who have contributed to the many different chapters and provided critical commentaries of the different sections of this volume. Without their experience and cooperation, this book could not have been possible. Once more, thanks must go to our hospital, the advanced technological support of which gave us the possibility to accomplish this new project; to the medical illustrator Mrs. Nadia Simeoni, who has realized the numerous artistic drawings; and to Mr. Fabrizio Giavenni, managing director of B-K Medical Italia and Bjørn Fortling, biomedical engineer – Denmark, for gathering much of the data and photographic material of the technological equipment. Finally, our sincere gratitude goes to Mrs. Antonella Cerri and Mrs. Angela Vanegas of the medical editorial staff of Springer-Verlag Italia, for their constant assistance throughout the development of the project, organizing every stage of the editorial work.

We are confident that this textbook will be met with great interest from colorectal surgeons and all other clinicians involved in the care of patients suffering from benign anorectal diseases.

Treviso, December 2005 **G.A. Santoro, G. Di Falco**

Contents

Contributors

Pier Francesco Almerigi, M.D.
Department of Surgery
and Anaesthesiology
University of Bologna
S. Orsola-Malpighi Hospital
Bologna, Italy

Donato F. Altomare, M.D.
Associate Professor of Surgery
Head of Coloproctological Unit
Department of Emergency and Organ
Transplantation, General Surgery and
Liver Transplantation Unit
University of Bari
Bari, Italy

David C.C. Bartolo, M.S., F.R.C.S.
Consultant Colorectal Surgeon
Colorectal Unit
Western General Hospital
Edinburgh, Scotland, United Kingdom

Gabriele Bazzocchi, M.D.
Chief, Rehabilitation for Visceral
Disorders Unit
Montecatone Rehabilitation Institute
University of Bologna
Imola, Italy

Marc Beer-Gabel, M.D.
Director of the Pelvic Floor Unit
Consultant Gastroenterologist
Tel Hashomer Hospital
Tel-Aviv, Israel

Geerard L. Beets, M.D., Ph.D.
Department of Surgery
University Hospital Maastricht
Maastricht, The Netherlands

Regina G.H. Beets-Tan, M.D., Ph.D.
Department of Radiology
University Hospital Maastricht
Maastricht, The Netherlands

Roberto Bellomo, M.D.
Department of Surgery
Ospedale "S. Maria dei Battuti"
S.Vito al Tagliamento
Pordenone, Italy

Nicolae Bolog, M.D.
Institute of Diagnostic Radiology
University Hospital
Zürich, Switzerland

Michael Camilleri, M.D.
Clinical Enteric Neuroscience
Translational and Epidemiological
Research (C.E.N.T.E.R.) Group
Mayo Clinic College of Medicine
Rochester, Minnesota, United States

Bruno Cola, M.D., F.A.C.S.
President of the European
Council of Coloproctology
Chairman, Department of Surgery and
Anaesthesiology
University of Bologna
S. Orsola-Malpighi Hospital
Bologna, Italy

Dajana Cuicchi, M.D.
Department of Surgery
and Anaesthesiology
University of Bologna
S. Orsola-Malpighi Hospital
Bologna, Italy

Richelle J.F. Felt-Bersma, M.D., Ph.D.
Department of Gastroenterology
and Hepatology
VU University Medical Center
Amsterdam, The Netherlands

Bjørn Fortling
Engineer
B-K Medical
Herlev, Denmark

Franco Galanti, M.D.
Department of Surgery
Ospedale "S. Maria dei Battuti"
S.Vito al Tagliamento
Pordenone, Italy

Giuseppe Gizzi, M.D.
Associate Professor
Department of Medicine and
Gastroenterology
University of Bologna
S. Orsola-Malpighi Hospital
Bologna, Italy

Steve Halligan, M.B., B.S., M.D.,
F.R.C.P., F.R.C.R.
Professor of Gastrointestinal Radiology
Department of Specialist Radiology
University College Hospital
London, United Kingdom

Tracy L. Hull, M.D.
Head, Section of Anal Physiology
and Ultrasound
Department of Colorectal Surgery
The Cleveland Clinic Foundation
Cleveland, Ohio, United States

Michael Hünerbein, M.D., Ph.D.
Department of Surgery and Surgical
Oncology
Charité University Hospital
Campus Berlin Buch and Helios
Hospital
Berlin, Germany

Aldo Infantino, M.D.
Chief, Department of Surgery
Ospedale "S. Maria dei Battuti"
S.Vito al Tagliamento
Pordenone, Italy

Urban Karlbom, M.D., Ph.D.
Associate Professor
Department of Surgery
University Hospital
Uppsala, Sweden

Jonathan B. Kruskal, M.D., Ph.D.
Chief, Abdominal Imaging
Beth Israel Deaconess
Medical Center
Associate Professor of Radiology
Harvard Medical School
Boston, Massachussets, United States

Max J. Lahaye, M.D.
Department of Radiology
Department of Surgery
University Hospital Maastricht
Maastricht, The Netherlands

Wouter H. Lamers, M.D., Ph.D.
Department of Anatomy
& Embryology
University Hospital Maastricht
Maastricht, The Netherlands

Raffaele Lombardi, M.D.
Department of Surgery
and Anaesthesiology
University of Bologna
S. Orsola-Malpighi Hospital
Bologna, Italy

Borut Marincek, M.D.
Professor of Radiology
Chairman, Institute of Diagnostic
Radiology
University Hospital
Zürich, Switzerland

Klaus E. Matzel, M.D.
Chirurgische Klinik
mit Poliklinik
FAU Erlangen-Nurnberg
Erlangen, Germany

Lars Påhlman, M.D., Ph.D., F.R.C.S.,
F.R.C.S. (Glasg)
Professor of Surgery
Department of Surgery
University Hospital
Uppsala, Sweden

CLAUDIO PASTORE, M.D.
Coloproctology Service,
Department of Surgery
Regional Hospital
Treviso, Italy

LUCIANO PELLEGRINI, M.D.
Division of Gastroenterology
M.F. Toniolo Hospital
Bologna, Italy

LIA PISEGNA CERONE, M.D.
Department of Surgery
Ospedale "S. Maria dei Battuti"
S.Vito al Tagliamento
Pordenone, Italy

CARLO RATTO, M.D.
Department of Clinica Chirurgica
Catholic University
Rome, Italy

ALBERTO REALIS LUC, M.D.
Colorectal Unit
Colorectal Eporediensis Center
Policlinico of Monza
Monza, Italy

BEATRICE SALVIOLI, M.D., PH.D.
Department of Internal Medicine
University of Bologna
S. Orsola-Malpighi Hospital
Bologna, Italy

AHMED SHAFIK, M.D., PH.D.
Professor and Chairman
Department of Surgery
and Experimental Research,
Faculty of Medicine
Cairo University
Cairo, Egypt

JAAP STOKER, M.D., PH.D.
Professor of Radiology
Department of Radiology
Academic Medical Center
University of Amsterdam
Amsterdam, The Netherlands

ANGELO STUTO, M.D.
Department of Surgery
S.M.A. Hospital
Pordenone, Italy

STUART A. TAYLOR, M.D., M.R.C.P., F.R.C.R.
Consultant Radiologist and Honorary
Senior Lecturer
Department of Imaging
University College Hospital
London, United Kingdom

MAAIKE P. TERRA, M.D.
Department of Radiology
Academic Medical Center
University of Amsterdam
Amsterdam, The Netherlands

JOE J. TJANDRA, M.B.B.S., M.D., F.R.A.C.S.,
F.R.C.S., F.R.C.P.S., F.A.S.C.R.S
Associate Professor of Surgery
Department of Colorectal Surgery
Epworth and Royal Melbourne Hospital
University of Melbourne
Melbourne, Victoria, Australia

MARIO TROMPETTO, M.D.
Colorectal Unit
Colorectal Eporediensis Center
Policlinico of Monza
Monza, Italy

DOMINIK WEISHAUPT, M.D.
Institute of Diagnostic Radiology
University Hospital
Zürich, Switzerland

STEVEN D. WEXNER, F.A.C.S., F.R.C.S.,
F.R.C.S. (ED)
Chairman, Department of Colorectal
Surgery
Cleveland Clinic Florida
Weston, Florida, United States

ANDREW ZBAR, MD, FRCS (ED), FRCS
(GEN), FRACS, FCCS
Professor of Surgery
School of Clinical Medicine
and Research
University of the West Indies
Cave Hill Campus
St. Michael, Barbados

LUIGI ZORCOLO, M.D.
Assistant Professor
Colorectal Unit
University of Cagliari
Cagliari, Italy

SECTION I

Fundamental Principles of Ultrasound Imaging

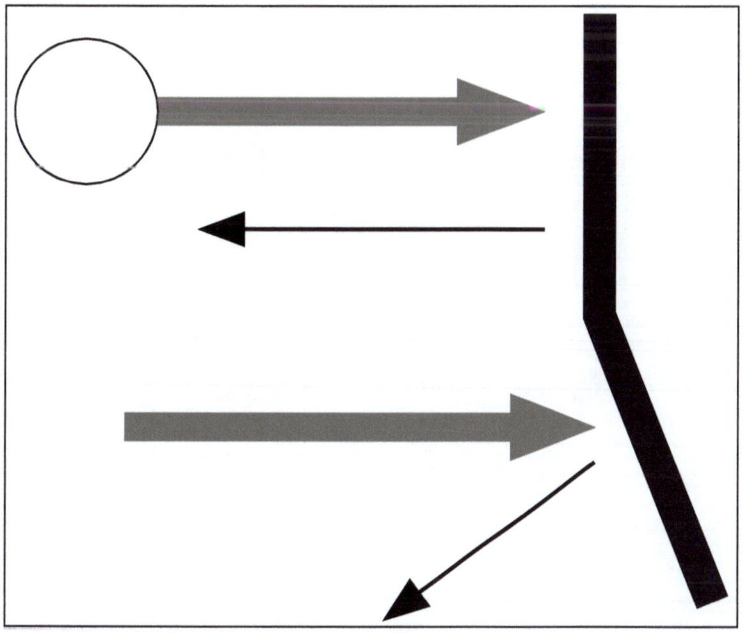

Fundamental Principles of Ultrasound Imaging

G.A. Santoro

In examinations using external energy sources such as X-rays, ultrasound, and injected radioactive substances, the information contained in the images is produced by the interaction between the energy and the organ under examination. This interaction can be visualized in two different ways: an image may be formed by the energy which manages to pass through the organ or its parts, or the energy reflected or scattered from portions of the structure under examination may be transferred into images. The two techniques are respectively termed visualization by transmission and visualization by reflection. In the visualization by transmission technique, the energy is propagated through the object, i.e., the biological tissues; the energy which is not absorbed, scattered, or reflected by the tissues is visualized. Traditional radiology makes use of this technique. The visualization by reflection method uses the energy which has been scattered back from or reflected by the tissues. Diagnostic ultrasound currently uses the technique of formation of images by reflection.

Nature of Ultrasound

The term ultrasound describes the general form of mechanical energy emitted at a frequency above the limit of human audibility. The maximum frequency audible to humans is in the range of 16–20,000 cycles per second, called Hertz (Hz), whereas in diagnostic applications frequencies in the 2.5–20 MHz (megahertz = million cycles per second) range are used, corresponding to wavelengths of 1–0.1 mm in tissue.

Ultrasonic Transducer

The ultrasonic energy required to form an image must be supplied from an external source which can be continuous or impulsive. The formation of images by reflection makes use of impulsive ultrasound energy. The basic transducer, also called probe, which transmits and receives the ultrasonic impulses is made up of a piezoelectric disk (which is a ceramic crystal, usually lead zirconate titanate) that after the application of an electrical current, vibrates and transmits these vibrations into the object in contact with it. The ultrasound frequency depends on the thickness of the crystal. The piezoelectric effect is symmetrical, so that the same crystal can be used as a receiver to produce small electrical signals when struck by an ultrasound wave.

Propagation in Tissue

Elastic waves at ultrasonic frequency are generated by a perturbation which causes the particles of a given medium to vibrate. The vibration of the particles of the medium is a basic characteristic of the propagation of elastic waves. It is therefore impossible for such waves to advance in a vacuum. Different modes of propagation are possible, and in diagnostic applications, longitudinal waves are used. The term means that the motion of the particles in the medium is parallel to the direction of wave propagation. The molecules move back and forth around their intermediate position producing bands of compression and rarefaction so that the energy is transmitted through the medi-

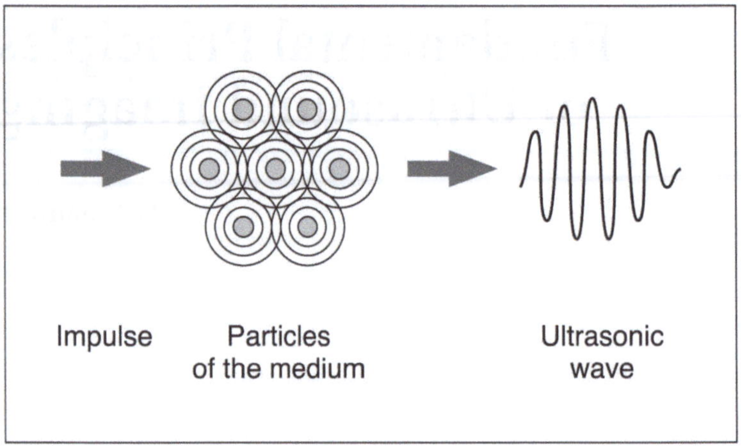

Fig. I.1. Elastic waves are generated by a perturbation which causes the particles of a medium to vibrate. The vibrations of the particles are in the direction of propagation of the wave

um as a perturbation without transfer of matter (Fig. I.1). Each repetition of this back-and-forth motion is called a cycle. The length of the wave (λ) is the distance between two bands of compression or rarefaction. The velocity at which the energy is transmitted through the medium, which coincides with the velocity of propagation v, depends on the strength of the elastic forces between particles (which relates to the elasticity of the tissue) and to the masses of the particles (which determines density of the medium). These two factors determine the acoustic impedance of the tissue. When the particles are heavy, a given ultrasound energy is transmitted with small movements of the particles; when they are light, larger excursions are involved. The velocity of propagation can be roughly considered constant in the frequency interval used in diagnostic applications. The wavelength λ and the frequency f are linked to the velocity of propagation v by the equation: $v=f \times \lambda$.

As a sound beam passes through the body, the beam is attenuated or reduced in intensity by a combination of absorption, reflection, refraction, and diffusion. The intensity at each point of a wave is defined as the energy flow per unit of time through the unit area perpendicular to the direction of propagation at the point considered. The amplitude of the ultrasound beam is expressed in decibels (dB). For average soft tissues, the loss amounts to approximately 1 dB per centimeter tissue depth for each megahertz. The acoustic absorption is mainly due to the transformation of the ultrasonic energy into thermal energy. Three factors determine the amount of absorption: (1) the frequency of the sound; (2) the viscosity of the conducting medium, mainly linked to the protein content; and (3) the relaxation time of the medium. The relaxation time is the time it takes for a molecule to return to its original position after it has been displaced. Absorption is very low in fluid media, intermediate in soft tissue, and very high in bone and gas at the frequencies used in diagnostics (Table I.1).

Ultrasound energy is also lost to the receiving transducer if it is reflected or refracted away from the returning line of sight or if the beam diverges. When an ultrasonic wave propagating in an acoustically uniform medium reaches an interface with a medium of differing characteristic mechanical impedance (Table I.2), reflection and refraction of the wave occurs. Image formation depends entirely on the returning echoes. The amount of reflection depends on the difference in the acoustic impedance of the two surfaces and on the angle of incidence of the beam. Acoustic impedance is the product of the density and velocity of sound in the conducting medium. Within soft tissues, only a few percent is reflected at each interface, but almost total reflection occurs at tissue/gas interfaces. For incidence of a wave over a theoretically plane surface, the reflec-

Table I.1. Absorption coefficients for various materials

Material	Absorption coefficient (dB/cm)
Water	0.002
Blood	0.2
Fat	0.6
Skeletal muscle	1-5–2.5
Bone	10
Air	35

Table I.2. Resonance coefficients for various interfaces

	Resonance coefficient
Interface between water and fat	3.5%
Interface between water and bone	68%
Interface between water and air	100%

tion obeys Snell's law for light, and waves are reflected at an angle equal to the angle of incidence (specular reflection). When the incidence of the ultrasound wave between two media is perpendicular to the surface (normal incidence) (Fig. I.2a), the reflection is optimal. When the incidence is oblique, the reception of the reflected ultrasound by the transducer depends on the angle of incidence (Fig. I.2b). Using a rotating endoprobe within mainly circular structures such as sphincters, most specular reflections will be at right angles and so maximal (Fig. I.3). Strength and directionality are the cardinal features of echoes from flat surfaces. Where the irregularities in the surface are of the same order of size as the ultrasound wavelength, a different mechanism – known as scattering – produces echoes. Here, each small interface is vibrated by the mechanical shock it has received from the incident ultrasound pulse. The vibratory energy is reradiated equally in all directions, each discontinuity behaving as an isolated point source of ultrasound (Fig. I.4). It is important to note that the texture in the image is an interference pattern and is not a one-to-one representation of the histological reality. Scattering within biological tissues reduces the propagating energy so that it contributes to attenuation together with reflection and absorption. Whatever the properties of biological tissues (the amount of collagen fibers is the dominant element in determining the value of characteristic

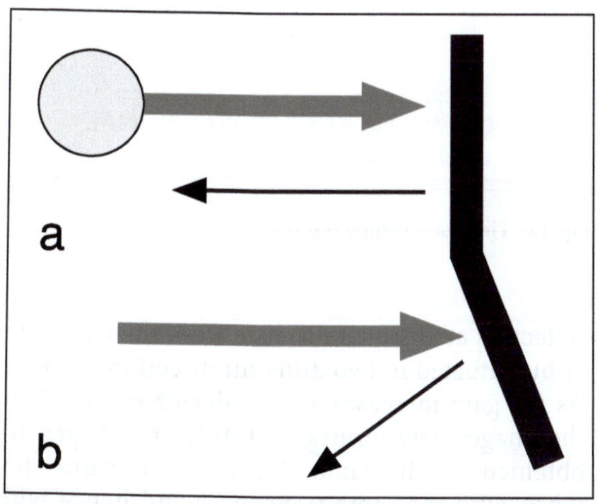

Fig. I.2. Specular reflection: normal incidence (**a**), oblique incidence (**b**)

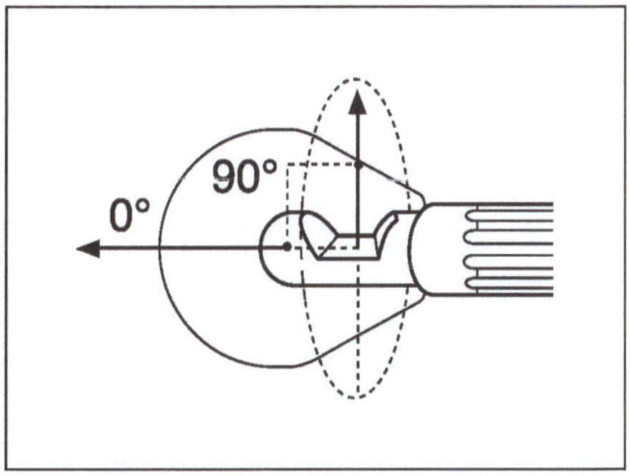

Fig. I.3. Using a rotating endoprobe within mainly circular structures, most specular reflections will be at right angles and so maximal

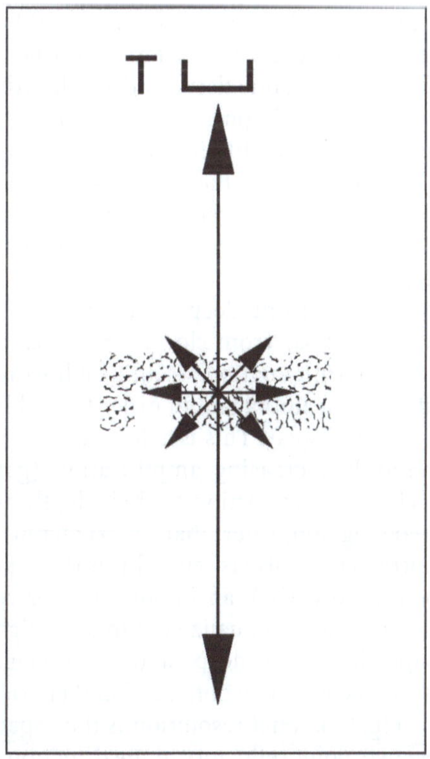

Fig. I.4. Diffraction develops when the interface is much smaller than the wavelength of the incident wave that is scattered uniformly in all directions (T = transducer)

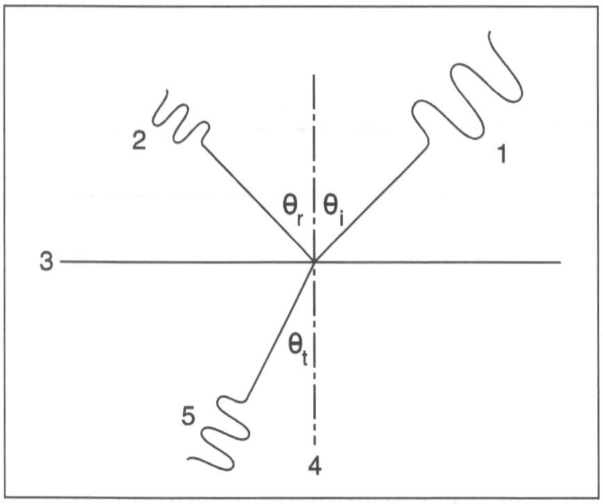

Fig. I.5. Refraction of the ultrasound wave along the pathway with oblique incidence between two media with different propagation velocities: incident wave (*1*), reflected wave (*2*), interface (*3*), normal line (*4*), refracted wave (*5*)

impedance) contribute to the formation of discontinuity of characteristic impedance and their variations, the physics of scattering or reflection of widespread structures is not yet possible to establish. Fat, gas, and bone have very different densities, but various soft tissues have very similar densities, and changes in impedance are due to alteration in the elasticity of the tissues. When the mechanical vibration encounters an obstacle (the interfaces between one tissue and another, discontinuity in the biological tissue, cavities full of fluid, air bubbles, or foreign bodies) as the wave front advances, part of the energy is reflected and the rest continues or is refracted, with an angle of refraction different from the angle of incidence (Fig. I.5).

The echoes from deep structures are much weaker than those from closer structures due to greater signal attenuation. Accurate adjustment of amplification is important in order to enable adequate screen display. This is achieved by applying progressively increasing amplification (gain) to later echoes in proportion to their depth using a time-varying amplifier that is triggered when each ultrasound pulse is sent. This is the time gain compensation (TGC), an important user control that must be set to equalize the image brightness for superficial and deep structures (Fig. I.6). Adjustments influence both axial and lateral resolution (Fig. I.7). Axial resolution is the capacity to resolve two-point reflectors in the direction of the axis of the ultrasound beam. Lateral resolution signifies the capacity for resolving two-point reflectors at an equal distance from the transducer but situated in two different directions from it. As the gain increases, the rendering of details in the images deteriorates, and different images are obtained for the same objects, at the same distance, with the same transducer and hence with the same potential lateral resolution (Fig. I.8).

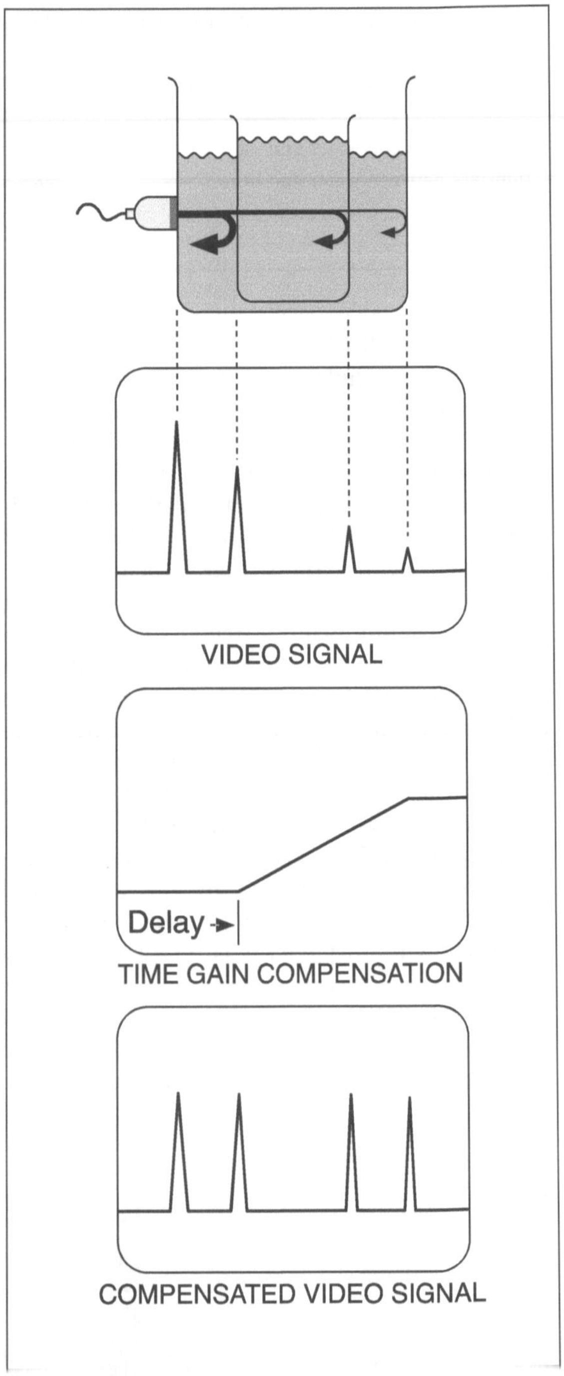

Fig. I.6. Time gain compensation

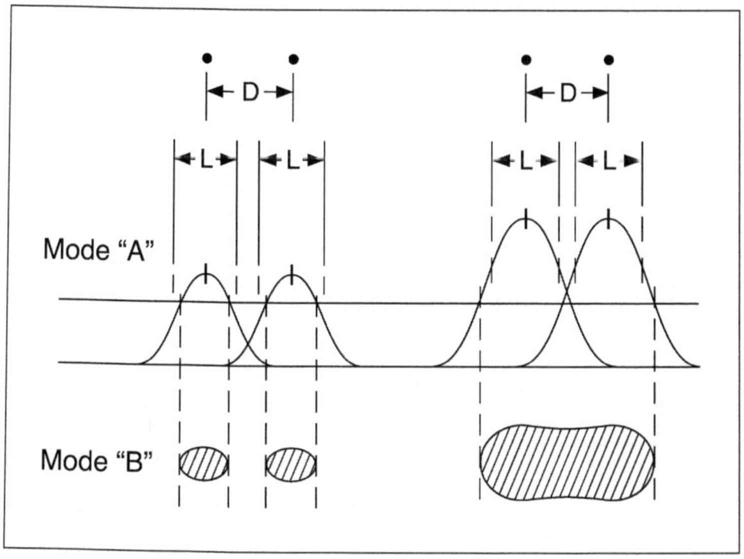

Fig. I.7. Influence of gain adjustment of echographic equipment on the resolution obtained in mode B display. As the gain increases (*right-hand figure*) the rendering of details in the images deteriorates

Scanning Methods

The same transducer used to emit the ultrasonic impulse responds to mechanical vibrations by generating a corresponding electrical signal. In the conventional pulse-echo ultrasound process, signals are recorded at a depth calculated from the time delay between transmission and receipt of the echoes using the value of the speed and sound in tissue to convert from time to depth. The signal is transmitted to a series of electronic circuits and frequently presented as a luminous signal on the screen of an oscilloscope (Fig. I.9). By making a correlation between the luminous point on the screen and the distance traveled by the ultrasonic waves advancing within the tissues, an image is formed of the organization of the layers encountered by the ultrasound beam in the direction in which the transducer is pointing. The images used in clinical echography may appear as images of the amplitude of the echo signals in relation to the

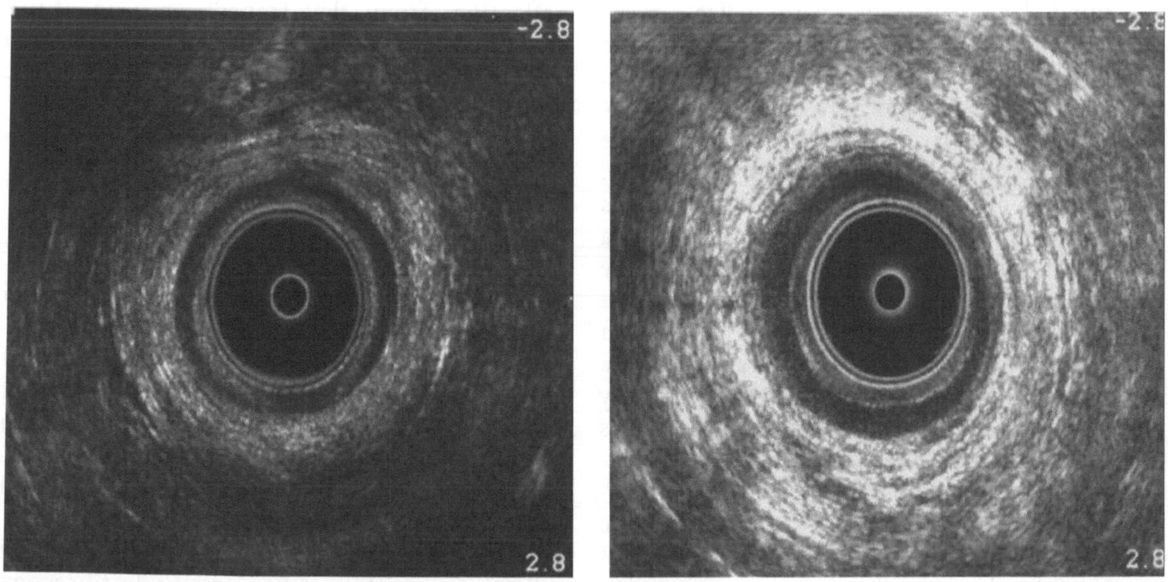

a b

Fig. I.8. The uniform time gain compensation makes the image in **b** brighter

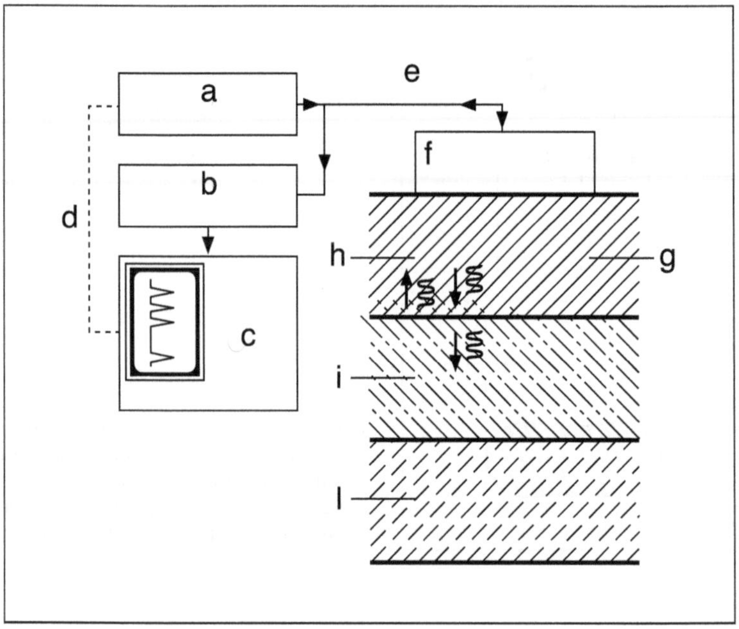

Fig. I.9. Diagram of echographic equipment with amplitude mode (A-mode) display: transmitter (*a*), receiver (*b*), oscilloscope (*c*), trigger signal (*d*), pulse electrical signal (*e*), piezoelectric transducer (*f*), pulse mechanical signal (*g*), medium 1 (*h*), medium 2 (*i*), medium 3 (*l*)

distance from the probe along a single observation direction (A-mode, or amplitude mode), or the return signals may be displayed as luminous dots on the screen (B-mode, or brightness mode), the brightness of which is amplitude dependent. Grey scale means that the brightness is assigned to one of a fixed series of shades of grey, usually 256 in number. The illuminate dots are displayed on the screen in the same sequence of time and geometry according to which the ultrasonic signal encounters a differing acoustic impedance along its path while the ultrasonic beam moves in the scanning plane. This system permits two-dimensional imaging of a section (tomography) in the scanning plane. If a sequence of scans is performed at a sufficiently high frequency, a continuous, real-time display is supplied of sections of the organ even though the organ is in motion. Information on the absorption of different tissues and the depth of the organ to be studied allow a choice of probes for various applications. The highest frequencies give better resolution and better display of detail, but the tradeoff for this is a short focal zone and limited penetration. With a mechanically rotated single crystal, this is fixed by the design of the transducer. Focusing describes the optimum range of resolution for the transducer to work at. For the B-K Medical 10-MHz transducer, the axial resolution is <0.05 mm and the lateral resolution 0.5–1 mm, with a focal range of 5–45 mm [1–2].

Artefacts

Reverberation is an artefact due to a gross mismatch of acoustic impedance at an interface, usually an air/tissue interface, causing a very strong reflection which is only partially absorbed by the transducer and which is reflected back to the interface where it is again reflected back to the transducer. The beam therefore reverberates back and forth from the interface and transducer, creating a series of reflections separated by a constant distance, which indicates the distance of the reflection from the transducer (Fig. I.10). Reverberation echoes are common in anal endosonography when there is loss of acoustic contact within the canal (Fig. I.11).

Interpretative Principles

The prime determinant of the strength of ultrasonic echoes is the impedance mismatch between adjacent tissue components. The larger the mismatch, the stronger the echo. The echogenicity of any structure may be characterized by the level of echoes within it (hyper- or hypoechoic). The echo pattern may be homogeneous or inhomogeneous. Water has the lowest reflectivity and appears black. Fat varies in reflectivity but is usually moderately reflective. Collagen is more reflective and whiter whereas muscle fibers are

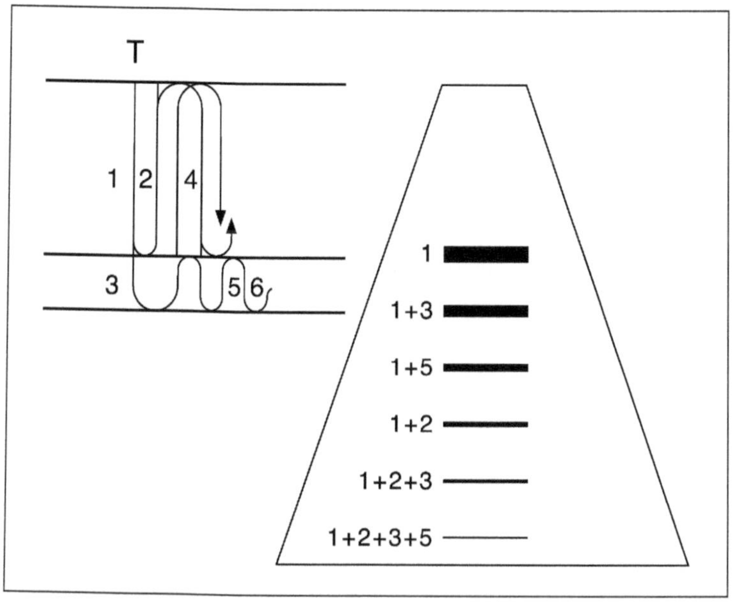

Fig. I.10. Reverberation echoes develop when there is a very strong reflection returning to the transducer. Part will be reflected from the transducer back into the tissue. This, in turn, will be reflected back to the transducer, and so on. This creates a series of equally spaced reflections. The *gap* indicates the distance between the transducer (T) and the initial reflection

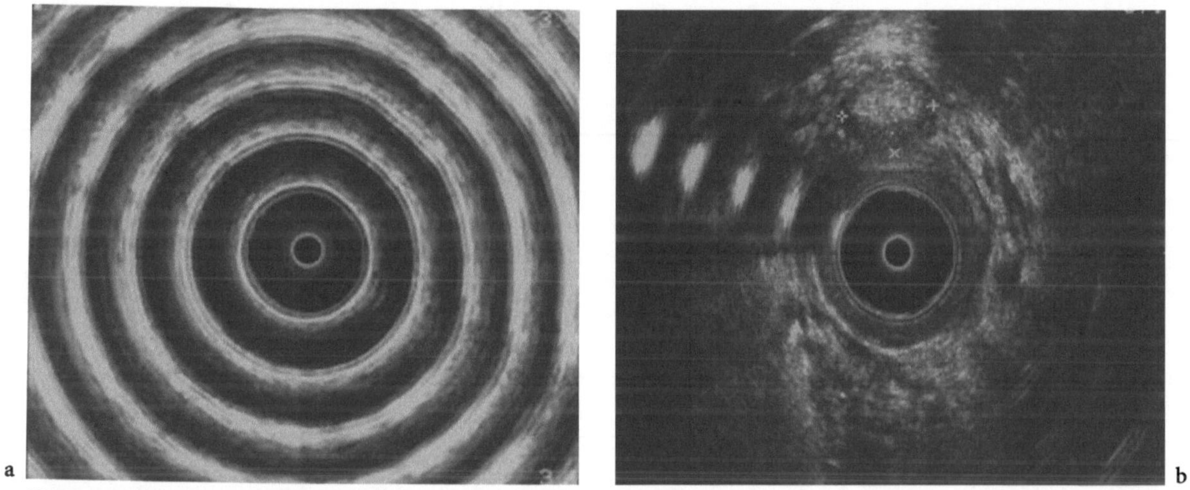

Fig. I.11. The image has been taken with the probe free standing in air. The gas impedance mismatch at the cone/air interface creates major reflection echo patterns with an equally spaced series of concentric rings (**a**). The probe has been inserted beyond the anal canal into the rectal ampulla. Acoustic contact has been lost from 9–11 o'clock, producing a reverberation echo (**b**)

poorly reflective and blacker. Solid tumors are usually poorly reflective and inhomogeneous. While uniform regions of fiber or fat are echo-poor, admixtures between them and watery tissues give stronger echoes. For a given impedance mismatch, a region that contains a large number of scatterers is more echogenic than one where they are spread out.

References

1. Bartram CI, Frudinger A (1997) Basic principles of ultrasonography. In: Bartram CI, Frudinger A. Handbook of anal endosonography. Wrightson Biomedical, Petersfield, UK
2. Santoro GA, Di Falco G (2004) Basic principles of ultrasonography. In: Santoro GA, Di Falco G. Atlas of endoanal and endorectal ultrasonography. Springer Italy, Milan

Section II

New Technical Developments in Endoanal and Endorectal Ultrasonography

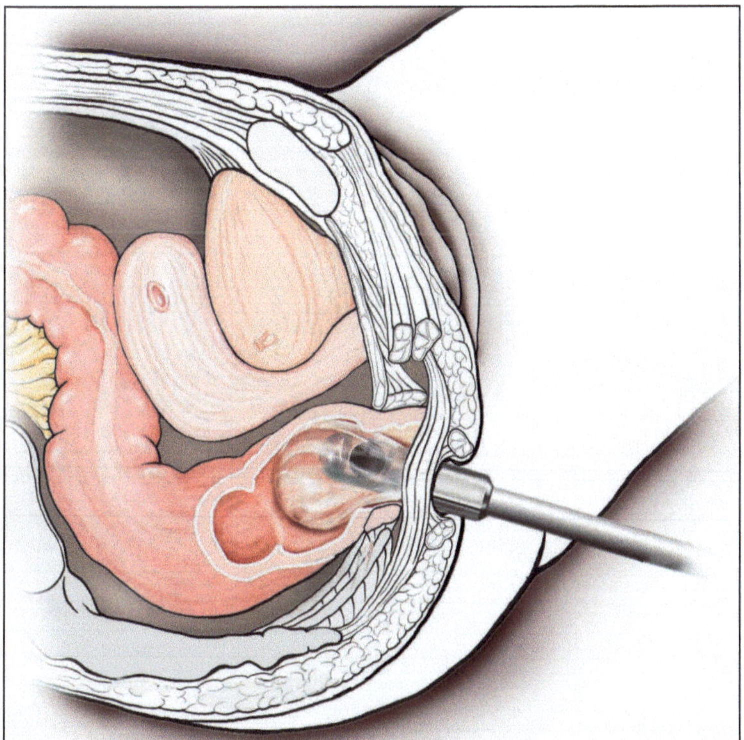

New Technical Developments in Endoanal and Endorectal Ultrasonography

G.A. Santoro, B. Fortling

In order to obtain meaningful ultrasonic images, the operator must have an overall understanding and therefore correct use of the controls available on the ultrasound device. In fact, unsuitable regulation of the equipment produces poor images and can lead to false positive or negative diagnosis.

Many types of ultrasound probes have been developed to evaluate the rectal wall and anal sphincter. Most of these have been made to examine the prostate gland and are not suitable for evaluating the wall of the anorectum and the immediately adjacent tissues. The types of endorectal probes include mechanical sector probes with a single transducer, which may have a limited field of view of 120–210° or may incorporate radial probes with a full 360° field of view and linear and curved array probes, which have a limited 120–210° field of view. Some of these probes are biplanar and can be changed from the axial plane to the longitudinal (sagittal, coronal) plane with the press of a button. All of these probes have a frequency range from 5 to 10 MHz. The focal range of a 7.0-MHz transducer is 2–5 cm whereas a 5.5-MHz transducer has a focal range of 1–4 cm. The longer focal length provides an advantage in examining perirectal structures. The 10.0-MHz transducer is preferred in the anal canal as it gives improved resolution of the sphincter mechanism over the 7.0-MHz transducer.

We currently use an Hawk 2102 EXL B-K Medical scanner (B-K Medical A/S, Mileparken 34, DK-2730 Herlev, Denmark) (Fig. II.1) with a 1850 radial array probe, which gives a 360° axial view of the rectal wall (Fig. II.2) [1–3]. The radial probe has a 24-cm metal shaft with a rotating transduc-

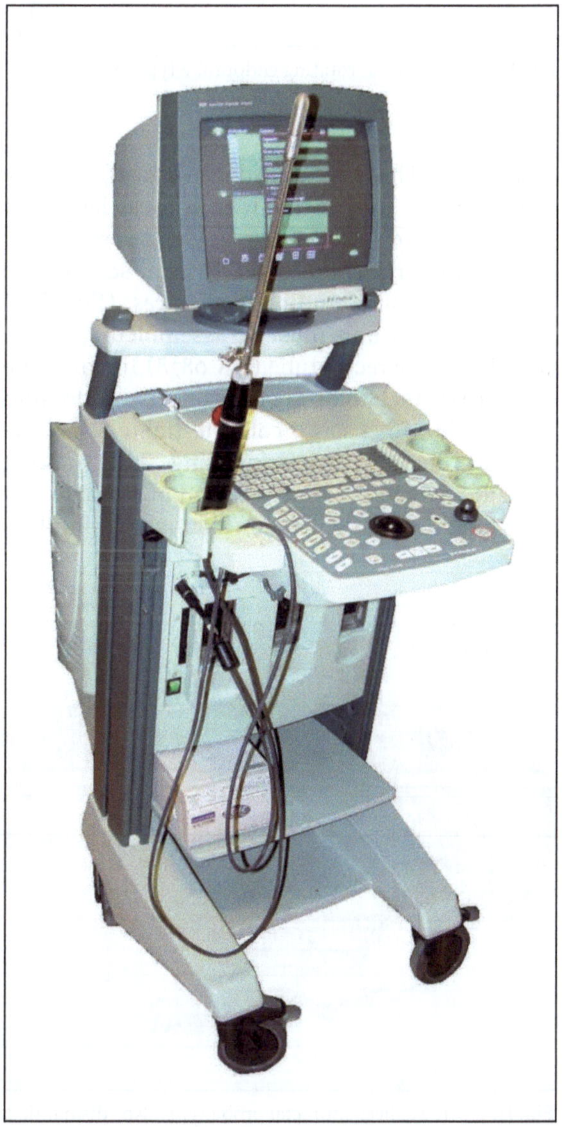

Fig. II.1. B-K Medical scanner: Hawk 2102 EXL

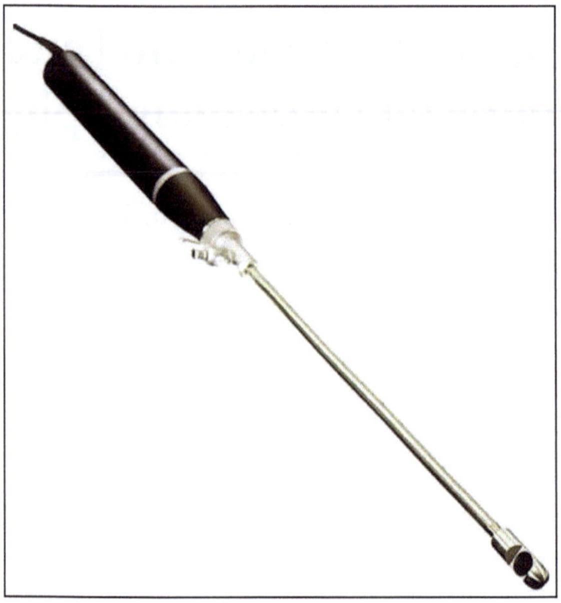

Fig. II.2. B-K Medical rotating endoprobe type 1850

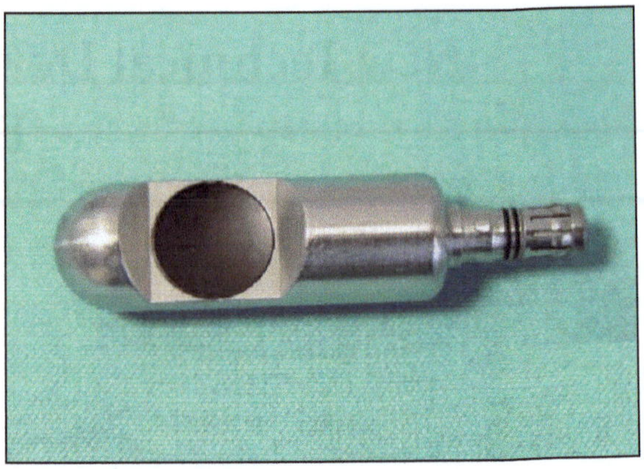

a

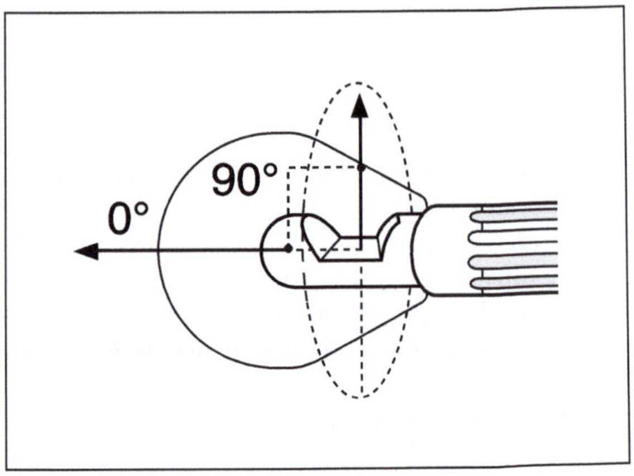

b

Fig. II.3. B-K Medical transducer type 8539 (a, b)

er at its tip. This 8539 transducer has a frequency range from 5 to 10 MHz with a focal length of 2–5 cm and a 90° scanning plane and is rotated at 4–6 cycles per second to get a radial scan of the rectum and surrounding structures (Fig. II.3) [4–5]. The B-K unit must be assembled carefully (Fig. II.4). The rectal tube (UA 0878) fits over the central axle that holds the transducer and slot into the handle with a screw collar to tighten the tube onto a rubber compression ring. The rotating transducer is pushed into the end of the axle and is covered by a latex balloon that is held in place by two metal rings, one of which screws onto the metal shaft (Fig. II.5). A syringe filled with 50 ml of tap water is manipulated to remove air bubbles then attached to a spigot at the base of the probe.

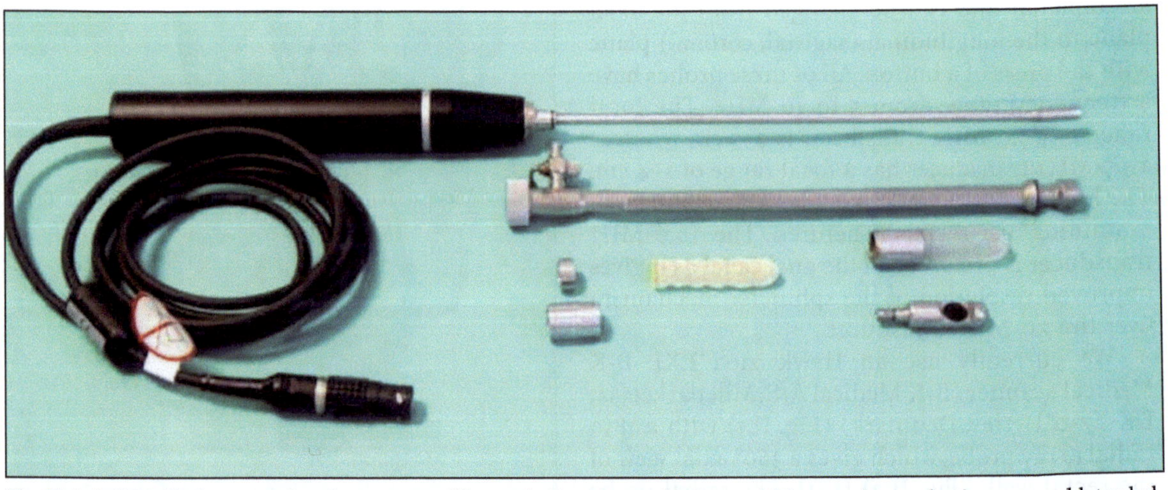

Fig. II.4. B-K Medical anorectal probe type 1850 (dismantled), with rectal tube, 10 MHz transducer, plastic cone, and latex balloon

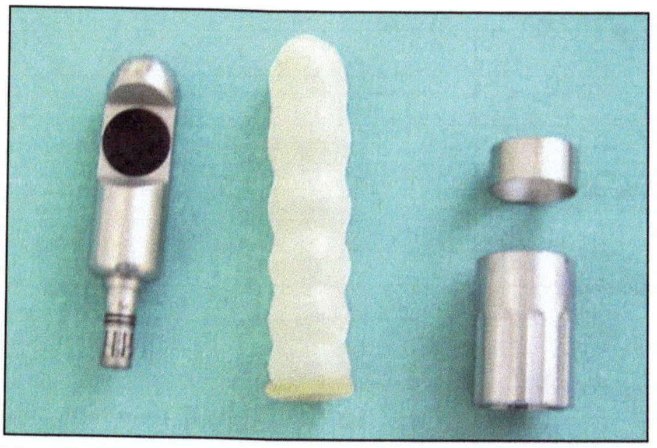

Fig. II.5. Transducer, metal rings, and latex balloon for endorectal ultrasound

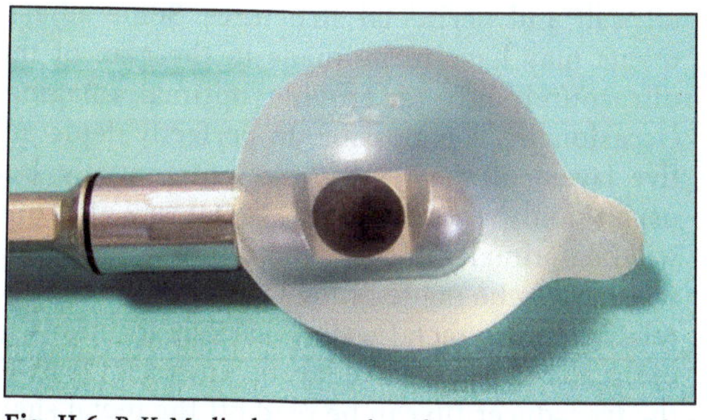

Fig. II.6. B-K Medical anorectal probe type 1850 assembled with latex balloon

Water is gently injected into the balloon; the water is then withdrawn again with the transducer tip in the dependent position. In this way, all of the air is removed from the water-filled balloon. This procedure may have to be repeated to remove all of the air (Fig. II.6). Latex balloon filled with degassed water allows acoustic coupling between the transducer and the rectal wall (Fig. II.7). The rectum can be of varying diameters and therefore the volume of water in the balloon may have to be adjusted intermittently.

Endoluminal ultrasound is usually performed with the patient in the left lateral decubitus position. Before the probe is inserted into the rectum, a digital rectal examination may be performed to identify the size, fixation, morphology, and location of the tumor, if it is low enough. If there is a stenotic annular lesion, the finger can check to determine whether it will allow easy passage of the probe [6–7]. The entire shaft of the probe is coated with a thin layer of warm gel using a paper towel. The probe tip is gently inserted through the anal canal and then angled posteriorly and advanced cephalad to as high a level as possible, with the bony sacrum used as a curved landmark. The patient should be instructed before the examination that no pain should be experienced. If

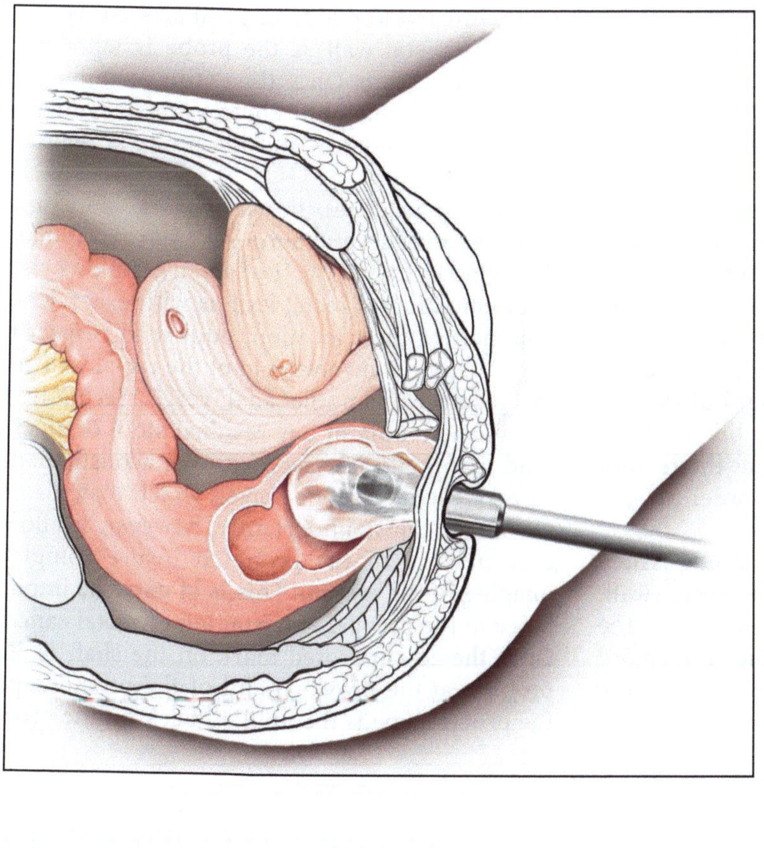

Fig. II.7. Diagrammatic representation of an endorectal ultrasonography

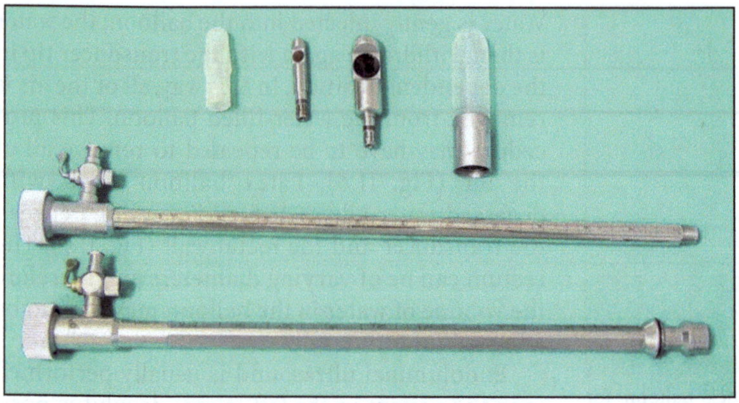

Fig. II.8. B-K Medical transducer type 6005

pain should occur, the study should be halted until the cause of the pain is elucidated. Under no circumstances should force be used to advance the probe. The examiner should never try to push the tip through a narrow stenotic lesion. However, in most instances, passage can be achieved although the volume of the fluid in the balloon will have to be substantially reduced in order to withdraw the probe through the stenotic portion. In some instances, a plastic cone filled with water will facilitate the imaging of a stenotic lesion, or it may be necessary to use a smaller probe, 7 mm in diameter (7 MHz, type 6005, focal range: 0.5-3 cm) (Fig. II.8). Once the tip is advanced to as high a level as possible, usually 10–14 cm from the anal verge, the balloon can be inflated with 50 ml of water. The amount of water may have to be increased to provide complete acoustic coupling with the rectal wall. The examiner should never distend the balloon with more than 80 ml of degassed water, as it may rupture. If this occurs, the probe must be removed from the rectum and cleaned, a new balloon installed, and the whole procedure started over. If air or stool gets between the balloon and rectal wall, it will prevent visualization of the wall. To avoid this, we administer an enema 2 h before the examination, but despite this, problems can arise, and it may be necessary to remove the probe and suction out the rectum with reintroduction of the probe in order to optimize the image.

With the probe at the highest level possible and with good visualization of the rectal wall, images are obtained at 1-cm intervals as the probe is withdrawn. The tip of the ultrasound probe should be maintained in the center of the rectal lumen to gain optimal imaging of the rectal wall and perirectal structures. Some adjustments may have to be made in the gain of the ultrasound unit to provide optimal imaging. Occasionally, it is possible to perfectly depict all five layers of the rectum circumferentially, but usually, only a portion of the rectal wall at a time will be optimally imaged, and minor adjustments will have to be made in the location of the probe relative to the rectal wall at various locations to optimally image all five layers. The exact level of the transducer tip can be read off the metal shaft of the ultrasound probe. More closely spaced images (0.5 cm) are obtained in the area of any abnormality. The balloon may have to be deflated and reinflated to maintain good acoustic contact with the rectal wall as the probe is withdrawn down the rectum. Once the entire rectum down to the anal sphincter has been evaluated, the balloon is fully deflated, and the probe is removed from the rectum.

In most instances, the use of a large-bore proctoscope serves several purposes (A.4522, Sapimed, Alessandria, Italy) (Fig. II.9). Firstly, it allows visual examination of rectal lesions with exact determination of their location, both with respect to circumferential involvement of the rectal wall and the distance from the anal verge. Secondly, it allows suctioning of any residual stool or enema fluid that might interfere with the acoustic pathways of the ultrasound waves, which may distort the image. Most importantly, however, it allows easy passage of the probe to insure complete imaging of the rectum. This is of extreme importance in the preoperative staging of rectal cancer. Once the 20-cm scored mark on the shaft of the probe is at the proximal end of the proctoscope, the proctoscope is then pulled back on the probe

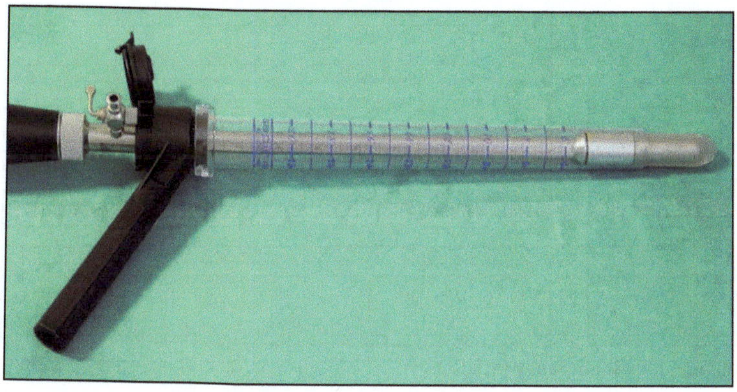

Fig. II.9. Rectosigmoidoscope for endorectal ultrasonography (A.4522, Sapimed)

as far as possible, thus exposing the transducer for 2 cm beyond the end of the proctoscope. The balloon is then instilled with 30–60 cc of water, the volume of fluid usually needed to gain optimal imaging.

If the anus is being evaluated, the same probe is used with a transducer that has a shorter focal zone of 1–4 cm. A water-filled, hard-plastic cone (WA 0543) made of sonolucent polymethyl pentene (TPX) plastic and 1.7 cm in outer diameter is used in place of the latex balloon (Fig. II.10) [8]. A hole at the top allows air to escape as the assembly is filled with degassed water. A gel-containing condom is then placed over the probe, and a thin layer of water-soluble lubricant is placed on the exterior of the condom. Any air interface will cause a major interference pattern. The probe is now ready for insertion. The outer walls of this cone are parallel so that the probe may be moved within the anal canal without causing any anatomical distortion (Fig. II.11). This is very important when assessing the canal at different levels. There does not appear to be any benefit from asking the patient to "squeeze" their pelvic floor to assess sphincter contraction. At the origin of the canal, the "U"-shaped sling of the puborectalis is the main landmark and should be used for final adjustment [9].

When the patient is in the left lateral position and the spigot for introducing water into the probe is pointing toward the ceiling, by convention, the anterior aspect of the anus will be superior (12 o'clock) on the screen, right lateral will be left (9 o'clock) on the screen, left lateral will be right (3 o'clock) on the screen, and posterior will be inferior (6 o'clock) on the screen (just as in the image on axial CT scan) (Fig. II.12).

Future Directions

When we display a normal two-dimensional (2-D) ultrasound cross-sectional view, there are many elements of the image that will not be correctly recognized as components of a three-dimensional (3-D) structure – or at least not perceived in their true spatial relationships. With ultrasound imaging, we are usually looking at a 3-D structure that contains a solid volume of echoes and that therefore does not readily translate onto a 2-D projection. In routine clinical scanning, the operator forms a mental representation of the 3-D anatomic or pathological structure while viewing a large series of 2-D slices interactively. In this case, the operator is using manual sense information about the physical location of the individual slices in building up 3-D subjective impressions. Three-dimensional and, indeed, four-dimensional (4-D) ultrasound has been promoted by different ultrasound companies for several years. The acquisition of a 3-D data volume and the underlying techniques are, however, different from application to application. Some areas of the human body require extremely high-resolution 3-D volumes of data for adequate and precise diagnostic evaluation (anal sphincter, rectal wall, fistula, urethral sphincter complex, etc.); other areas require less when it comes to sampling the 3-D data volume (baby face, kidney, pancreas). For endoanal and endorectal ultrasound in general, the problems will be in assessing anatomy and in characterizing tissue structure and type.

Three-dimensional reconstruction of 2-D images is possible by connecting the ultrasound apparatus to a computer equipped with special software (BK 3Di) (Fig. II.13) [10]. A normal dig-

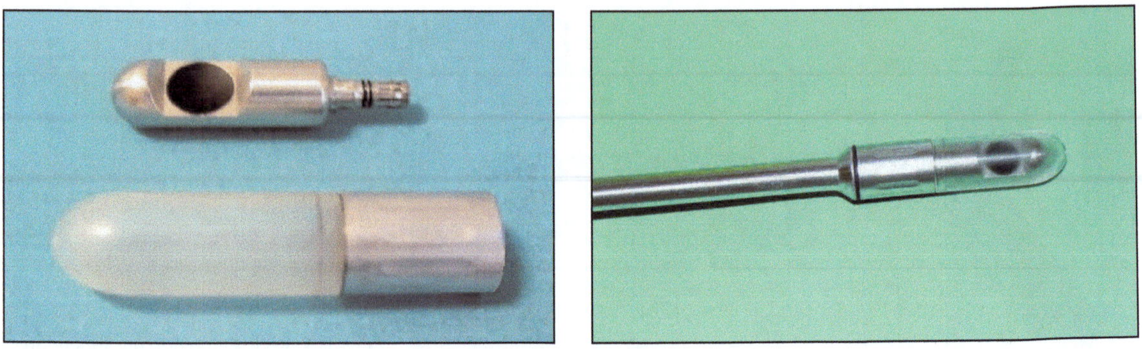

a b

Fig. II.10. Transducer and plastic cone for endoanal ultrasonography (a, b)

ital ultrasound image is displayed using a display matrix of around 700×700 pixel elements, with each pixel assigned a value between 0 and 255 (256 levels of grey). The result seen on the ultrasound monitor is a 2-D image with no depth information. Adding the third dimension to the pixels means that the pixels are transformed to voxels (voxel is a pixel, X- and Y-plane only, in the ultrasound image with an added Z-plane), each of which also will have an assigned value between 0 and 255. The depth of the voxel is critical to the resolution of the 3-D image, and this depth is directly related to the spacing between two adjacent images. Ideally, the voxel should form an exact cube, but because generally sampling with slightly lesser resolution in the Z-plane (due to acquisition speed considerations) compared with the 700×700 matrix, the resolution in Z-plane is marginally lower. High-resolution data volumes may consist of typical voxel sizes around 0.15×0.15×0.2 mm (or 0.25 mm). This means that an acquisition based upon, for

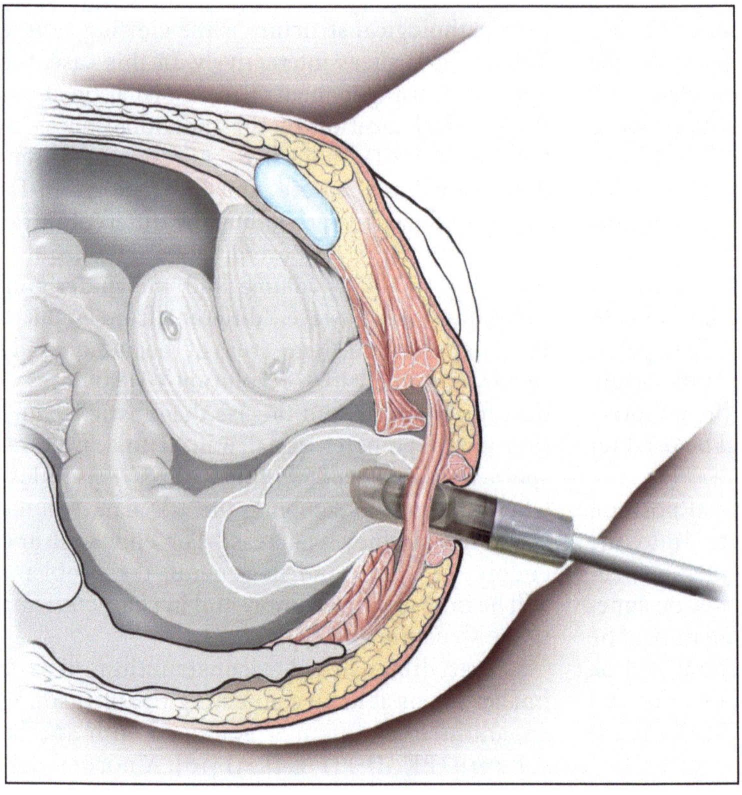

Fig. II.11. Diagrammatic representation of an endoanal ultrasonography

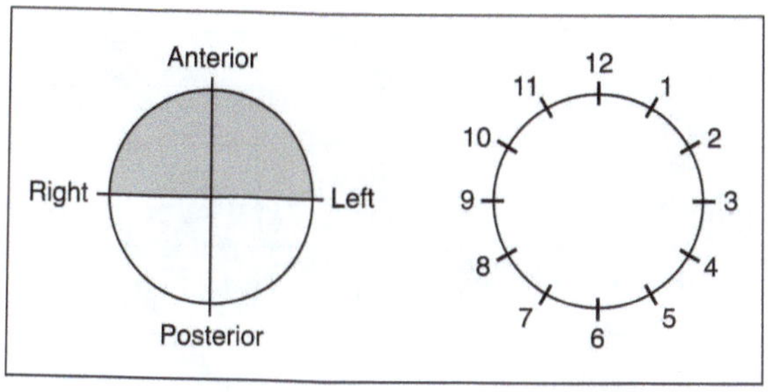

a

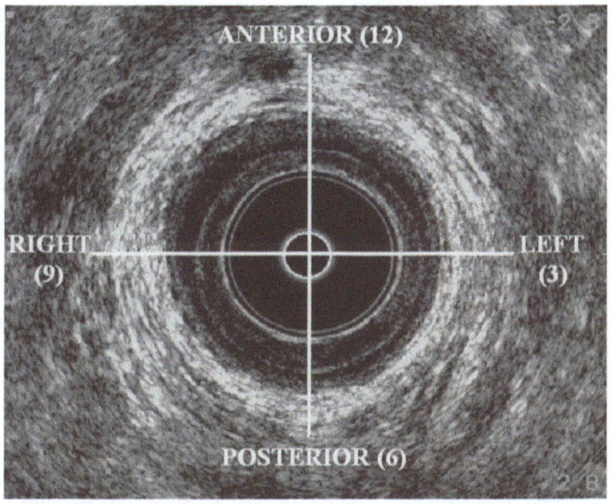

b

Fig. II.12. Lesion localization with patient in left lateral position when the spigot for introducing water into the balloon is pointing toward the ceiling (**a**, **b**)

example, sampling of transaxial images over a distance of 60 mm in the human body will result in a data volume block consisting of between 240 and 300 transaxial images. This is far more than any 4-D technique can handle using computer power as we know it today. High-resolution 3-D technique and consequently much slower acquisition speed does not function in 4-D mode. Four to five transaxial images are, as mentioned, sampled per 1-mm distance (in the Z-plane). Acquisition of a high number of parallel transaxial images can be performed using a special colorectal pullback mover (UA0552) with the B-K Medical ultrasound probe type 1850 (Fig. II.14). The colorectal pullback mover is a computer-controlled, motor-driven device that can be operated at different levels of resolution. For the endoanal application, the usual setting is 0.2–0.3 mm between adjacent transaxial images. Scanning the anal canal with these settings over a pullback distance of 35 mm will typically yield 175 parallel images (Fig. II.15). This approach provides a neat way of uniformly scanning a solid volume, the acquisition taking typically 60 s. However, it is subject to the important limitation of being rather bulky. An alternative approach is to use a manual technique. In the case of manual acquisition, the samples will not be uniform, and they may be anisotropic in the sense that a voxel gives different values. Extreme cases will result in voxels either having no samples, that is, having data gaps, or having multiple samples. Gaps cause visually distracting artefacts in the resulting displays. The new B-K Medical 2050 anorectal transducer solves most

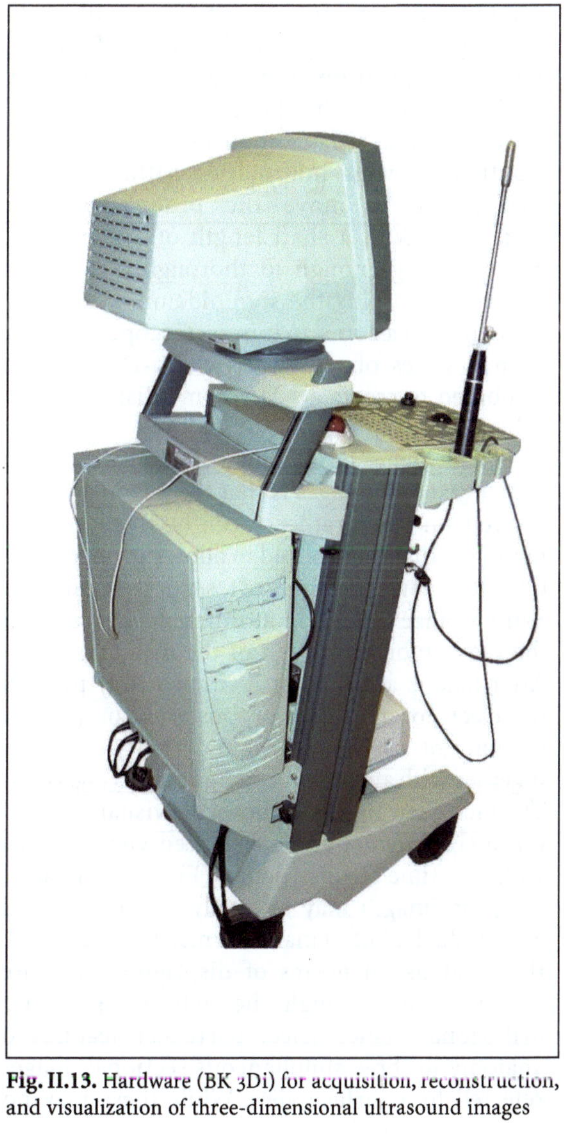

Fig. II.13. Hardware (BK 3Di) for acquisition, reconstruction, and visualization of three-dimensional ultrasound images

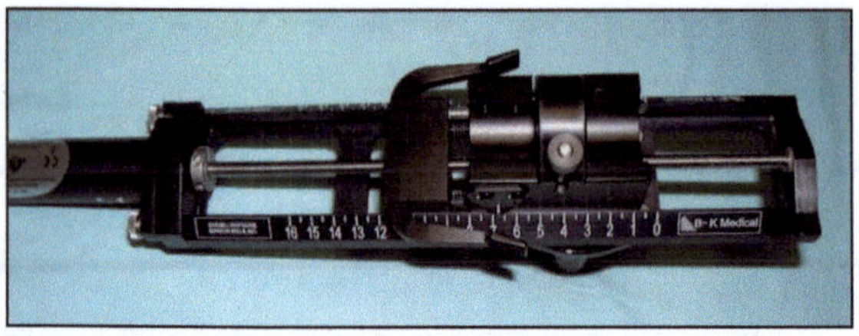
a

Fig. II.14. Ultrasound probe type 1850 and colorectal pull-back mover (UA0552) used to acquire three-dimensional anorectal endo images (**a**, **b**)

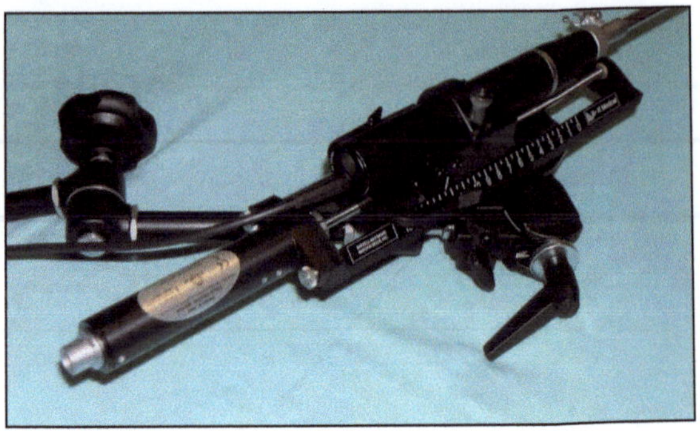
b

of these problems. It is designed so that no moving parts come in contact with human tissue. The transducer's 360° rotating head, the proximal–distal actuation mechanism, and the electronic mover are fully enclosed within the housing of the slim probe (Fig. II.16). Both 3-D data-set acquisition and high-precision positioning of the scan head over a longitudinal distance of 60 mm are accomplished at the touch of a button, allowing information gathering without having to move the probe's position (Fig. II.17). With a shaft length of 270 mm, the probe is long enough to thoroughly cover the entire rectum plus the sigmoideum. It also can pass through a 200 x 20 mm rectoscope. The data from a series of closely spaced 2-D images is combined to create a 3-D volume displayed as a cube (Fig. II.18).

An advantage of working with high-resolution 3-D ultrasound images is that the 3-D image does not remain fixed; rather, it can be freely rotated, rendered, tilted, and sliced to allow the operator to infinitely vary the different section parameters and visualize the lesion at different angles to get the most information out of the data (Fig. II.19). After data is acquired, it is immediately possible to select coronal anterior–posterior or posterior–anterior as well as sagittal right–left views, together with any oblique image plane (Fig. II.20). The multiview function allows the visualization of up to six different and specialized views at once with real-time reconstruction (Fig. II.21). In addition, the images may be easily saved, reviewed, and studied. Multiplanar reformatting is probably the most useful means of displaying structure. Multiple cuts through the data along regular orthogonal planes select particular features of anatomy in three simultaneous sectional images, referred to a surface view. While these may not appear obviously 3-D, they are a valid and extremely useful way of interactively viewing a 3-D tissue image.

If one wants to see the internal structure, a volume representation may be chosen. In this, one allows the ray to pass through the data, and contributions from different depths are added together in some way and used to construct the image pixel on the screen (volume rendering) (Fig. II.22). The most commonly known version is "Surface Render Mode," extensively used by some medical centers in producing perhaps the very first images of an unborn baby's facial contours. Surface Render Mode is, by its requirements, mainly a superficial postprocessed topographical presentation of an often rapidly (4-D) acquired data set, with a lesser degree of information inside

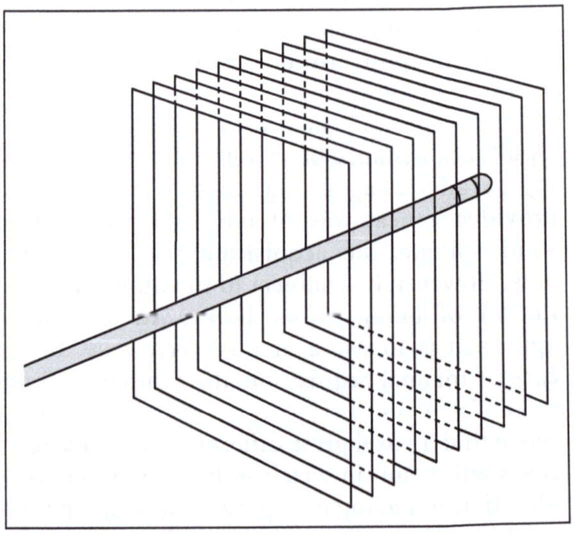

Fig. II.15. Schematic model for acquisition of three-dimensional anorectal endo image as parallel transverse two-dimensional images

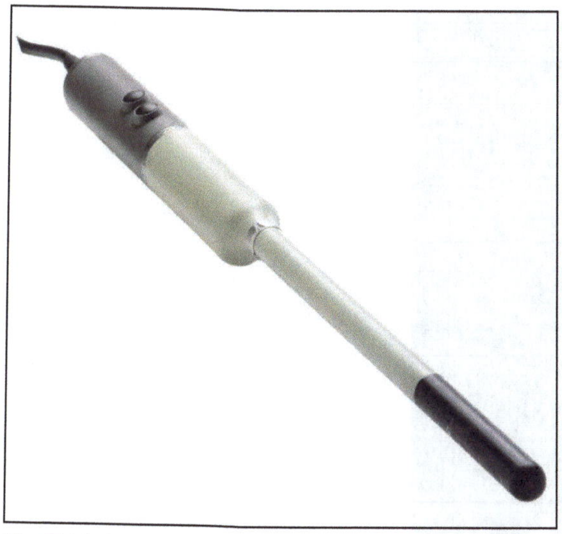

Fig. II.16. B-K Medical anorectal transducer type 2050

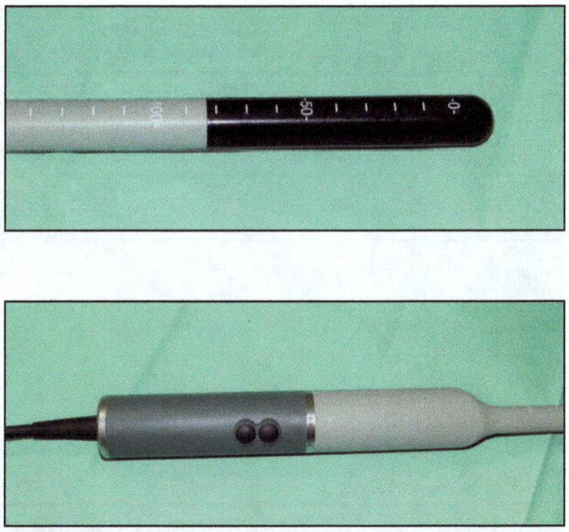

a

b

Fig. II.17. Three-dimensional acquisition is controlled by two buttons on the probe (**a, b**)

the depth of the 3-D volume of data compared with high-resolution 3-D data volumes. An ultrasound image has under normal circumstances no depth information due to the fact that the lateral resolution of the image must be kept as high as possible. The image may be compared to looking at a photographic image on a piece of paper. Three-dimensional ultrasound does not change this fact. The three surfaces visible on the screen when viewing a 3-D volume all have no depth information. This can be compared to looking at a cardboard box from the outside. The content inside the box remains unknown. "Volume Render Mode" is a special feature that successfully can be applied to high-resolution 3-D data volumes. Imaging processing includes maximum intensity, minimum intensity, and summed voxel projections combined with positional or intensity weighting. This technique changes the depth information of 3-D data volume so information inside the cube to some extend is reconstructed. Most processes, particularly smoothing, decrease the information. This may be desirable in some cases. If an image is cluttered with noise, the observer's visual perception may be overloaded, and detail may consequently be missed. The loss of information may not be apparent at first. It may turn out, however, that after smoothing, there are details missing or geometric accuracy is reduced. The effect may be particularly dramatic if a number of voxels in the Z-plane originate from scanning hypoechoic structures. A rupture of the otherwise hyperechoic external sphincter complex in the anal canal is a good example because tears normally appear hypoechoic compared with the competent segments of this striated muscle. Another example is voxel values behind, for example, a strongly reflective interface, such as a fistula enhanced by introduction of contrast agent (i.e., hydrogen peroxide). Following a tortuous fis-

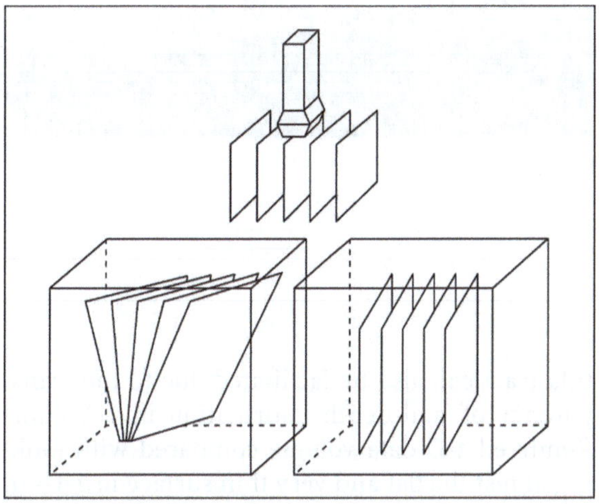

Fig. II.18. Schematic model for reconstruction of the acquired set of two dimensional images into a three dimensional volume displayed as a cube

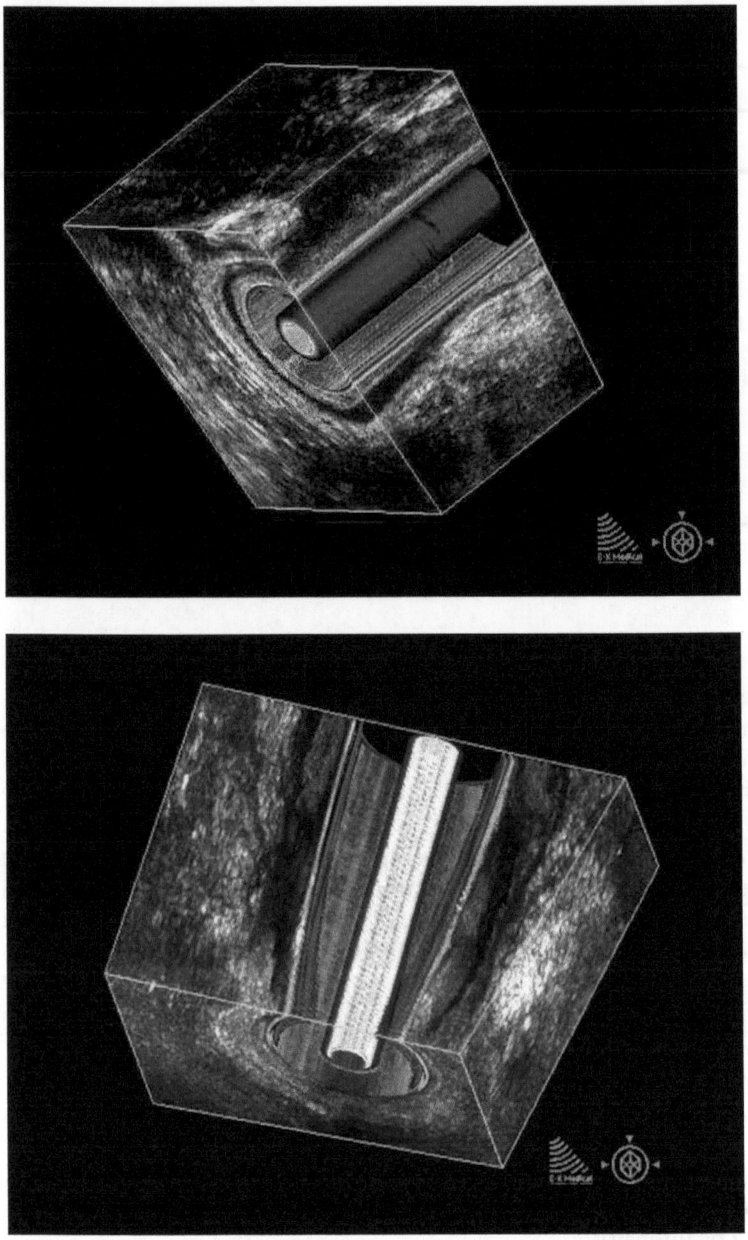

a

b

Fig. II.19. Three-dimensional ultrasound images (a, b)

tula tract can also be facilitated due to the transparency of, and depth information in, a Volume Rendered 3-D data volume compared with looking at just the flat and very thin surface in 2-D- or conventional 3-D-mode images (Fig. II.23). It is always essential, however, to display unprocessed images together with processed images in order that misinterpretations do not occur as a result of image processing. Recently, a new computerized system has been introduced that could allow significant improvements to the 3-D image on post-processing (Fig. II.24). The acquisition and storage of a 3-D volume allows the possibility of rescanning this recorded data at a later stage, providing in principle all the information available at the scan.

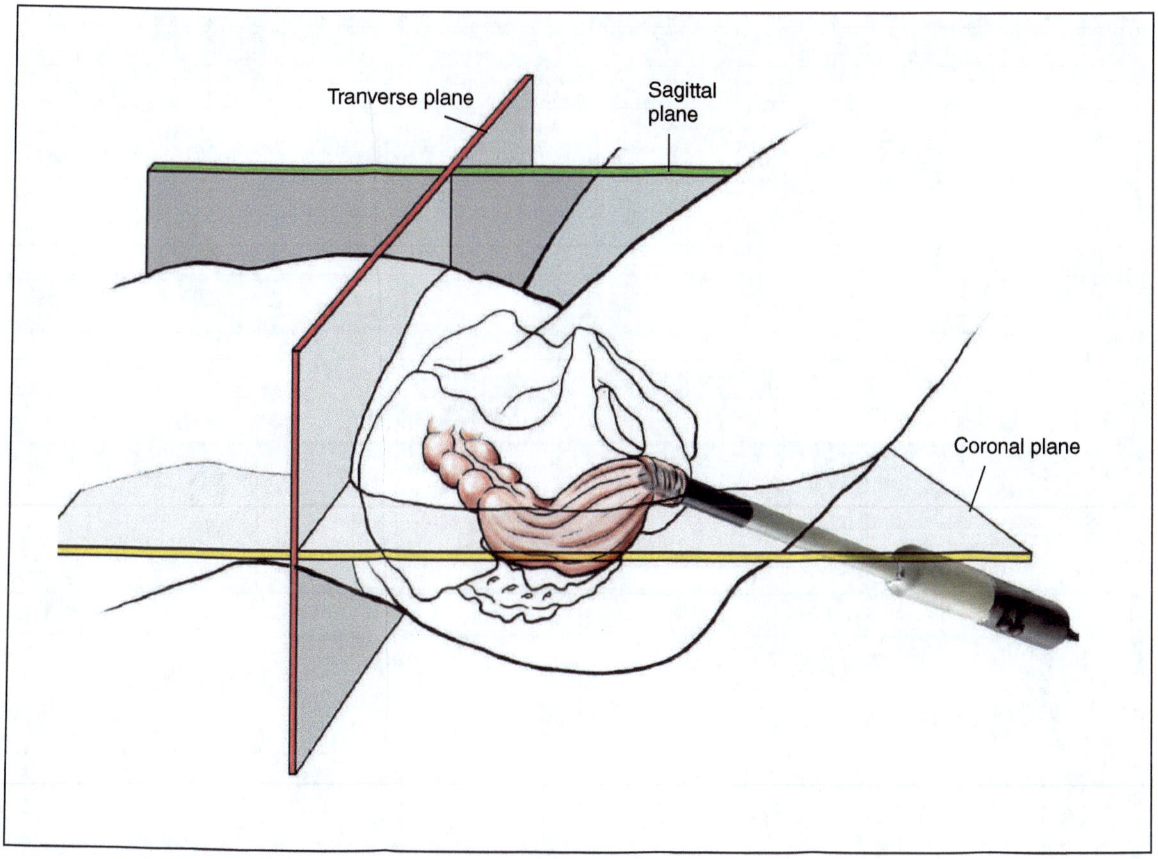

a

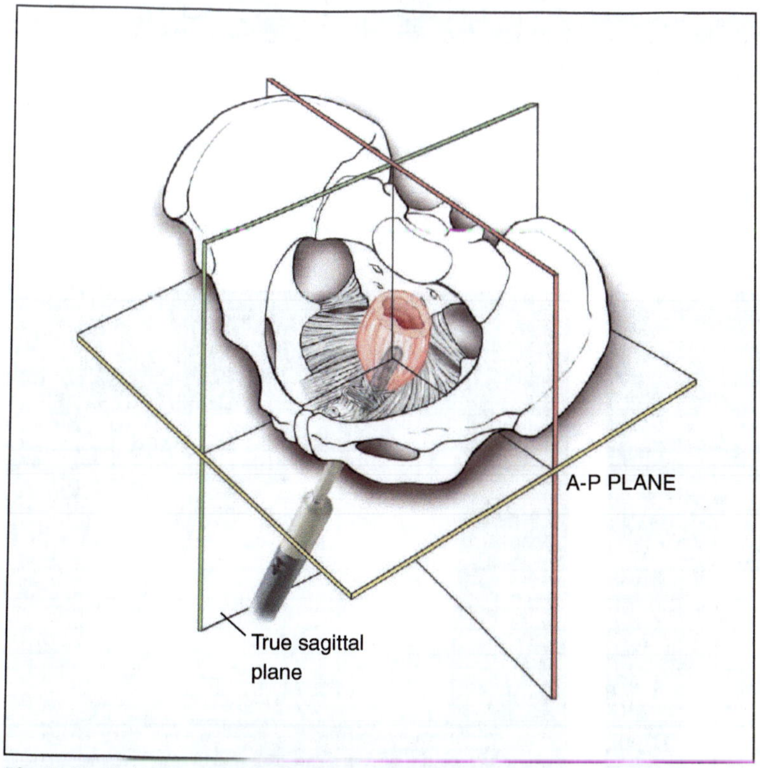

b

Fig. II.20. Schematic representation of the acquired volume and planimetric display of the transverse, sagittal, and coronal planes (**a, b**)

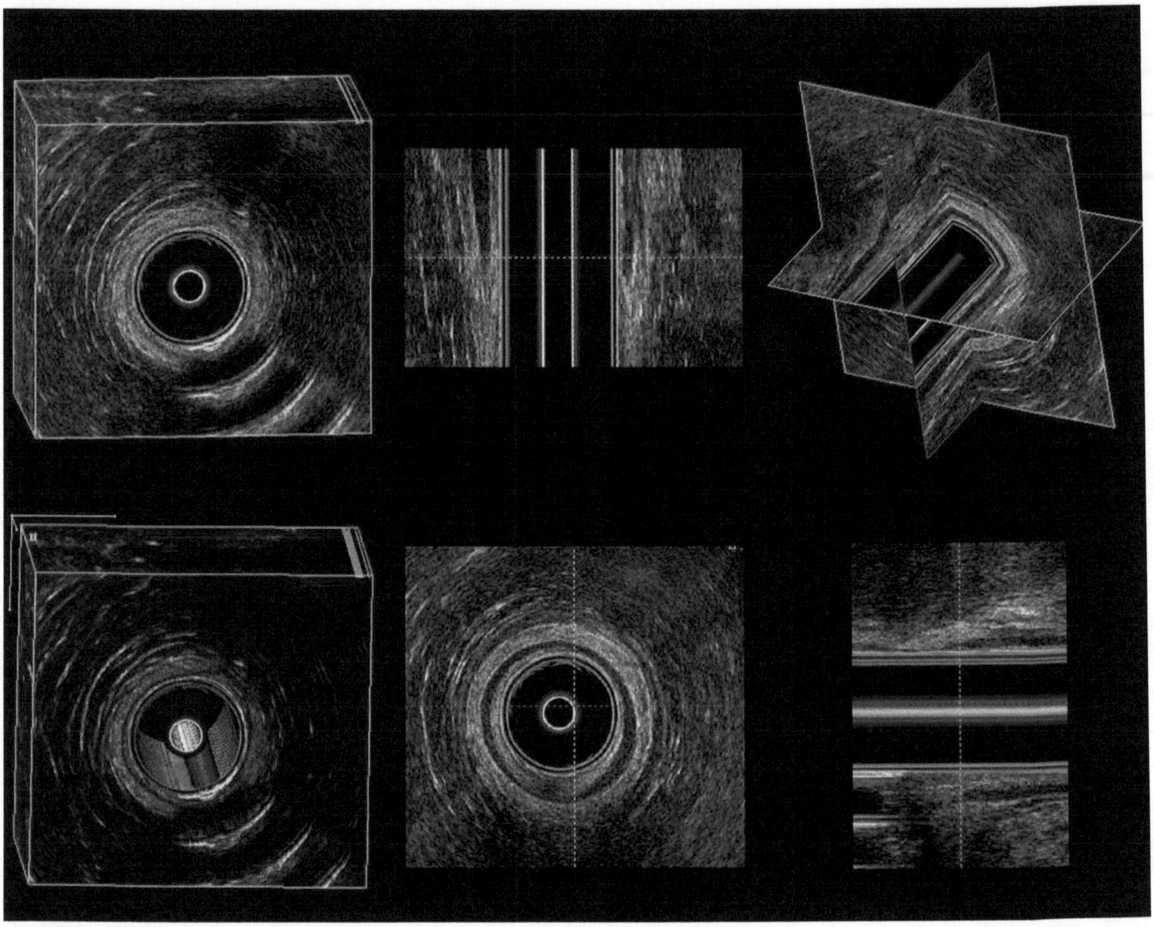

Fig. II.21. Scan image in multiview with six types of cube image presentation

a

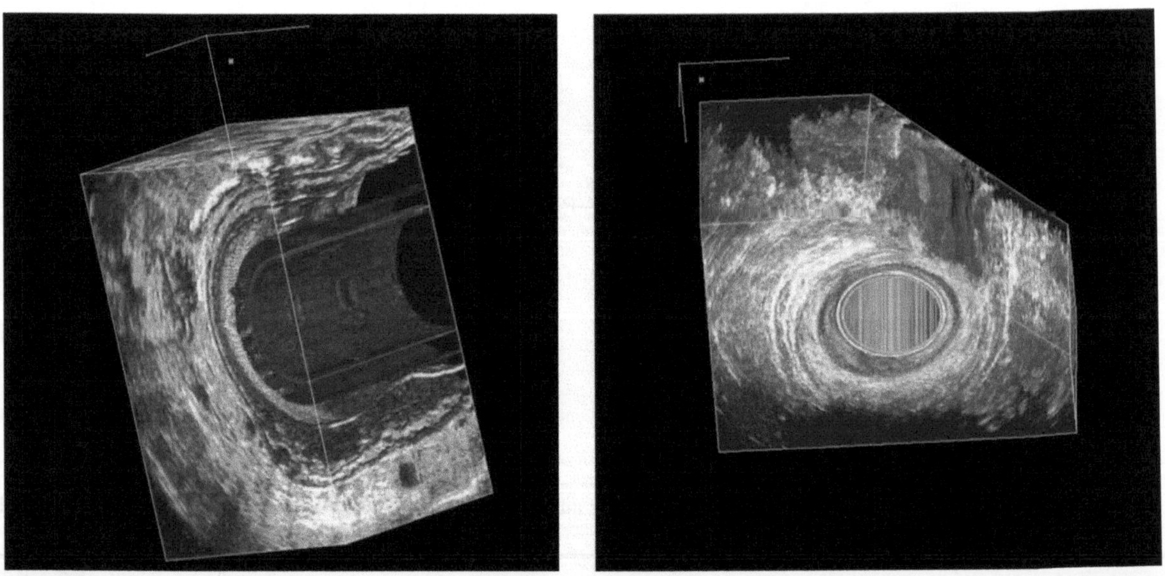

b

Fig. II.22. Volume render mode (**a, b**)

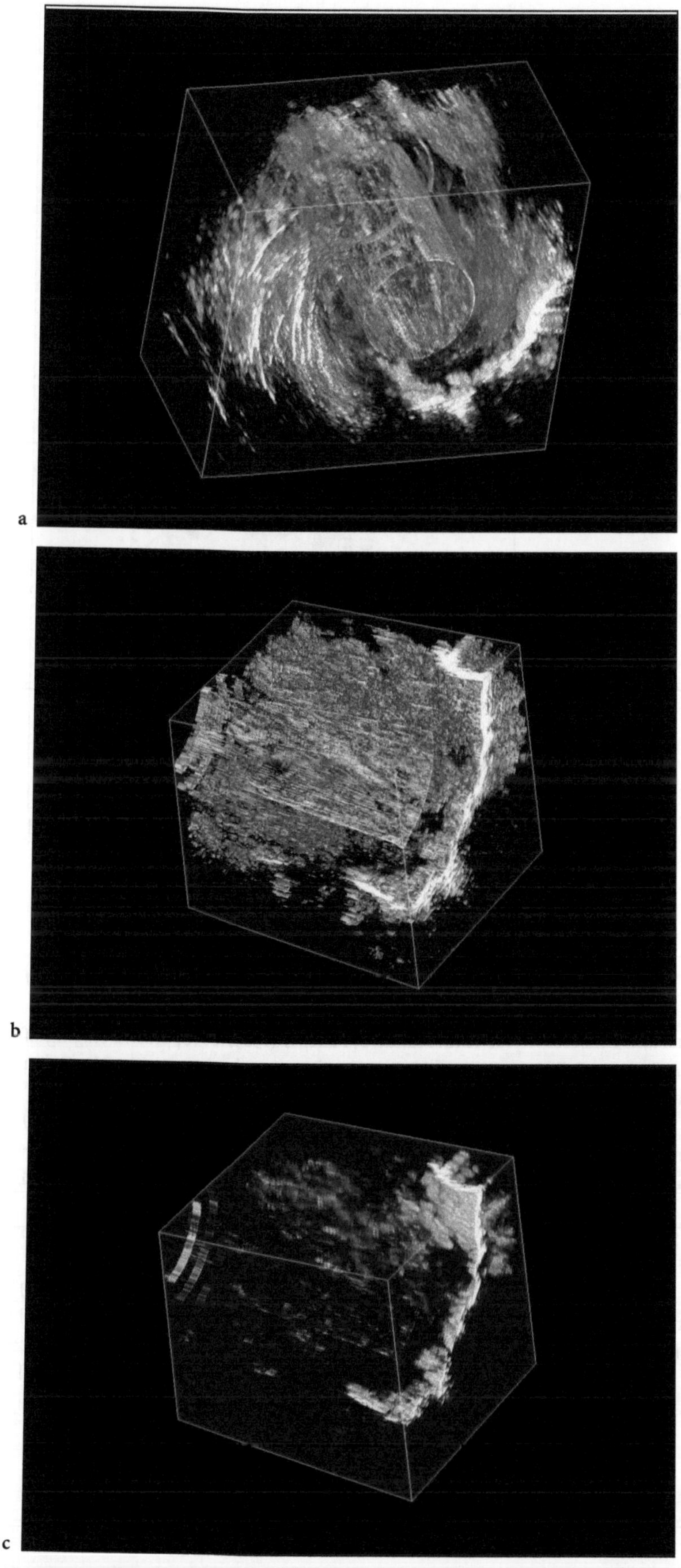

Fig. II.23. Effects of imaging processing on fistula tract views (**a–c**)

A fundamental development of the new probe type 2050 is that the double crystal covers a frequency range from 6 to 16 MHz. This means that higher frequencies may be used, with the associated improved resolution. The images obtained are therefore usually of a higher quality than those obtained with conventional probes.

The most common applications for the 3-D facilities are in surgery planning, assessment of complex anatomy and pathology, measurement in three dimensions, and better diagnosis.

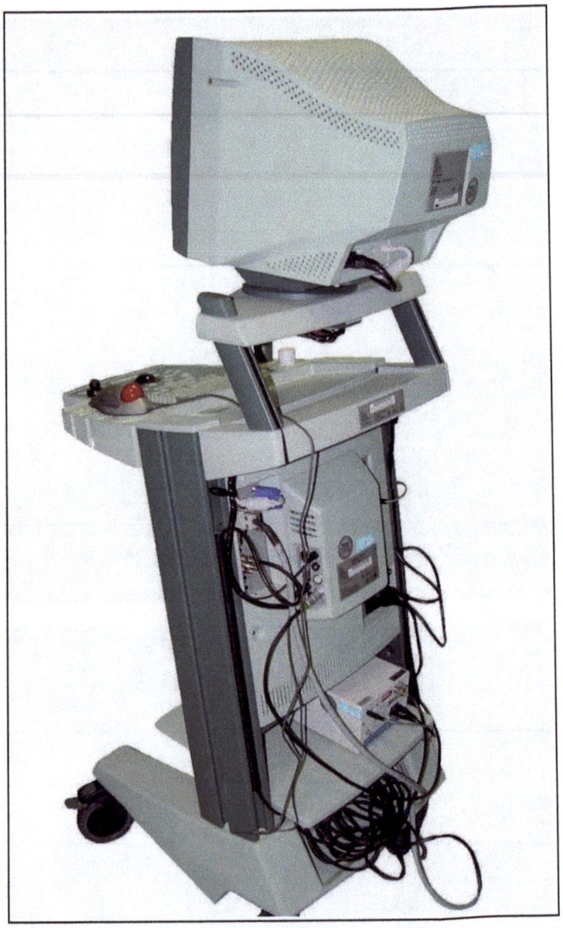

Fig. II.24. New hardware for acquisition, reconstruction, and visualization of three-dimensional ultrasound images

References

1. Santoro GA, Di Falco G (2004) Endoanal and endorectal ultrasonographic techniques. In: G.A. Santoro, G. Di Falco. Atlas of endoanal and endorectal ultrasonography. Springer Italy, Milan
2. Bartram CI, Frudinger A (1997) Handbook of anal endosonography. Wrightson Biomedical, Petersfield, UK
3. Hildebrandt U, Feifel G, Schwarz HP, Scherr O (1986) Endorectal ultrasound: instrumentation and clinical aspects. Int J Colorectal Dis 1:203–207
4. Law PJ, Bartram CI (1989) Anal endosonography: technique and normal anatomy. Gastrointest Radiol 14:349–353
5. Kumar A, Scholefield JH (2000) Endosonography of the anal canal and rectum. World J Surg 24:208–215
6. Hildebrandt U, Feifel G (1985) Preoperative staging of rectal cancer by intrarectal ultrasound. Dis Colon Rectum 28:42–46
7. Lohnert MSS, Doniec JM, Henne-Bruns D (2000) Effectiveness of endoluminal sonography in the identification of occult local rectal cancer recurrences. Dis Colon Rectum 43:483–491
8. Saclarides TJ (1998) Endorectal ultrasound. Surg Clin North Am 78:237–249
9. Hussain SM, Stoker J, Schutte HE, Lameris JS (1996) Imaging of the anorectal region. Europ J Radiol 22:116–122
10. Giovannini M (2000) Three-dimensional endorectal ultrasound: gadget or technology of future? Acta Endoscopica 30:19–25

Invited Commentary

M. Hünerbein

Endoscopic ultrasound (EUS) remains the most sensitive imaging modality for evaluation of the rectum and the anal canal. Although most publications deal with the staging of rectal cancer, endorectal ultrasound also plays a major role in the diagnosis of benign anorectal disease, especially fistula and sphincter defects.

Recently, several new ultrasound techniques have been developed that could significantly improve the diagnostic value of endorectal ultrasound. These new methods include power Doppler sonography, a variety of harmonic imaging techniques, electronic compounding, and pulse-sequencing methods that improve the signal-to-noise relation as well as structural conspicuity.

The introduction of contrast agents has changed the diagnostic potential of Doppler ultrasonography dramatically. Since the concentration of the contrast agent can be determined as a function of time, a measure for the actual blood flow can now be obtained that provides quantitative information. By using these technological advances, it is now possible to assess blood flow in very small vessels that feed normal or abnormal tissues and to assess changes in flow and vascularity that occur in response to therapeutic efforts.

Elastography has been developed as a new EUS technique that differentiates the tissue stiffness similar to palpation. The prototypic elasticity imaging technique consists of a device for generating shear waves in tissue, an EUS-based method for imaging propagation of these waves, and an algorithm for processing the wave images to generate quantitative images, depicting tissue stiffness. During the examination, a sequence of ultrasonic images is acquired while the tissue is slightly compressed by the ultrasound probe [1]. Using numerical analysis of image pairs for the acquired sequence, the tissue strain is calculated that represents the spatial elasticity distribution of a specific cross-section of the organ.

However, the techniques mentioned above appear to be most valuable for pre- and postoperative evaluation of anorectal malignancy. The most promising new technique for the diagnosis of benign anorectal diseases, such as fistulas and sphincter tears, is three-dimensional (3-D) endorectal ultrasound. Three-dimensional imaging overcomes some of the difficulties and problems associated with conventional two-dimensional (2-D) endorectal ultrasound, which is usually done by real-time interpretation of 2-D cross-sectional images. Although these images may provide valuable information, it is often difficult to interpret the images because the 3-D anatomy must be reconstructed mentally from multiple sectional images. Consequently, major efforts have been made to develop techniques for the generation of 3-D images. Regardless of the imaging technique, these methods involve acquisition of serial cross-sectional images that are subjected to computer processing to produce a 3-D data set. It must be emphasized that the quality of 3-D images is dependent on the resolution of the probe used to acquire the individual 2-D images. Currently, only probes with 10 MHz or, better, 16 MHz, as described by Santoro and Fortling, can be considered to provide adequate resolution. Other factors influencing the quality of the images include the number of acquired scan planes and acquisition time (motion artifacts).

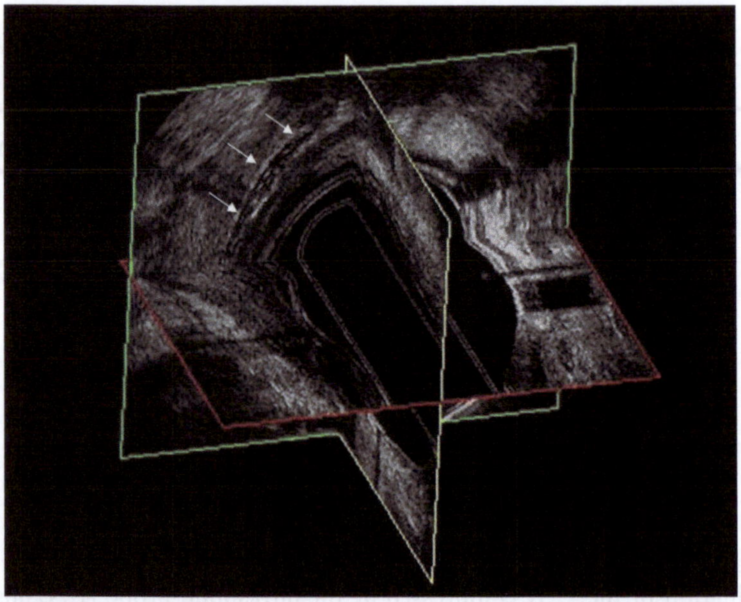

a

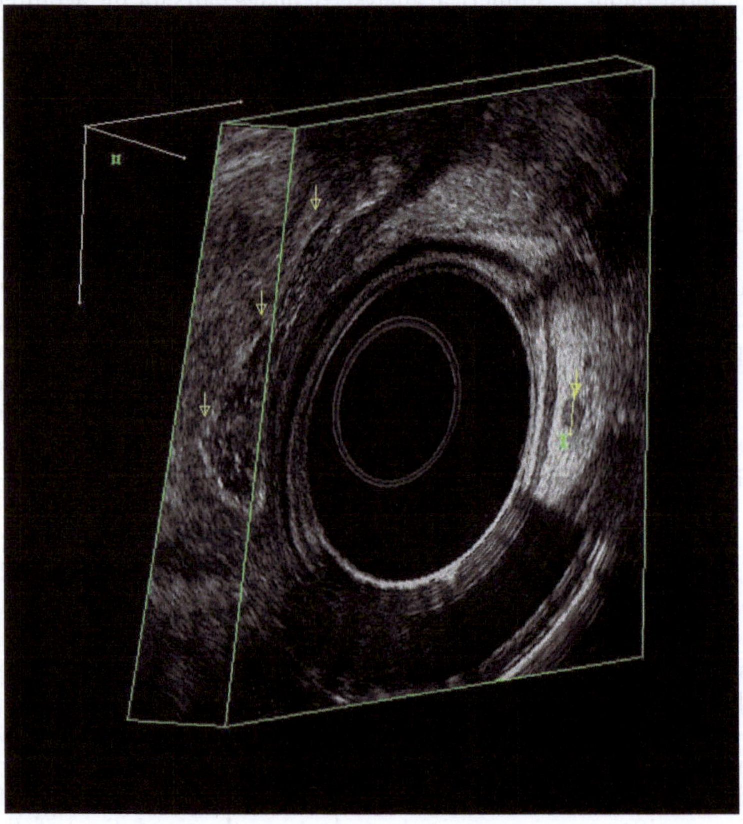

b

Fig. II.25. Perirectal fistula: multiplanar image (**a**), three-dimensional reconstruction (**b**)

The 3-D data can then be displayed in multiple planes (multiplanar reformatting) or as 3-D reconstruction (Fig. II.25). The data can be subjected to rendering algorithms that display only selected pixels, depending on the brightness. Various rendering modes, such as maximum, minimum, transparency mode, or combinations thereof, are available. Although these modes are helpful to enhance some information, other details may be lost. It is very important to realize that too much manipulation of the data can destroy any information and may lead to confusion and misinterpretation of the data. Similar to conventional endoscopic ultrasound, this new technique requires training and experience.

Three-dimensional reconstructions may closely resemble the real 3-D anatomy and can therefore significantly improve the assessment of normal and pathologic anatomy. Complex information on the exact location, extent, and relation of the tumor to relevant structures can be displayed in a single 3-D image. Although hard copies are valuable, interactive manipulation of the data on the computer will even increase the ability of the surgeon to assess critical details.

Interactive analysis of the 3-D data, also referred to as virtual operation planning, allows the display of data according to the clinical requirements. Various 3-D views, including rotating cine loops, can be visualized. Selected structures can be marked by colors, and measurements can be made. Computer animation techniques can be performed to simulate surgical procedures, for example, tumor resections (Fig. II.26). It seems likely that these new diagnostic tools will be increasingly used in the future to facilitate planning of operations and for surgical training.

Until now, only a limited number of studies have been available that have investigated the clinical relevance of 3-D endorectal ultrasound. In a pilot study, Müller et al. performed 3-D endorectal ultrasound in three patients with rectal cancer [2]. More recently, a comprehensive study involving 100 patients demonstrated encouraging results of 3-D endorectal ultrasound in the evaluation of rectal cancer [3]. Three-dimensional ultrasound facilitated the interpretation of ultrasound scans and improved the diagnostic confidence in approximately 60% of examinations.

Comparable preliminary experience has also been reported for 3-D endoanal ultrasound imaging of perianal fistulas and sphincter defects. West et al. performed preoperative 3-D endoanal ultrasound and endoanal magnetic resonance imaging (MRI) in 40 patients with symptoms of a perianal fistula and a visible external opening [4]. The results were assessed separately by experienced observers. Fistulas were described according to the following characteristics: classification of the primary fistula tract according to Parks, location of the internal opening, presence of secondary tracts, and fluid collection [5]. The methods agreed in 88% of cases for primary fistula tracts, in 90% for location of the internal opening, in 78% for secondary tracts, and in 88% for fluid collection.

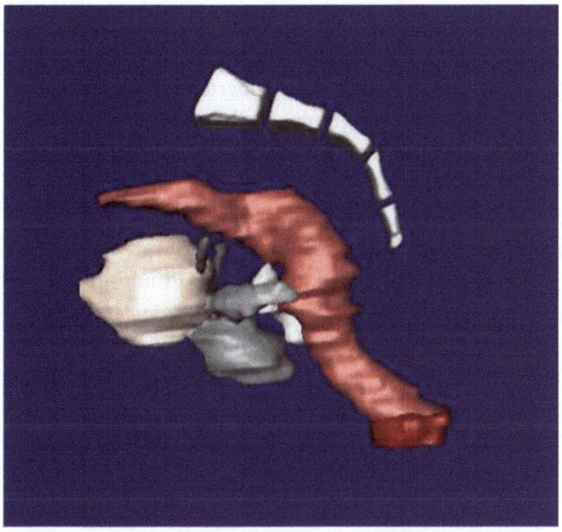

Fig. II.26. Computer-generated three-dimensional (3-D) model of anal canal, rectum, prostate, pelvis, bladder, and spine based on 3-D endorectal ultrasonography data

Recently, the group of Bartram conducted a prospective study to compare the accuracy of 3-D endoanal ultrasound with that of hydrogen-peroxide-enhanced 3-D endoanal ultrasound in diagnosing fistula in ano in 19 patients [6]. The accuracy of 3-D endoanal ultrasound and that of hydrogen-peroxide-enhanced 3-D endoanal ultrasound were compared with a reference standard derived from surgical findings, MRI, and follow-up. There were 21 internal openings and primary tracks in 19 patients: one superficial, one intersphincteric, 18 transsphincteric, and one extrasphincteric. Fourteen patients had 19 secondary tracks. Both techniques detected fistula tracks in 19 of 21 (90%) patients. Hydrogen peroxide improved conspicuity of some tracks and internal openings and so may be helpful in difficult cases although no overall diagnostic benefit was demonstrated.

In conclusion, 3-D endosonography is capable of improving diagnostic evaluation of benign anorectal disease. This technique facilitates the interpretation of transrectal ultrasound images by displaying previously unattainable scan planes, multiplanar images, and 3-D views. Accurate depiction of the anatomy can be enhanced by various rendering techniques. Future perspectives include the application of 3-D color Doppler techniques, four-dimensional (4-D) endorectal ultrasound, and 3-D-ultrasound-based systems for intraoperative navigation.

References

1. Lorenz A, Ermert H, Sommerfeld HJ et al (2000) Ultrasound elastography of the prostate. A new technique for tumor detection. Ultraschall Med 21:8–15
2. Mueller MP, Stamos MJ, Cavaye DM et al (1992) Three-dimensional transrectal ultrasound: preliminary patient evaluation. J Laparoendosc Surg 2:223–227
3. Hünerbein M, Schlag PM (1997) 3D-Endosonography for staging of rectal cancer. Ann Surg 225:432–438
4. West RL, Dwarkasing S, Felt-Bersma RJF et al (2005) Hydrogen-peroxide-enhanced three dimensional endoanal ultrasonography and endoanal magnetic resonance imaging in evaluating perianal fistulas: agreement and patient preference. Eur J Gastroenterol Hepatol 16:1319–1324
5. Parks AG, Gordon PH, Hardcastle JD (1976) A classification of fistula-in-ano. Br J Surg 63:1–12
6. Buchanan GN, Bartram CI, Williams AB et al (2005) Value of hydrogen peroxide enhancement of three-dimensional endoanal ultrasound in fistula-in-ano. Dis Colon Rectum 48:141–147

SECTION III

State of the Art in Pelvic Floor Imaging

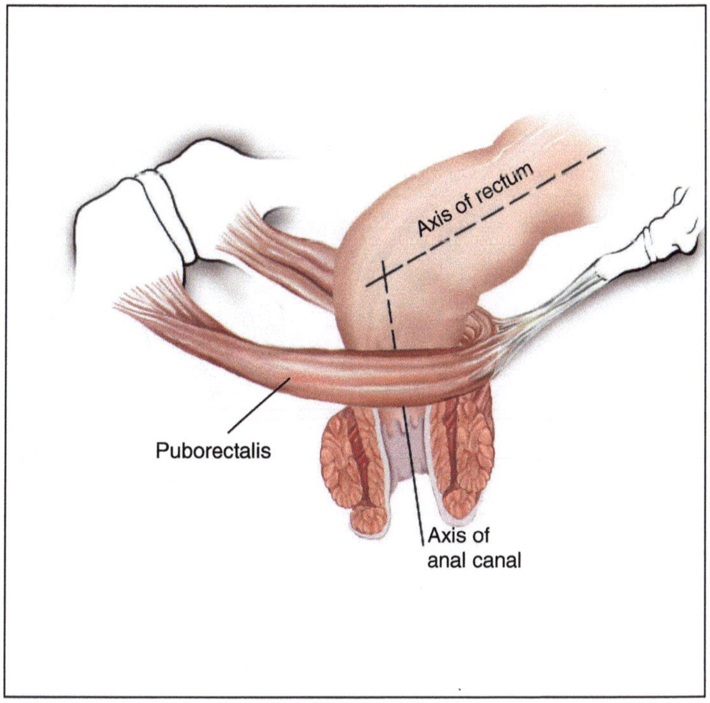

III.1.
Introduction

G.A. Santoro, G. Di Falco

The imaging of pelvic floor structures is presently of great interest. In the last two decades, growing attention has been dedicated to increasing both understanding on the pelvic floor anatomy (particularly related to physiology and pathophysiology) and improving technologies for diagnosis. Endoluminal ultrasonography (EUS) and magnetic resonance imaging (MRI) have become an important part of the diagnostic workup in pelvic floor dysfunction [1, 2]. Their contributions should be effectively integrated with other techniques (i.e., endoscopy, anorectal manometry and electromyography, evacuation proctography) for a complete assessment of the main pathologic conditions of the pelvic floor and to plan the best form of treatment.

The advantage of EUS is that it is inexpensive and widely available; however, similar to all ultrasound methods, EUS is operator dependent. Despite the fact that intraobserver and interobserver agreement has been reported in the literature as good or very good [3], measurement of the different anal structures did not provide homogeneous morphometric results [4, 5]. Many debates have centered around who should perform EUS examinations: colorectal surgeons, gastroenterologists, or radiologists. We are persuaded that the operator's experience is the most relevant factor, irrespective of specialty.

The current 360° rotating endoprobe, specifically designed for anorectal scanning, has provided important information to a detailed understanding of the anatomy of this region [6]. The increasing interest in endoanal (EAUS) and endorectal (ERUS) ultrasonography, accomplished with a wider spread in using these procedures, has allowed the definition of clinical indications and the field of applications. The ambitious aim of this diagnostic tool is to correctly identify very small and thin structures, with no precise interfaces and limits with the adjacent structures, which often cannot be visualized or measured with conventional techniques. The influence of age, gender, parity, obstetric trauma, body weight, height, and a number of other incompletely understood factors on variability of anorectal anatomy has for a long time led to significant confusion and conflicting results. Both EUS and MRI have contributed to modify previous knowledge of anorectal anatomy and adequately correlate imaging with pelvic floor dysfunction [7–9]. Significant improvement in reducing investigational problems has been recently obtained by using more sophisticated devices [i.e., three-dimensional (3-D) acquisition systems, probe pull-through systems, and the newer probe with integrated 3-D and pull-through devices], which allow evaluation of the anal canal and rectum in a variety of projections, including the transverse, sagittal, and coronal planes, and all the possible diagonal views. Measurement of linear distance, thickness, and volume are readily available.

However, considering both diagnostic applications and potential pitfalls of EAUS and ERUS, it is mandatory to standardize as much as possible the equipment used, technique of examination, manner of performing measurements, and definitions and subjective interpretations. By minimizing the effect of these confounding variables, different investigators will be able to communicate and compare results.

The purpose of this section is to describe the normal anatomy of the anal canal and rectum by means of EUS and MRI. Attention will be given to the more recent acquisition in pelvic floor imaging.

References

1. Stoker J, Halligan S, Bartram CI (2001) Pelvic floor imaging. Radiology 218:621-641
2. Stoker J, Rociu E, Zwamborn AW et al (1999) Endoluminal MR imaging of the rectum and anus: technique, applications and pitfalls. Radiographics 19:383–398
3. Gold DM, Halligan S, Kmiot WA, Bartram CI (1999) Intraobserver and interobserver agreement in anal endosonography. Br J Surg 86:371–375
4. Enck P, Heyer T, Gantke B, Schmidt WU et al (1997) How reproducible are measures of the anal sphincter muscle diameter by endoanal ultrasound? Am J Gastroenterol 92:293–296
5. Beets-Tan RGH, Morren GL, Betts GL, Kessels AGH et al (2001) Measurement of anal sphincter muscles: endoanal US, endoanal MR imaging, or phased-array MR imaging? A study with healthy volunteers. Radiology 220:81–89
6. Dalley AF (1987) The riddle of the sphincters. The morphophysiology of the anorectal mechanism reviewed. Am Surg 53:298–306
7. Sultan AH, Kamm MA, Hudson CN et al (1993) Anal-sphincter disruption during vaginal delivery. N Engl J Med 329:1905–1911
8. Hussain SM, Stoker J, Lameris JS (1995) Anal sphincter complex: endoanal MR imaging of normal anatomy. Radiology 197:671–677
9. Schafer A, Enck P, Furst G, Kahn T et al (1994) Anatomy of the anal sphincters. Comparison of anal endosonography to magnetic resonance imaging. Dis Colon Rectum 37:777–781

III.2. Endosonographic Anatomy of the Normal Anal Canal

G.A. Santoro, G. Di Falco

The anal canal is 2- to 4-cm long. The dentate line of the mucosa denotes the squamocolumnar junction. The circular smooth muscle of the rectal wall continues downward as the internal anal sphincter (IAS) that extends from the anorectal junction to approximately 1 cm below the dentate line (Fig. III.1) [1]. The outer longitudinal component of the muscularis propria conjoined with striated muscle fibers from the levator ani, particularly the puboanalis (Fig. III.2), and a large fibroelastic ele-

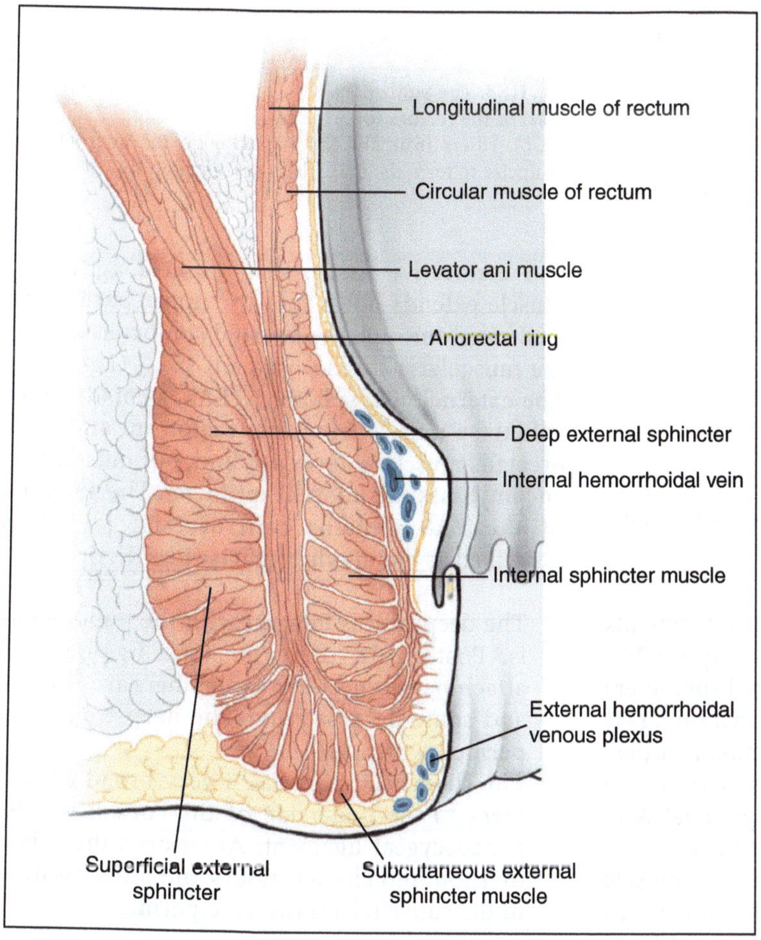

Fig. III.1. Normal anatomy of the anal canal. The muscularis propria of the rectal wall consists of both circular and longitudinal smooth muscle fibers. The circular layer is in continuity with the circular internal anal sphincter muscle. The longitudinal layer extends into the intersphincteric space of the anal canal. The external sphincter extends further down than the internal sphincter

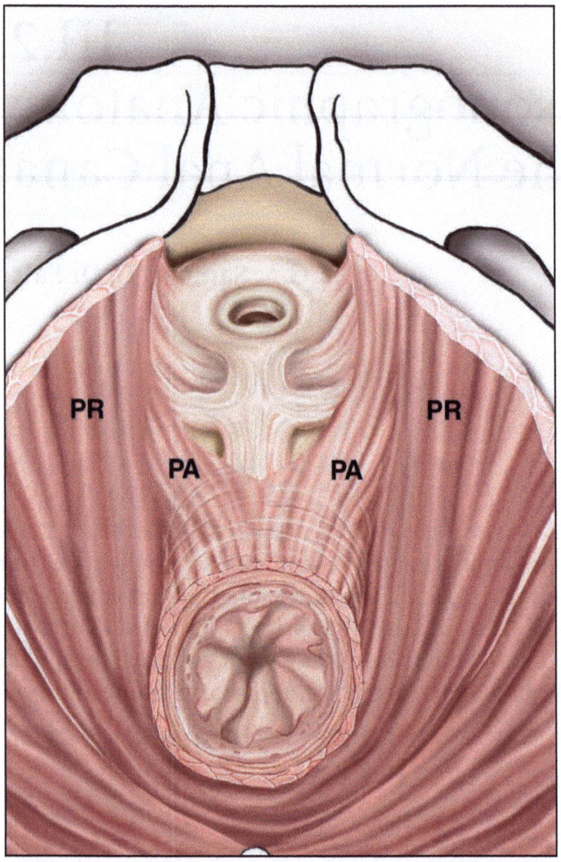

a

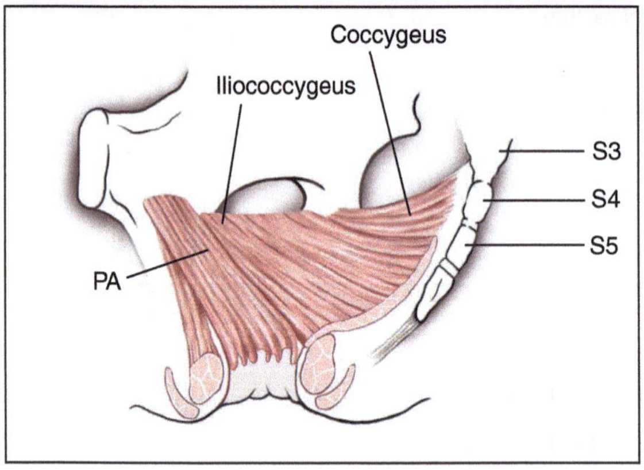

b

Fig. III.2. The puboanalis (*PA*) rises from the medial border of the puborectalis (*PR*)

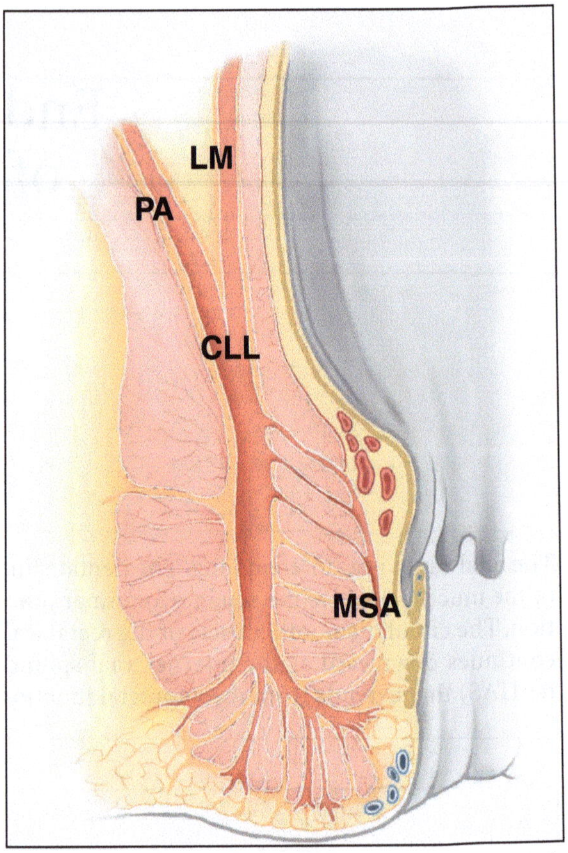

Fig. III.3. The puboanalis (*PA*) joins the longitudinal muscle (*LM*) of the rectum to form the conjoined longitudinal layer (*CCL*). Fibers from the LM run through the internal anal sphincter to form the muscularis submucosae ani (*MSA*)

ment derived from the endopelvic fascia, extends caudally as the conjoined longitudinal layer (CLL) between the external and internal anal sphincters and terminates at the anorectal junction [2–5] (Figs. III.3 and 4). Its fibroelastic component permeating through the subcutaneous part of the external sphincter terminates in the perianal skin. Konerding et al. [6], however, failed to detect striated muscle fibers within the longitudinal muscle that was solely composed of smooth muscle cells and connective tissue. Part of the longitudinal muscle extends down into the upper part of the anal canal through the internal sphincter to form the muscularis submucosae ani [2–4] (Fig. III.3). The external anal sphincter (EAS) is made up of voluntary muscle from the levator ani and puborectalis muscle to form a cylinder of muscle that encompasses the internal sphincter. The anatomy of the EAS remains controversial [7]. It is described as having three parts (Fig. III.5):

1. The deep part is integral with the puborectalis. Posteriorly, there is some ligamentous attachment; anteriorly, some fibers are circular and some decussate into the deep transverse perineii.
2. The superficial part has a very broad attachment to the underside of the coccyx via the anococcygeal ligament. Anteriorly, there is a division into circular fibers and a decussation to the superficial transverse perineii.

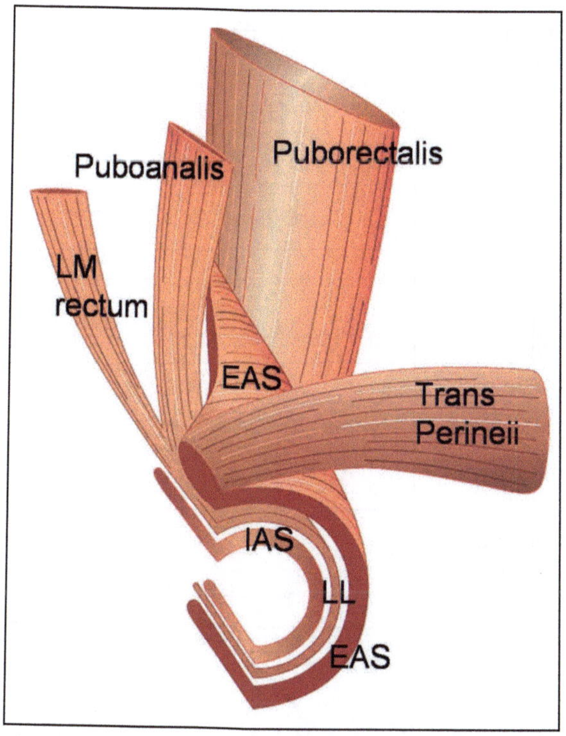

Fig. III.4. Diagram of the perineal muscles. *IAS* internal anal sphincter, *EAS* external anal sphincter, *LM* longitudinal muscle, *LL* longitudinal layer (with permission from [3])

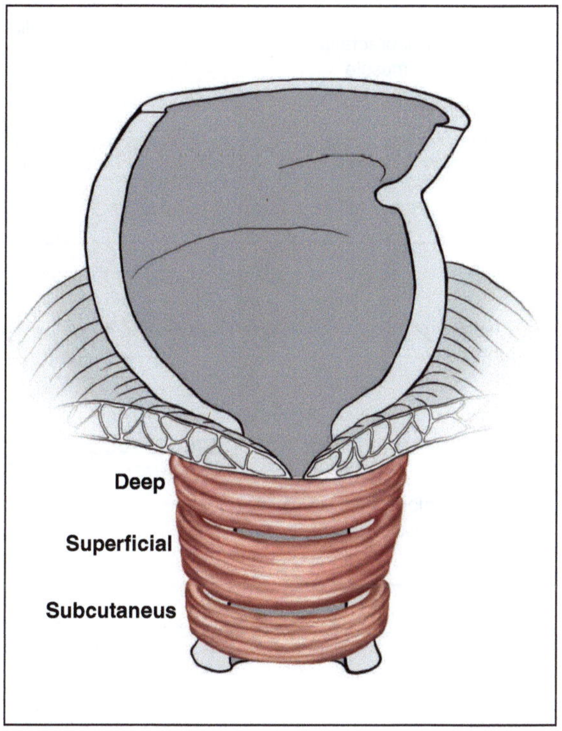

Fig. III.5. The external anal sphincter is subdivided into three parts: deep, superficial, and subcutaneous

3. The subcutaneous part lies below the IAS.
The anterior part of the external sphincter differs between genders. In males, it is symmetrical at all levels; in females, it is shorter anteriorly, and there is no evidence of anterior ring high in the canal [8] (Fig. III.6).

a 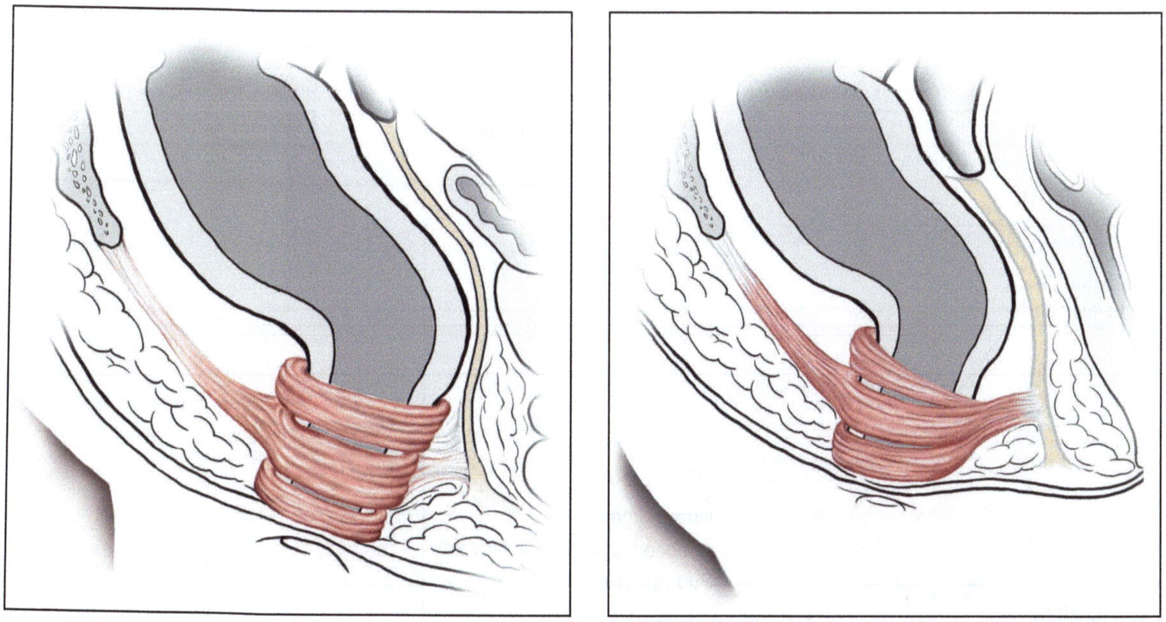 b

Fig. III.6. Schematic representation of the external anal sphincter in male (**a**) and female (**b**). Anteriorly, the sphincter is shorter in the female

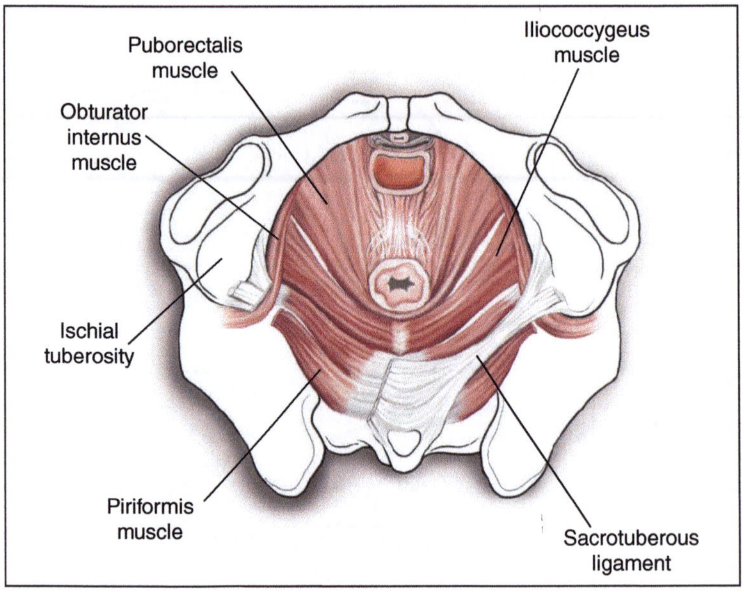

a

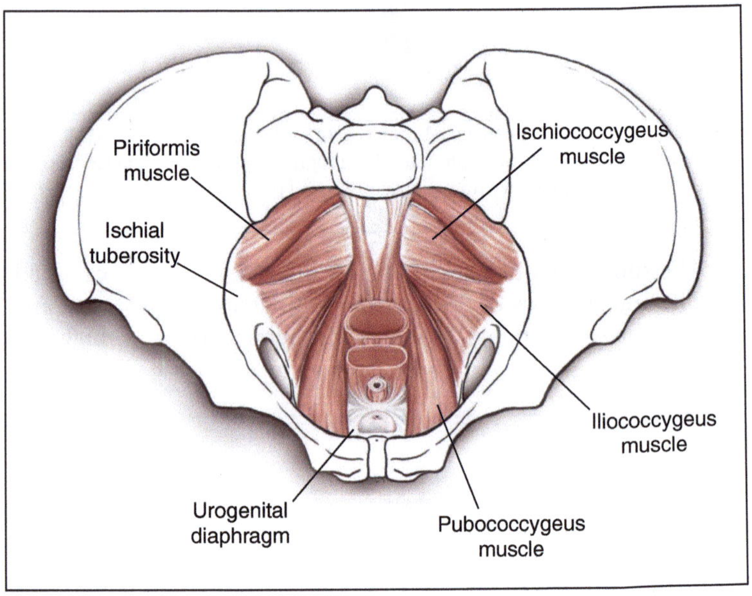

b

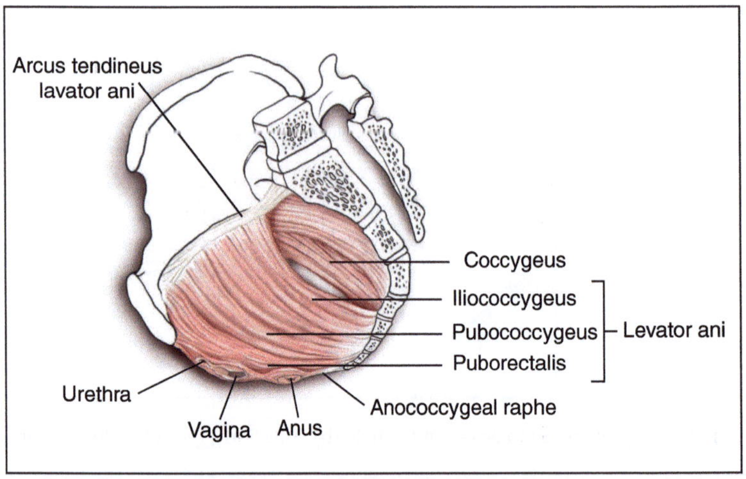

c

Fig. III.7. Schematic representation of the pelvic anatomy (**a-c**)

The levator ani, subdivided in the iliococcygeus, pubococcygeus, and puborectalis muscles, is the fundamental structure of the pelvic floor, arising from the side wall of the pelvis, supporting the pelvic contents, and separating the ischioanal fossa below from the supralevator space above [9] (Fig. III.7). The iliococcygeus lies posterolaterally, arising from the ischial spine to insert into the coccyx and anococcygeal ligament. The ischiococcygeus is a small, often rudimentary, subdivision of this. The pubococcygeus arises from the pubic bone, along with the puborectalis, and from a tendinous arch formed by obturator fascia running posteriorly toward the ischial spine (Fig. III.7). Pubococcygeal fibers run posteriorly toward the coccyx in a plane just cranial to the iliococcygeus. Fibers also cross the midline to form rectal and vaginal hiatus. The puborectalis arises from the pubis forming a distinct sling around the anorectal junction (Fig. III.8).

The perineal body (also named the central perineal tendon) anatomically is a junctional zone where fibers from the puborectalis, the external sphincter, the longitudinal muscle, and the internal sphincter decussate and fuse into muscles of the anterior urogenital triangle, notably, the deep and superficial transverse perineii and bulbospongiosus muscles (Fig. III.9). Such anatomic configuration gives to the perineal body a fundamental function to support all musculoligamentous components of the pelvis, anchoring the anal canal to the ischial and pubic bones [10] (Fig. III.10). The lack of these connections could be one of the most important reasons of a perineal descent, determining also damage to the pelvic nerves (i.e., pudendal nerves) and muscles (i.e., levator ani) and disconnecting functionally the anterior from posterior perineum. Perineal body damage could predispose to anterior or posterior perineal prolapse of the pelvic organs [11]. The anatomy of the perineal body differs between genders. In males, it is smaller and posterior to the spongious bodies; in females, it lies within the anovaginal septum [10] (Fig. III.10).

The area around the anorectum is divided into spaces (Fig. III.11). The perianal space surrounds the lower anal canal. Lateral to the sphincter is the ischioanal fossa, which is bounded laterally by the obturator internus muscle and superiorly by the levator ani muscle. The intersphincteric space is not a recognized anatomical term but is used to describe the area between the internal and the external sphincter. The supralevator space lies above the levator ani muscle and is demarcated superiorly by the pelvic peritoneum.

Endosonographic Anatomy

Most studies that highlighted a better comprehension of the sonographic anatomy of the anal canal and pelvic floor have emerged from Professor Clive Bartram and his group from the Intestinal Imaging Centre at St. Mark's Hospital in London. According to these studies, the anus is fundamentally a four-layer structure (Fig. III.12) [3, 4, 12–17]. From inner to outer, these are:

1. *Subepithelial tissues: moderately reflective.* The mucosa as well the level of dentate line is not visualized. The muscularis submucosae ani can be sonographically identified in the upper part of the anal canal as a low reflective band (Fig. III.13).
2. *Internal anal sphincter: hypoechoic* (Fig. III.14). The sphincter is not completely symmetric, either in thickness or termination (Fig. III.15). In older age groups, the sphincter becomes thicker and loses its uniform low-level echogenicity, which is characteristic of smooth muscle throughout the gut, to become more echogenic and inhomogeneous in texture [3, 13] (Fig. III.16). Although it seems normal and without lesions, sometimes the IAS has differences in echogenicity and thickness. Recently, an increasing interest in IAS degeneration has occurred. In such a condition (first described by using EAUS), the IAS appears intact but thinner than normal and hyperechoic; it has been regarded as a cause of passive fecal incontinence [14].
3. *Longitudinal muscle: hyperechoic.* This muscle is moderately echogenic, which is surprising, as it is mainly smooth muscle. However, an increased fibrous stroma may account for this (Fig. III.17). The intersphincteric space, in which the longitudinal muscle is located, presents a wide variability in thickness and is not always distinctly visible along the entire anal canal. However, the ability to identify this structure in normal subjects, differentiating it from the IAS and EAS, could be useful in assessing diseases involving the intersphincteric space. The puboanalis is seen as a low-reflective, triangular-shaped band of muscle

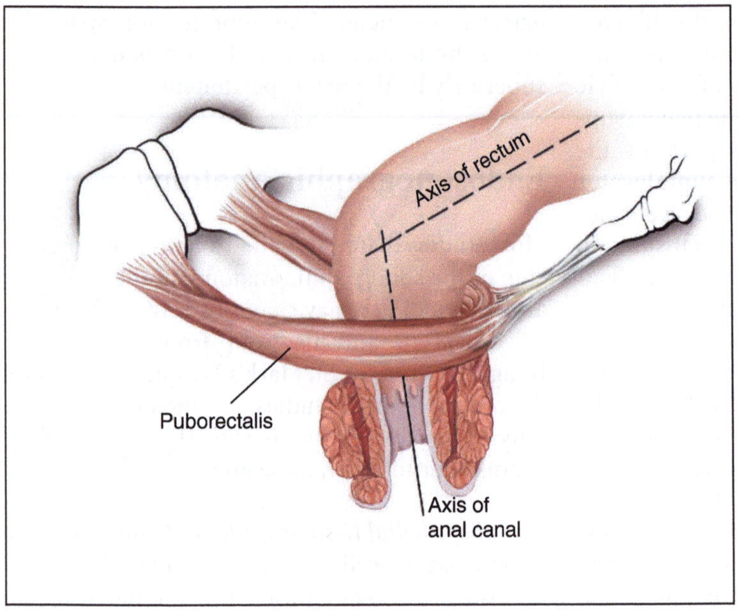

Fig. III.8. The puborectalis muscle swings behind the anal canal at its most proximal limit to encircle the sphincter posteriorly

just medial to the puborectalis [3, 4, 13] (Fig. III.18). By using three-dimensional EAUS, it is possible to obtain excellent images of the conjoined longitudinal layer (Fig. III.19).

4. *External anal sphincter: mixed echogenicity.* Endosonography largely overestimates the size of the EAS due to its failure to recognize and separate the CLL. The EAS and the CLL contain large amounts of fat and fibrous tissue, which lead to similar echogenicities of both structures [18] (Fig. III.20).

Ultrasound imaging of the anus can be divided into three levels: high, mid, and low portions [3, 19] (Fig. III.21). The level refers to the following anatomical structures:

1. *High*: the sling of the puborectalis and the deep part of the external sphincter;

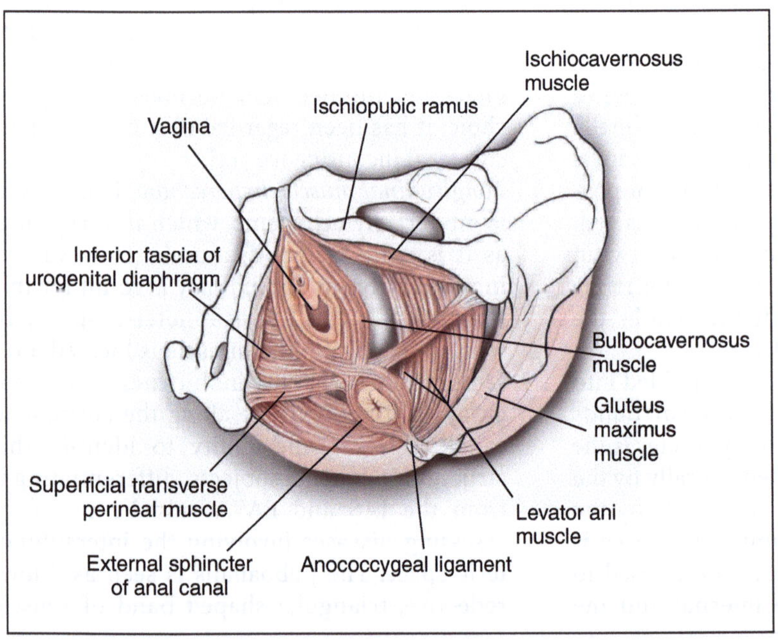

Fig. III.9. Bulbospongiosus muscle, transverse perineal muscles, and external anal sphincter meet in the perineal body

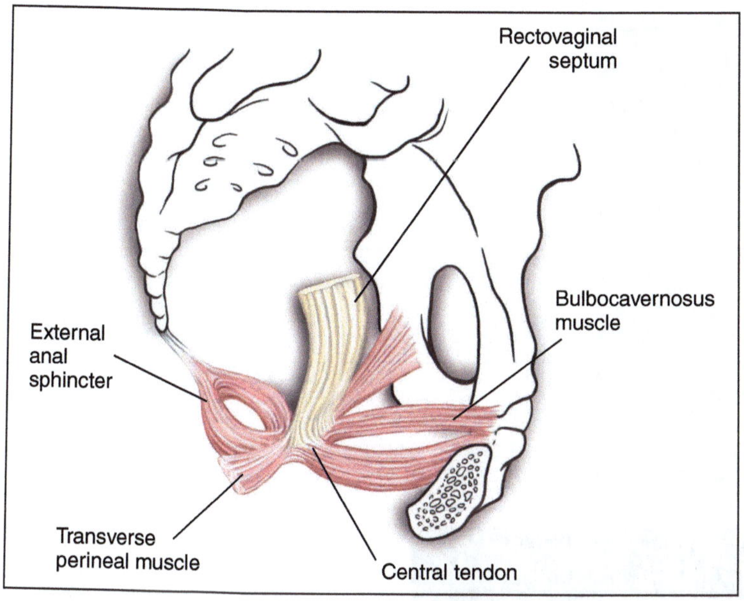

Fig. III.10. The perineal body lies within the rectovaginal septum in the female

2. *Mid*: the anococcygeal ligament, superficial part of the external sphincter, internal sphincter, perineal body, and vagina in females;
3. *Low*: the subcutaneous part of the external sphincter.

The muscles of the lower and the upper part of the anal canal are different. The first US image recorded is normally at the puborectalis level and labeled *high* (Fig. III.22). The puborectalis muscle slings the anal canal instead of completely surrounding it. At its upper end, the puborectalis is attached to the funnel-shaped levator ani muscle, and the levator ani anchors the sphincter complex to the inner side of the pelvis [10]. The deep part of the external sphincter is similar in echogenicity to the puborectalis and so is indistinguishable from it. Anteriorly, the circular fibers of the deep part of the external sphincter are not recognizable in females whereas in males, thin arcs of muscle from the deeper part of the sphincter may be seen extending anteriorly (Fig. III.22). This is particularly frequent in middle-aged to older women, especially if multiparous. Anatomic studies detailed the lower length of the ventral EAS in females, showing that the differences with males are already present in the fetus [20]. Three-dimensional longitudinal imaging can offer suggestive features of these anatomic characteristics of EAS [15, 21, 22] (Fig. III.23). In examining a female subject, the ultrasonographic differences between the natural gaps (hypoechoic areas with smooth, regular edges) and sphincter ruptures (mixed echogenicity, due to scarring, with irregu-

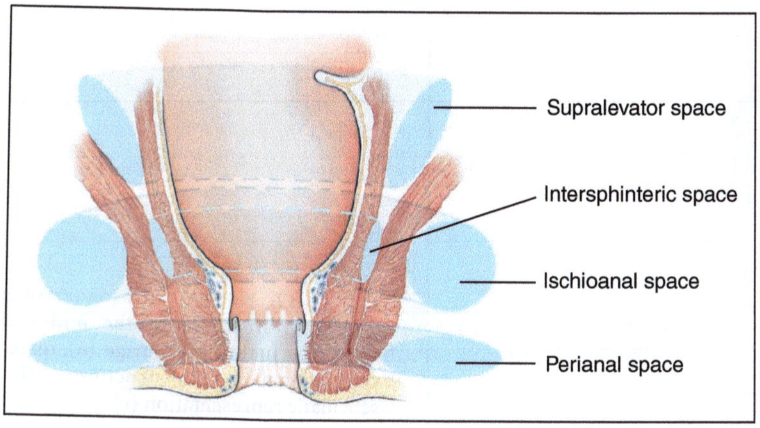

Fig. III.11. Schematic representation of the different perianal spaces

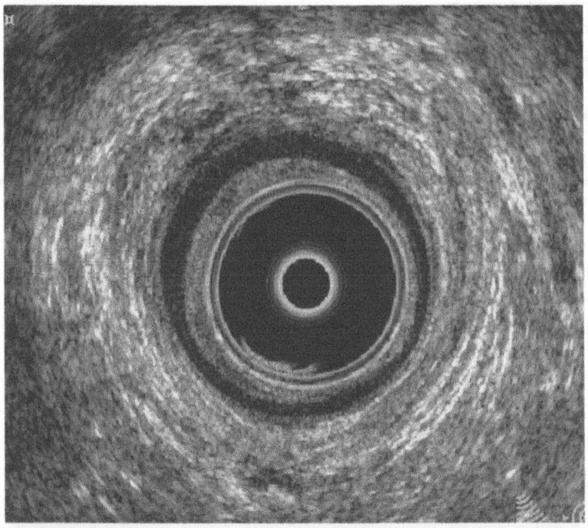
a

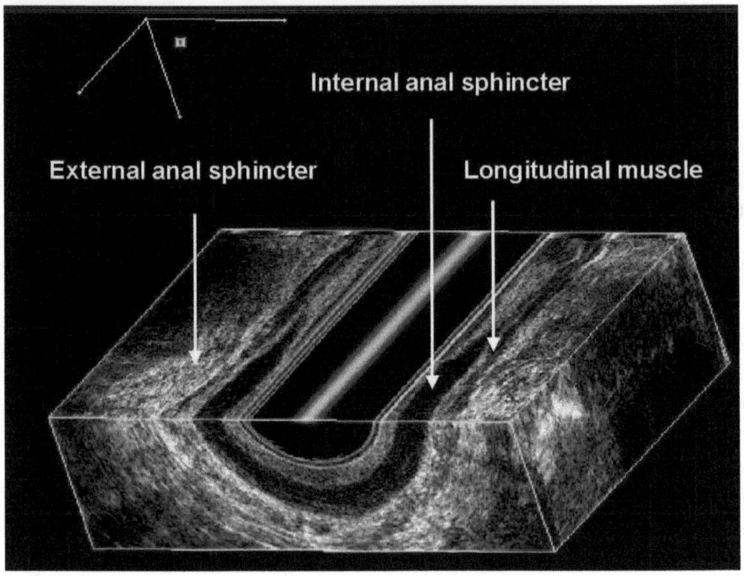

b

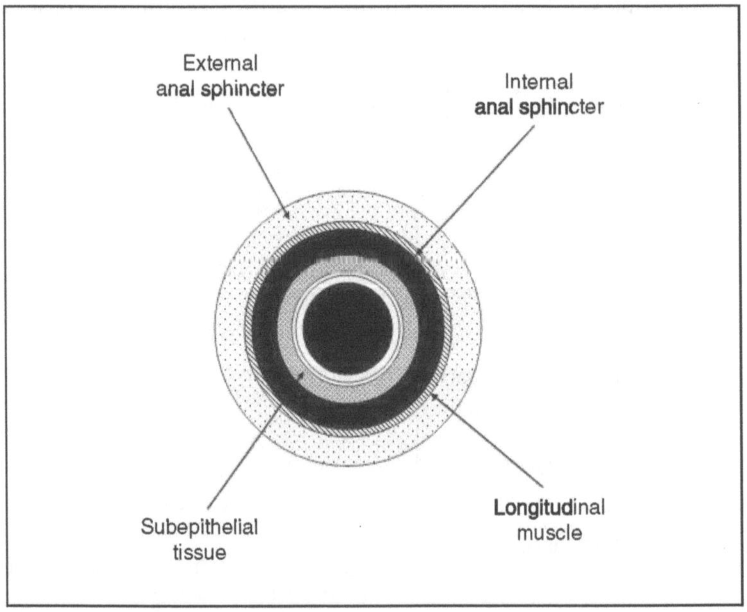

c

Fig. III.12. Normal ultrasonographic four-layer structure of the mid-anal canal in a male. Axial image (**a**), three-dimensional reconstruction (**b**), schematic representation (**c**)

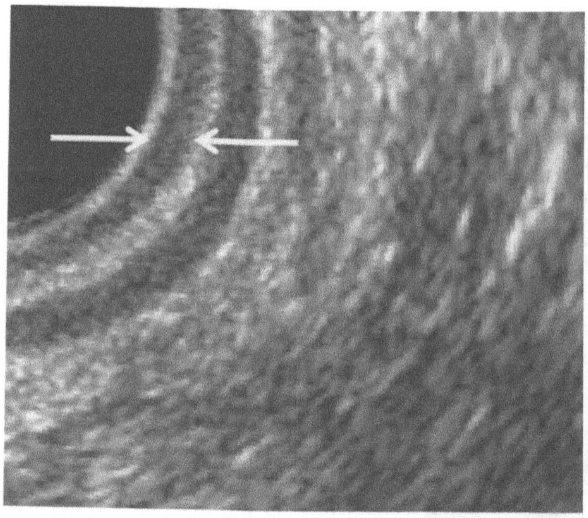

Fig. III.13. The muscularis submucosae ani can be sonographically identified as a low reflective band within the moderately reflective subepithelium (*arrows*)

lar edges) occurring at the upper anterior part of the anal canal must be kept in mind [8]. Bollard et al. [23] found manometric confirmation of the EAS gaps identified by EAUS.

Moving the probe a few millimeters in the distal direction will appear an intact anterior EAS (Fig. III.24), forming just below the superficial transverse perineal muscles, imaged at 11 and 1 o'clock (Fig. III.25). This image is a mid-canal projection in which the IAS, conjoining longitudinal muscle, and superficial EAS all are identified. This image will be labeled *mid*. As reported by Bartram [3], in females, fibers between the transverse perineii fuse with the external sphincter so that there is no plane of dissection between these two structures. In males, a plane of fat persists between the transverse perineii and the external sphincter (Fig. III.25). The perineal body is seen as a complex structure of concentric rings with a hypoechoic or hyperechoic center. It is the central portion of the perineum where the EAS, the bulbospongiosus, and the transverse perineal muscles meet (Fig. III.25). EAUS is able to precisely identify differences of the perineal body between males and females. However, it remains difficult to reliably measure this structure because of the lack of clear limits. Also, the proposed use of a finger introduced into the vagina as a landmark seems to be of poor benefit, altering its normal configuration due to the digital compression on the central perineum [24, 25].

Three-dimensional endosonography may provide accurate imaging of the perineal body in females and more accurate measurement (Fig. III.26).

The anococcygeal raphe is seen as a posterior hypoechoic triangle (Fig. III.27).

When the probe is pulled further out, the image of the IAS will disappear, and only the subepithelium and the subcutaneous segment of the longitudinal muscle plus the EAS will be seen. This last image will be labeled *low* (Fig. III.28).

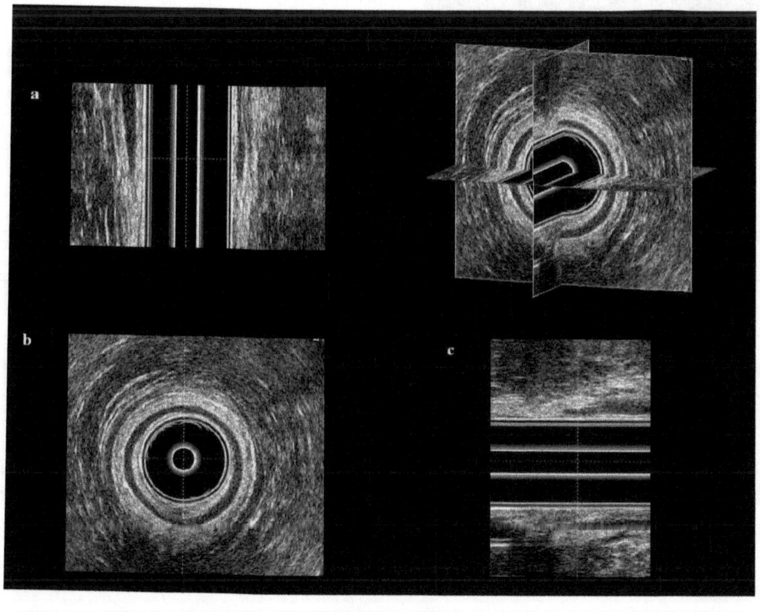

Fig. III.14. The internal sphincter in the coronal (**a**), transverse (**b**), and sagittal (**c**) planes

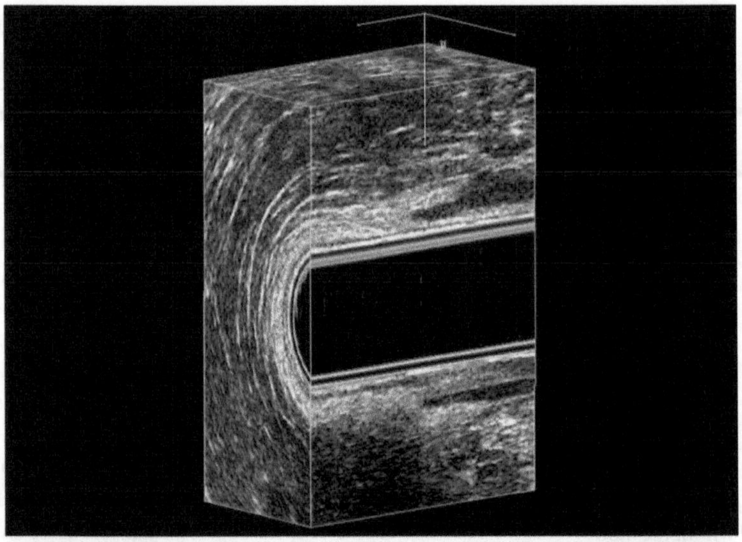

a

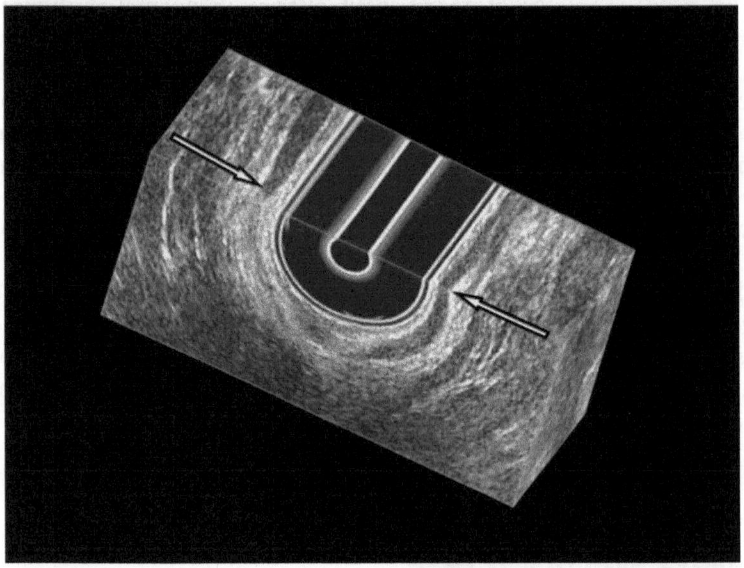

b

Fig. III.15. The internal sphincter ends at the level of the junction between the superficial and subcutaneous external sphincter. Its termination can be is symmetric (**a**) or not completely symmetric (**b**) (*arrows*)

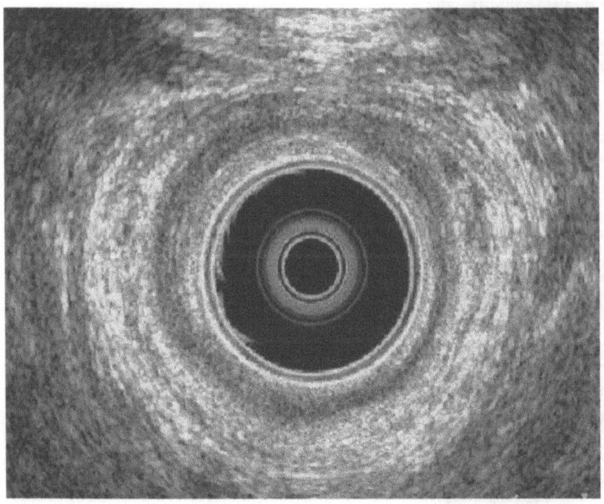

Fig. III.16. The sphincter is intact but more echogenic and inhomogeneous in texture in this 67-year-old man with a minor degree of incontinence

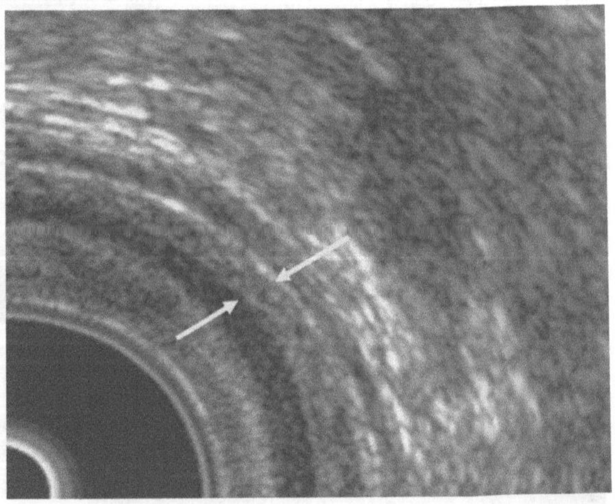

Fig. III.17. The longitudinal layer can be sonographically identified as a moderately echogenic structure (*arrows*)

a
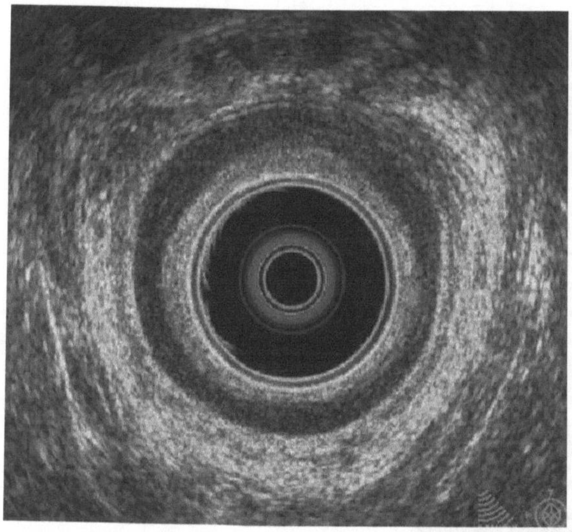

b
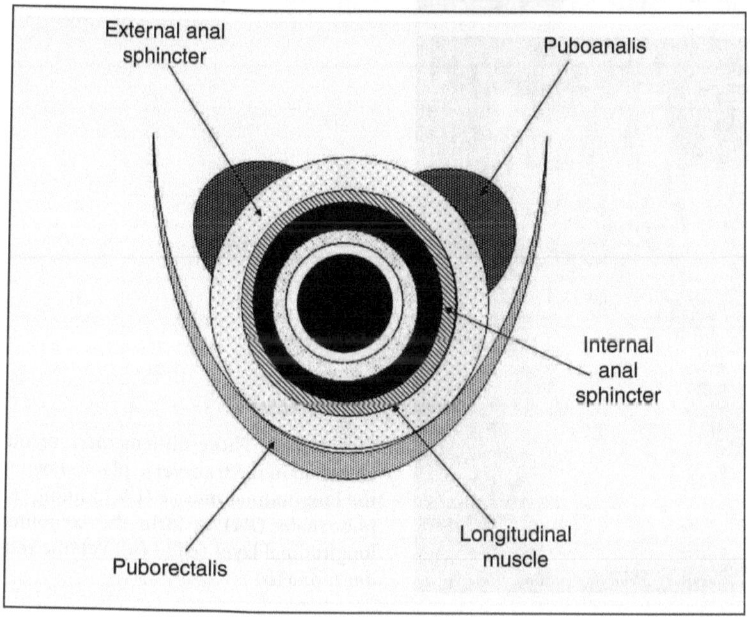

Fig. III.18. The puboanalis is seen as a low-reflective, triangular-shaped band of muscle just medial to the puborectalis (a). Schematic representation (b)

Normal Values

The anal canal length is the distance measured between the proximal canal, where the puborectalis muscle is identified, and the lower border of the subcutaneous external sphincter. It is significantly longer in males than in females as a result of a longer EAS whereas there is no difference in puborectalis length. In males, the anterior part of the external sphincter is present along the entire length of the canal (Fig. III.29). In females, the anterior ring of the external sphincter is shorter. Williams et al. [21] reported that the anterior EAS occupied 58% of the male anal canal compared with 38% of the female canal (p <0.01). In females, the puborectalis occupied a significantly larger proportion of the canal than in males (61% versus 45%; p=0.02). There was no difference in the length of the IAS between males and females (34.4 mm versus 33.2 mm) or the proportion of the anal canal that it occupied (67% versus 73%; p=0.12).

Normal values for sphincter dimensions differ between techniques. The importance of defining the true values of sphincter muscle thickness is not relevant because the purpose of measuring anal sphincters is to distinguish a normal versus abnormal measurement, regardless of the absolute values. Measurement should be taken at the 3 and 9 o'clock positions in the midlevel of the anal canal. The thickness of IAS varies from 1.8±0.5

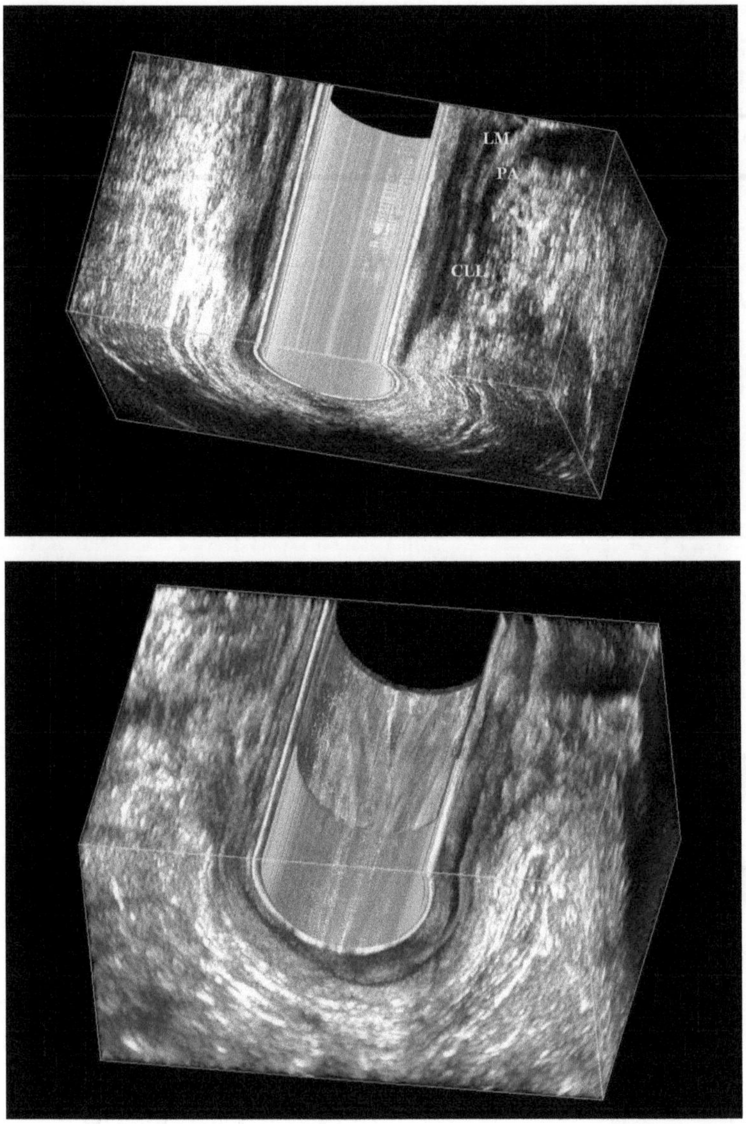

a

b

Fig. III.19. Three-dimensional reconstruction in the transverse plane showing the longitudinal muscle (*LM*) joining the puboanalis (*PA*) to form the conjoined longitudinal layer (*CLL*) (**a**). Volume render mode (**b**)

mm and increases with age owing to the presence of more fibrous tissue as the absolute amount of muscle decreases [3], measuring 2.4–2.7 mm <55 years and 2.8–3.5 mm >55 years. Any IAS >4 mm thick should be considered abnormal whatever the patient's age; conversely, a sphincter of 2 mm is normal in a young patient but abnormal in an elderly one. The longitudinal muscle is 2.5±0.6 mm in males and 2.9±0.6 mm in females. The average thickness of the EAS is 8.6±1.1 mm in males and 7.7±1.1 mm in females.

Many studies have specifically addressed the problems of the reproducibility of EAUS sphincter measurements [17, 18, 26–28]. Enck et al. [27]

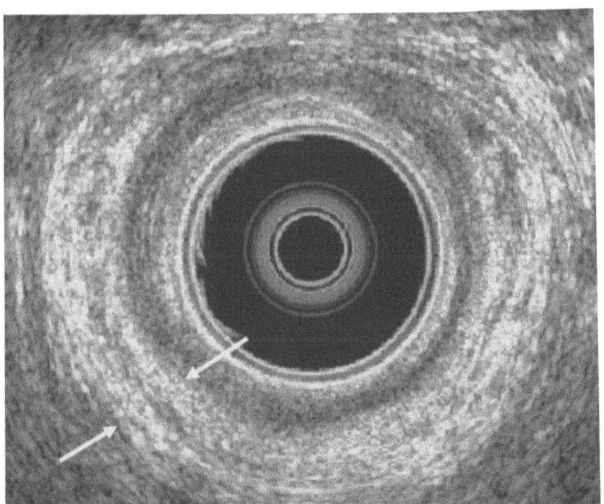

Fig. III.20. The external sphincter can be sonographically identified as a structure with mixed echogenicity (*arrows*)

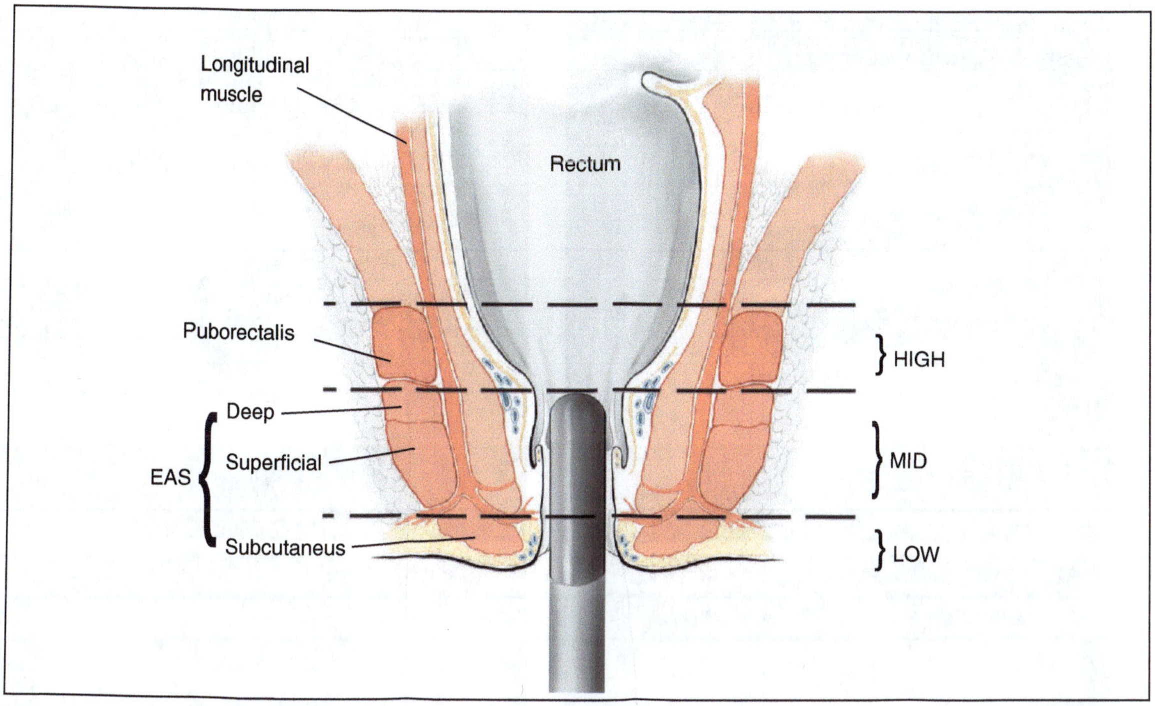

Fig. III.21. Schematic representation of the three levels (high, mid and low) of the anal canal with the probe in situ. *EAS* external anal sphincter, *IAS* internal anal sphincter

examined a small group of healthy volunteers and concluded that EAUS did not provide reliable measurements of internal and external sphincter thicknesses. Gold et al. [28] examined 51 patients and found that measurements of the internal sphincter were more reproducible than those of the external sphincter. These findings are consistent with results from Beets-Tan et al. [18], which compared EAUS, endoanal MRI, and phased-array MRI for anal sphincter measurement in healthy volunteers. EAUS enabled reliable measurement of only internal sphincter thickness

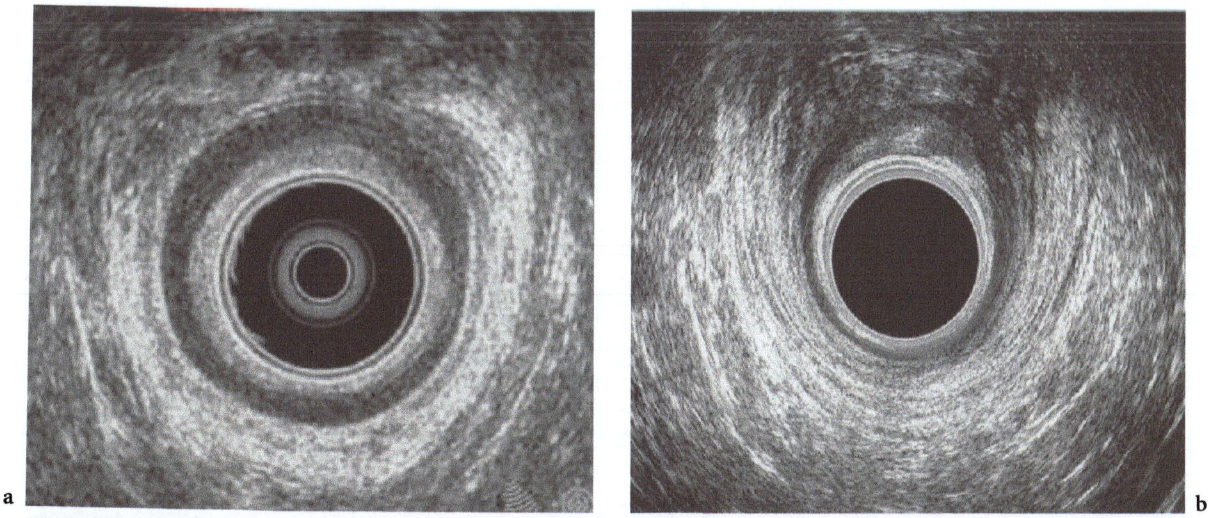

Fig. III.22. Normal ultrasound anatomy of the deep level of the anal canal demonstrating the puborectalis (*PR*). Anteriorly, a thin arc of muscle from the deeper part of the sphincter may be seen in males (**a**) whereas the deep part of the external sphincter is not recognizable in females (**b**)

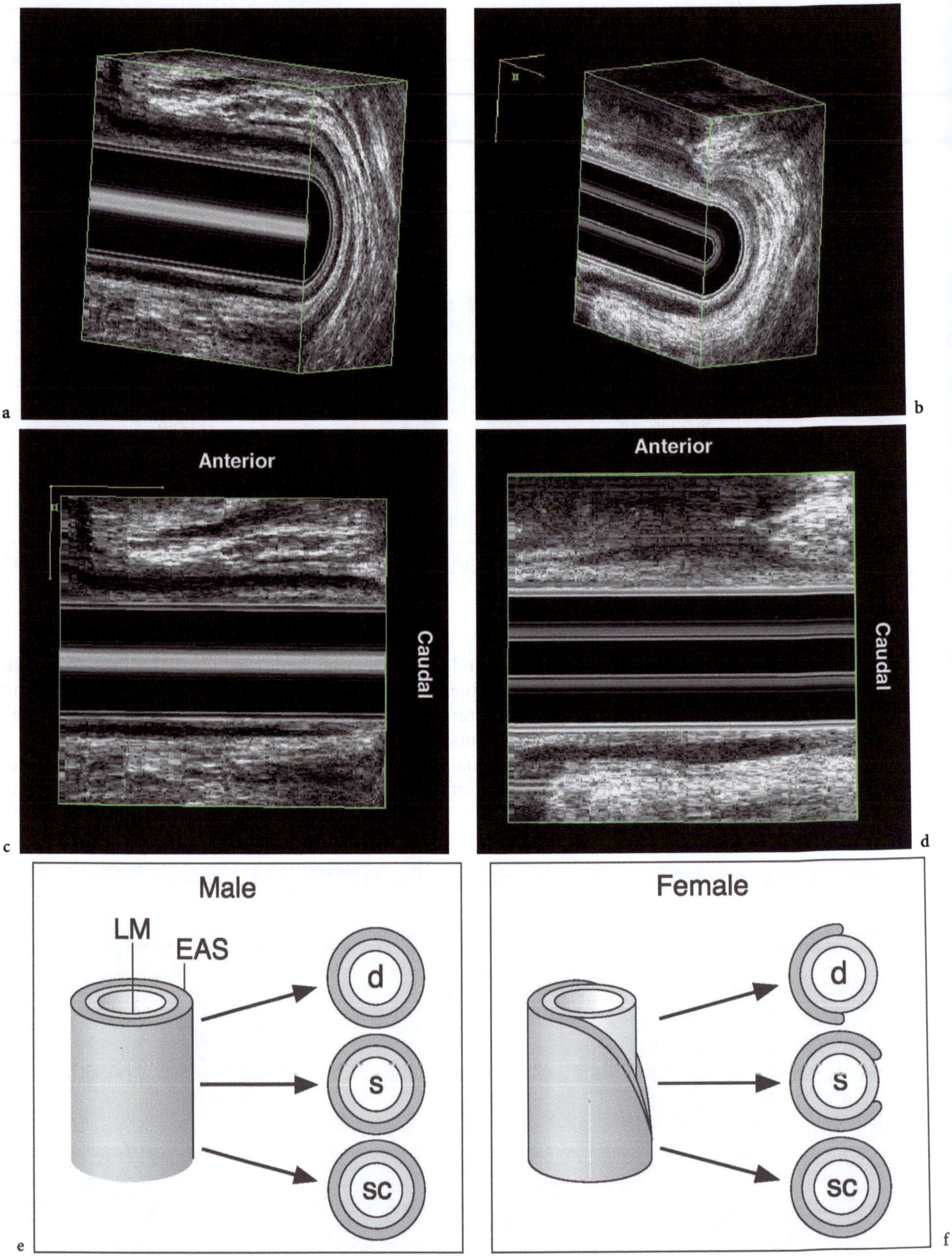

Fig. III.23. Three-dimensional endosonographic reconstruction demonstrating that the anterior anal sphincter is shorter in the female: male (**a**), female (**b**). Sagittal images: male (**c**), female (**d**). Schematic representation: (**e, f**). *LM* longitudinal muscle, *EAS* external anal sphincter, (**d** = deep; **s** = superficial; **sc** = subcutaneous)

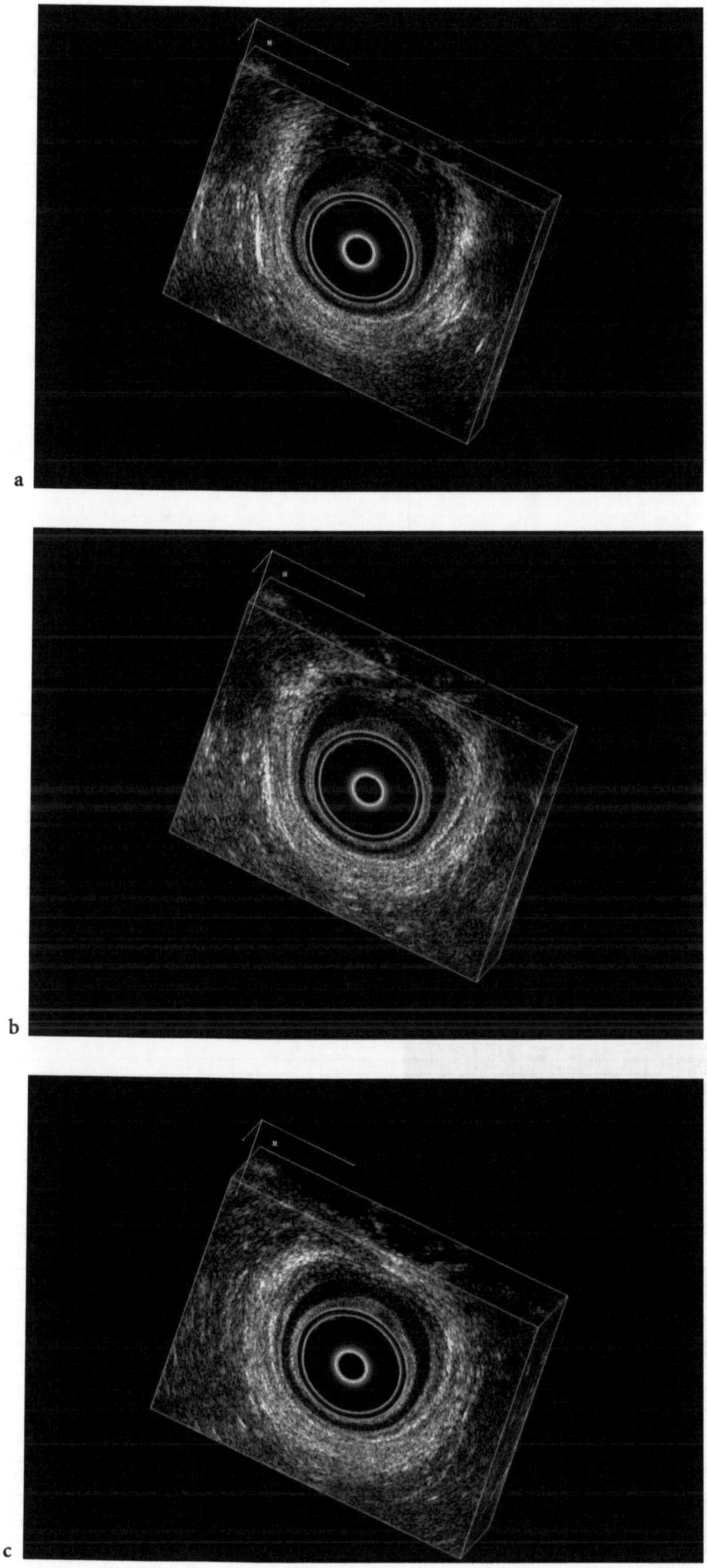

Fig. III.24. Formation of the anterior ring of the external sphincter in females: upper anal canal (a), junction between upper and mid-anal canal (b), mid-anal canal (c)

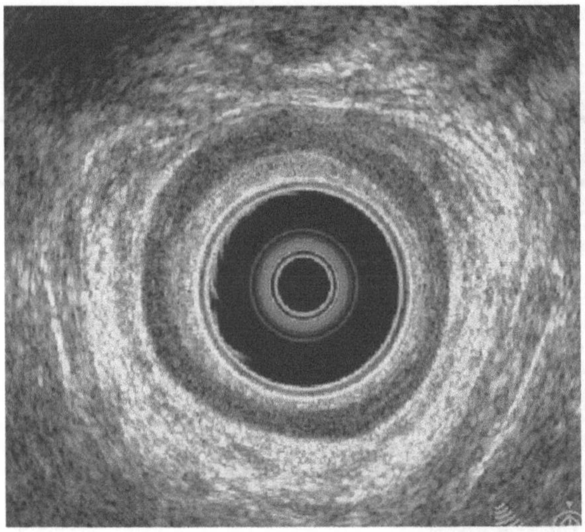
a

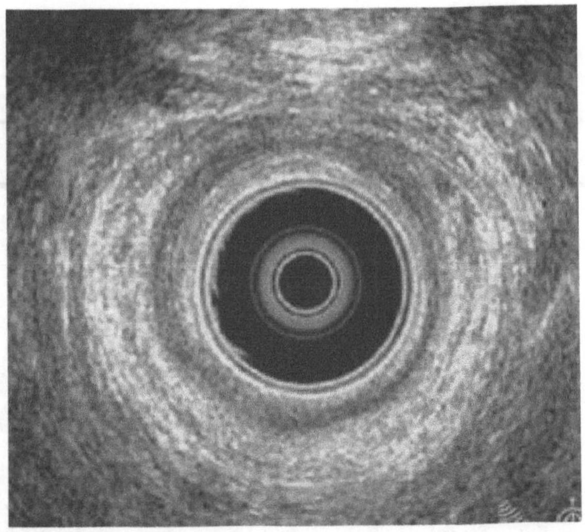
b

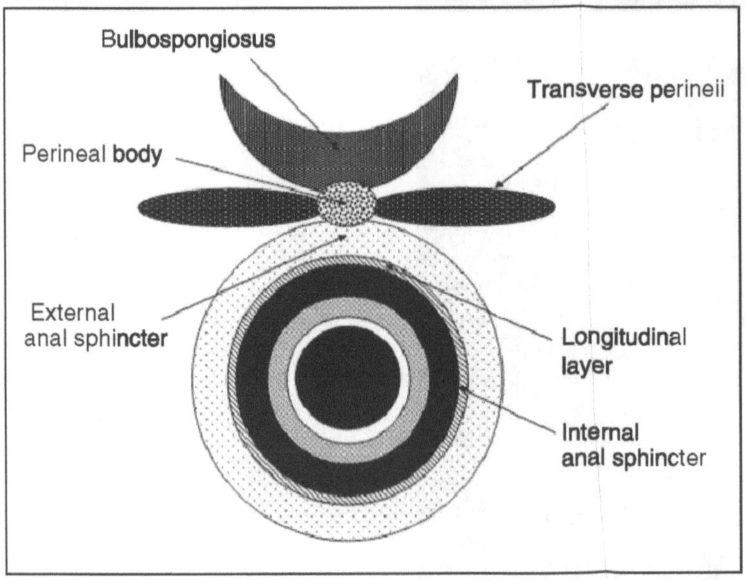

c

Fig. III.25. Bulbospongiosus muscle, transverse perineal muscles, and external anal sphincter meet in the perineal body. In males (**a**), a plane of fat persists between the transverse perineii and the external sphincter whereas in female (**b**), the transverse perineii fuse with the external sphincter. Schematic representation (**c**)

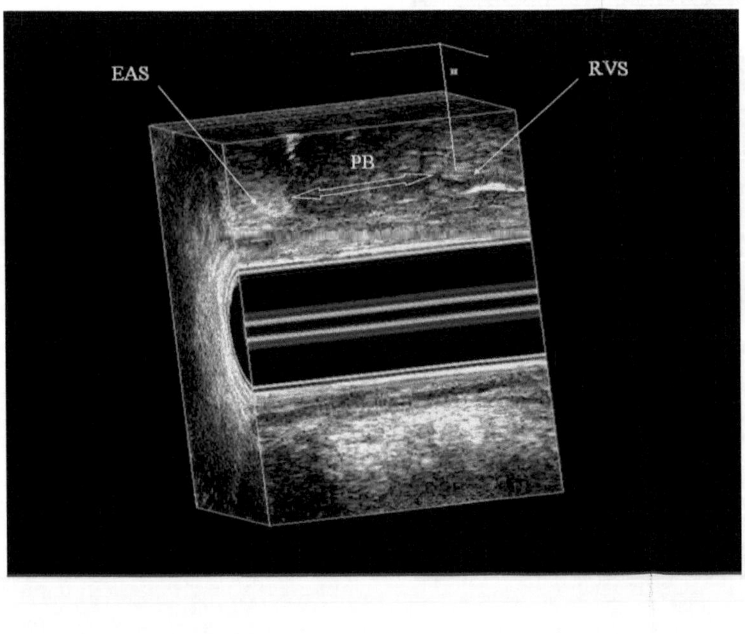

Fig. III.26. Sagittal image demonstrating the length of the perineal body (*PB*) that extends from the rectovaginal septum (*RVS*) to the external sphincter (*EAS*)

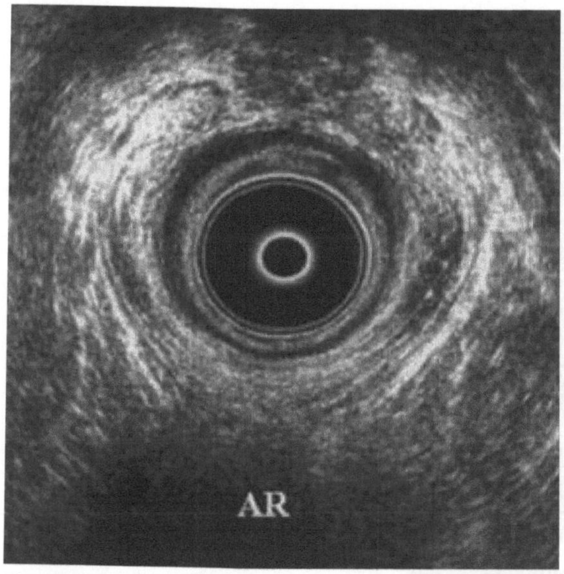

Fig. III.27. The anococcygeal raphe (*AR*) is seen as a posterior hypoechoic triangle

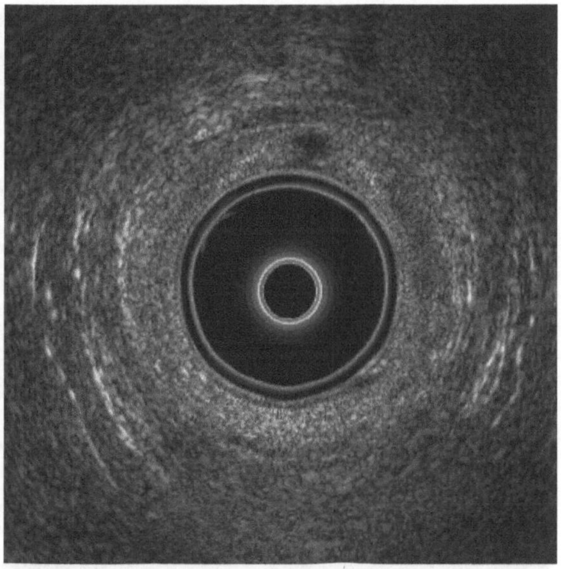

Fig. III.28. Image at the superficial level demonstrating the subcutaneous external anal sphincter. The internal sphincter is absent at this level

whereas both MRI methods enabled reliable measurement of all sphincter components. Measurement errors of the longitudinal muscle and external sphincter are related to the US features of these muscles, which show low contrast with the surrounding hyperechoic fatty tissue. Both the inner and outer borders of the external sphincter are more difficult to define, leading to less reliable measurement. In contrast, the internal sphincter is easy to define because it is a hypoechoic structure that is highlighted against hyperechoic fatty tissues. Williams et al. [21] reported different results. They found an excellent correlation for the interobserver measurement of the external and internal sphincters and submucosal width on endosonography and poor correlation only for the longitudinal muscle. Frudinger et al. [17] also reported that the EAS thickness was difficult to define in only 2% of patients at all three levels examined and in 3% at the subcutaneous level only. A significant negative correlation with patient age was also demonstrated in this study at all anal canal levels. In particular, the anterior EAS part was found significantly thinner in older subjects.

The high inherent soft-tissue contrast makes MRI a more reliable imaging method to measure anal sphincter components [29–35]. It is important to realize, however, that this limitation of EAUS does not apply in the detection of localized sphincter defects, where its benefit has been proved [36–39]. It has been suggested that measuring sphincter thickness is important when EAUS cannot depict any sphincter damage in order to exclude diffuse structural sphincter changes associated with idiopathic fecal incontinence, passive fecal incontinence, or obstructive defecation disorders [40–43].

A postulated association between manometric function of the sphincters and their sonographic appearance, however, remained controversial in the literature. Some authors found no correlation between muscle thickness and muscle performance, neither resting nor squeeze pressure. Scanning anal sphincter muscles may allow for determination of their integrity but not for their morphometric properties.

Multiplanar EAS has enabled detailed longitudinal measurement of the components of the anal canal [44, 45] (Fig. III.29). Williams et al. [44] reported that the anterior EAS was significantly longer in males than in females (30.1 mm versus 16.9 mm; p <0.001). There was no difference in the length of the puborectalis between males and females, indicating that the gender difference in anal canal length is solely due to the longer male EAS. The IAS did not differ in length between males and females. West et al. [45] reported similar results, with IAS and EAS volumes found larger in males than in females.

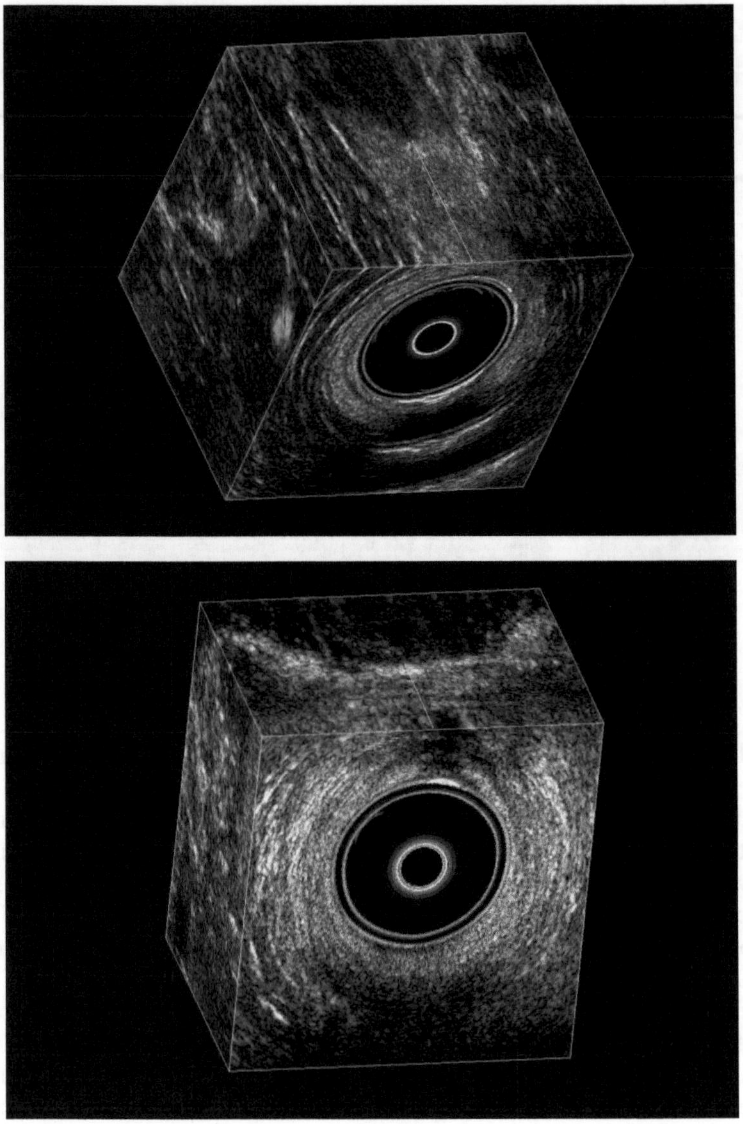

a

b

Fig. III.29. Three-dimensional view demonstrating that the anal canal is longer in male (**a**) than in female (**b**) as a result of a longer external anal sphincter

References

1. Uz A, Elhan A, Ersoy M, Tekdemir I (2004) Internal anal sphincter: an anatomic study. Clin Anat 17:17–20
2. Lunniss PJ, Phillips RKS (1992) Anatomy and function of the anal longitudinal muscle. Br J Surg 79:882–884
3. Bartram CI (2003) Ultrasound. In: Bartram CI, DeLancy JOL. Imaging Pelvic Floor Disorders. Springer, Berlin Heidelberg New York
4. Williams AB, Bartram CI, Halligan S et al (2002) Endosonographic anatomy of the normal anal canal compared with endocoil magnetic resonance imaging. Dis Colon Rectum 45:176–183
5. Shafik A (1976) A new concept of the anatomy of the anal sphincter mechanism and the physiology of defecation III. The longitudinal anal muscle: anatomy and role in sphincter mechanism. Invest Urol 13:271–277
6. Konerding MA, Dzemali O, Gaumann A et al (1999) Correlation of endoanal sonography with cross-sectional anatomy of the anal sphincter. Gastrointest Endosc 50:804–810
7. Shafik A (1975) A new concept of the anatomy of the anal sphincter mechanism and the physiology of defecation. The external anal sphincter: a triple-loop system. Invest Urol 12:412–419
8. Thakar R, Sultan A (2004) Anal endosonography and its role in assessing the incontinent patient. Best Pract Res Clinic Obstet Gynaec 18:157–173

9. Santoro GA, Di Falco G (2004) Basic anatomy. In: Santoro GA, Di Falco G. Atlas of endoanal and endorectal ultrasonography. Springer Italy, Milan
10. Stoker J (2003) The anatomy of the pelvic floor and sphincters. In: Bartram CI, DeLancy JOL. Imaging Pelvic Floor Disorders. Springer, Berlin Heidelberg New York
11. Woodman PJ, Graney DO (2002) Anatomy and physiology of the female perineal body with relevance to obstetrical injury and repair. Clin Anat 15:321–334
12. Bartram CI, Frudinger A (1997) Handbook of anal endosonography. Wrightson Biomedical, Petersfield
13. Burnett SJD, Bartram CI (1991) Endosonographic variations in the normal internal anal sphincter. Int J Colorectal Dis 6:2
14. Vaizey CJ, Kamm MA, Bartram CI (1997) Primary degeneration of the internal anal sphincter as a cause of passive faecal incontinence. Lancet 349:612–615
15. Williams AB, Bartram CI, Halligan S et al (2001) Multiplanar anal endosonography – normal anal canal anatomy. Colorectal Disease 3:169–174
16. Sultan AH, Kamm MA, Talbot IC et al (1994) Anal endosonography for identifying external sphincter defects confirmed histologically. Br J Surg 81:463–465
17. Frudinger A, Halligan S, Bartram CI et al (2002) Female anal sphincter: age-related differences in asymptomatic volunteers with high-frequency endoanal US. Radiology 224:417–423
18. Beets-Tan RGH, Morren GL, Beets GL et al (2001) Measurement of anal sphincter muscles: endoanal US, endoanal MR imaging, or phased-array MR imaging? A study with healthy volunteers. Radiology 220:81–89
19. Stoker J, Halligan S, Bartram CI (2001) Pelvic floor imaging. Radiology 218:621–641
20. Fritsch H, Brenner E, Lienemann A, Ludwikowski B (2002) Anal sphincter complex: reinterpreted morphology and its clinical relevance. Dis Colon Rectum 45:188–194
21. Williams AB, Cheetham MJ, Bartram CI et al (2000) Gender differences in the longitudinal pressure profile of the anal canal related to anatomical structure as demonstrated on three-dimensional anal endosonography. Br J Surg 87:1674–1679
22. Gold DM, Bartram CI, Halligan S et al (1999) Three-dimensional endoanal sonography in assessing anal canal injury. Br J Surg 86:365–370
23. Bollard RC, Gardiner A, Lindow S et al (2002) Normal female anal sphincter: difficulties in interpretation explained. Dis Colon Rectum 45:171–175
24. Zetterstrom JP, Mellgren A, Madoff RD et al (1998) Perineal body measurement improves evaluation of anterior sphincter lesions during endoanal ultrasonography. Dis Colon Rectum 41:705–713
25. Oberwalder M, Thaler K, Baig MK et al (2004) Anal ultrasound and endosonographic measurement of perineal body thickness. A new evaluation for fecal incontinence in females. Surg Endosc 18:650–654
26. Nielsen MB, Hauge C, Rasmussen OO et al (1992) Anal sphincter size measured by endosonography in healthy volunteers. Effect of age, sex and parity. Acta Radiol 33:453–456
27. Enck P, Heyer T, Gantke B et al (1997) How reproducible are measures of the anal sphincter muscle diameter by endoanal ultrasound? Am J Gastroenterol 92:293–296
28. Gold DM, Halligan S, Kmiot WA, Bartram CI (1999) Intraobserver and interobserver agreement in anal endosonography. Br J Surg 86:371–375
29. Williams AB, Bartram CI, Modhwadia D et al (2001) Endocoil magnetic resonance imaging quantification of external sphincter atrophy. Br J Surg 88:853–859
30. Williams AB, Malouf AJ, Bartram CI et al (2001) Assessment of external anal sphincter morphology in idiopathic fecal incontinence with endocoil magnetic resonance imaging. Dig Dis Sci 46:1466–1471
31. Hussain SM, Stoker J, Zwamborn AW et al (1996) Endoanal MR imaging of the anal sphincter complex: correlation with cross-sectional anatomy and histology. J Anat 189:677–682
32. Rociu E, Stoker J, Eijkemans MJC, Lameris JS (2000) Normal anal sphincter anatomy and age- and sex-related variations at high-spatial-resolution endoanal MR imaging. Radiology 217:395–401
33. Morren GL, Beets-Tan GH, van Engelshoven MA (2001) Anatomy of the anal canal and perianal structures as defined by phase-array magnetic resonance imaging. Br J Surg 88:1506–1512
34. DeSouza NM, Puni R, Zbar A et al (1996) MR imaging of the anal sphincter in multiparous women using an enoanal coil: correlation with in vitro anatomy and appearances in fecal incontinence. Am J Roentgenol 167:1465–1471
35. Stoker J, Rociu E, Zwamborn AW et al (1999) Endoluminal MR imaging of the rectum and anus: technique, applications and pitfalls. Radiographics 19:383–398
36. Sentovich SM, Wong WD, Blatchford GJ (1998) Accuracy and reliability of transanal ultrasound for anterior anal sphincter injury. Dis Colon Rectum 41:1000–1014
37. Kumar A, Scholefield JH (2000) Endosonography of the anal canal and rectum. World J Surg 24:208–215
38. Hussain SM, Stoker J, Schutte HE, Lameris JS (1996) Imaging of the anorectal region. Europ J Radiol 22:116–122
39. Sultan AH, Kamm MA, Hudson CN et al (1993) Anal-

sphincter disruption during vaginal delivery. N Engl J Med 329:1905–1911
40. Zetterstrom JP, Mellgren A, Jensen LL et al (1999) Effect of delivery on anal sphincter morphology and function. Dis Colon Rectum 42:1253–1260
41. Burnett SJ, Spence-Jones C, Speakman CT et al (1991) Unsuspected sphincter damage following childbirth revealed by anal endosonography. Br J Radiol 64:225–227
42. Tjandra JJ, Milsom JW, Stolfi VM et al (1992) Endoluminal ultrasound defines anatomy of the anal canal and pelvic floor. Dis Colon Rectum 35:465–470
43. Nielsen MB, Rasmussen OO, Pedersen JF, Christiansen J (1993) Anal endosonographic findings in patients with obstructed defecation. Acta Radiol 34:35–38
44. Williams AB, Bartram CI, Halligan S et al (2001) Multiplanar anal endosonography-normal anal canal anatomy. Colorectal Dis 3:169–174
45. West RL, Felt-Bersma RJF, Hansen BE et al (2005) Volume measurement of the anal sphincter complex in healthy controls and fecal-incontinent patients with a three-dimensional reconstruction of endoanal ultrasonography images. Dis Colon Rectum 48:540–548

III.3. Endosonographic Anatomy of the Normal Rectum

G.A. Santoro, G. Di Falco

The normal rectum is 11- to 15-cm long and has a maximum diameter of 4 cm. It is continuous with the sigmoid colon superiorly at the level of the third sacral segment and courses inferiorly along the curve of the sacrum to pass through the pelvic diaphragm and become the anal canal (Fig. III.30). It is surrounded by fibrofatty tissue that contains blood vessels, nerves, lymphatics, and small lymph nodes. The superior one third is covered anteriorly and laterally by the pelvic peritoneum. The middle one third is only covered with peritoneum anteriorly, where it curves anteriorly onto the bladder in males and onto the uterus in females. The lower one third of the rectum is below the peritoneal reflection and is related anteriorly to the bladder base, ureters, seminal vesicles, and prostate in males (Fig. III.31a) and to the lower uterus, cervix, and vagina in females (Fig. III.31b). The rectal wall consists of five layers surrounded by perirectal fat or serosa (Fig. III.32).

On ultrasound, the normal rectal wall is 2- to 3-mm thick and is composed of a five-layer structure [1, 2]. There is some debate as to what the actual layers represent anatomically. Hildebrandt and Feifel [3] believe that three layers are anatomical while the other layers represent interfaces between the anatomical layers. Beynon et al. [4], however, have produced both experimental and

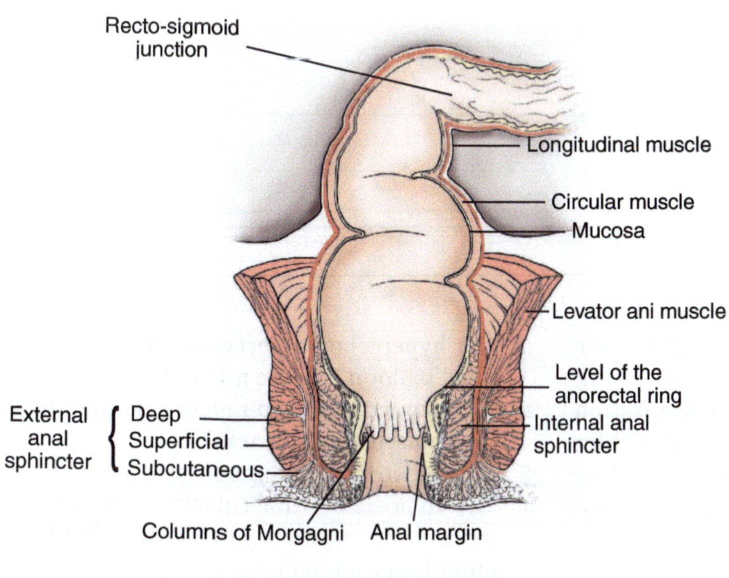

Fig. III.30. Coronal anatomy of the anorectum

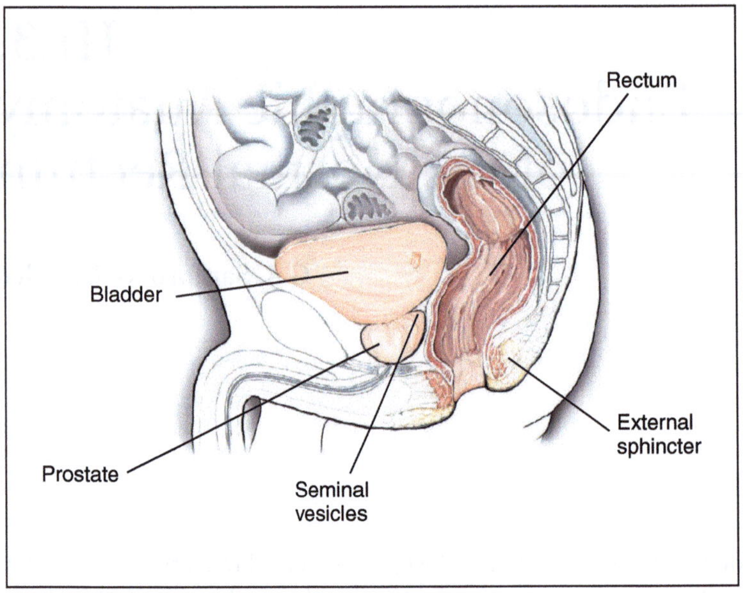

a

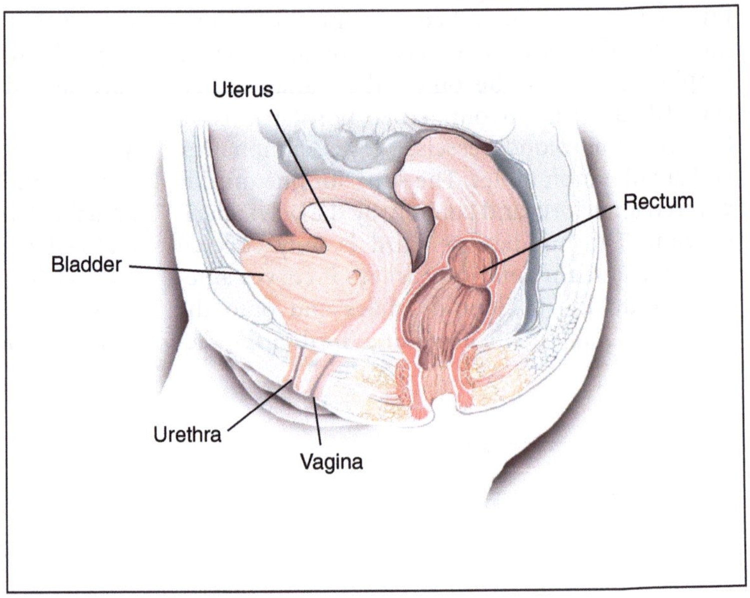

b

Fig. III.31. Sagittal anatomy of the anorectum in males (**a**) and females (**b**)

clinical evidence that the five anatomic layers are recognizable. These five layers cannot be seen in all patients and at all levels. Good visualization depends on maintaining the probe in the center lumen of the rectum and having adequate distension of the water-filled balloon with good acoustic contact with rectal wall.

The layers represent (Fig. III.33):

1. The hyperechoic interface between the water-filled balloon and the mucosa;
2. The hypoechoic deep mucosa (lamina propria plus muscularis mucosae);
3. The hyperechoic submucosa;
4. The hypoechoic muscularis propria (in rare cases seen as two layers: inner circular and outer longitudinal layer);

a 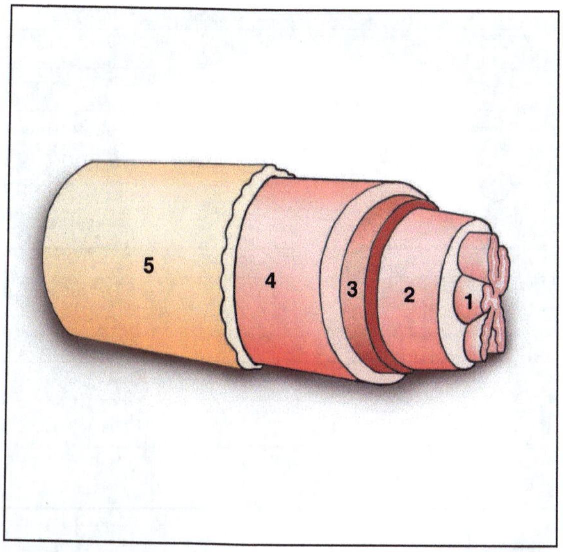

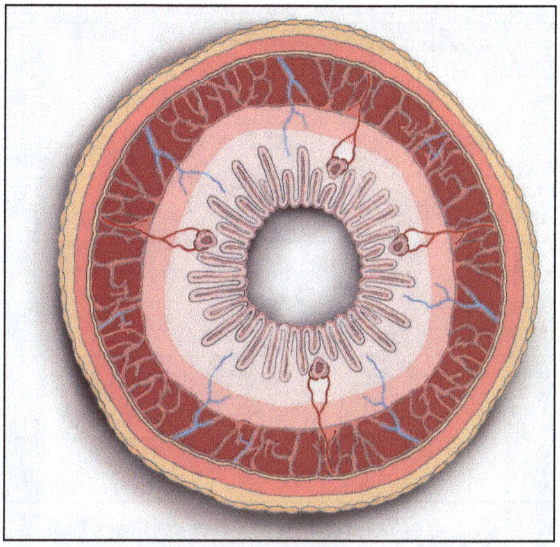 b

Fig. III.32. Diagrammatic representation of five-layer structure of the normal rectal wall (a, b): *1* mucosa, *2* submucosa, *3* muscularis propria-circular layer, *4* muscularis propria-longitudinal layer; *5* serosa/perirectal fat

a 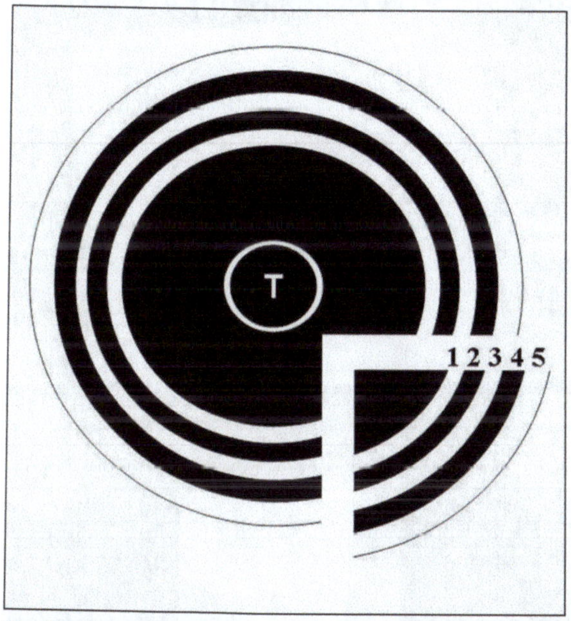

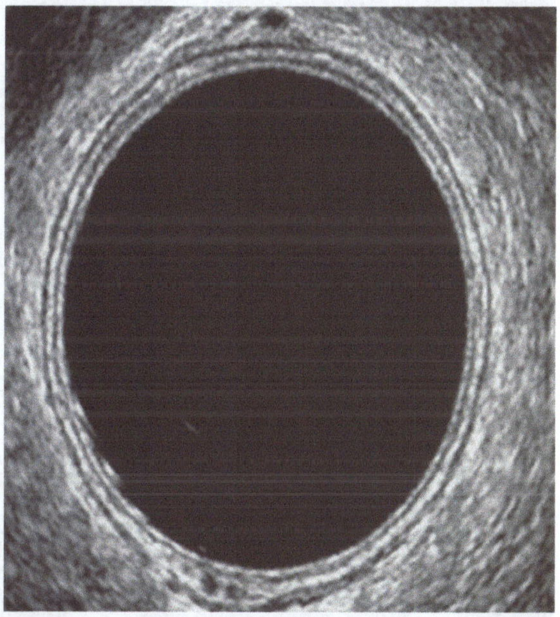 b

Fig. III.33. Schematic ultrasound representation of rectal wall (**a**). Layers: *1* acoustic interface with mucosal surfaces, *2* mucosa, *3* submucosa, *4* muscularis propria, *5* perirectal fat interface. Normal pattern of rectal wall (**b**). T = Transducer

5. The hyperechoic interface between the rectal wall and the perirectal fat tissue or serosa.

The ultrasonographer must have a clear understanding of what each of these five lines represent anatomically [5]. When staging a rectal cancer, various levels of the tumor must be optimally imaged and the integrity of the lines carefully assessed [6]. Attention must be focused on the third hyperechoic layer. Once it has been ascertained that the middle hyperechoic line is broken, then an invasive lesion is recognized, and attention is then turned to the thickness of the muscularis propria and the integrity of the outer hyperechoic line to see if the perirectal fat is invaded.

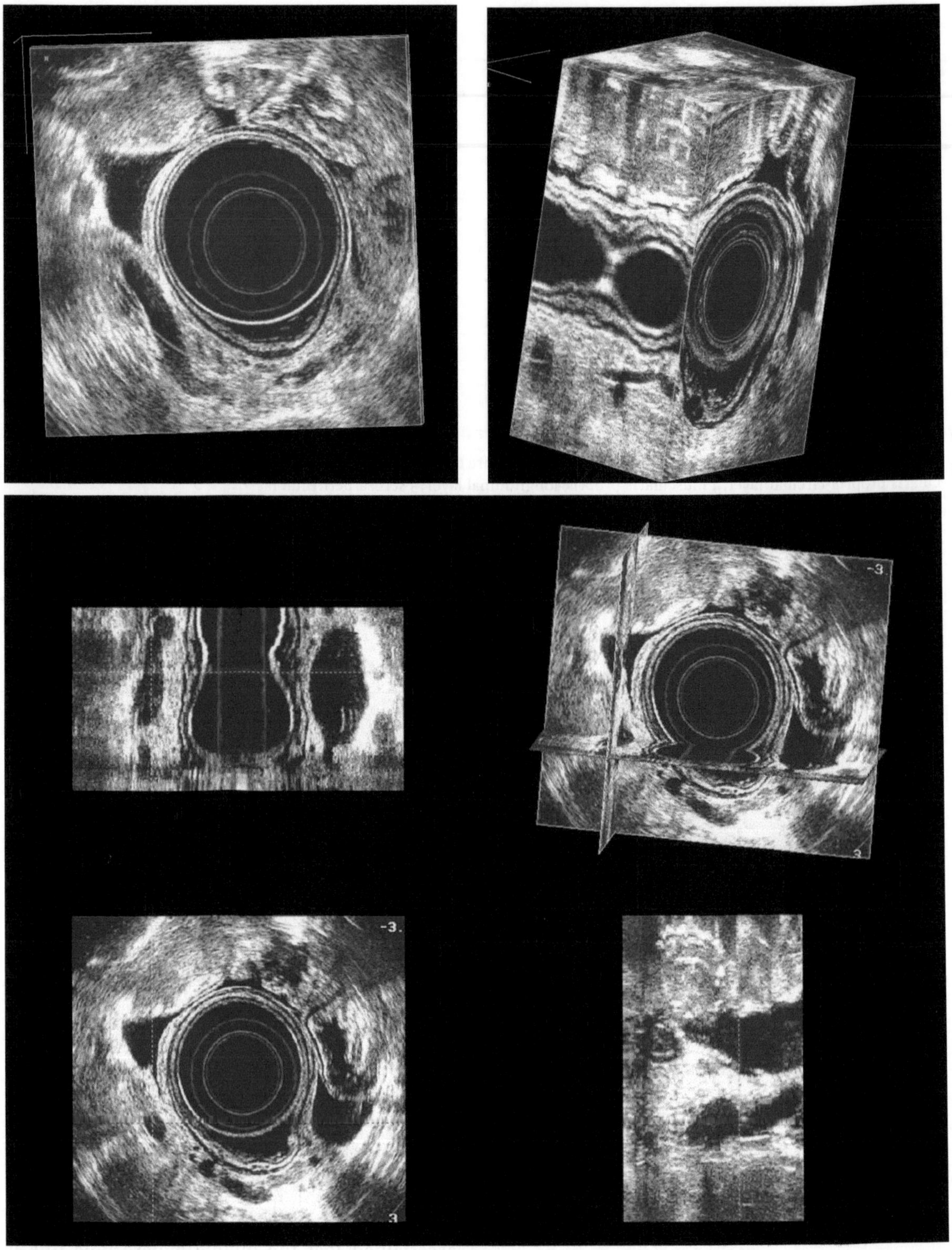

a b c

Fig. III.34. Sonographic view of blood vessels (**a**). Three-dimensional reconstruction (**b**) and multiview image presentation (**c**) showing the elongated pattern of vasculare structure

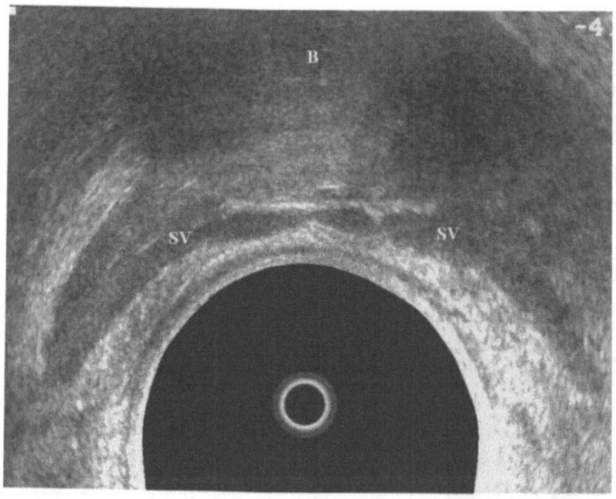

Fig. III.35. Sonographic view of the bladder (*B*) and seminal vesicles (*SV*)

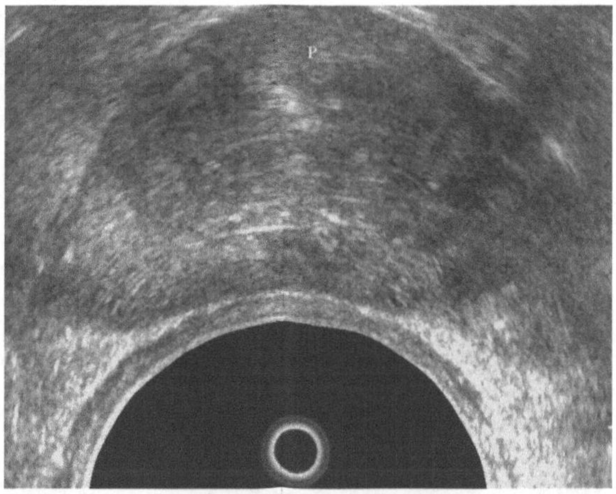

Fig. III.36. Sonographic view of the prostate (*P*)

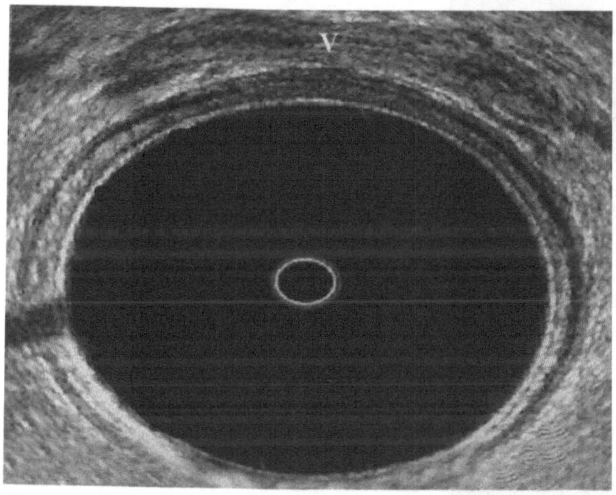

Fig. III.37. Sonographic view of the vagina (*V*)

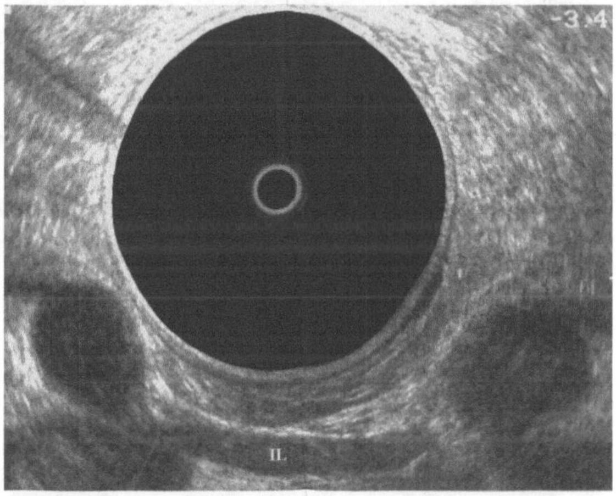

Fig. III.38. Sonographic view of the intestinal loops (*IL*)

The fibrofatty tissue surrounding the rectum contains blood vessels, nerves, and lymphatics and has an inhomogeneous echo pattern. Very small 2–3 mm, round to oval, hypoechoic lymph nodes may be seen and must be distinguished from blood vessels, which are also circular hypoechoic areas but when followed longitudinally, they seem to extend further than the corresponding diameter and can often be seen to branch and to elongate in a longitudinal fashion, confirming that this is a blood vessel and not a node (Fig. III.34) [7]. Anteriorly, the bladder, seminal vesicles, (Fig. III.35) and prostate (Fig. III.36) can be identified in males and the uterus, cervix, and vagina in females (Fig. III.37). Intestinal loops can also easily identified as elongate structures (Fig. III.38).

Technology progress has allowed an increased resolution of the five distinct layers of the rectal wall. Three-dimensional (3-D) rectal ultrasound offers images of the rectal wall in the coronal plane as well as in the transaxial and the longitudinal planes (Fig. III.39) [1, 8]. Moreover, with the new, high-frequency probes the five layers are more clearly distinguished.

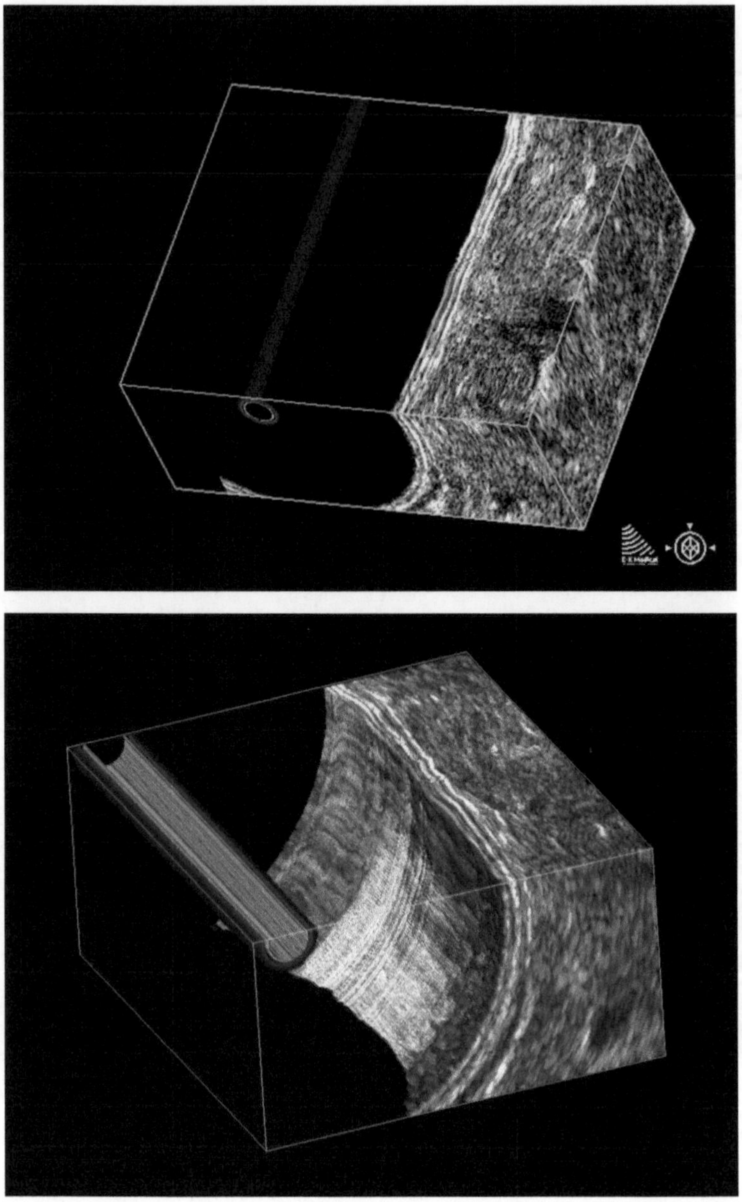

a

b

Fig. III.39. Normal ultrasound anatomy of the rectal wall in three-dimensional images (**a**, **b**)

References

1. Santoro GA, Di Falco G (2004) Basic anatomy In: Santoro GA, Di Falco G. Atlas of endoanal and endorectal ultrasonography. Springer Italy, Milan
2. Bartram CI, Frudinger A (1997) Handbook of anal endosonography. Wrightson Biomedical, Petersfield
3. Hildebrandt U, Feifel G, Schwarz HP, Scherr O (1986) Endorectal ultrasound: instrumentation and clinical aspects. Int J Colorectal Dis 1:203–207
4. Benyon J, Foy DM, Temple LN, et al (1986) The endoscopic appearance of normal colon and rectum. Dis Colon Rectum 29:810–813
5. Kumar A, Scholefield JH (2000) Endosonography of the anal canal and rectum. World J Surg 24:208–215
6. Hildebrandt U, Feifel G (1985) Preoperative staging of rectal cancer by intrarectal ultrasound. Dis Colon Rectum 28:42–46
7. Hussain SM, Stoker J, Schutte HE, Lameris JS (1996) Imaging of the anorectal region. Europ J Radiol 22:116–122
8. Hunerbein M, Schlag PM (1997) 3D-endosonography for staging of rectal cancer. Ann Surg 225:432–438

III.4. Endoanal Magnetic Resonance Imaging: Anatomy of the Normal Anal Sphincter

J. Stoker

Introduction

Magnetic resonance imaging (MRI) gives detailed insight into the anatomy of the anal sphincter, especially when high spatial resolution imaging is performed. The MRI figures in this chapter have been obtained at a field strength of 1.5 T with the use of an endoanal coil and in one figure with an endovaginal coil. All are T2-weighted images (turbo spin-echo sequences) where the fat-containing marrow of the bony pelvis is relatively hyperintense (bright) with a very hypointense (black) cortex. Striated muscles (e.g., external sphincter) have a relatively low signal intensity. Smooth muscles (e.g., internal anal sphincter) are relatively hyperintense. Fat and most vessels are relatively hyperintense.

Anatomy

The anal sphincter is a cylindrical, multilayered complex that is tilted in the sagittal plane, with the superior part more anteriorly than the inferior part. The canal is 4–6 cm (average 5 cm) in length [1, 2].

Innermost is the anal lining [(sub)mucosa/(sub)epithelium], and subsequent layers comprise the internal anal sphincter, intersphincteric space with longitudinal layer, and the external sphincter and puborectalis (pubovisceralis) muscle.

Lining of the Anal Canal

The lining of the anal canal varies along the longitudinal axis, but only some of these differences are appreciated at imaging. These differences primarily concern the presence of hypointense muscularis submucosae ani (Figs. III.40 and 41) and relevant abundant presence of veins in the submucosa (including three specialized vascular engorgements (anal cushions) sealing off the anal canal) at the upper part of the anal canal.

Internal Sphincter

The internal sphincter is a circular smooth muscle that is the continuation of the circular layer of the muscularis propria of the rectum. This layer increases in thickness below the anorectal junction to form the internal sphincter. The sphincter has an important role in maintaining continence and is the main contributor to anal rest pressure. The internal sphincter is approximately 2.8-mm thick at endoluminal imaging [2]. The inferior border of the internal sphincter is approximately 1 cm above the inferior edge of the sphincter complex (Figs. III.42 and 43). The internal sphincter is relatively hyperintense at T2-weighted sequences with a homogeneous, uniform architecture (Fig. III.40). In the coronal plane, often a multilayered appearance, is appreciated at endoluminal MRI (Figs. III 42 and 43). When intravenous contrast medium is administrated, avid enhancement of the internal sphincter is seen at T1-weighted sequences.

Intersphincteric Space

The intersphincteric space is the plane of surgical

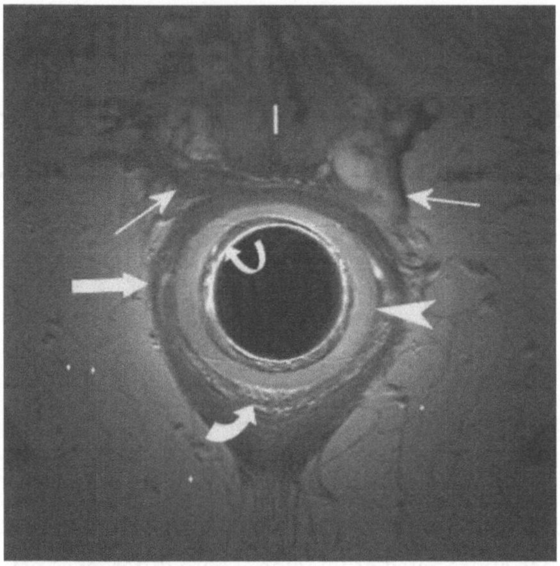

Fig. III.40. Endoanal axial oblique T2-weighted turbo spin-echo through the lower half of the anal sphincter of a woman. Imaging plane orthogonal to the axis of the anal canal. Relatively hyperintense mucosa/submucosa with hypointense muscularis submucosae ani (*thin curved arrow*). The internal anal sphincter (*arrowhead*) is relatively hyperintense and forms a ring of uniform thickness. The external sphincter (*arrow*) ring is relatively hypointense. The hyperintense fat-containing intersphincteric space is between the internal and external anal sphincters. This space contains the relatively hypointense longitudinal layer that often has a beaded appearance at cross-section (*thick curved arrow*). Vaginal introitus (*I*), bulbospongiosus muscle (*thin arrow*)

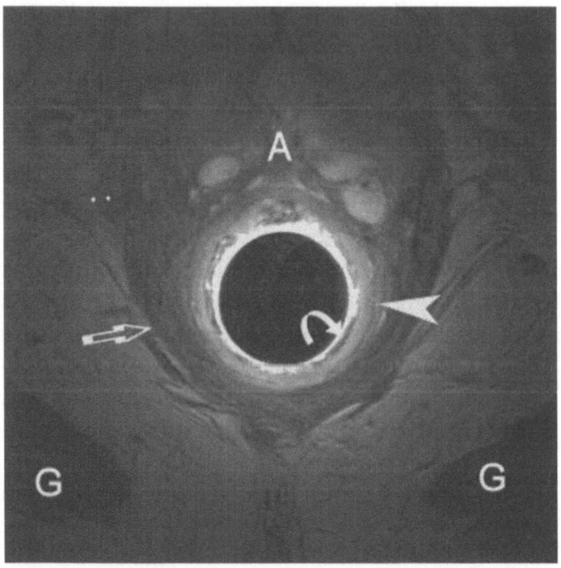

Fig. III.41. Endoanal axial oblique T2-weighted turbo spin-echo though the upper half of the anal canal of a woman. Muscularis submucosae ani (*thin curved arrow*), internal sphincter (*arrowhead*), puborectal (pubovisceral) muscle (*open arrow*). Anovaginal septum (*A*), gluteal musculature (*G*)

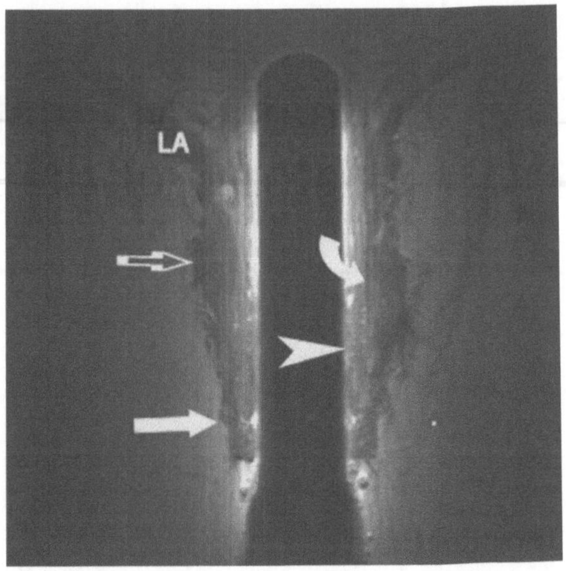

Fig. III.42. Endoanal coronal oblique T2-weighted turbo spin-echo in a woman. The internal anal sphincter (*arrowhead*) has a multilayered appearance. Longitudinal muscle (*thick curved arrow*) in intersphincteric space, external sphincter (*arrow*), puborectal (pubovisceral) muscle (*open arrow*), iliococcygeal part of the levator ani (*LA*)

dissection between the sphincters. Within this space is loose areolar tissue, seen as a bright line on T2-weighted sequences (Fig. III.40). The relative hypointense longitudinal layer courses through this space (Figs. III.40 and 42) and lies either close to the internal sphincter or the external sphincter and puborectal muscle. The bright signal areolar tissue can be hardly discerned, and in these cases, the intersphincteric space is filled by the longitudinal layer.

Longitudinal Layer

The longitudinal layer (conjoint longitudinal layer, or longitudinal muscle) is a sheet of fibroelastic and muscular tissue. This layer is the continuation of the smooth muscle longitudinal layer of the rectum with contribution of levator ani striated muscle (puboanalis) (Fig. III.44) [3] and endopelvic fascia fibroelastic components. Cranially it is predominantly muscular and caudally fibroelastic although this difference is not discernible at imaging. The fibroelastic tissue forms a network throughout the sphincter and passes through the subcutaneous external sphincter as bundles or fibers to insert into the perianal skin. At T2-weighted sequences, the longitudinal

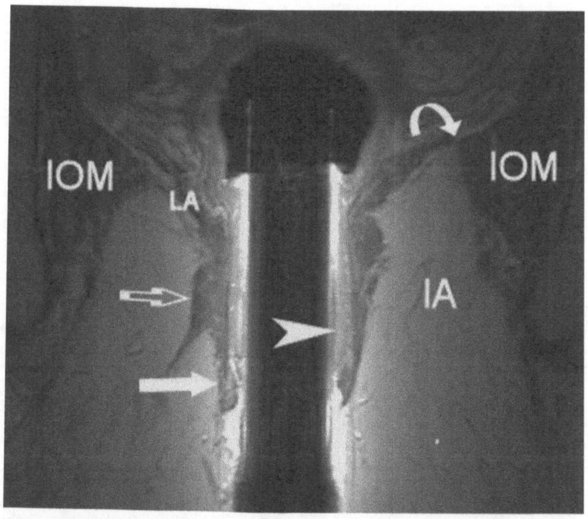

Fig. III.43. Endoanal coronal oblique T2-weighted turbo spin-echo in a woman. The iliococcygeal part of the levator ani (*LA*) is attached to the fascia of the internal obturator muscle (*IOM*) at the arcus tendineus levator ani (*curved arrow*). Internal sphincter (*arrowhead*), external sphincter (*arrow*), puborectal (pubovisceral) muscle (*open arrow*), ischioanal space (*IA*)

muscle layer is seen as a relatively hypointense layer within the hyperintense intersphincteric space (Figs. III.40 and 42), with its termination into multiple bundles in the lower sphincter and perineal body. In cross-section, the longitudinal layer can have a beaded appearance (Fig. III.40). The longitudinal layer is 2.5-mm thick [2].

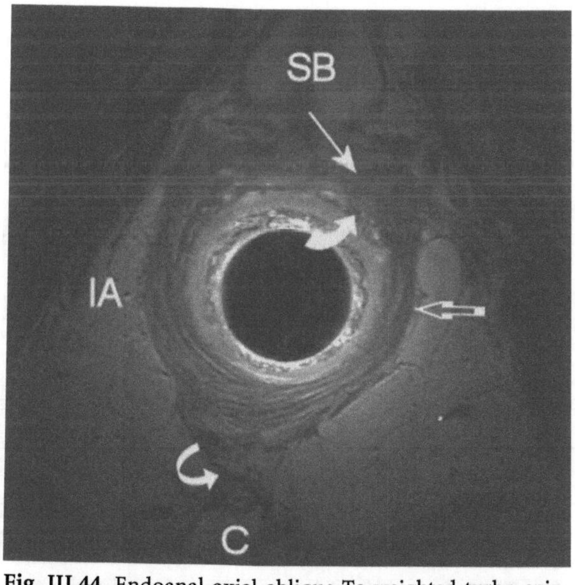

Fig. III.44. Endoanal axial oblique T2-weighted turbo spin-echo in a man. The oblique orientated puboanalis (*thin arrow*) – part of the puborectal (pubovisceral) muscle – contributing to the longitudinal layer (*thick curved arrow*). Puborectal (pubovisceral) muscle (*open arrow*), spongiose body (*SB*), coccyx (*C*), anococcygeal ligament (*thin curved arrow*), ischioanal space (*IA*)

External Anal Sphincter

The inferior outer aspect of the anal sphincter is formed by the cylindrical external sphincter. The muscle is a striated muscle under voluntary control, and action of the external sphincter is voluntary closure and reflex closure of the anal canal. Thereby it contributes to the sphincter tonus to some extent. The external sphincter is relatively hypointense at T2-weighted sequences (Figs. III.40, 42, and 43) and does not show much enhancement after intravenous contrast medium.

The external sphincter is approximately 2.7-cm high while it is shorter anteriorly in women, approximately 1.5 cm [2]. The lateral part of the external sphincter is approximately 2.7-cm high. The external sphincter has a thickness of 4 mm at endoluminal imaging. The external sphincter extends approximately 1 cm beyond the internal sphincter (Figs. III.42 and 43) and envelops the lower part of the intersphincteric space.

MRI has given further insight into the concept of the anatomy of the external sphincter and puborectal/puboanal muscle although this is not fully elucidated yet. The external sphincter comprises approximately the lower outer half of the anal sphincter and the puborectal (pubovisceral) muscle the upper, outer half [2, 4] (Figs. III.42 and 43). Often at MRI, different parts of the external sphincter can be identified at certain levels, which to some extent supports a multilayer anatomy [2]. Often, several bundles can be identified, sometimes divided by a small cleft.

Fibers of the anterior part of the external sphincter decussate into the transverse perineal muscle and perineal body. The deep part of the external sphincter is intimately related to the puborectal muscle (Figs. III.42 and 43). Posterior fibers are continues with the anococcygeal ligament (Fig. III.44).

Puborectal (Pubovisceral) Muscle

The levator ani comprises the puborectal muscle, pubococcygeus muscle, and iliococcygeus muscle. The latter two constitute the major part of the pelvic diaphragm while the puborectal muscle forms the upper, outer part of the anal sphincter. The muscle adds to the resting tone and contracts in response to sudden increases in intra-abdominal pressure to prevent incontinence. The urogenital hiatus with urethra, vagina, and anus and supportive structures is bordered and supported by the puborectal muscle.

The puborectal muscle is also named the pubovisceral muscle, as this better reflects the anatomical location and attachments of this muscle. The name puborectal muscle is somewhat confusing, as this muscle is part of the anal sphincter and is only related to the rectum at the anorectal junction. The muscle has contributions to other structures that can be named separately (e.g., pubovaginalis). The puborectal muscle is approximately 2.8-cm high and 5.6-mm thick when measured at endoanal MRI [2] (Fig. III.41). The sling-like puborectal muscle has a somewhat tilted transverse orientation with the open ends attached to the pubic bone (Fig. III.45). Because of the sling form, no striated muscle is present anteriorly at this level of the anal sphincter. Posteriorly, the muscle has attachments to the anococcygeal ligament. Attachments have been identified to other structures, such as the vagina in females, where the pubovaginalis passes along the vagina to the perineal body with attachments to the lateral vaginal walls [5, 6]. A part of the muscle (puboanalis) contributes to the longitudinal muscle (Fig. III.44).

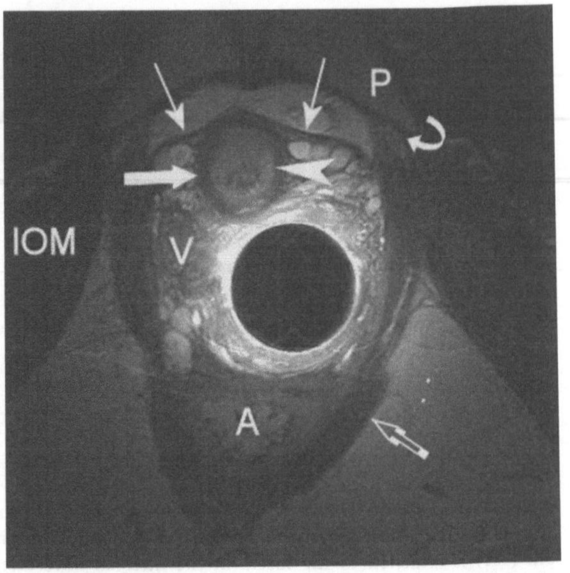

Fig. III.45. Endovaginal axial oblique T2-weighted turbo spin-echo through the superior part of the urethra of a woman. The urethra has a multilayered appearance with central the mucosa/submucosa, bordered by the hyperintense smooth muscle lissosphincter (*arrowhead*) and the striated rhabdosphincter (*arrow*). The compressor urethrae (*thin arrows*) is anterior to the urethra and attaches to the levator ani [at this level, puborectal (pubovisceral) muscle]. The puborectal muscle (*open arrow*) is attached (*curved arrow*) to the pubic bone (*P*). Vaginal wall (*V*), anus (*A*), internal obturator muscle (*IOM*)

Surrounding Structures

Anal Sphincter Support

Support to the anal sphincter is given by numerous attachments to surrounding structures. Anteriorly, the attachment to the perineal body is important, as well as other supportive structures in the anovaginal septum in females and the Denonvilliers' fascia in males. The perineal body (central perineal tendon) is a pyramidal fibromuscular node located midline between the urogenital region and the anal sphincter. At this center, numerous striated muscles and fascia converge and interlace: the longitudinal muscle of the anorectum, the pubovaginal (puboprostatic) part of the pubococcygeus muscle, the bulbospongiosus muscle, the transverse perineal muscle, and the external anal sphincter (Figs. III.40 and 46). In

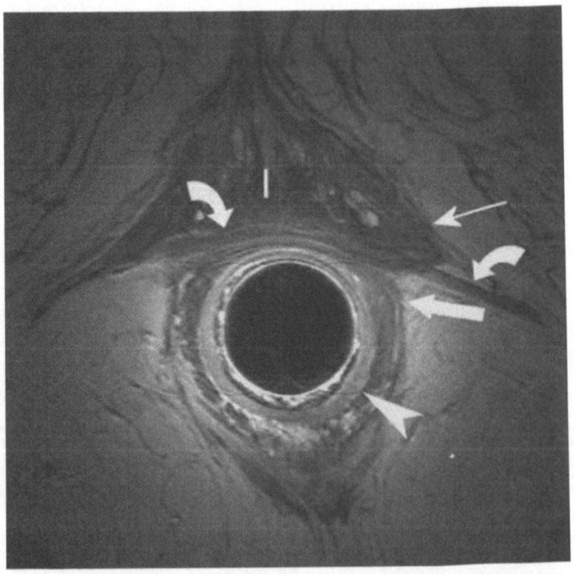

Fig. III.46. Endoanal axial oblique T2-weighted turbo spin-echo in a woman demonstrates the transverse perineal muscle (*curved arrows*) that is in close relationship to the external sphincter (*arrow*) and the bulbospongiosus muscle (*thin arrow*). External sphincter (*arrow*) and internal sphincter (*arrowhead*) show a variable degree of atrophy. Vaginal introitus (*I*)

males, this structure is more like a central point and may be named the central perineal tendon. In females, the insertion is larger, and the imbrication of the muscle fibers is more pronounced; therefore, it is often described as the perineal body.

Lateral support is given by the levator ani muscle (puborectal/pubovisceral muscle) and transverse perineal muscle. Posterior support is given by the attachment of the anococcygeal ligament to the coccyx and superior support by the continuity with the rectum (Figs. III.42–44). The fibroelastic network surrounding and involving the anal sphincter gives more general support.

Pelvic Diaphragm

The pelvic diaphragm is a major constituent of the pelvic floor and comprises the levator ani muscle and coccygeus muscle. The diaphragm is a musculotendinous structure with a constant muscle tone resulting in a dome-like structure supporting the pelvic organs (Figs. III.42 and 43) and closing the urogenital hiatus.

The levator ani muscle comprises three parts: the iliococcygeus, the pubococcygeus, and the puborectalis (pubovisceralis), with the former two being part of the pelvic diaphragm. The iliococcygeus muscle and pubococcygeus muscle arise from the ischial spine, the tendineus arc of the levator ani muscle at the internal obturator fascia (Fig. III.43), and the lower border pubic bone near the pubic symphysis. The pubococcygeus has a more anterior origin than the iliococcygeus muscle. Insertion is posteriorly into the midline anococcygeal raphe and coccyx. Based on the origin and attachments, the parts of the levator ani can be identified at MRI. The coccygeus muscle (ischiococcygeus muscle) forms the posterior part of the pelvic diaphragm. This shelf-like musculotendinous structure spans from the tip of the ischial spine, along the posterior margin of the internal obturator muscle, to the lateral side of the coccyx and the lowest part of the sacrum. The posterior edge of the coccygeus muscle includes the sacrospinous ligament.

Pelvic Sidewall

The internal obturator muscle forms the major constituent of the pelvic sidewall (Figs. III.43 and 45). A tendineus ridge of the obturator fascia, the arcus tendineus levator ani, forms the pelvic sidewall attachment for the iliococcygeus part of the levator ani (Fig. III.43). Posteriorly is the triangular shaped piriform muscle, lying directly superior to the pelvic floor and the largest structure in the greater sciatic foramen. The fascia of the pelvic wall is a strong membrane covering the surface of the internal obturator and piriform muscles with firm attachments to the periosteum [7].

Bony Pelvis

The bony pelvis is important for support and is the site of attachment of multiple pelvic floor structures. The anal sphincter has direct connection to the bony pelvis by the puborectal muscle (Fig. III.45) and is further connected by ligaments (e.g., the anococcygeal ligament) (Fig. III.44) or interconnections (e.g., via attachment to the pelvic diaphragm).

Vagina

The vagina is visualized as an H-shaped structure anterior to the anus while the vestibular entrance is a sagittal cleft (Figs. III.40 and 46). Depending on age, the vagina has a low signal intensity outer muscular layer and relative hyperintense inner epithelium/submucosal layer. There are abundant hyperintense venous structures surrounding the vagina, forming part of the anovaginal septum.

Urethra and Urethra-Supporting Structures

The urethra is identifiable as a multilayer structure anterior to the vagina with central mucosa/submucosa, concentric hyperintense smooth muscle lissosphincter, and outer striated rhabdosphincter (Fig. III.45). Multiple urethral support structures can be identified, but detailed description is beyond the scope of this chapter [8]. Most easily identifiable at both endoluminal and external MRI is a sling-like structure anterior to the urethra, most likely the compressor urethrae [8] (Fig. III.45). This structure courses just anterior to the urethra and has lateral attachments to the levator ani muscle [9, 10].

Perineal Region

The transverse perineal muscle (formerly named superficial transverse perineal muscle), the bulbospongiosus muscle, and the ischiocavernous muscle are the external genital muscles, also named perineal muscles (Figs. III.40 and 46). Especially the transverse perineal muscle (Fig. III.46) has a supportive function. This muscle inserts into the perineal body and external sphincter. There is considerable variance in presence.

The superficial perineal fascia envelops a pad of fat tissue filling a large part of the ischioanal space (Figs. III.43 and 44). A network of fibroelastic connective tissue fibers traverses the perianal fat continuous with the longitudinal layer [11].

References

1. Beets-Tan RGH, Morren GL, Beets G et al (2001) Measurement of anal sphincter muscles: endoanal US, endoanal MR imaging, or phased array MR imaging? A study with healthy volunteers. Radiology 220:81–89
2. Rociu E, Stoker J, Eijkemans MJC, Laméris JS (2000) Normal anal sphincter anatomy and age- and sex-related variations at high spatial resolution endoanal MR imaging. Radiology 217:395–401
3. Lunniss PJ, Phillips RKS (1992) Anatomy and function of the anal longitudinal muscle. Br J Surg 79:882–884
4. Hussain SM, Stoker J, Laméris JS (1995) Anal sphincter complex: endoanal MR imaging of normal anatomy. Radiology 197:671–677
5. Sampselle CM, DeLancey JOL (1998) Anatomy of female continence. J Wound Ostomy Continence Nurs 25:63–74
6. DeLancey JOL, Richardson AC (1992) Anatomy of genital support. In: Benson, JT (ed) Female pelvic floor disorders: investigation and management, 1st edn. Norton Medical Books, New York
7. Last RJ (1978) Anatomy. Regional and applied, 6th edn. Churchill Livingstone, Edinburgh
8. Stoker J (2003) Anatomy of the pelvic floor and sphincters. In: Bartram CI, DeLancey JOL (eds) Imaging pelvic floor disorders. Springer, Berlin Heidelberg New York
9. Tan IL, Stoker J, Zwamborn AW et al (1998) Female pelvic floor. Endovaginal MR imaging of normal anatomy. Radiology 206:777–783
10. Tunn R, DeLancey JOL, Quint EE (2001) Visibility of pelvic organ support system structures in magnetic resonance images without an endovaginal coil. Am J Obstet Gynecol 184:1156–1163
11. Haas PA, Fox TA (1977) The importance of the perianal connective tissue in the surgical anatomy and function of the anus. Dis Colon Rectum 20:303–313

III.5. MR Anatomy of the Rectum and the Mesorectum

M.J. Lahaye, W.H. Lamers, G.L. Beets, R.G.H. Beets-Tan

Magnetic resonance imaging (MRI) of rectal cancer is gradually becoming more important in the management of this disease. Knowledge of relevant MR anatomy of the rectum and mesorectum is important for radiologists, surgeons, and radiation oncologists involved in the multidisciplinary approach of rectal cancer.

Total mesorectal excision (TME), first described by Heald in 1979 [1], has become the standard surgical procedure for curative resection of rectal cancer. Previously, surgeons often bluntly worked their way through the fat surrounding the rectal wall, with a considerable likelihood of leaving tumor tissue behind in the fat. With a TME, the rectum is removed en bloc with the complete mesorectal compartment, including the surrounding mesorectal fat and lymph nodes. The border of this compartment is formed by the mesorectal fascia. In a TME procedure, this fascia constitutes the ideal resection plane to remove, through sharp dissection, the complete mesorectal compartment within its fascia (Fig. III.47). The

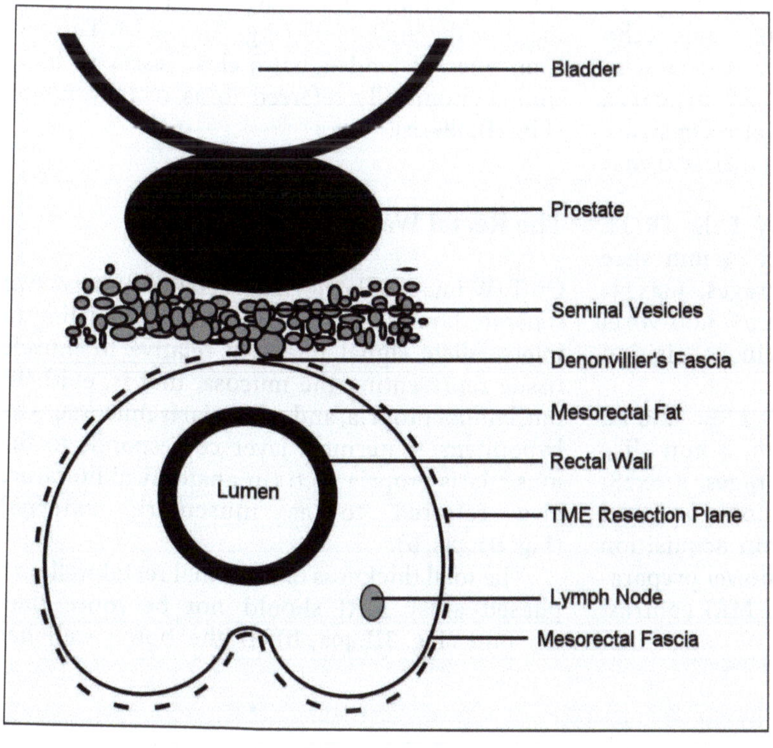

Fig. III.47. A total mesorectal excision (TME) radically removes en bloc the tumor-bearing part of the rectum together with the associated mesorectal compartment, including surrounding mesorectal fat, mesorectal lymph nodes, and its border, the mesorectal fascia. The mesorectal fascia is used as the resection plane during the TME procedure distance of the tumor to the circumferential resection margin (CRM) is an important prognostic variable: the closer the tumor, the higher the risk for a local recurrence [2].

A preoperative pelvic MRI can visualize the rectal tumor, the mesorectum, and the surrounding mesorectal fascia [3]. By understanding the MR pelvic anatomy, the distance of the tumor to the mesorectal fascia can be accurately identified [4], and an involved or close circumferential resection margin of a standard TME specimen can be anticipated. Rather than proceeding with a standard resection and putting the patient at risk for a local recurrence, the clinician can choose for neoadjuvant (chemo)radiotherapy and/or a more extensive resection.

Techniques

Imaging Sequences

MRI of the rectum were performed at 3.0 Tesla (T) (Intera Achieva 3.0T Release 1.2.1.3. Quasar Dual, maximum gradient strength 30 mT/m, maximum slew rate 200 T/m/s, Philips Medical System, Best, The Netherlands).

The male and female volunteers were positioned supine, in feet-first position, and a six-element synergy phased array coil was used. Sequences used were a sagittal T2-weighted (T2W), two-dimensional (2-D), fast spin echo (FSE) [T2W FSE: TR/TE 4,598/150 ms, 34-echo train length, 4-mm slice thickness, 0.8 mm gap, 2 signal averages, 432x272 matrix, 512 reconstruction, 0.58/0.92/4.00-voxel MPS (mm), 250-mm FOV, 5:13 min acquisition time].

An axial T2W, 2-D, FSE [T2W FSE: TR/TE 5,312/150 ms, 28-echo train length, 4-mm slice thickness, 0.80 gap, 2 signal averages, 384x235 matrix, 512 reconstruction, 0.65/1.06/4.00-voxel MPS (mm), 250-mm FOV, 5:19 min acquisition time].

A coronal T2W FSE [T2W FSE: TR/TE 5,952/150 ms, 29-echo train length, 4-mm slice thickness, 0.80 gap, 2 signal averages, 416x281 matrix, 512 reconstruction, 0.67/1.07/4.00-voxel MPS (mm), 280-mm FOV, 5:39 min acquisition time]. Volunteers did not receive bowel preparation or intravenous or intrarectal MRI contrast agents.

Anatomical Preparations

Male and female human hemipelvic preparations were obtained from the collection of the Department of Anatomy and Embryology, Maastricht University. Images of axial sections of the pelvis were acquired from the male and female specimens of the Visible Human Data Set. These anatomical data sets were developed under a contract from the National Library of Medicine by the Departments of Cellular and Structural Biology, and Radiology, University of Colorado School of Medicine, Denver, USA.

MR Anatomy of the Rectum and the Rectal Wall

The Rectum

The rectum extends from the anorectal junction to the rectosigmoid junction. For practical purposes, the rectosigmoid junction is arbitrarily defined, most often, as 15 cm from the anal verge. Other definitions use a length of 12 cm or the dentate line or anorectal junction as a starting point. The most common definition of 15 cm from the anal verge corresponds to the level of the third sacral vertebrae (Fig. III.48a, b), which is lower than often thought. At the anorectal junction, the rectum bends sharply posterior and caudal into the anal canal (Fig. III.48a, b). The rectum, when distended, has a clear reservoir function, anatomically referred to as rectal ampulla (Fig. III.48a, b).

The Rectal Wall

On T2W images, the normal rectal wall shows two separate layers. The innermost layer is a line of intermediate signal intensity relative to muscle tissue representing the mucosa, that is, epithelium, lamina propria, and muscularis mucosae. The hypointense outermost layer corresponds to the muscularis propria recti (in anatomical literature also referred to as muscularis externa) (Fig. III.48a, b).

The total thickness of a normal rectal wall on a phased array MRI should not be more than 1–3 mm (Fig. III.49a, b). If the bowel wall has

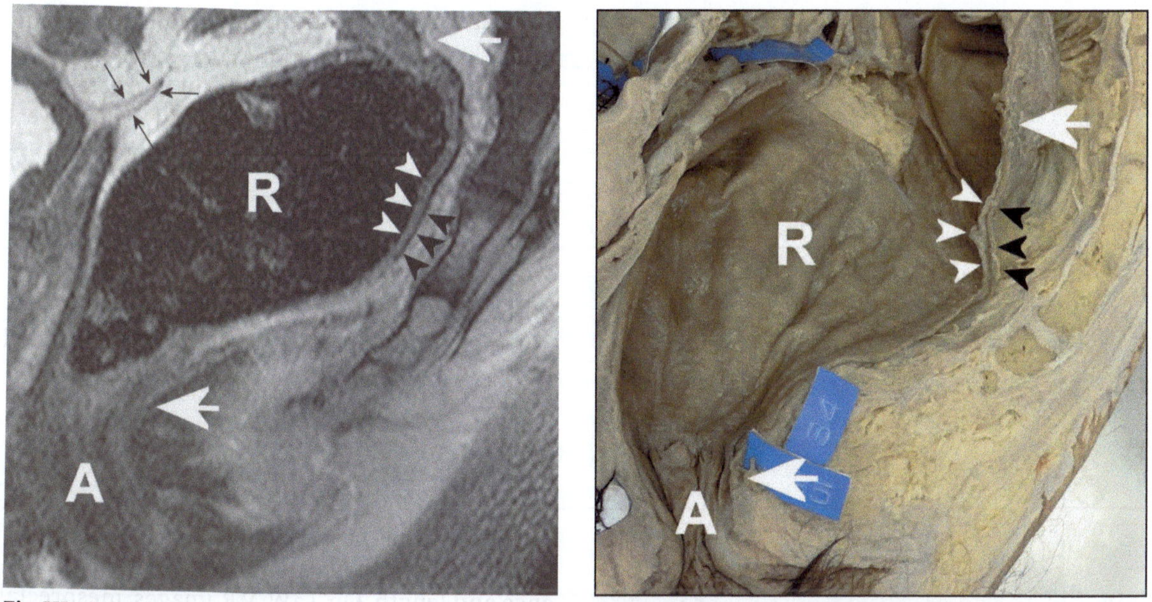

a b

Fig. III.48. Sagittal T2-weighted fast spin echo (TR/TE 4,598/150 ms) magnetic resonance image of a healthy male volunteer (**a**) shows the rectosigmoid transition and end of the rectum (*white arrows*) in the anal canal (*A*). The rectal ampulla (*R*) is evident. The inner layer of the rectal wall can be visualized as a line of intermediate signal intensity relative to muscle tissue representing the mucosa (*white arrowheads*). The outside layer of the rectal wall, a hypointense line, corresponds to the muscularis propria recti (*black arrowheads*). The peritoneal reflection appears as a low signal intensity V-shaped structure ("seagull sign", *black arrows*). Midsagittal rectum seen from the left of the male pelvis (**b**) shows the whole rectum (*between the white arrows*); rectal ampulla (*R*), anal canal (*A*), mucosae (*white arrowheads*), and muscularis propria (*black arrowheads*)

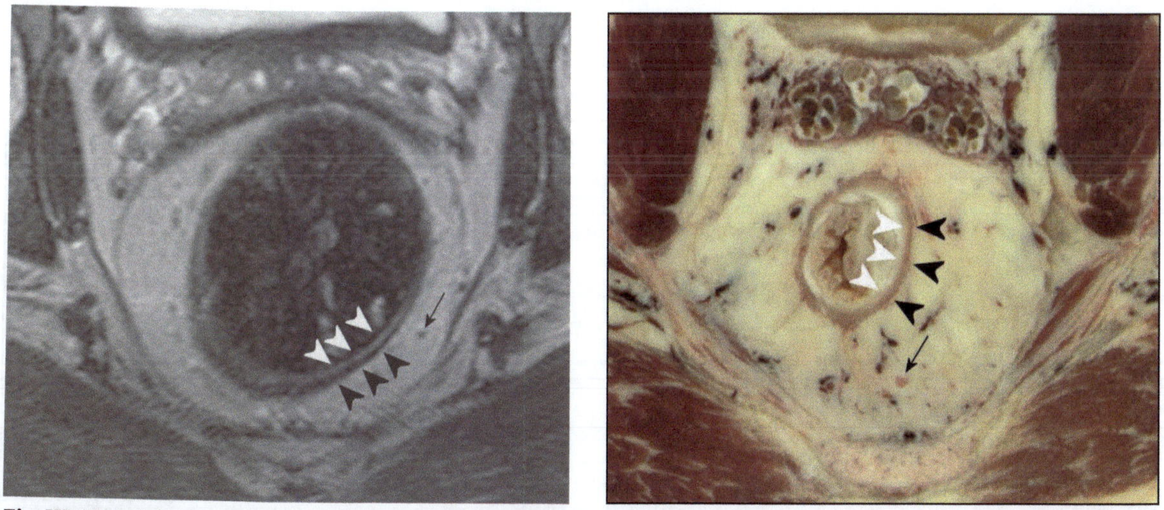

a b

Fig. III.49. Axial T2-weighted fast spin echo (TR/TE 5,312/150 ms) magnetic resonance image (**a**) shows the inner layer of the rectal wall as a line of intermediate signal intensity relative to muscle tissue representing the mucosae (*white arrowheads*). The outside layer of the rectal wall, a hypointensity line, corresponds to the muscularis propria recti (*black arrowheads*). A small lymph node is visible as a low signal intensity round structure (*black arrow*). Axial section of the male pelvis (**b**) shows the inner layer of the rectal wall, the mucosae (*white arrowheads*), and the outside layer of the rectal wall, the muscularis propria recti (*black arrowheads*). A small lymph node is also visible (*black arrow*)

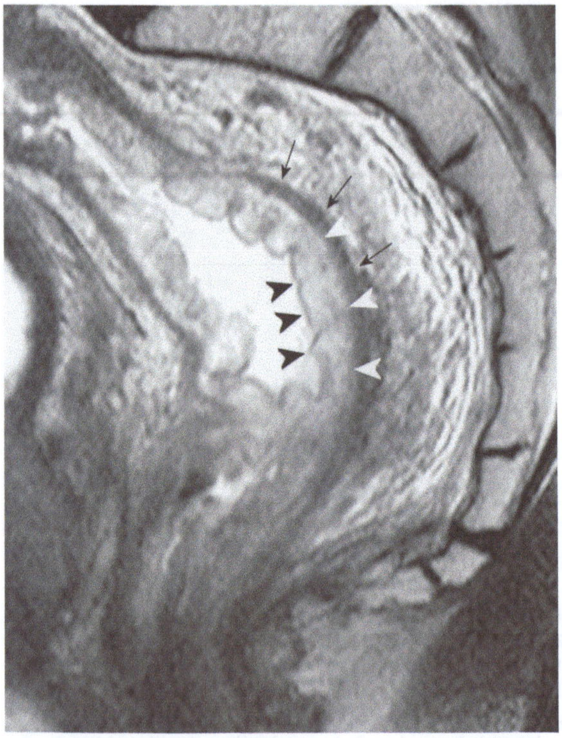

Fig. III.50. Sagittal T2-weighted fast spin echo (TR/TE 3,427/150 ms) magnetic resonance image of a male patient with rectal cancer shows a layer of high signal intensity (*white arrowheads*) corresponding to the edematous submucosal layer between the inner mucosal layer (*black arrowheads*) and outer layer, the muscularis propria recti (*black arrows*)

become edematous (i.e., inflammatory conditions), a third layer of high signal intensity corresponding to the thickened submucosal layer appears in between the inner and outer layers (Fig. III.50).

MR anatomy of the Mesorectum

The mesorectum is enclosed by the mesorectal fascia and contains the rectum, mesorectal fat, blood vessels, lymphatic vessels, and lymph nodes.

The Mesorectal Fat

The mesorectal fat surrounds the rectal wall but is not equally thick along its entire circumference and length. On T2W MR images, mesorectal fat is seen as a high-intensity structure surrounding the rectum. Anteriorly, the rectum is close to the genital organs – the vagina and cervix in females and the prostate and seminal vesicles in males. Anteriorly, the mesorectal fat is much thinner than on the lateral and posterior aspect (Fig. III.51a, b). This results in a closer distance of the anterior rectal wall to the vagina and cervix in women and the prostate and seminal vesicles in men. A low anteriorly located rectal

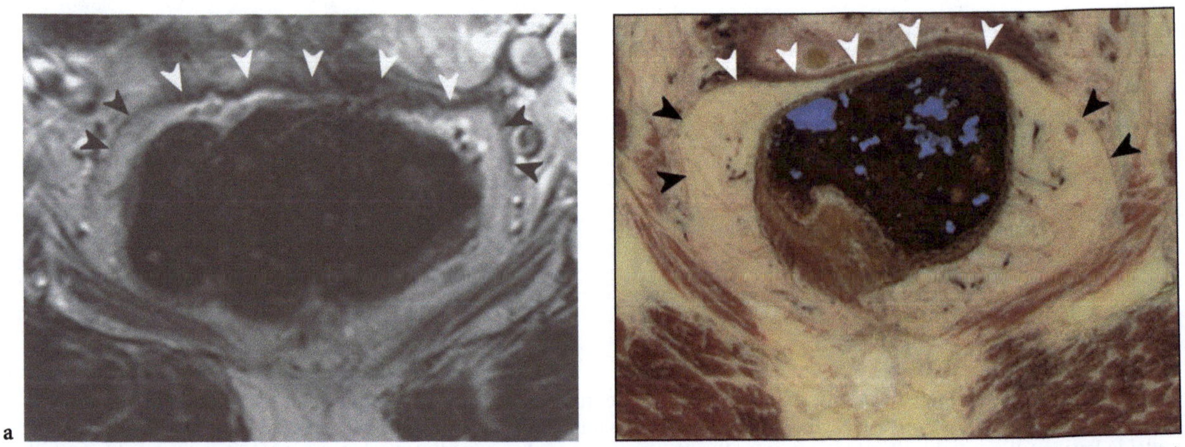

Fig. III.51. Axial T2-weighted fast spin echo (TR/TE 5,312/150 ms) magnetic resonance image of a healthy male volunteer (**a**) shows the mesorectal fascia (*black arrowheads*) as a fine line of low signal intensity surrounding the mesorectal fat. The Denonvilliers' fascia is also visualized (*white arrowheads*) posterior to the seminal vesicles. Axial section of the male pelvis (**b**) shows the mesorectal fascia (*black arrowheads*). The Denonvilliers' fascia is also visualized (*white arrowheads*) posterior to the seminal vesicles

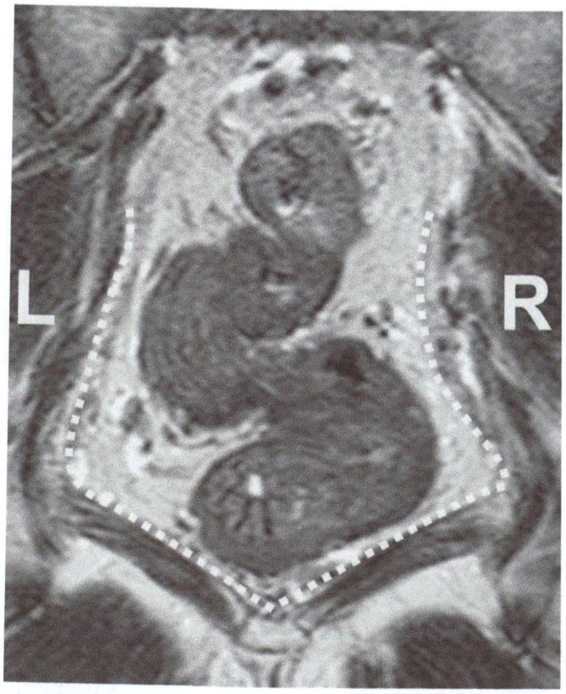

Fig. III.52. A coronal T2-weighted fast spin echo (TR/TE 3,427/150 ms) magnetic resonance image of a patient with rectal cancer shows the distal tapering or coning of the mesorectum, which entails a close topographical relationship of the distal rectal wall and the muscles of the pelvic floor (*white dotted line*). L = left; R = right

cancer has therefore a shorter distance to the mesorectal fascia, with a higher risk for a positive or close CRM. Furthermore, the distal tapering or coning of the mesorectum entails a close topographical relationship of the distal rectal wall and the muscles of the pelvic floor (Fig. III.52). At the anorectal junction, the mesorectal fat has all but disappeared, and the mesorectal fascia can no longer be distinguished from the pelvic floor muscles.

The Mesorectal Fascia

The mesorectum is bounded by the mesorectal fascia (Fig. III.53a, b). On both T1- and T2W images, the mesorectal fascia is seen as a fine line of low signal intensity surrounding the mesorectal fat.

In the literature, the mesorectal fascia is also referred to as the fascia propria or the perirectal fascia. Sometimes it is erroneously described as Denonvilliers' fascia and even Waldeyer's fascia. Denonvilliers' fascia is the thickened anterior part of the mesorectal fascia that separates the mesorectal fat from the vagina or seminal vesicles. On T2W MR images, the Denonvilliers' fascia

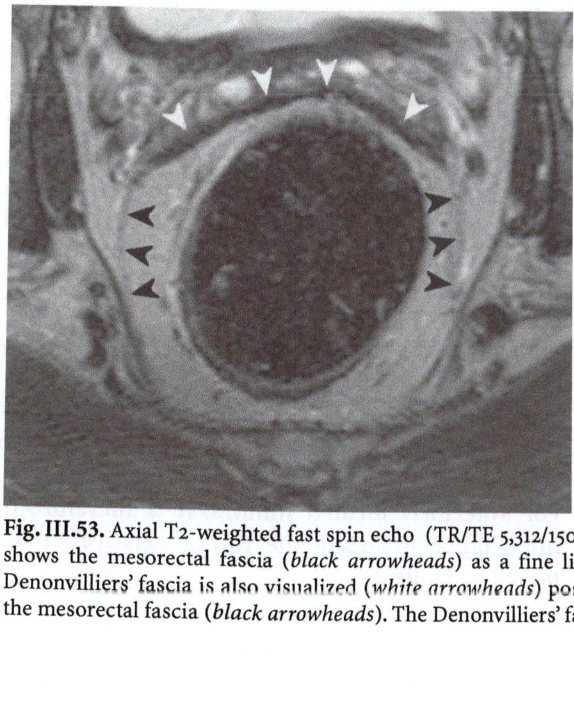

a

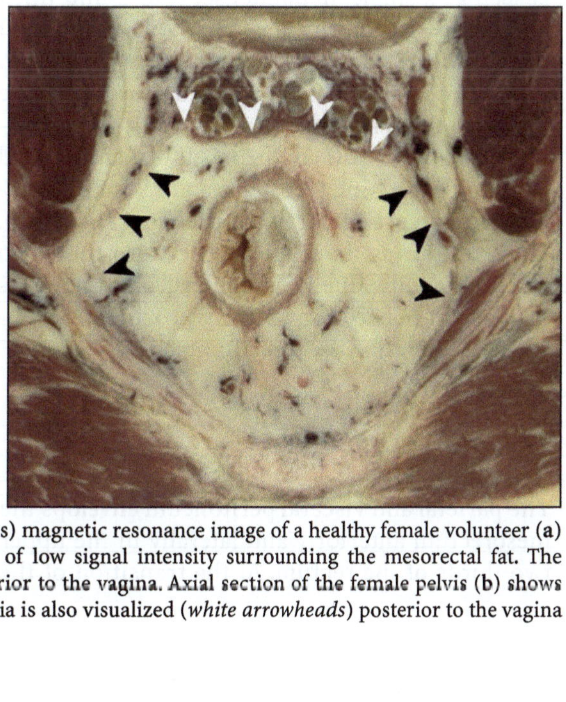

b

Fig. III.53. Axial T2-weighted fast spin echo (TR/TE 5,312/150 ms) magnetic resonance image of a healthy female volunteer (**a**) shows the mesorectal fascia (*black arrowheads*) as a fine line of low signal intensity surrounding the mesorectal fat. The Denonvilliers' fascia is also visualized (*white arrowheads*) posterior to the vagina. Axial section of the female pelvis (**b**) shows the mesorectal fascia (*black arrowheads*). The Denonvilliers' fascia is also visualized (*white arrowheads*) posterior to the vagina

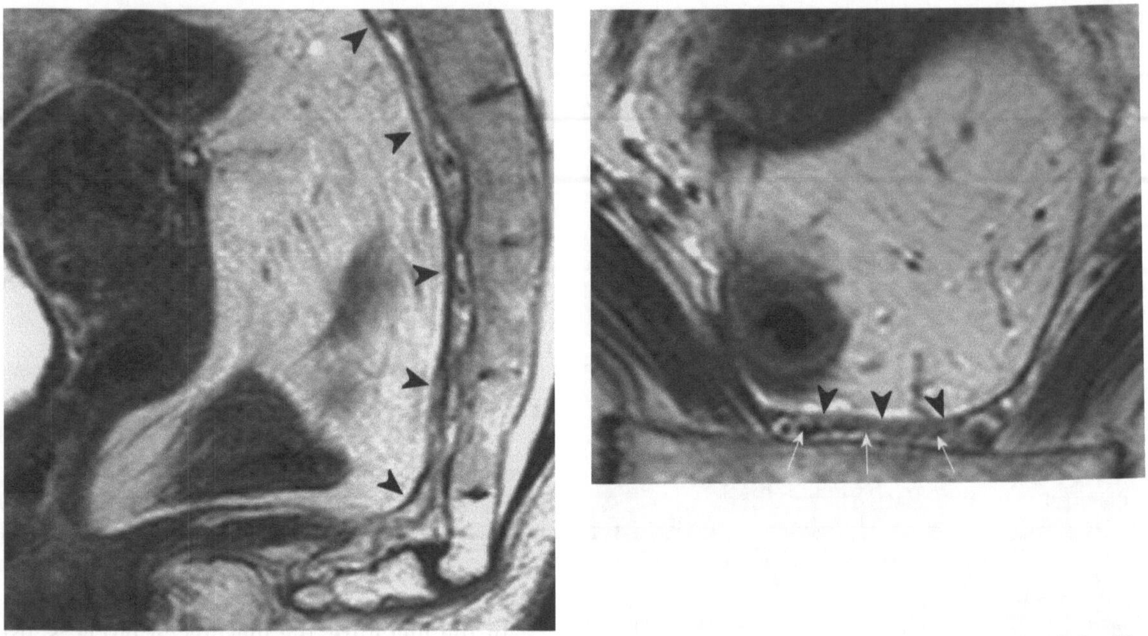

a b

Fig. III.54. Sagittal T2-weighted (T2W) fast spin echo (FSE) (TR/TE 4,598/150 ms) magnetic resonance (MR) image of a healthy female volunteer (**a**) shows the Waldeyer's fascia as a hypointense linear presacral structure of low signal intensity close to the sacrum (*black arrowheads*). Axial T2W FSE (TR/TE 5,312/150 ms) MR image of a healthy female volunteer (**b**) shows the Waldeyer's fascia as a hypointense linear presacral structure (*black arrowheads*). The presacral venous plexus and the lateral sacral veins are visualized as round, tubular, structures of low signal intensity (*white arrows*)

is seen as a single, hypointense, 1- to 2-mm thick anatomical structure (Figs. III.51a, b and 53a, b) The Waldeyer's fascia is the presacral fascia [5]. This presacral fascia is located dorsal to the mesorectal fascia and is thus anatomically a separate entity. On MRI, both the dorsal mesorectal fascia and the Waldeyer's fascia are seen as a single hypointense linear structure (Fig. III.54a, b). However, during the surgical procedure, these two fascias are individually recognized, and the virtual space in between the fascias provides an optimal landmark for the resection plane.

The Peritoneum

The parietal and visceral peritoneum envelops the mesorectum anteriorly and laterally in the upper two thirds of the rectum. At the transition of the middle and lower third of the rectum, just above the pelvic floor, the peritoneum reflects onto the seminal vesicles in males to form the rectovesical pouch and the posterior vaginal wall in females to form the rectouterine pouch (of Douglas). The height of the rectovesical excavation is about 6.5 cm and that of the rectouterine excavation about 7.5 cm from the dentate line. The peritoneal reflection appears as a low-signal-intensity V-shaped structure ("seagull sign") on sagittal T2W MR images (Fig. III.48a).

Whereas a tumor that comes close to or invades the mesorectal fascia may lead the clinician to a change in management, a tumor that comes close to or invades the visceral peritoneum above the pouch of Douglas is less likely to do so. For anteriorly located tumors, it is therefore of importance to locate the tumor relative to the pouch of Douglas.

Neurovascular and Lymphatic Anatomy

Vascular Supply

The hindgut, and thus the rectum, is embryologically supplied by the inferior mesenteric artery. It arises from the aorta at the level of the third lumbar vertebra (L3). One of its branches, the superior rectal artery, is the main feeding artery of the rectum. Once the superior rectal artery reaches the posterior wall of the rectum, it splits into left and right branches that feed both sides of the rectum via their fine peripheral branches. On axial T2W MR images, the superior rectal artery and its branches can be detected as low-intensity, tubular structures in the presacral region. The superior rectal vein runs on the dorsal and left side from the artery (Figs. III.55, 56, and 57).

The distal part of the rectum receives addi-

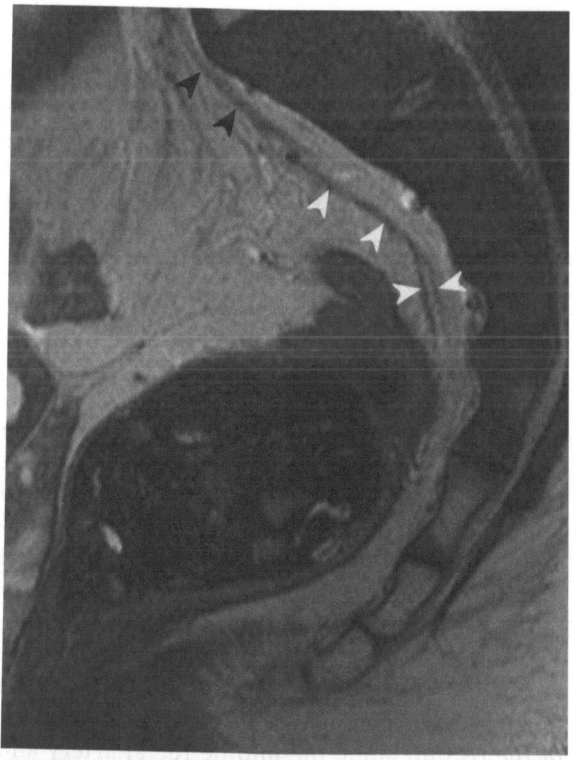

Fig. III.55. On sagittal T2-weighted fast spin echo (TR/TE 4,598/150 ms) magnetic resonance image the superior rectal artery and its branches can be detected as low signal intensity, tubular structures in the presacral region (*white arrowheads*). The superior rectal vein runs on the dorsal and left side of the artery (*black arrowheads*)

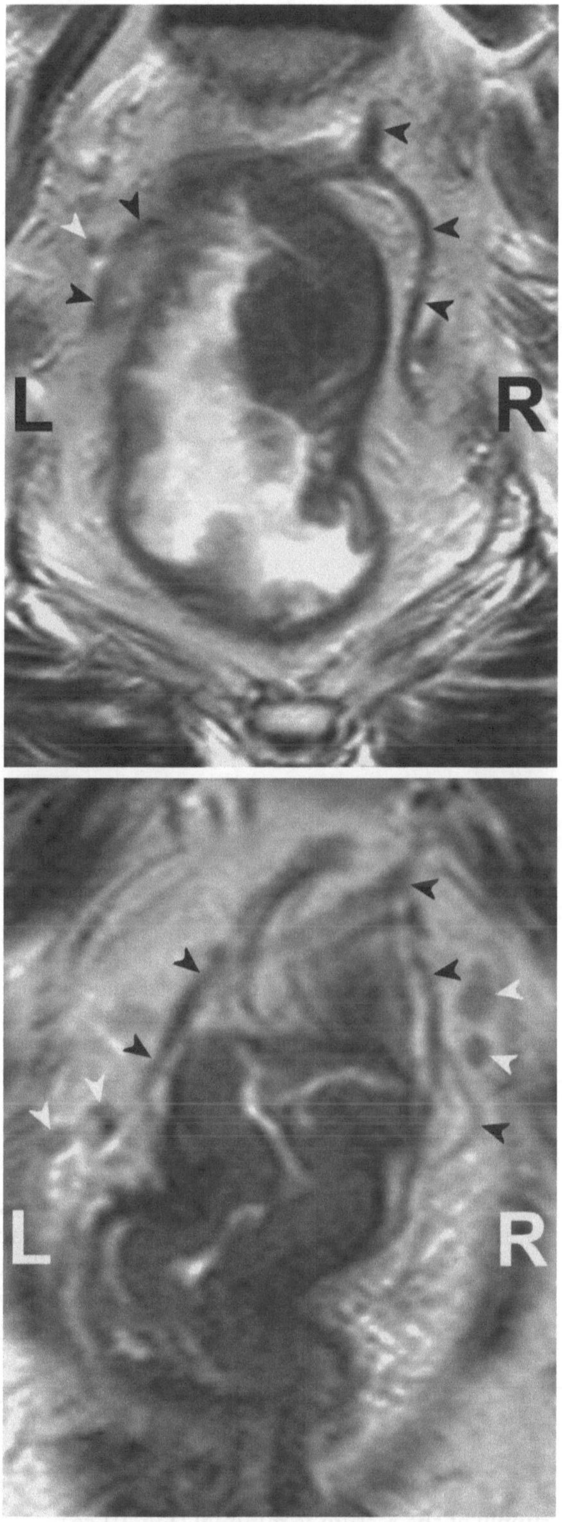

Figs. III.56 and 57. Coronal T2-weighted fast spin echo (TR/TE 3,427/150 ms) magnetic resonance images of a patient with rectal cancer shows the superior rectal artery and its branches (*black arrowheads*). Also, small hypointense lymph nodes are depicted (*white arrowheads*). L = left; R = right

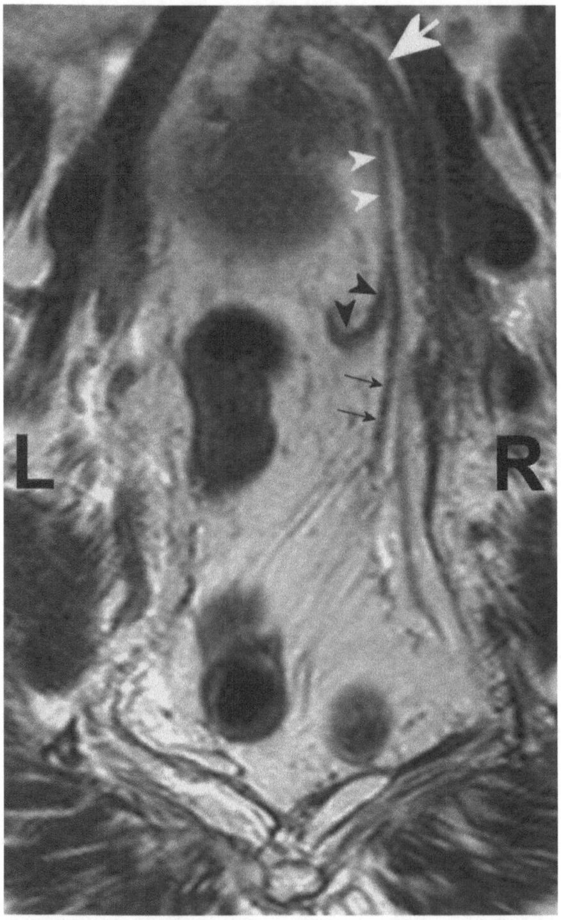

Fig. III.58. On the coronal T2-weighted fast spin echo (TR/TE 3,427/150 ms) magnetic resonance image the common iliac artery (*white arrow*) and its first branch – the internal iliac artery (*white arrowheads*) – are depicted. Both the pudendal artery (*black arrows*) and the middle rectal artery (*black arrowheads*) originate from the internal iliac artery. L = left; R = right

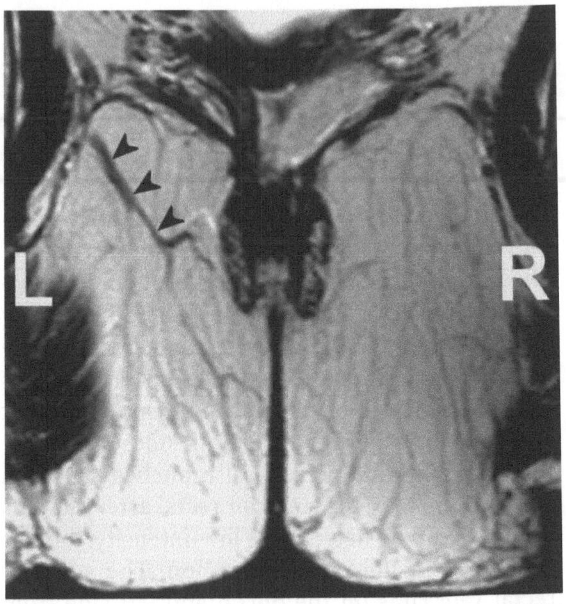

Fig. III.59. Coronal T2-weighted fast spin echo (TR/TE 5,952/150 ms) magnetic resonance image shows the inferior rectal artery (*black arrowheads*). It courses through the ischiosacral fossa, under the pelvic floor, toward the lower part of the rectum and anal canal. L = left; R = right

tional blood supply from the middle rectal artery, an inconsistent branch from the internal iliac artery (Fig. III.58), accompanied by a parallel, small, middle rectal vein. The internal iliac artery and vein course together with the ureter on the lateral pelvic side wall close to the mesorectal fascia. The inferior rectal artery comes off the pudendal artery, a branch of the internal iliac artery. The inferior rectal artery is situated below the pelvic floor muscles, and its relevance in blood supply of the rectum is minimal (Fig. III.59).

Anastomoses between the lateral and median sacral veins, which accompany the corresponding arteries, often form the so-called "presacral venous plexus" behind Waldeyer's fascia. On T2W MR images, they are seen as low-intensity tubular structures (Fig. III.54b). The presacral venous plexus can bleed profusely, and hemostasis may be difficult to achieve if it is accidentally injured during rectal surgery.

Lymph Drainage

The main lymphatic drainage of the rectum follows the superior rectal artery and vein to the inferior mesenteric vein and further up the paraaortic nodes (Fig. III.60a, b). Most of the lymph nodes in the mesorectum are situated along these vessels in the posterior and lateral part of the mesorectum [6]. Only a few lymph nodes are situated anteriorly in the mesorectum. These lymph nodes are situated inside the mesorectum. There is some controversy on the incidence and importance of lymphatic drainage of the rectum along the middle rectal artery and vein into the so-called lateral lymph pelvic nodes. These lymph nodes are situated outside the mesorectum. Through the efforts of Japanese sur-

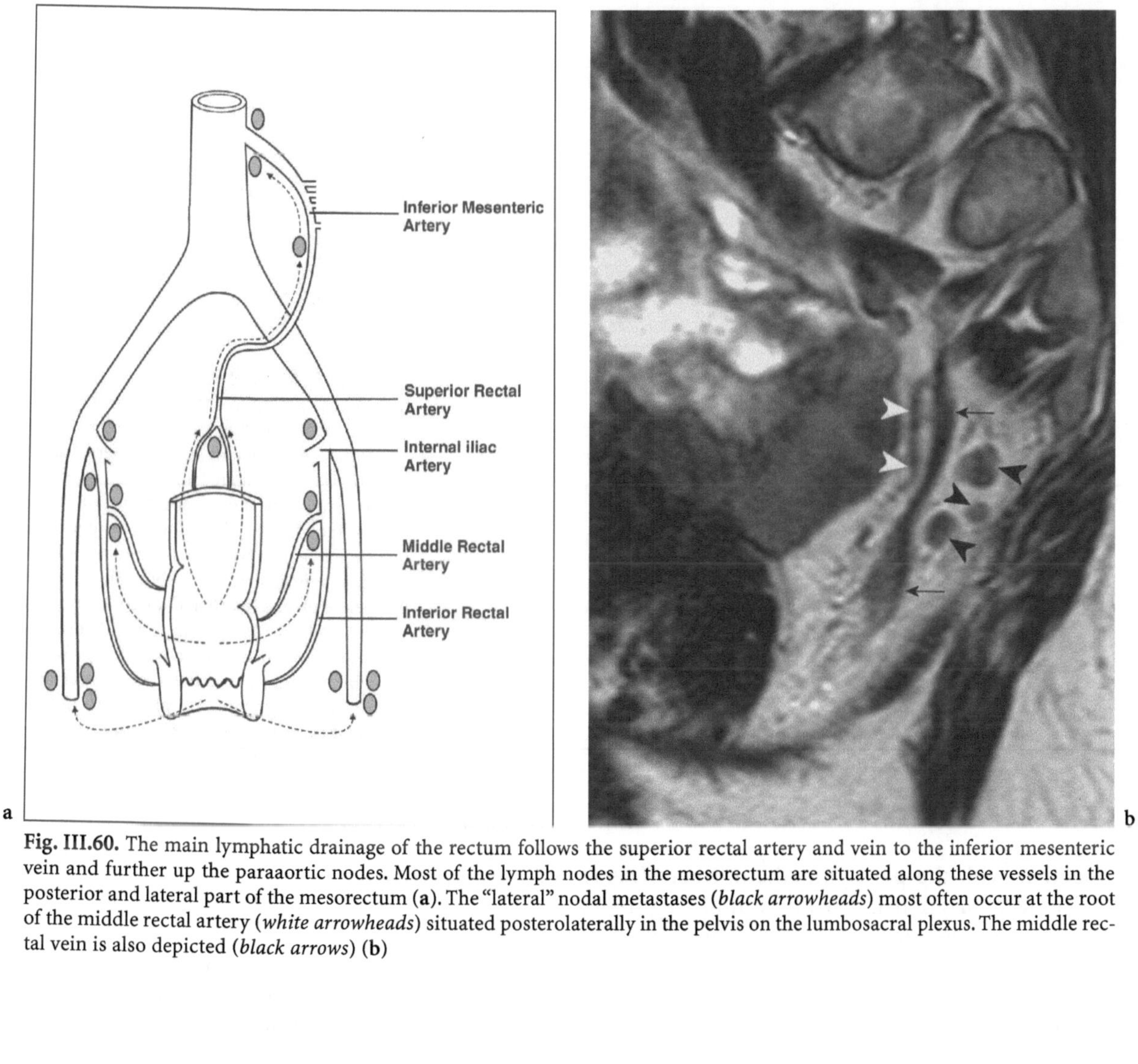

Fig. III.60. The main lymphatic drainage of the rectum follows the superior rectal artery and vein to the inferior mesenteric vein and further up the paraaortic nodes. Most of the lymph nodes in the mesorectum are situated along these vessels in the posterior and lateral part of the mesorectum (**a**). The "lateral" nodal metastases (*black arrowheads*) most often occur at the root of the middle rectal artery (*white arrowheads*) situated posterolaterally in the pelvis on the lumbosacral plexus. The middle rectal vein is also depicted (*black arrows*) (**b**)

geons, it is clear that lymph node metastases do occur in these lateral lymph nodes, usually in patients with distal rectal cancer and in the presence of mesorectal nodal metastases [7]. The "lateral" nodal metastases are often thought to be situated close to the obturator muscle while in reality, they most often occur at the root of the middle rectal artery situated posterolaterally in the pelvis on the lumbosacral plexus (Figs. III.56 and 57). On T2W MR images of healthy volunteers, small lymph nodes less than 4 mm in diameter and of hypointense signal intensity can sometimes be seen. In rectal cancer, it is known that size alone is not a good indicator for nodal metastases, as small nodes can harbor metastases [8].

Nerves

The relevant visceral nervous anatomy concerns sympathic and parasympathetic innervation for anorectal, urinary, and sexual functions. Because of its close relationship with the mesorectum, the nerves and plexuses can be invaded by a locally advanced tumor and easily injured when the rectum is mobilized during surgery [9, 10].

At the level of the promontory, just below the aortic bifurcation, presacral sympathic nerve fibers form the superior hypogastric plexus. The superior hypogastric plexus splits into left and right hypogastric nerves that, at a lower level,

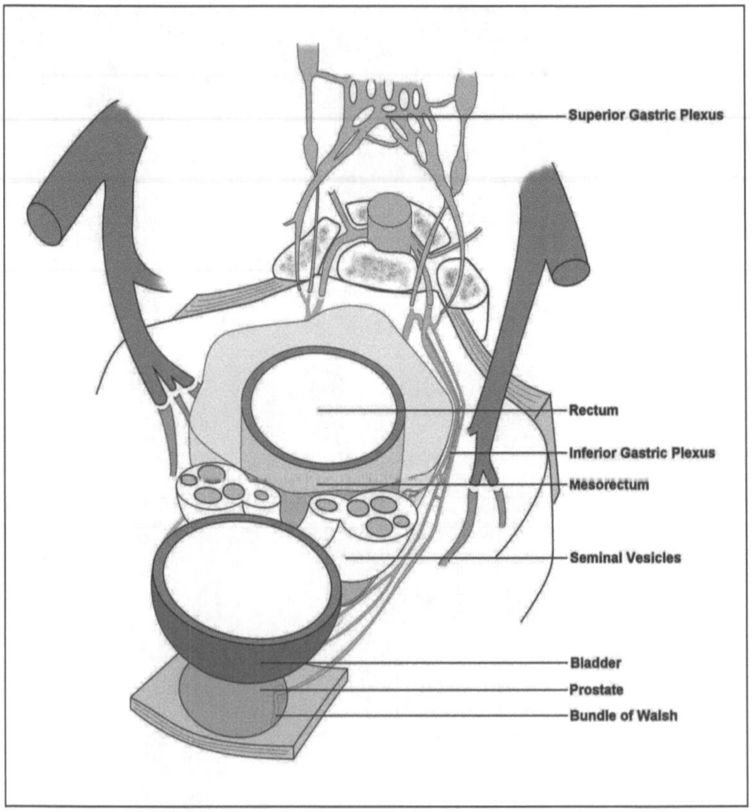

Fig. III.61. The superior hypogastric plexus splits into left and right hypogastric nerves that, at a lower level, together with the parasympathetic fibers (*nervi erigentes*) originate from spinal segments S2–S5, clasp the mesorectum on their course to the bladder and genitals. Together they form the left and right inferior hypogastric, or pelvic plexus. The pelvic plexus is situated anterolaterally of the rectum. The pelvic plexus continues into the neurovascular bundle of Walsh, which courses medially and inferiorly along the posterolateral aspect of the prostate gland. (Figure by courtesy of F. Köckerling [11])

together with the parasympathetic fibers (*nervi erigentes*) originating from spinal segments S2–S5, clasp the mesorectum on their course to the bladder and genitals. Together they form the left and right inferior hypogastric, or pelvic plexus. The pelvic plexus is situated anterolaterally of the rectum and continues into the neurovascular bundle of Walsh, which courses medially and caudally along the posterolateral aspect of the prostate gland (Fig. III.61). On T2W FSE MR images, the pelvic plexus can not be discerned.

Conclusion

MRI is becoming important in the management of rectal cancer patients. Knowledge of relevant MR anatomy of the rectum and mesorectum is mandatory for radiologists, surgeons, and radiation oncologists involved in the multidisciplinary approach of rectal cancer. This chapter aimed at providing detailed information on the MR anatomy of clinically relevant structures.

References

1. Heald RJ (1974) A new approach to rectal cancer. Br J Hosp Med: 22:277–281
2. Nagtegaal ID, Marijnen CA, Kranenbarg EK et al (2002) Circumferential margin involvement is still an important predictor of local recurrence in rectal carcinoma: not one millimeter but two millimeters is the limit. Am J Surg Pathol 26:350–357
3. Bissett IP, Fernando CC, Hough DM et al (2001) Identification of the fascia propria by magnetic resonance imaging and its relevance to preoperative assessment of rectal cancer. Dis Colon Rectum 44:259–265
4. Beets-Tan RG, Beets GL, Vliegen RF et al (2001) Accuracy of magnetic resonance imaging in prediction of tumour-free resection margin in rectal cancer surgery. Lancet 357:497–504

5. Heald RJ, Moran BJ (1998) Embryology and anatomy of the rectum. Semin Surg Oncol 15:66–71
6. Dworak O (1991) Morphology of lymph nodes in the resected rectum of patients with rectal carcinoma. Pathol Res Pract 187:1020–1024
7. Moriya Y, Sugihara K, Akasu T, Fujita J (1997) Importance of extended lymphadenectomy with lateral node dissection for advanced lower rectal cancer. World J Surg 21:728–732
8. Brown G, Richards CJ, Bourne MW et al (2003) Morphologic predictors of lymph node status in rectal cancer with use of high-spatial-resolution MR imaging with histopathologic comparison. Radiology: 227:371–377
9. Church JM, Raudkivi PJ, Hill GL (1987) The surgical anatomy of the rectum – a review with particular relevance to the hazards of rectal mobilisation. Int J Colorectal Dis 2:158–166
10. Havenga K, DeRuiter MC, Enker WE, Welvaart K (1996) Anatomical basis of autonomic nerve-preserving total mesorectal excision for rectal cancer. Br J Surg 83:384–388
11. Köckerling F (2002) Total Mesorectal Excision with the Water-Jet. Science Med Dr. Sperber, Hannover

Invited Commentary

J. Kruskal

Imaging advances continue to be made in depicting the anatomy of the anal canal and rectum. The preceding chapters have highlighted the exquisite detail that is provided by contemporary ultrasound, including volumetric imaging and magnetic resonance imaging (MRI). Recent MR advances have been made possible by the wide availability of 3T magnets that provide superior anatomic detail and resolution. These high-field-strength magnets, coupled with improved engineering and the increased use of endorectal coils, are being used with increased frequency in centers specializing in management of anorectal disorders. Such high resolution multiplanar MRI of the anorectal region now provides detailed resolution capable of evaluating the spectrum of inflammatory and neoplastic disorders that are known to occur. At this stage of technical development, one anticipated focus is correlating imaging findings with subsequent management of different anorectal diseases. Many surgeons and gastroenterologists remain unfamiliar with the anatomic detail provided by contemporary MRI coupled with the exquisite delineation and characterization of different disease entities. Another focus will be to familiarize physicians with the capabilities of anorectal MRI such that these can be fully taken advantage of when evaluating disease processes and planning treatment, including surgical management. Another anticipated focus of research will be imaging for the evaluation of postoperative anatomy, especially dynamic changes that occur following surgery.

The ability to image dynamic pelvic floor anatomy has been covered in another chapter. While endoanal sonography remains widely used for depicting the anatomy of the anal canal, sonography is not routinely used for imaging the rectum. Since rectal imaging requires distention of a water-filled balloon to obtain acoustic coupling, the technique has found its widest application for staging of rectal cancers. For rigid endoscopes, which still provide superior anatomic detail compared with flexible systems, insertion above the rectosigmoid junction is unlikely to occur and is thus a limitation of this technology.

Two areas that are garnering increased attention are positron emission tomography/computed tomography (PET/CT) and the use of multiplanar high-resolution CT scanning for imaging rectal anatomy and evaluating rectal tumors (Fig. III.62). PET/CT is now routinely used for the

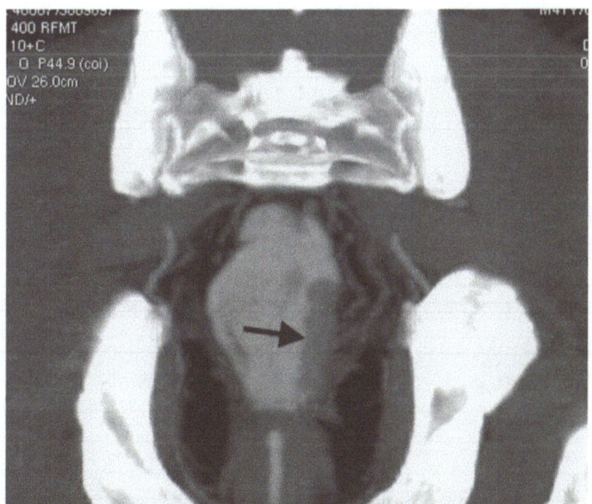

Fig. III.62. Thick-slab coronal maximum intensity projection (MIP) image of a T3 rectal cancer (*arrow*) growing up the left lateral rectal wall demonstrates tumor extension beyond the rectal wall

staging of colorectal tumors, especially during postoperative surveillance when other modalities are unlikely to confidently distinguish scarring from recurrence, but the anatomic detail provided by this modality is limited purely by the resolution of the CT scanner being used. Since CT scanning remains the current standard for exclusion of liver, lung, and intraperitoneal metastases in patients with rectal cancer, it is a logical extension to develop CT techniques aimed at local staging of rectal tumors. The superb submillimeter resolution now provided by 64-row multidetector CT (MDCT) scanners allows images to be reconstructed in multiple planes without loss of anatomic detail. For rectal imaging, this so-called isotropic imaging technique permits exquisite detail in the sagittal and coronal planes during different phases of contrast administration. In this way, CT scanning can now be used to show the extent of transmural tumor extension coupled with vascular anatomy for surgical planning. It must be emphasized that this is still being used in an experimental manner and that the detail provided by 3T MRI and transrectal ultrasound is still recognized as being the most accurate for purposes of tumor staging.

Section IV

Endoanal Ultrasonography in the Assessment of Patients with Fecal Incontinence

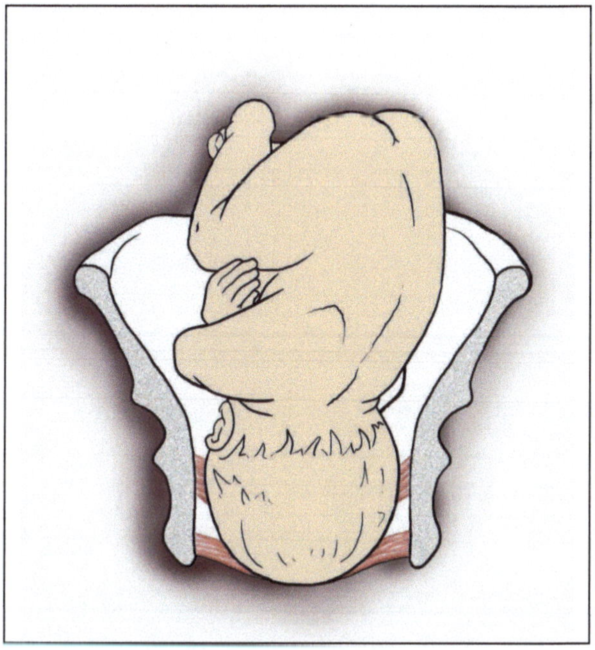

IV.1. Introduction

G.A. Santoro, G. Di Falco

Continence depends on a number of factor that include stool consistency, the capacity of the sigmoid colon to retard progress of stool, the compliance and sensation of the urgency of the rectum, the phasic contractions of the puborectalis muscle to form a normal anorectal angle, a normal internal (IAS) and external (EAS) sphincter function, and normal sensation in the anal canal [1] (Fig. IV.1). The etiology of fecal incontinence can be subdivided into three main groups (Table IV.1): (1) functional, (2) sphincter weakness, and (3) sensory loss. The majority of patients with incontinence are women with an obstetric injury, and symptoms can occur even in an elderly population who had experienced vaginal deliveries earlier in life [2].

Accurate evaluation of patients with fecal incontinence is crucial for the treatment plan. Physiology of defecation and continence has been traditionally studied with anorectal

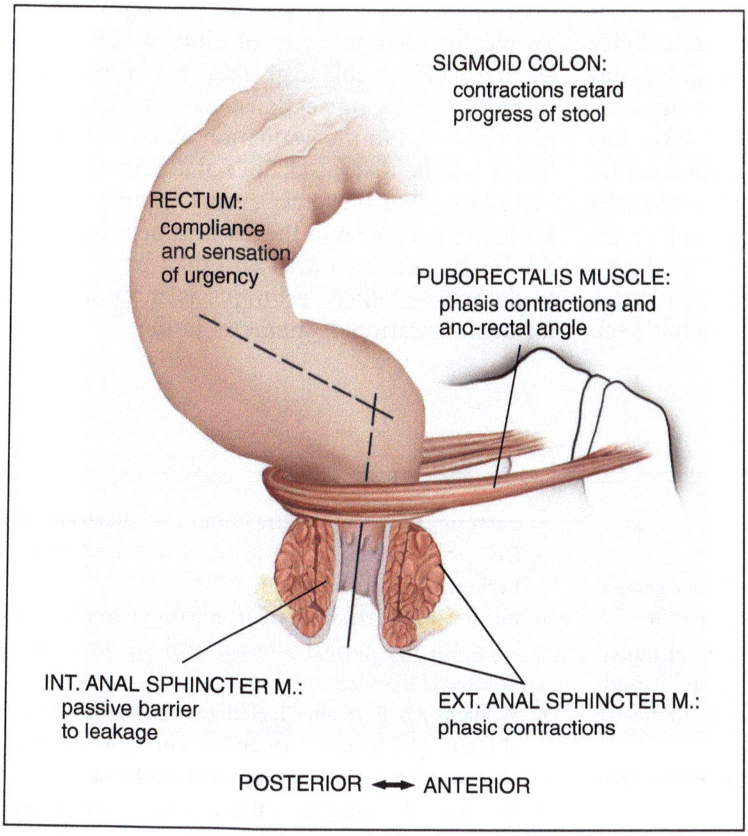

Fig. IV.1. Schematic representation of the different mechanisms of continence to stool

Table IV.1. Etiology of fecal incontinence

Category	Mechanism	Common causes
Functional	Rapid transit	Irritable bowel syndrome, inflammatory bowel disease, tumors
	Pelvic floor dyssynergia	Idiopathic, spinal cord injury
	Psychological	Dementia, psychosis, behavioral
Sphincter weakness	Sphincter muscle injury	Obstetrical trauma, accidental trauma, surgical trauma
	Pudendal nerve injury	Obstetrical trauma, idiopathic, peripheral neuropathy
	Central nervous system injury	Spina bifida, spinal cord injury, cerebrovascolar accident
Sensory loss	Afferent nerve injury	Diabetic neuropathy, spinal cord injury

manometry. This procedure, however, is able to give a number of useful clinical data but can offer only indirect and not very reliable information on the integrity of anal sphincters based on registration of the resting pressure, squeeze pressure, and rectoanal inhibitory reflex. The importance of endoanal ultrasound (EAUS) in delineating the different structures of the anal canal and the pelvic floor has been confirmed in numerous studies [3–10]. The ultrasonographic images of the IAS and EAS are realistic, and their modifications are well correlated to anorectal function [11–16]. EAUS has better diagnostic specificity and sensitivity when compared with digital examination and computerized tomography (CT). Magnetic resonance imaging (MRI) has been suggested as a better diagnostic procedure. However, differences in definition of anal canal anatomy have been described in relation to the technique used. Endoanal coil has been used for a long time; however, it could distort the anatomy and, recently, a phased-array technique has been preferred [17–20]. With this procedure, all the main features of the anal canal morphology showed with EAUS are similarly confirmed: good resolution of the IAS; shorter EAS at the anterior anal canal in females; no precise subdivision of the EAS into two or three parts; difficulty measuring the perineal body. The only significant advantage of phase-array MRI over endoanal MR and EAUS is the imaging of a wider field of view [21–22]. Considering technical characteristics, time consumption, costs, and availability of instruments in hospitals, in our opinion MR should be used in cases of clinical complexity when EAUS is unable to give reliable information.

In the following sections, accuracy and reliability of EAUS in the evaluation of anal sphincter injury will be discussed. Special attention will be focused on the obstetric events leading to anal sphincter damage and their assessment by EAUS. EAUS and endoanal MRI will then be compared to determine which technique is more accurate for demonstration of sphincter lesions.

References

1. Jorge JM, Wexner SD (1993) Etiology and management of fecal incontinence. Dis Colon Rectum 36:77–97
2. Oberwalder M, Dinnewitzer A, Baig K et al (2004) The association between late-onset fecal incontinence and obstetric anal sphincter defects. Arch Surg 139:429–432
3. Stoker J, Halligan S, Bartram CI (2001) Pelvic floor imaging. Radiology 218:621–641
4. Bartram CI (2003) Ultrasound. In: Bartram CI, DeLancy. JOL Imaging pelvic floor disorders. Springer, Berlin Heidelberg New York
5. Burnett SJD, Bartram CI (1991) Endosonographic variations in the normal internal anal sphincter. Int J Colorectal Dis 6:2
6. Williams AB, Bartram CI, Halligan S, Marshall MM et al (2001) Multiplanar anal endosonography – normal anal canal anatomy. Colorectal Dis 3:169–174
7. Frudinger A, Halligan S, Bartram CI (2002) Female

anal sphincter: age-related differences in asymptomatic volunteers with high-frequency endoanal US. Radiology 224:417–423
8. Williams AB, Cheetham MJ, Bartram CI et al (2000) Gender differences in the longitudinal pressure profile of the anal canal related to anatomical structure as demonstrated on three-dimensional anal endosonography. Br J Surg 87:1674–1679
9. Nielsen MB, Hauge C, Rasmussen OO (1992) Anal sphincter size measured by endosonography in healthy volunteers. Effect of age, sex, and parity. Acta Radiol 33:453–456
10. Kumar A, Scholefield JH (2000) Endosonography of the anal canal and rectum. World J Surg 24:208–215
11. Gold DM, Halligan S, Kmiot WA, Bartram CI (1999) Intraobserver and interobserver agreement in anal endosonography. Br J Surg 86: 371–375
12. Enck P, Heyer T, Gantke B, Schmidt WU (1997) How reproducible are measures of the anal sphincter muscle diameter by endoanal ultrasound? Am J Gastroenterol 92: 293–296
13. Thakar R, Sultan A (2004) Anal endosonography and its role in assessing the incontinent patient. Best Pract Res Clinic Obstet Gynaec 18:157–173
14. Sultan AH, Kamm MA, Talbot IC et al (1994) Anal endosonography for identifying external sphincter defects confirmed histologically. Br J Surg 81: 463–465
15. Gold DM, Bartram CI, Halligan S (1999) Three-dimensional endoanal sonography in assessing anal canal injury. Br J Surg 86:365–370
16. Bollard RC, Gardiner A, Lindow S et al (2002) Normale female anal sphincter: difficulties in interpretation explained. Dis Colon Rectum 45:171–175
17. Stoker J, Rociu E, Zwamborn AW et al (1999) Endoluminal MR imaging of the rectum and anus: technique, applications and pitfalls. Radiographics 19:383–398
18. Hussain SM, Stoker J, Lameris JS (1995) Anal sphincter complex: endoanal MR imaging of normal anatomy. Radiology 197:671–677
19. Williams AB, Malouf AJ, Bartram CI et al (2001) Assessment of external anal sphincter morphology in idiopathic fecal incontinence with endocoil magnetic resonance imaging. Dig Dis Sci 46:1466–1471
20. Morren GL, Beets-Tan GH, van Engelshoven MA (2001) Anatomy of the anal canal and perianal structures as defined by phase-array magnetic resonance imaging. Br J Surg 88:1506–1512
21. Rociu E, Stoker J, Eijkemans MJC et al (1999) Fecal incontinence: endoanal US versus endoanal MR imaging. Radiology 212:453–458
22. Beets-Tan RGH, Morren GL, Betts GL et al (2001). Measurement of anal sphincter muscles: endoanal US, endoanal MR imaging, or phased-array MR imaging? A study with healthy volunteers. Radiology 220: 81–89

IV.2. Accuracy and Reliability of Endoanal Ultrasonography in the Evaluation of Anal Sphincter Injury

G.A. Santoro, G. Gizzi

Endoanal ultrasonography (EAUS) remains the gold standard in delineating the anatomy of the sphincter complex [1–8]. Features shown by EAUS can help to differentiate between incontinent patients with intact anal sphincters and those with sphincter lesions [9–14]. The operator should identify if there is a combined lesion of both internal (IAS) and external (EAS) sphincter or if the lesion involves just one muscle. Number, site, axial (in hours of the clock) and longitudinal extension, radial angle of the defect, presence of scarring, differences in echogenicity and thickness of the sphincters, and other local alteration should be carefully assessed and should always be reported. If a clear break is detected, it should be graded on the basis of the degree of circumferential involvement (<25% or >25%). Tears are defined by an interruption of the fibrillar echotexture. Scarring is characterized by loss of normal architecture, with an area of amorphous texture that usually has low reflectiveness [15].

This procedure has a key role in choosing the correct therapeutic option and has almost completely replaced the invasive and painful electromyography in mapping sphincter defects. However, finding a sphincter defect does not necessarily mean that it is the cause of fecal incontinence [16] whereas an anal sphincter that looks normal, without lesion, can have degeneration or atrophy [17]. The size of defect correlates with the severity of fecal incontinence [18]; however, a recent study failed to demonstrate a relationship between muscle injuries and the severity of clinical symptoms [19]. EAUS should, therefore, be complementary to anorectal manometry and neurophysiologic studies [20, 21].

Internal Anal Sphincter Abnormalities

The majority of lesions to the IAS are due to obstetric or iatrogenic injuries. Minor degrees of fecal incontinence (soiling) due to IAS injuries have been reported in 29% of patients after hemorrhoidectomy or mucoprolapsectomy [22]. Manual anal dilatation [23] or lateral internal sphincterotomy [24] for the treatment anal fissure have been associated with anal incontinence in 27% and 50% of patients, respectively. Up to 60% of patients can be rendered incontinent following fistula surgery [25].

Defects of the IAS are easily recognized given the prominent appearance of the IAS in the mid anal canal, and they appear as hyperechoic breaks in the normally hypoechoic ring. The pattern of sphincter disruption is related to the type of surgery [26]. Patients incontinent following manual dilatation exhibit a diffuse thinning of the IAS or disruption of the IAS at more than one site (Fig. IV.2). Patients incontinent after sphincterotomy have a single defect in the IAS associated with a thickening of the remaining muscle for a retraction phenomenon (Fig. IV.3). Patients who become incontinent following hemorrhoidectomy have defects in the site of the hemorrhoidal cush-

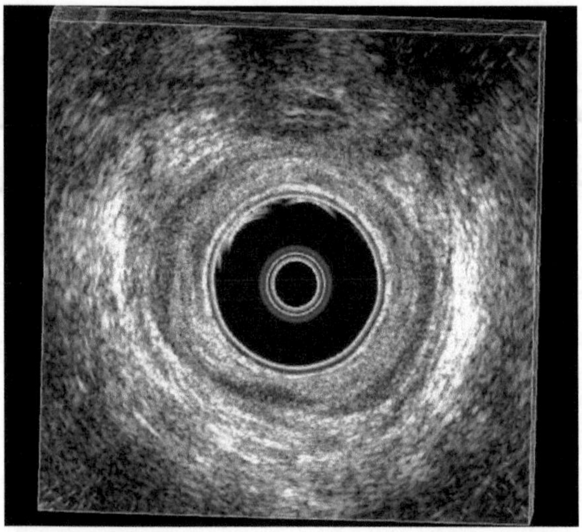

Fig. IV.2. Fragmentation of the internal anal sphincter following manual dilatation

fecal incontinence and intact anal sphincter. The IAS appeared thinner than normal and hyperechoic, and these conditions were combined with reduced resting pressure and normal squeeze pressure, rectal sensitivity, and pudendal latency. Incontinent patients with IAS degeneration were found to be older than those with obstetric trauma incontinence [5].

An apparently opposite EAUS condition is an abnormal thickness of the IAS (Fig. IV.10). It seems typical of older ages without differences of anal canal levels [5, 17, 27]. Interestingly, decreased thickness of the IAS can be frequently observed in patients with chronic anal fissure, a sign of an increased sphincter tone. Imaging of an IAS break following internal sphincterotomy for a fissure can help to follow-up clinical results of the operation or the unexpected sequelae (persistence of anal fissure and pain or, on the other hand, fecal incontinence).

ions (Figs. IV.4 and 5). Fistula surgery or obstetric trauma is associated with combined internal and external sphincter injuries (Figs. IV.6–8).

A thinning of IAS of less than 2 mm in a patient more than 50 years old is abnormal, and the term "primary degeneration of IAS" has been used to describe this (Fig. IV.9). Vaizey et al. [17] reviewed the EAUS examinations of 38 patients with passive

External Anal Sphincter Abnormalities

One of the most important contribute of EAUS has been in the correct imaging of the EAS [1–8], which is of major importance for continence. The most frequent cause of fecal incontinence is an obstetric injury to the EAS. The appearance of

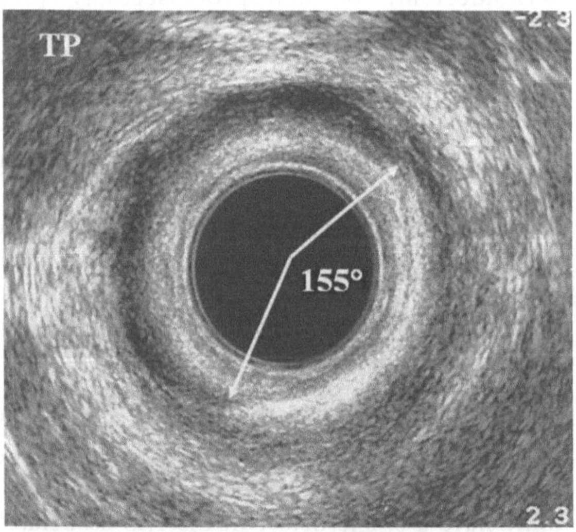

Fig. IV.3. Complete division of the internal anal sphincter (*arrows*) at the level of the transverse perineii (*TP*) following a left lateral internal sphincterotomy for fissure. The remaining muscle appears slightly thicker for a retraction phenomenon

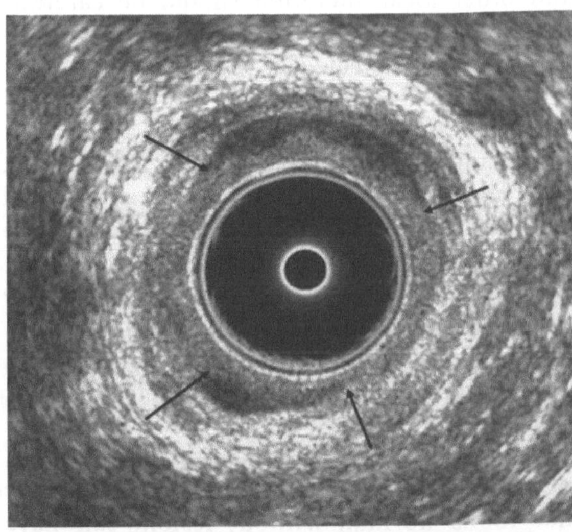

Fig. IV.4. Two complete defects of the internal anal sphincter between 2 and 6 o'clock (120°) and between 7 and 10 o'clock (90°) (*black arrows*) following hemorrhoidectomy

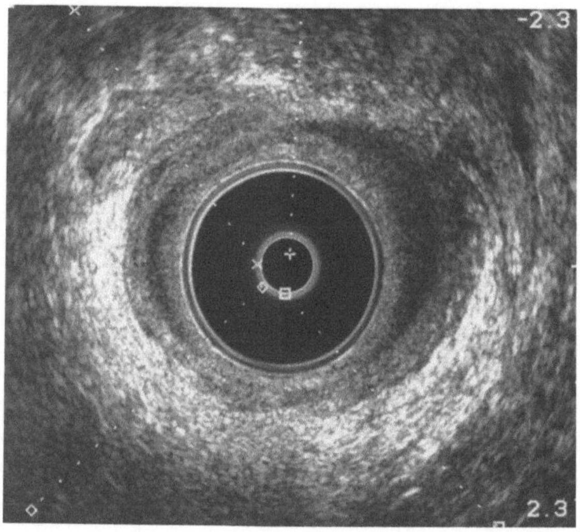

Fig. IV.5. Two complete defects of the internal anal sphincter between 5 and 7 o'clock (60°) and between 10 and 12 o'clock (60°) (*dots*) following hemorrhoidectomy

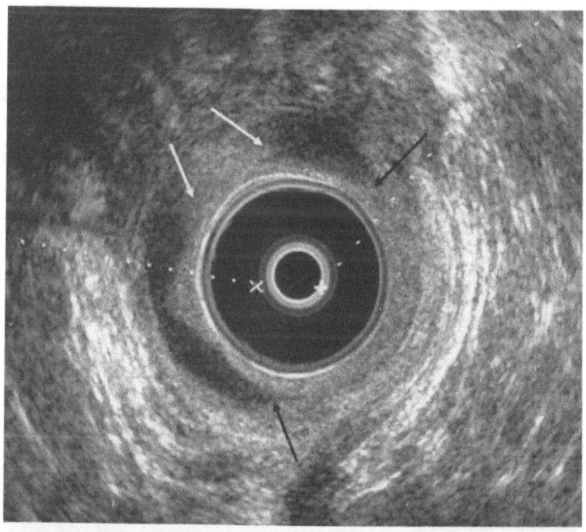
a

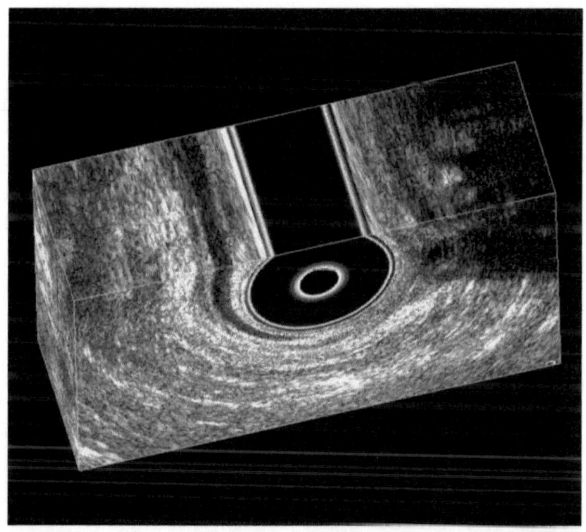
b

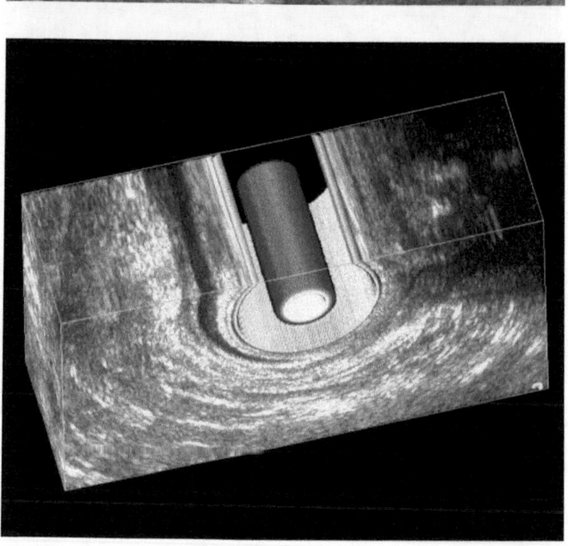
c

Fig. IV.6. Combined internal (between 1 and 6 o'clock, *black arrows*, and between 10 and 11 o'clock, *white arrows*) and external (between 10 and 2 o'clock, *dots*) anal sphincter defects following multiple operations for a recurrent high fistula (**a**). Three-dimensional coronal images showing the absence of the internal sphincter in the left side of the anal canal (**b, c**)

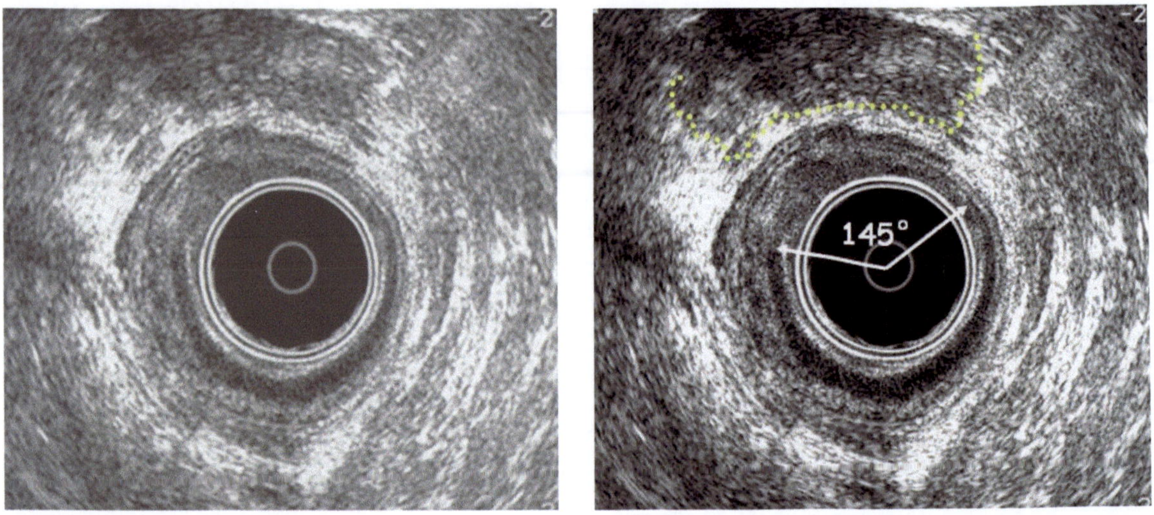

a b

Fig. IV.7. Obstetric trauma with an internal sphincter defect anteriorly (*arrows*) and scarring in the external sphincter between 11 and 1 o'clock (*dots*) (**a, b**)

an EAS defect is a break in the circumferential integrity of the mixed hyperechoic band (Figs. IV.11 and 12). A defect can have either a hypoechoic or a hyperechoic density pattern. This corresponds to replacement of the normal striated muscle with granulation tissue and fibrosis (Fig. IV.13). The majority of obstetric injuries are associated with a single, large, defect in the EAS anterior to the anal canal that can be combined to an additional division of the IAS (Fig. IV.14). In examining a female subject, it is important to remember the ultrasonographic

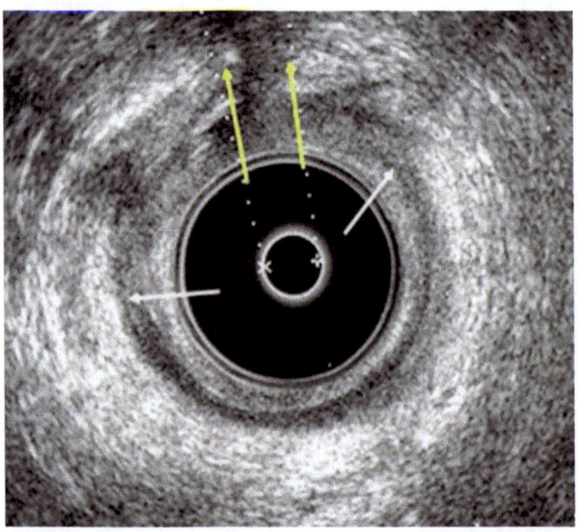

Fig. IV.8. Obstetric trauma with a well-defined defect of the external sphincter at 12 o'clock (*yellow arrows*) due to an episiotomy and an internal sphincter division between 10 and 2 o'clock (*white arrows*)

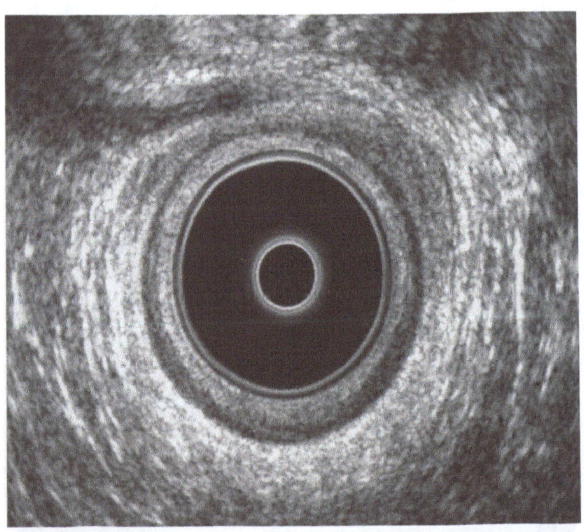

Fig. IV.9. A 68-year-old woman with passive fecal incontinence. The internal sphincter is intact but thinner than normal for this age (1.3 mm), indicative of primary degeneration

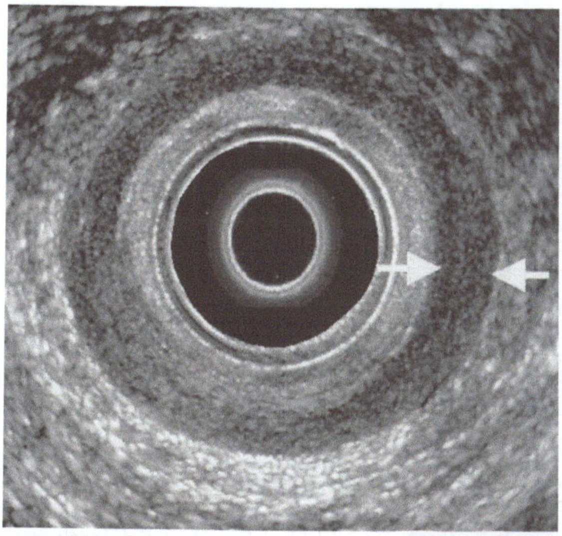

Fig. IV.10. Abnormal thickness of the internal anal sphincter (4.1 mm) in a 42-year-old woman with intra-anal prolapse (*arrows*)

differences between the natural gaps (hypoechoic areas with smooth, regular edges, occurring in the upper part of the anal canal) and the sphincter ruptures (mixed echogenicity due to scarring, with irregular edges) occurring at the upper anterior part of the anal canal [6, 14] (Fig. IV.15). Surgery for a fistula can also be responsible for damage to the EAS. This can more likely occur during treatment of complex, high fistulas or in patients who have undergone multiple operations for a recurrent or persistent fistula (Fig. IV.6).

A limitation of EAUS is the definition of EAS atrophy in patients with idiopathic fecal incontinence because of the vague contours of the mus-

a 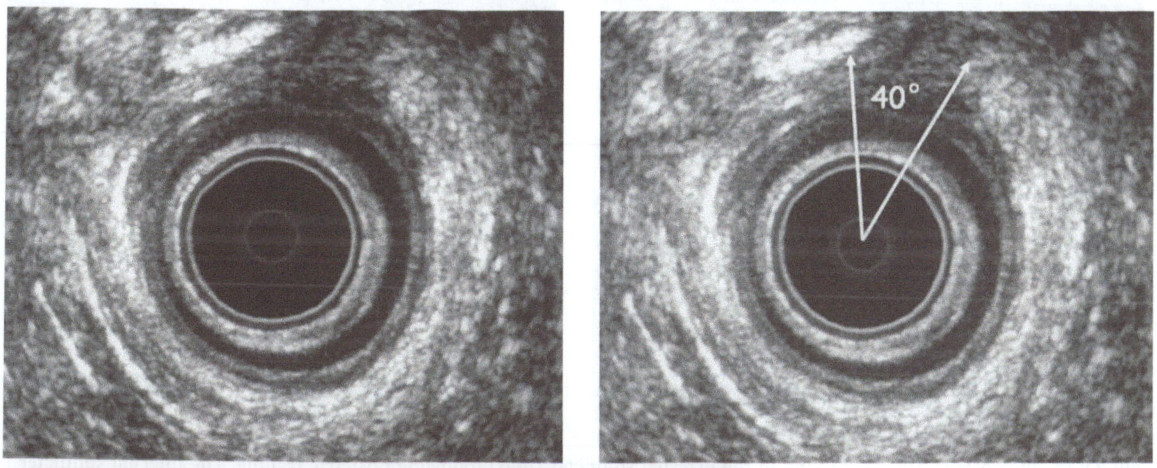 b

c 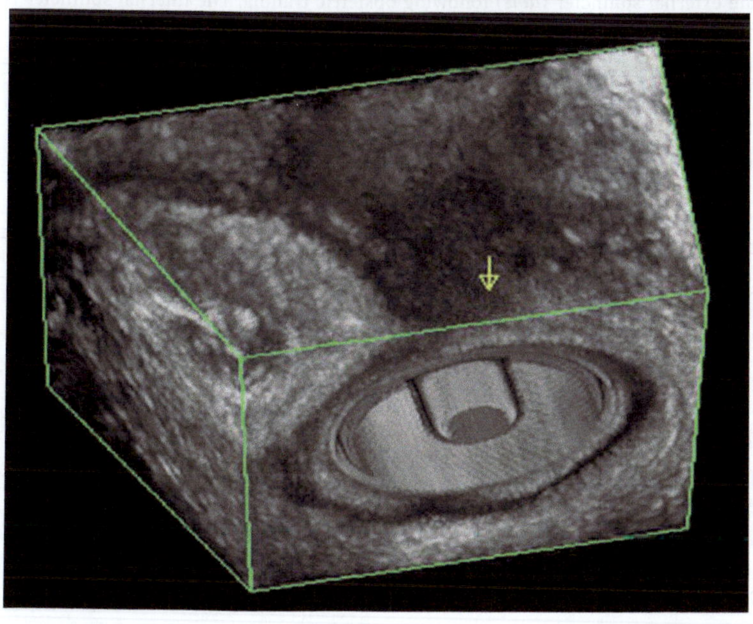

Fig. IV.11. The appearance of an external anal sphincter defect is a break in the circumferential integrity of the mixed hyperechoic band (**a**). The extent of the defect is measured in the axial plane as an angle (**b**). Three-dimensional image demonstrating the defect (*arrow*) in the coronal plane (**c**)

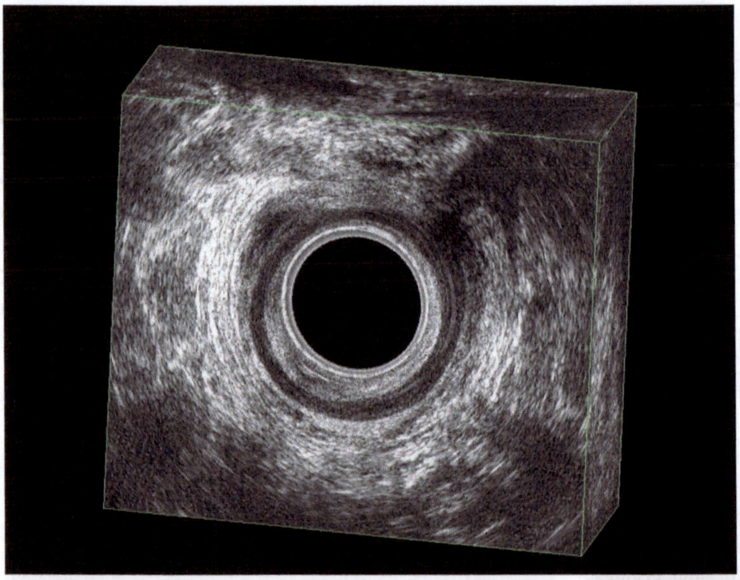

Fig. IV.12. Obstetric trauma with a well-defined defect of the external sphincter at 1 o'clock (circumferential involvement <25%)

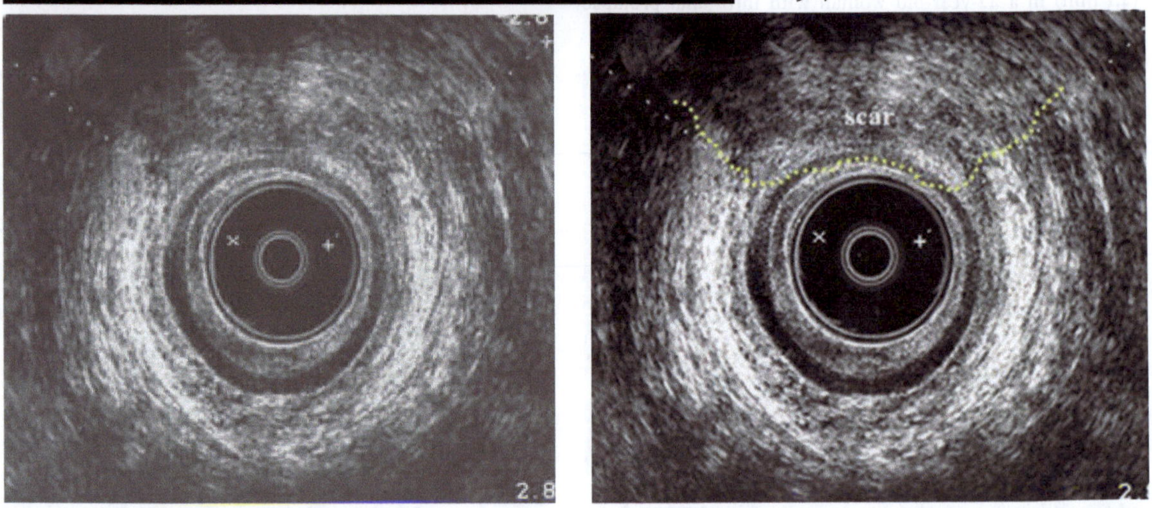

a b

Fig. IV.13. Hypoechoic area of scarring in the external sphincter (*dots*) following obstetric trauma. The internal sphincter is thinned anteriorly but is intact (**a, b**)

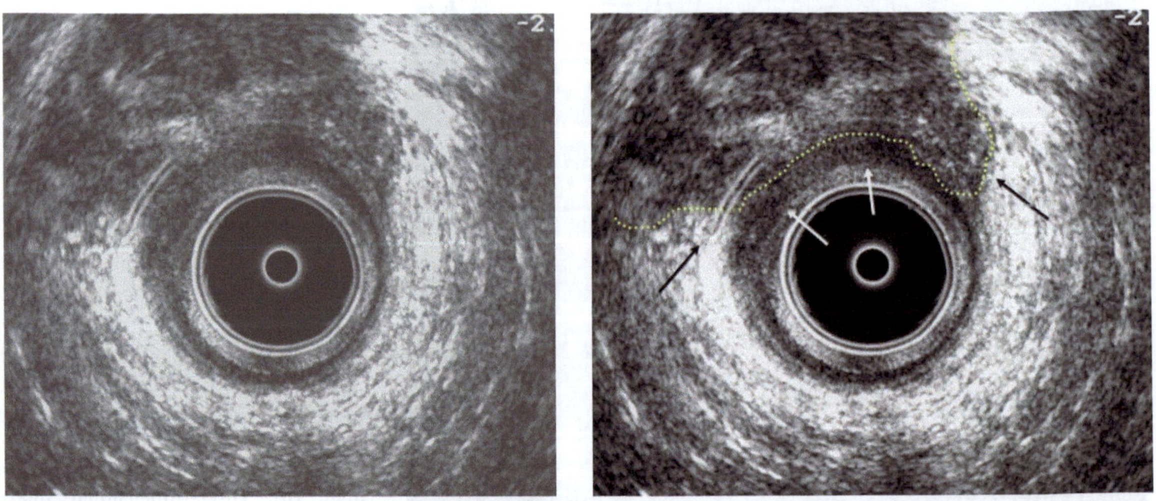

a b

Fig. IV.14. Obstetric external sphincter tear between 10 and 2 o'clock (*black arrows*) with a small defect of the internal sphincter from 11 to 12 o'clock (*white arrows*) (**a, b**)

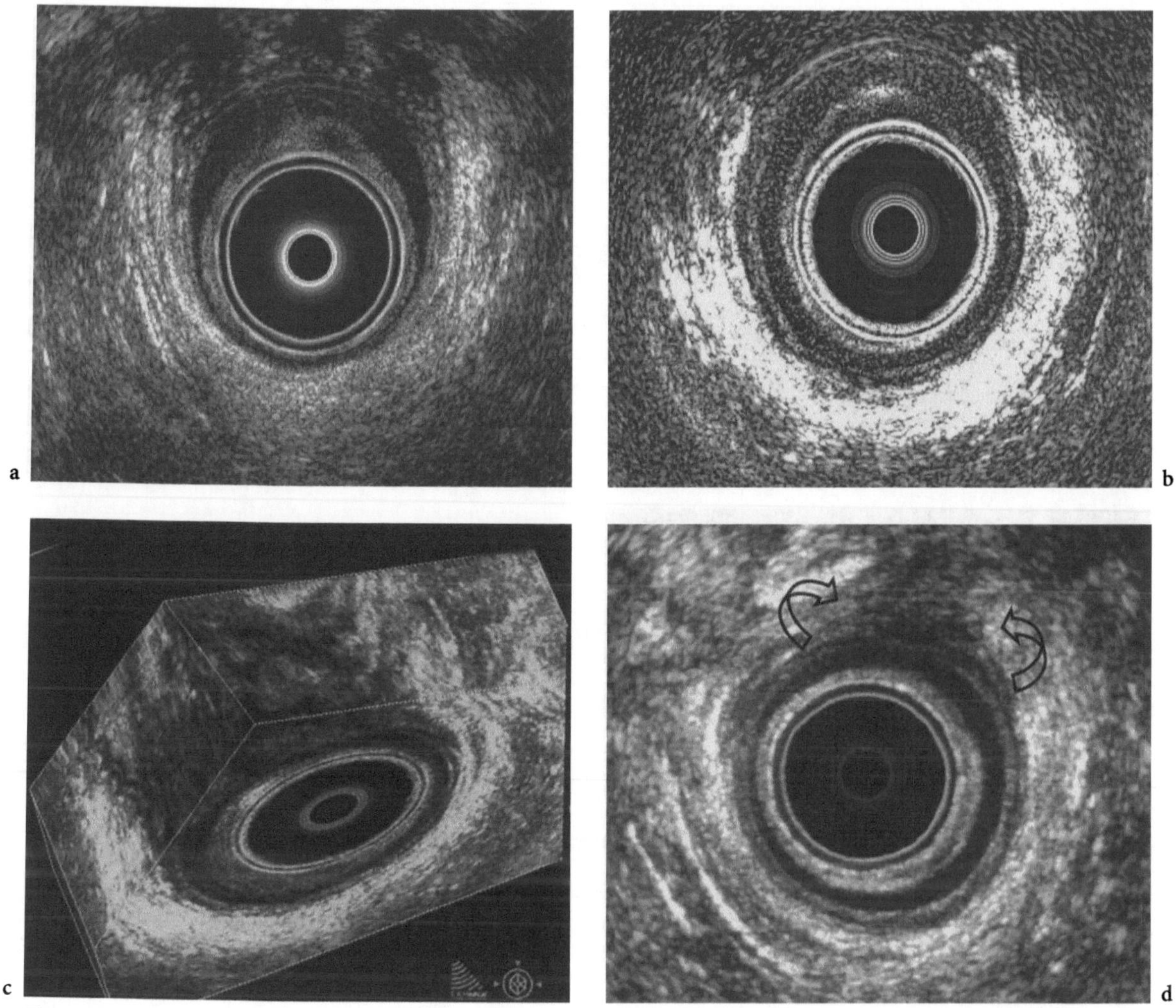

Fig. IV.15. Differences between a natural gap (hypoechoic areas with smooth, regular edges, occurring in the upper part of the anal canal) (**a**) and a ruptured external sphincter (mixed echogenicity, due to scarring, with irregular edges) (**b–d**)

cle ring [15, 28]. Endoanal magnetic resonance imaging (MRI) is more accurate in detecting atrophy as a thinner EAS, with replacement of muscle by fat [15, 29, 30]. EAUS also serves as a surveillance tool to monitor results following sphincteroplasty [17, 31] (Fig. IV.16). Savoye-Collet et al. [32] reported that in the 21 patients in whom EAUS documented closure of the EAS defect, 18 (86%) noted improvement in fecal incontinence. In contrast, eight of the ten patients who had a persistent defect in the EAS still had significant fecal incontinence.

Accuracy and Reliability

The accuracy of EAUS in the evaluation of incontinence has been supported by surgical findings. Gold et al. [9] and Enck et al. [10] reported that sensitivity and specificity in locating the defect was 100% and accuracy in the topographic detection of the defect was 90%. Deen et al. [33] investigated 44 incontinent patients with EAUS. All sonographically detected EAS defects were confirmed at operation, and 21 of 22 IAS defects were also confirmed at surgery. The sensitivity

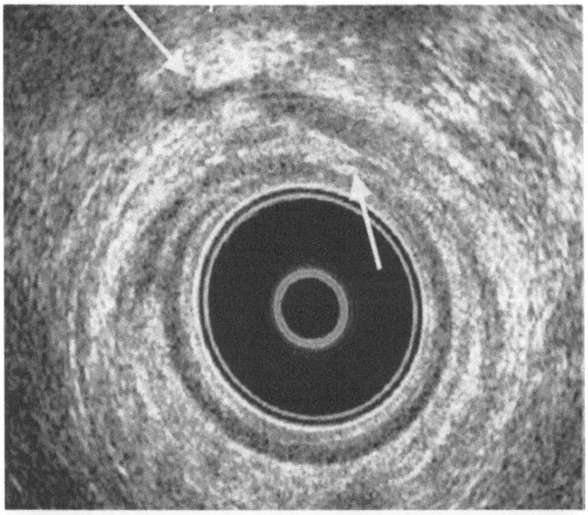

a

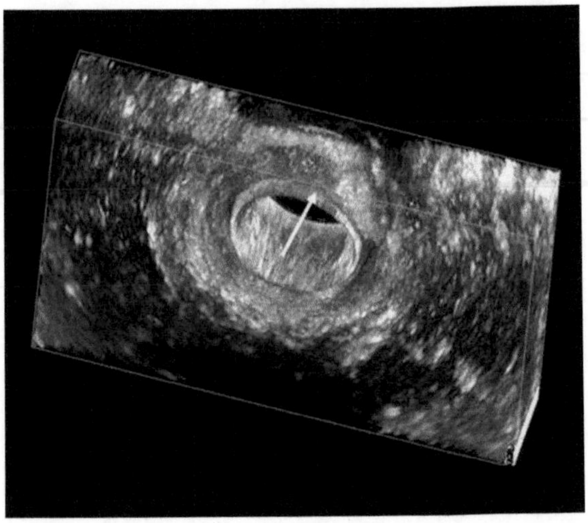

b

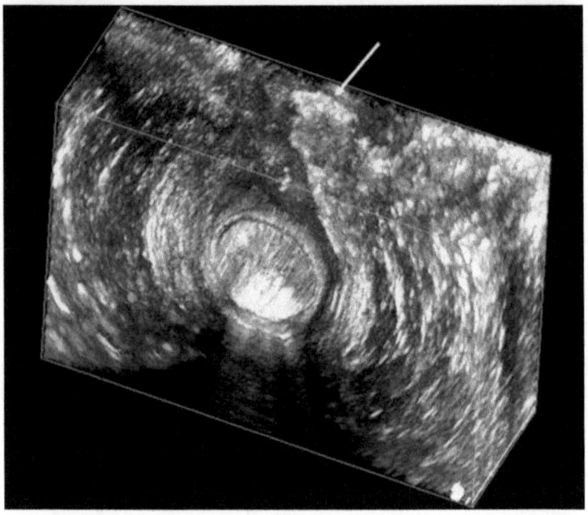

c

Fig. IV.16. Anterior external sphincter repair (**a**). Three-dimensional images in the coronal plane demonstrating the lower (**b**) and the upper (**c**) sling of the overlap

and specificity of EAUS was 100% for EAS defects and 100% and 95.5%, respectively, for IAS lesions. Sultan et al. [12] compared preoperative ultrasonographic findings with intraoperative results in 12 consecutive patients who underwent surgical repair for fecal incontinence. EAUS correctly identified all sphincters defects at time of surgery. Sentovich et al. [34] examined the accuracy and reliability of EAUS. In 22 incontinent women with known anal sphincter injury, the accuracy was 100%. However, in nulliparous women, EAUS falsely identified sphincter injury in 5–25% of normal anal sphincters. In this group, intact internal sphincters were more accurately predicted than intact external sphincters (95% vs. 85%). Overall, clinical agreement in the interpretation of the ultrasound between experienced ultrasonographers (interobserver reliability) was good (81% agreement). Agreement was significantly better for the IAS (74%, fair) than the EAS (61%, poor; p=0.0002) and in evaluating the distal anal canal (0–1.5cm) (78%) than the proximal anal canal (2.0–2.5cm from the anal verge) (48% agreement; p <0.0001). However, Gold et al. [35] reported that interobserver agreement for diagnosis of sphincter disruption was very good (k=0.80). There was no disagreement with respect to combined or isolated IAS tears although there was some disagreement regarding isolated EAS tears. Abramowitz et al. [36] demonstrated interobserver concordance in 98.9% of cases.

Three-dimensional (3-D) EAUS may improve diagnostic confidence of detecting damage to the

a

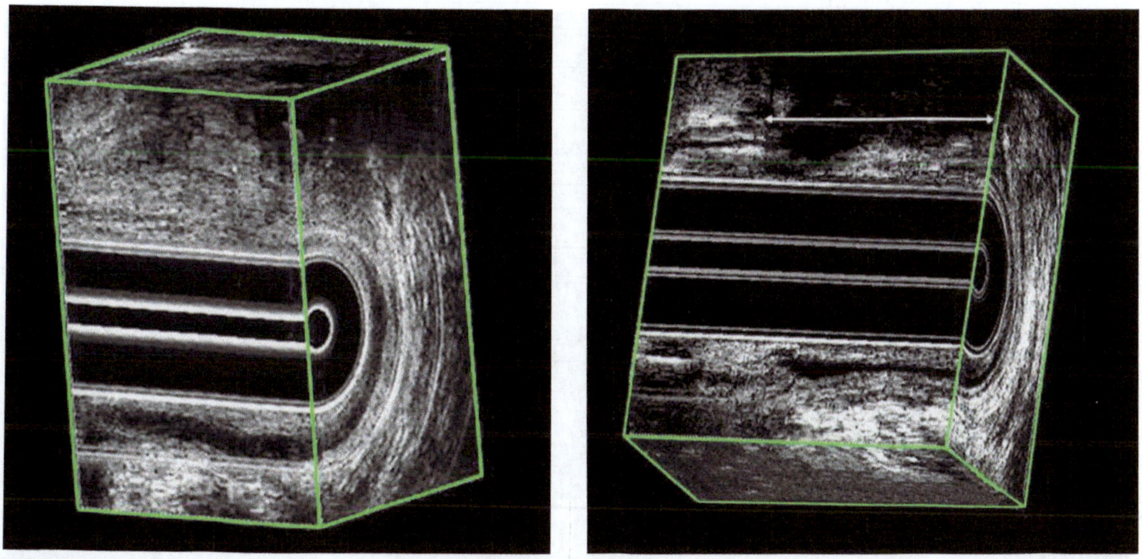

b

Fig. IV.17. Large internal sphincter defect in the anterior part of the anal canal (**a**). Three-dimensional sagittal view showing that this extends the full length of the internal sphincter, with a length of 29 mm (*arrow*) (**b**)

anal sphincter complex, and the relationship between the radial angle and longitudinal extent of a sphincter tear can be assessed [13] (Figs. IV.17–20). An additional advantage of 3-D reconstructions is the possibility of measuring the length of the remaining intact sphincter muscle. Christensen et al. [37] investigated the differences between 3-D and two-dimensional (2-D) EAUS in visualizing damage to the anal sphincter complex. The overall agreement between two observers was 98.2% using 3-D and 87.9% using 2-D. In our institution (unpublished data), we assessed the differences between 2-D and 3-D EAUS in defining the longitudinal extent of a sphincter defect in 33 patients with fecal incontinence due to obstetrical injury. The longitudinal extent of an EAS tear was graded as either proximal, central, or distal only, or a combination of two levels or full-length involvement. Two-dimensional EAUS localized the defect in the mid anal canal in most patients (94%), and in two patients, the defect was localized in the upper plus mid or mid plus distal anal canal, respectively. After 3-D reconstruction, the defects were localized the upper plus mid anal canal in four patients (12%), in the mid anal canal only in 22

a

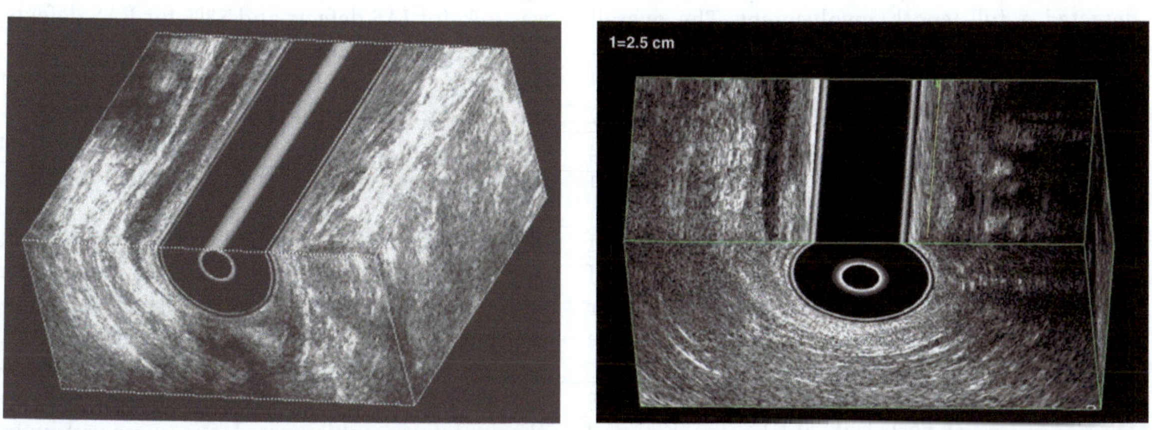

b

Fig. IV.18. Large internal sphincter defect in the left side of the anal canal (**a**). Three-dimensional coronal view showing that this extends the full length of the internal sphincter, with a length of 25 mm (**b**)

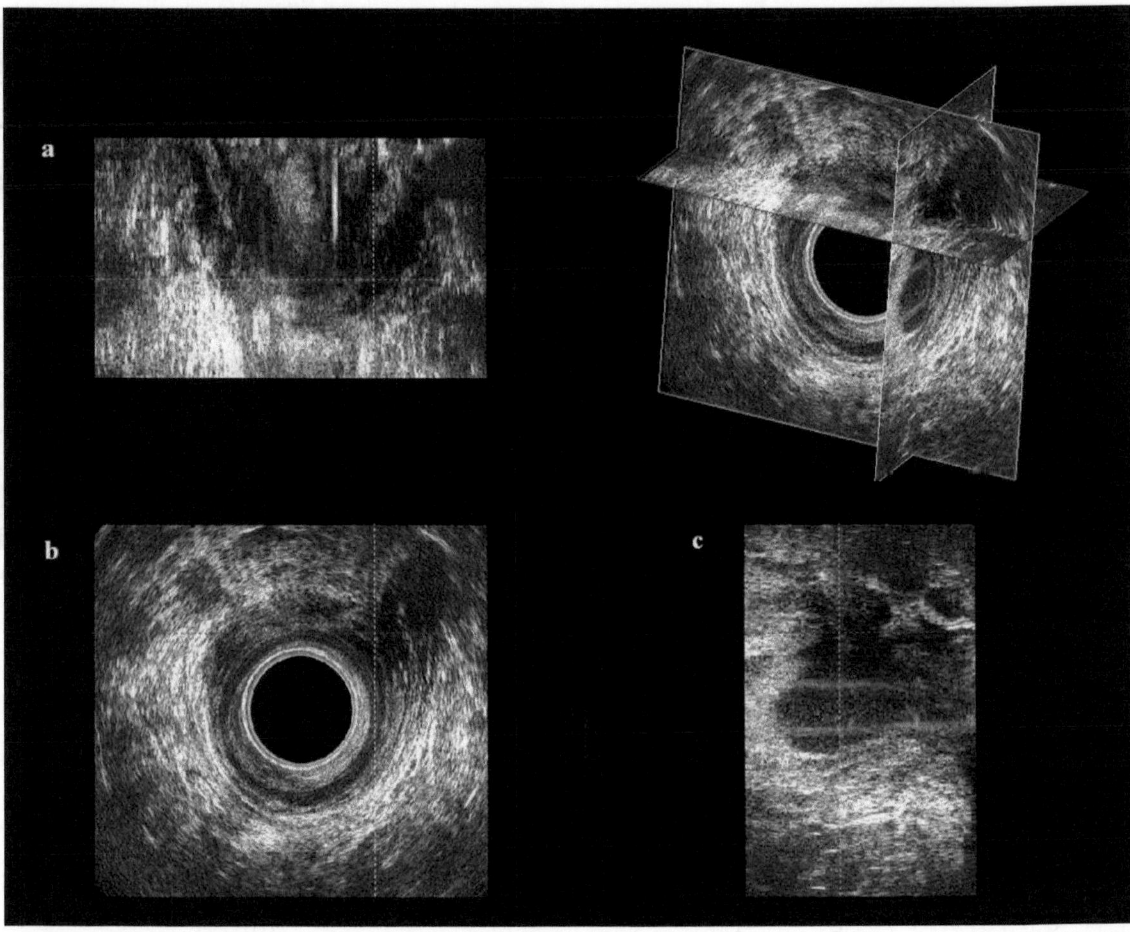

Fig. IV.19. Obstetric trauma with a well-defined defect of the external sphincter at 2 o'clock. Multiview reconstruction showing the defect in the coronal (**a**), axial (**b**), and sagittal (**c**) planes

patients (67%), and in the mid plus distal anal canal in six patients (18%). In one patient (3%), it detected a full-length involvement. The overall agreement between 2-D and 3-D EAUS was moderate (k=0.25) for EAS tears in the upper plus mid anal canal, good (k=0.71) for mid anal canal only lesions, and poor (k=0.14) for defects extending to the mid plus distal anal canal or for full-length involvement. Three-dimensional EAUS allows a better evaluation of the longitudinal extent of EAS defects and may improve the selection of patients for surgical repair of the anal sphincter complex, helping the surgeon to judge how far the repair should extend.

West et al. [38] examined whether 3-D EAUS measurements (EAS length, thickness, area, and volume) can be used to detect EAS atrophy and compared the results with MRI measurements. Agreement between 3-D EAUS and endoanal MRI was 61% for IAS defects and 88% for EAS defects. However, correlation was poor for EAS atrophy, suggesting that 3-D EAUS measurements are not suitable parameters for assessing EAS atrophy.

EAUS is the anorectal physiology study most likely to change a patient's management plan. Liberman et al. [20] reported that EAUS detected anal sphincter defects in five (11%) of 45 patients within the medical group of fecal incontinence who changed from medical to surgical management. In the surgical management group, 7% of patients changed from surgical to medical therapy because of normal EAUS findings, and 2% changed from sphincteroplasty to neosphincter surgery.

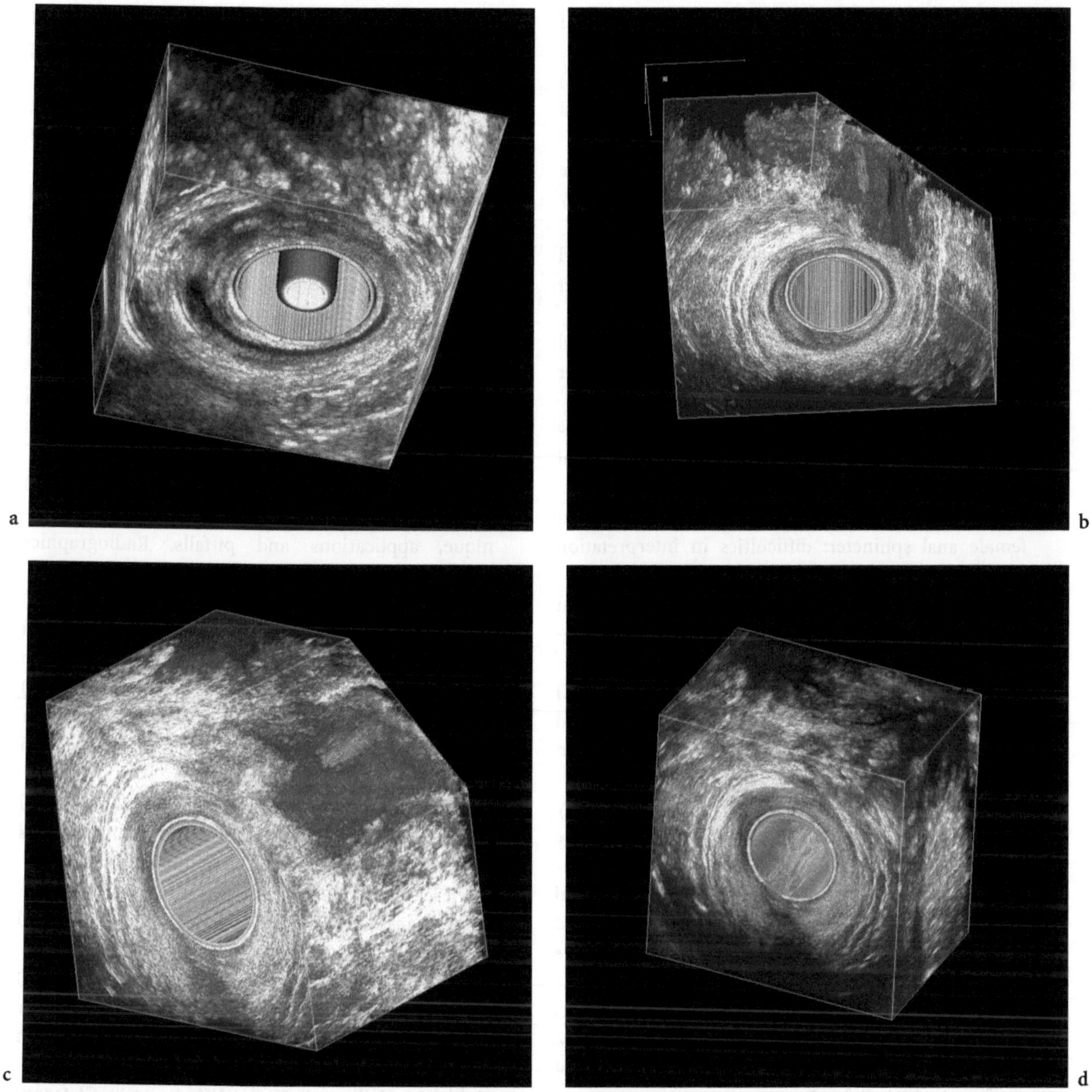

Fig. IV.20. Three-dimensional images with volume render mode showing the extent of a sphincter tear in different planes (**a–d**)

References

1. Stoker J, Halligan S, Bartram CI (2001) Pelvic floor imaging. Radiology 218:621–641
2. Bartram CI (2003) Ultrasound. In: Bartram CI, DeLancy JOL. Imaging pelvic floor disorders. Springer, Berlin Heidelberg New York
3. Burnett SJD, Bartram CI (1991) Endosonographic variations in the normal internal anal sphincter. Int J Colorect Dis 6:2
4. Williams AB, Bartram CI, Halligan S et al (2001) Multiplanar anal endosonography – normal anal canal anatomy. Colorectal Dis 3:169–174
5. Frudinger A, Halligan S, Bartram CI et al (2002) Female anal sphincter: age-related differences in asymptomatic volunteers with high-frequency endoanal US. Radiology 224:417–423
6. Williams AB, Cheetham MJ, Bartram CI et al (2000) Gender differences in the longitudinal pressure profile of the anal canal related to anatomical structure as demonstrated on three-dimensional anal endosonography. Br J Surg 87:1674–1679
7. Nielsen MB, Hauge C, Rasmussen OO et al (1992) Anal sphincter size measured by endosonography in healthy volunteers. Effect of age, sex and parity. Acta Radiol 33:453–456

8. Kumar A, Scholefield JH (2000) Endosonography of the anal canal and rectum. World J Surg 24:208–215
9. Gold DM, Halligan S, Kmiot WA, Bartram CI (1999) Intraobserver and interobserver agreement in anal endosonography. Br J Surg 86:371–375
10. Enck P, Heyer T, Gantke B et al (1997) How reproducible are measures of the anal sphincter muscle diameter by endoanal ultrasound? Am J Gastroenterol 92:293–296
11. Thakar R, Sultan A (2004) Anal endosonography and its role in assessing the incontinent patient. Best Pract Res Clinic Obstet Gynaec 18:157–173
12. Sultan AH, Kamm MA, Talbot IC et al (1994) Anal endosonography for identifying external sphincter defects confirmed histologically. Br J Surg 81:463–465
13. Gold DM, Bartram CI, Halligan S et al (1999) Three-dimensional endoanal sonography in assessing anal canal injury. Br J Surg 86:365–370
14. Bollard RC, Gardiner A, Lindow S et al (2002) Normal female anal sphincter: difficulties in interpretation explained. Dis Colon Rectum 45:171–175
15. Rociu E, Stoker J, Eijkemans MJC et al (1999) Fecal incontinence: endoanal US versus endoanal MR imaging. Radiology 212:453–458
16. Felt-Bersma RJ, van Baren R, Koorevaar M et al (1995) Unsuspected sphincter defects shown by anal endosonography after anorectal surgery. Dis Colon Rectum 38:249–253
17. Vaizey CJ, Kamm MA, Bartram CI (1997) Primary degeneration of the internal anal sphincter as a cause of passive faecal incontinence. Lancet 349:612–615
18. Felt-Bersma RJ, Cuesta MA, Koorevaar M (1996) Anal sphincter repair improves anorectal function and endosonographic image: a prospective study. Dis Colon Rectum 39:878–885
19. Voyvodic F, Rieger NA, Skinner S et al (2003) Endosonographic imaging of anal sphincter injury. Does the size of the tear correlate with the degree of dysfunction? Dis Colon Rectum 46:735–741
20. Liberman H, Faria J, Ternent CA et al (2001) A prospective evaluation of the value of anorectal physiology in the management of fecal incontinence. Dis Colon Rectum 44:1567–1574
21. Gantke B, Schafer A, Enck P, Lubke H (1993) Sonographic, manometric and myographic evaluation of the anal sphincters morphology and function. Dis Colon Rectum 36:1037–1041
22. Bennett RC, Friedman MHW, Goligher JC (1963) Late results of haemorrhoidectomy by ligature and excision. BMJ 2:216–219
23. Speakman CT, Burnett SJ, Kamm MA, Bartram CI (1991) Sphincter injury after anal dilatation demonstrated by anal endosonography. Br J Surg 78:1429–1430
24. Khubchandani IT, Reed JF (1989) Sequelae of internal sphincterotomy for chronic fissure in ano. Br J Surg 76:431–434
25. Kennedy HL, Zegarra JP (1990) Fistulotomy without external sphincter division for high anal fistula. Br J Surg 77:898–901
26. Farouk R, Bartolo DCC (1994) The use of endoluminal ultrasound in the assessment of patients with fecal incontinence. J R Coll Surg Edinb 39:312–318
27. Burnett SJ, Spence-Jones C, Speakman CT et al (1991) Unsuspected sphincter damage following childbirth revealed by anal endosonography. Br J Radiol 64:225–227
28. Nielsen MB, Rasmussen OO, Pedersen JF, Christiansen J (1993) Anal endosonographic findings in patients with obstructed defecation. Acta Radiol 34:35–38
29. Stoker J, Rociu E, Zwamborn AW et al (1999) Endoluminal MR imaging of the rectum and anus: technique, applications and pitfalls. Radiographics 19:383–398
30. Williams AB, Bartram CI, Modhwadia D et al (2001) Endocoil magnetic resonance imaging quantifictaion of external anal sphincter atrophy. Br J Surg 88:853–859
31. Nielsen MB, Dammegaard L, Pedersen JF (1994) Endosonographic assessment of the anal sphincter after surgical reconstruction. Dis Colon Rectum 37:434–438
32. Savoye-Collet C, Savoye G, Koning E et al (1999) Anal endosonography after sphincter repair: specific patterns related to clinical outcome. Abdom Imaging 24:569–573
33. Deen KI, Kumar D, Williams JG (1993) Anal sphincter defects: correlation between endoanal ultrasound and surgery. Ann Surg 218:201–205
34. Sentovich SM, Wong WD, Blatchford GJ (1998) Accuracy and reliability of transanal ultrasound for anterior anal sphincter injury. Dis Colon Rectum 41:1000–1004
35. Gold DM, Halligan S, Kmiot WA, Bartram CI (1999) Intraobserver and interobserver agreement in anal endosonography. Br J Surg 86:371–375
36. Abramowitz L, Sobhani I, Ganansia R et al (2000) Are sphincter defects the cause of anal incontinence after vaginal delivery? Results of a prospective study. Dis Colon Rectum 43:590–598
37. Christensen AF, Nyhuus B, Nielsen MB, Christensen H (2005) Three-dimensional anal endosonography may improve diagnostic confidence of detecting damage to the anal sphincter complex. Br J Rad 78:308–311
38. West RL, Dwarkasing S, Briel JW et al (2005) Can three-dimensional endoanal ultrasonography detect external anal sphincter atrophy? A comparison with endoanal magnetic resonance imaging. Int J Colorectal Dis 20:328–333

IV.3. Update in Perineal Anatomy and its Relevance to Obstetric Trauma

G.A. Santoro, L. Pellegrini, G. Di Falco

The prevalence of anal incontinence in women is strongly associated with obstetric history [1–5]. However, the mechanisms by which obstetrical events induce anal incontinence remain controversial [6–10]. The etiology of fecal incontinence has largely been attributed to damage to the innervation of the anal sphincter musculature sustained during vaginal childbirth, and Snooks et al. [11] could demonstrate the existence of pudendal nerve injury in 60% of patients with anal incontinence due to obstetric tearing. Sultan et al. [5] found that although pudendal nerve terminal motor latency (PNTML) was significantly prolonged after vaginal delivery, it was not associated with the defecatory symptoms, and Lee et al. [10] reported that pathologic postpartum PNTML recovers to the predelivery level within 2 months.

With the introduction of endoanal ultrasonography (EAUS), the role of anal sphincter disruption emerged, and the effect of pudendal nerve injury during vaginal delivery became less important [5, 6, 12–20]. Anal sphincter lacerations should be considered the main cause of fecal incontinence in women after vaginal delivery [5, 6, 12–20] and are strongly associated with primiparity, macrosomia, abnormal presentation, prolonged second-stage labor, and operative vaginal delivery [1, 2, 6–8, 21, 22]. Prospective studies [5, 6] before and after childbirth have also shown that up to one third of women sustain a sphincter defect that is not recognized after delivery but will be the primary cause of anal incontinence in later life. This late-onset incontinence is due to the compensation of pelvic floor muscles in younger women. With aging and weakening of these adjuvant pelvic supports, however, these defects become clinically evident [10, 22–24].

This chapter focuses on the mechanism of delivery and its relevance to pelvic floor injuries. We also review the role of EAUS in the assessment of anal sphincter injuries following obstetric trauma.

Mechanism of Delivery and its Relevance to Pelvic Floor Injuries

The natural process of childbirth carries inherent risks to the perineum. However, the precise mechanisms of anal sphincter injury during deliveries have still to be elucidated [6–10]. Labor is divided into three stages: (1) first stage – start to full dilatation of the cervix, (2) second stage – full dilatation to birth of baby, and (3) third stage – birth of baby to delivery of placenta. The fetus is descending during first and second stages of labor. The birth canal is formed by dilatation of the cervix and vagina and by stretching and displacement of the muscles of the pelvic floor and perineum. The bladder is pulled above the pubis because of its attachment to the uterus; the urethra is stretched and the bowel is compressed. By the end of the second stage, the birth canal has been fully formed (Fig. IV.21). Descent continues, and the occiput reaches the pelvic floor (Fig. IV.22). The occiput rotates to the front (internal rotation) and the head become occipitoanterior (Fig. IV.23). This process of pushing the head through the vaginal introitus results in downward descent of the pelvic floor, and most of the uterine pressure is direct toward the perineal body and

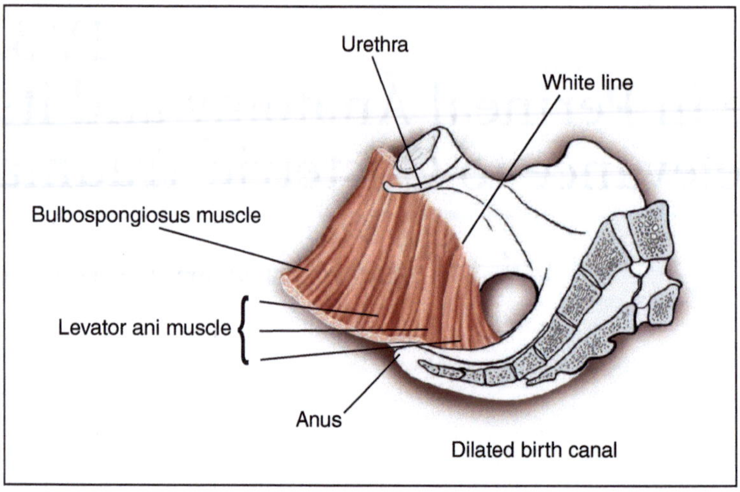

a

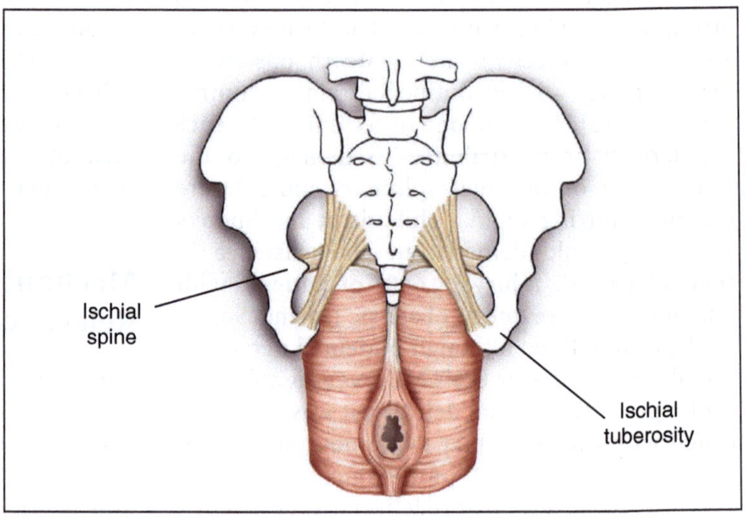

b

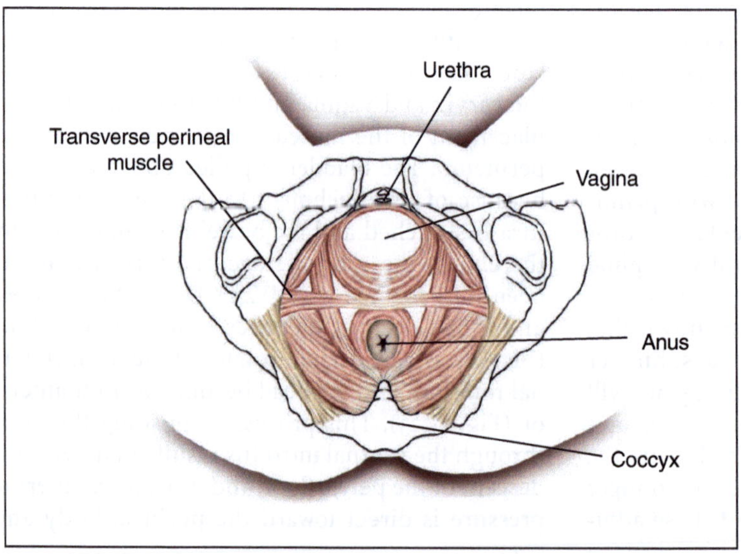

c

Fig. IV.21. Schematic representation of the birth canal at the end of the second stage of labor (**a**). Canal from the outside (**b**), and from hereback (**c**)

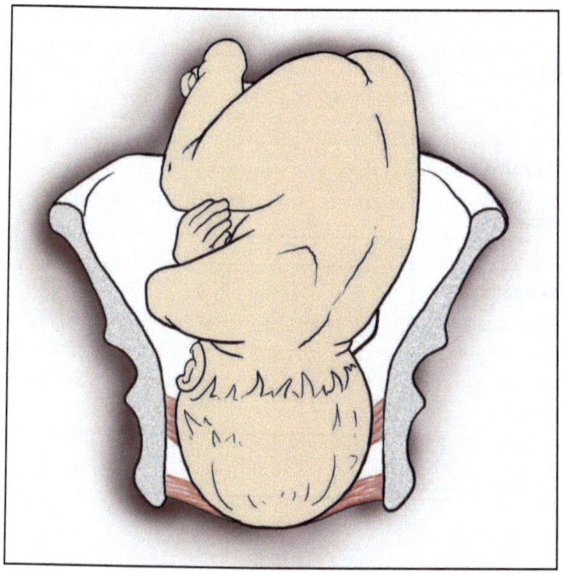

Fig. IV.22. Schematic representation showing mechanism of labor in left occipitoanterior position: the occiput reaches the pelvic floor

anorectum (Fig. IV.24). During the second stage of labor, the structures of pelvic floor are at highest risk of injury. Further descent of the fetus pushes the head forward with a movement of extension, and the occiput is delivered. Increasing extension round the pubis delivers the bregma, brow, and face (Fig. IV.24). Descent and delivery of the head has brought the shoulders into the pelvic cavity. The head on delivery is oblique to the line of the shoulders and rotates to the natural position relative to the shoulders with a movement known as "restitution" (Fig. IV.25a, b). Descent continues, and the shoulders rotate to bring the bisacromial diameter into the anteroposterior diameter of the pelvic outlet. This descent and rotation causes the head to rotate so that the occiput lies next to the left maternal thigh (external rotation) (Fig. IV.25c). The anterior shoulder now slips

a

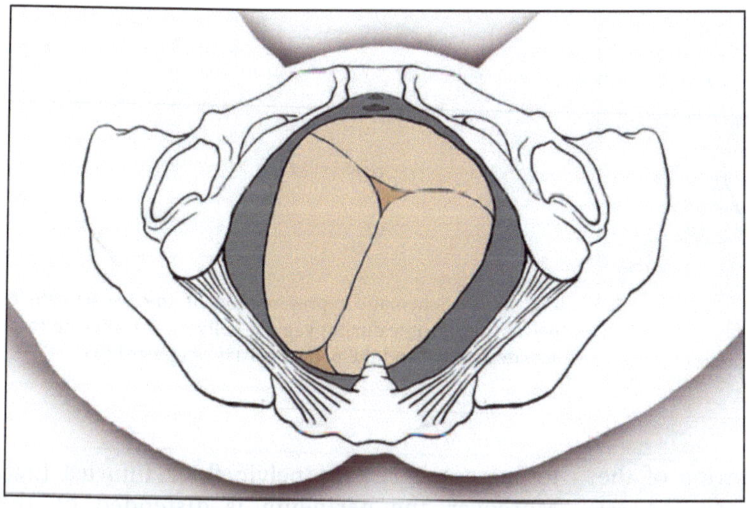

b

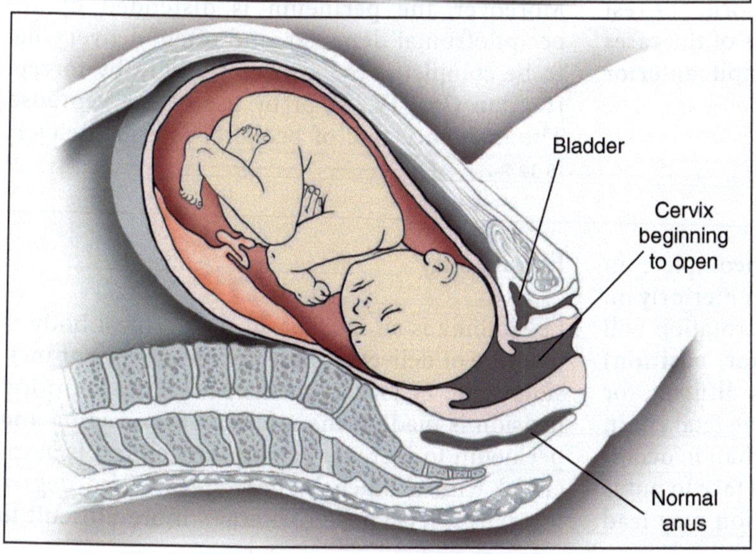

Fig. IV.23. Schematic representation showing mechanism of labor in left occipitoanterior position: descent and flexion (**a**); internal rotation (**b**)

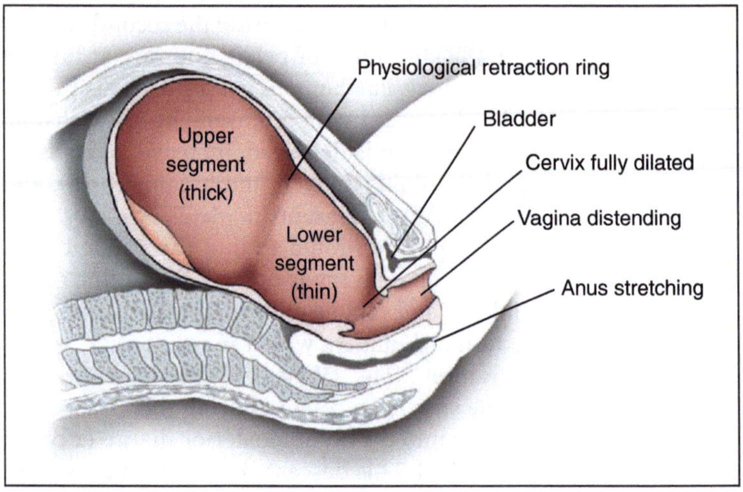

a

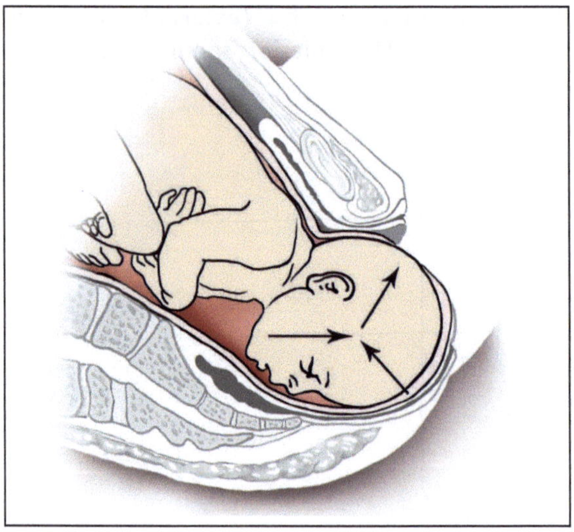
b

Fig. IV.24. Schematic representation of the mechanism of pelvic floor injury during vaginal delivery (**a**). Uterine force acts downward and the pelvic resistance upward (**b**)

under the pubis, and with lateral flexion of the fetal body, the posterior shoulder is born. The rest of the body follows easily. Two thirds of the cases will deliver spontaneously as occipitoanterior (Fig. IV.26).

Abnormal Presentation

If flexion of the head remains incomplete in descent, then rotation of the occiput anteriorly on the pelvic floor may not occur, and rotation will occur posteriorly (occipitoposterior position) (Fig. IV.27). The mechanism now is difficult, for flexion of the head is restricted by the fetal chest. The soft tissues are stretched more than in occipitoanterior, and the fetus is delivered face to pubis (Fig. IV.28). Occipitoposterior position may lead to increased risk of pelvic floor injuries [22]. Moreover, the perineum is distended by the occipitofrontal diameter, and often, delivery has to be completed by large episiotomy, by forceps rotation (Fig. IV.29), or by use of the ventouse. The incidence rate of occipitoposterior delivery is 12%.

Episiotomy

Episiotomy is an incision in the perineal body at the time of delivery. There are three types of incisions (Fig. IV.30): (1) median – a linear surgical incision is made is the midline of the vagina and perineum to increase vaginal capacity; it is associated with a much higher rate of third-degree injury [2, 7], (2) posterolateral – more difficult to

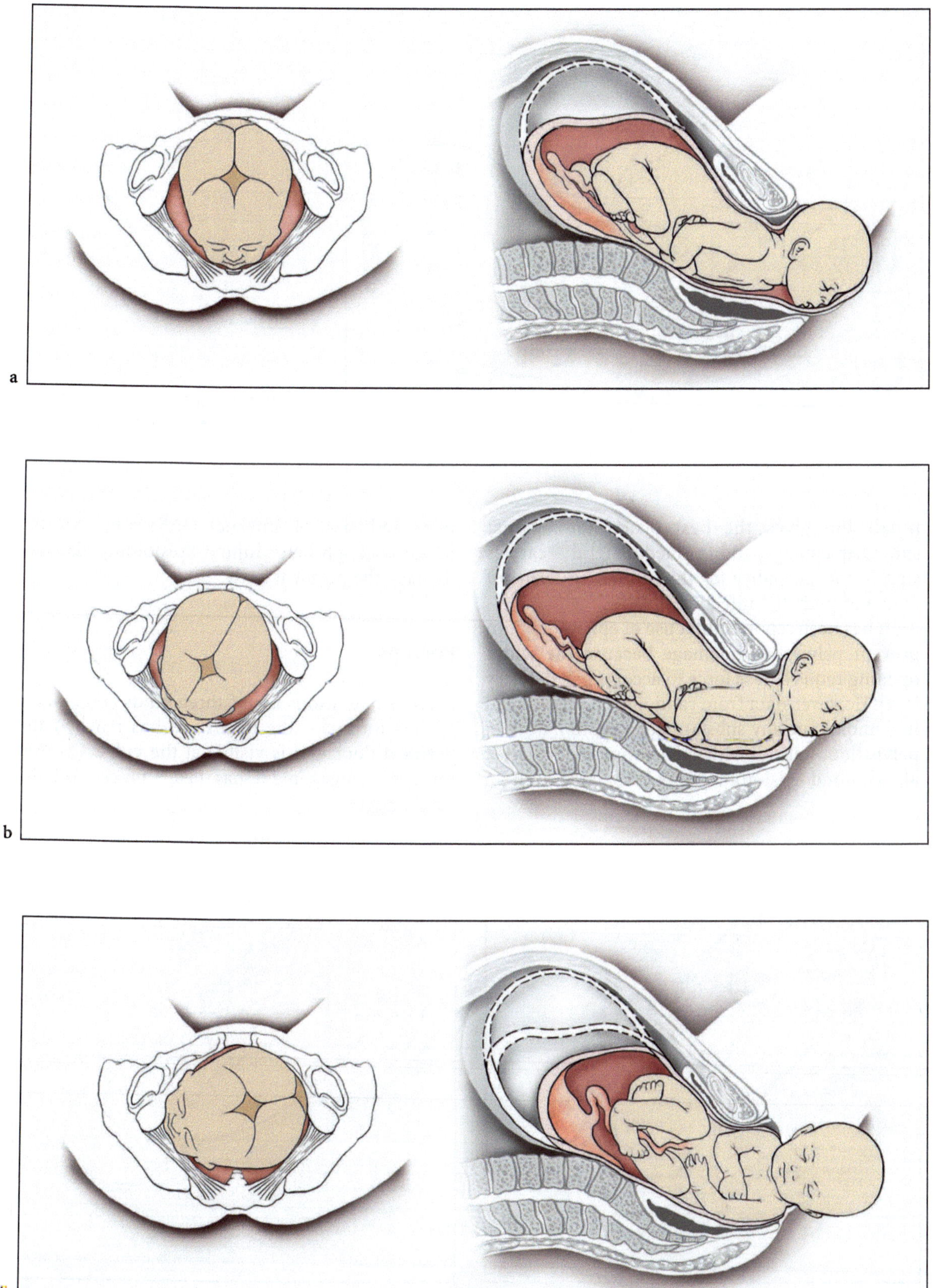

Fig. IV.25. Schematic representation showing mechanism of labor in left occipitoanterior position: delivery of head (**a**); restitution (**b**); external rotation (**c**)

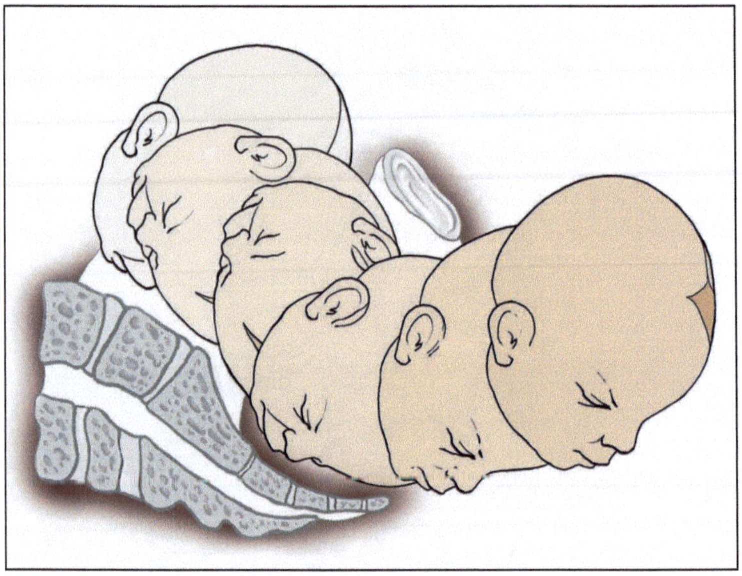

Fig. IV.26. Normal mechanism of labor in left occipitoanterior position from beginning to end

repair but gives the best protection against sphincter damage, and (3) mediolateral – carries significant morbidity for the mother in terms of pain and potential infection.

It has been reported that use of episiotomy can prevent pelvic floor damage because the wider opening requires less force to accomplish delivery [1, 2]. However, data from randomized trials failed to demonstrate any substantial protection against pelvic floor injuries with episiotomy, and Sultan et al. [5] found episiotomy to be associated with an increased risk of internal (IAS) and external (EAS) anal sphincter injury. Episiotomy also can damage the perineal body.

Forceps

Forceps operations are of three kinds (Fig. IV.31): (1) low forceps – the fetal head has reached the perineal floor and is visible at the vulva, (2) mid forceps – engagement has taken place, and the

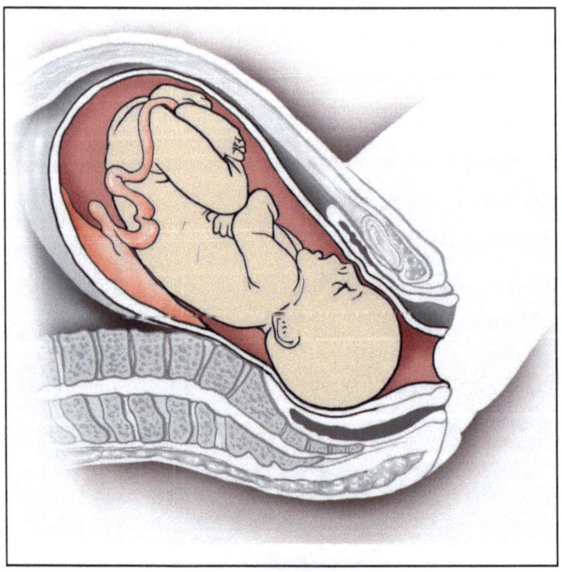

Fig. IV.27. Schematic representation showing mechanism of labor in occipitoposterior position

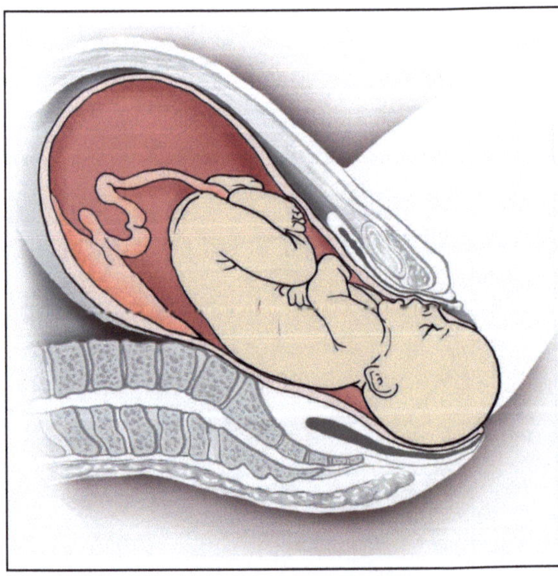

Fig. IV.28. During delivery in occipitoposterior position, the pelvic floor structures are stretched more than in occipitoanterior position

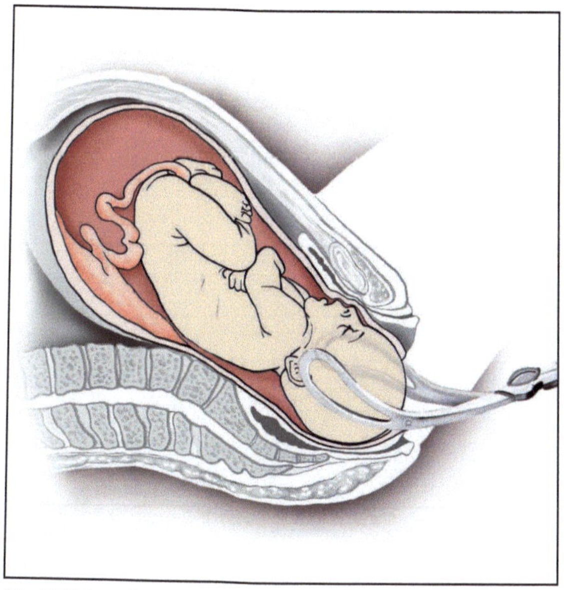

Fig. IV.29. Delivery in occipitoposterior position often has to be completed by forcepst

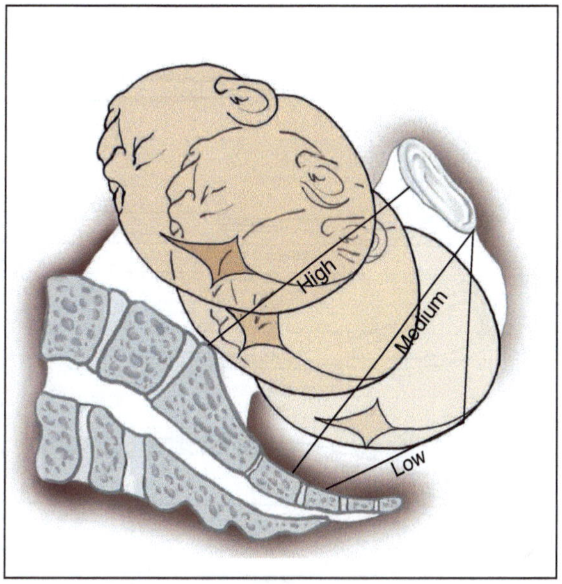

Fig. IV.31. Different forceps applications

leading part of the head is below the level of the ischial spines, and (3) high forceps – application of the forceps when the head is not engaged. There are many different patterns of forceps, and they are identified with three main operations (Fig. IV.32). Donnelly et al. [6] reported that use of forceps was associated with an eight-fold increase in risk of anal sphincter injury.

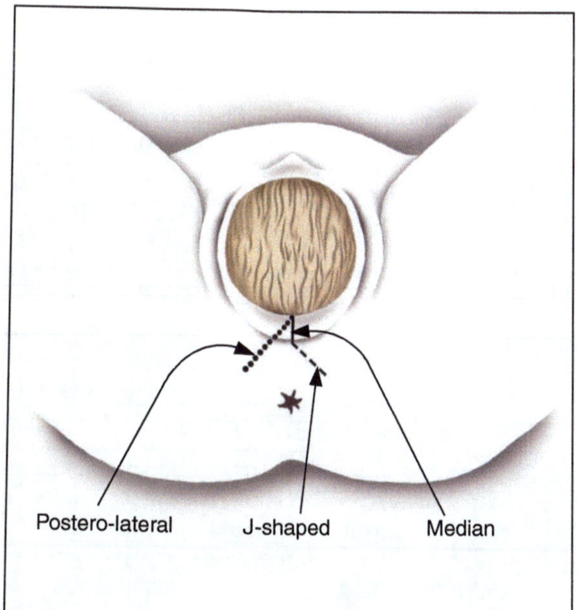

Fig. IV.30. Episiotomy incisions

Perineal Tears

These are more common in primigravid patients where the perineum is more rigid. The most important factors are the width of the pubic arch and the size and position of the fetal head. All malpresentations increase the amount of perineal distension. Perineal tears are classified in four degrees (Fig. IV.33): (1) first degree – vaginal mucosa and perineal skin, (2) second degree – extending into the perineal muscles, (3) third degree – involving the IAS and EAS sphincters, and (4) fourth degree – extending into the rectal mucosa. The most significant risk factor for third-degree perineal injury is the first vaginal delivery [6].

Primiparity

The most important risk factor for mechanical injury to the anal sphincters and to the pelvic floor muscles is first vaginal delivery. In contrast, pudendal nerve injury is more common with successive vaginal deliveries. A meta-analysis of the literature [21] estimated a 27% incidence of sphincter defects in primiparous women, an 8% incidence of new sphincter defects in multiparous women, and a 30% incidence of symptomatic defects postpartum. The probability of fecal incontinence due to a sphincter defect is 77–83%.

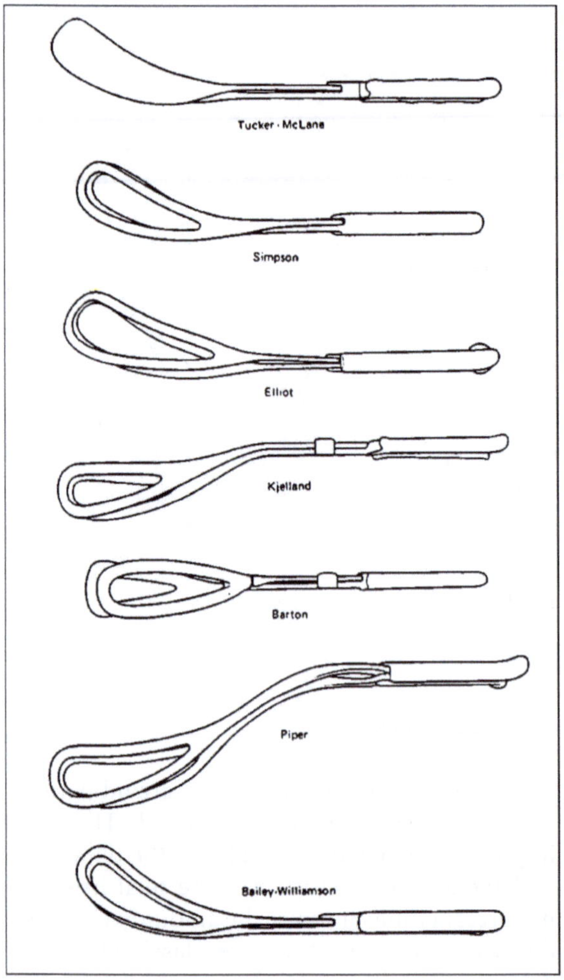

a

Fig. IV.32. Different patterns of forceps (**a**). Exposition of old forceps at Science Museum in London (**b**)

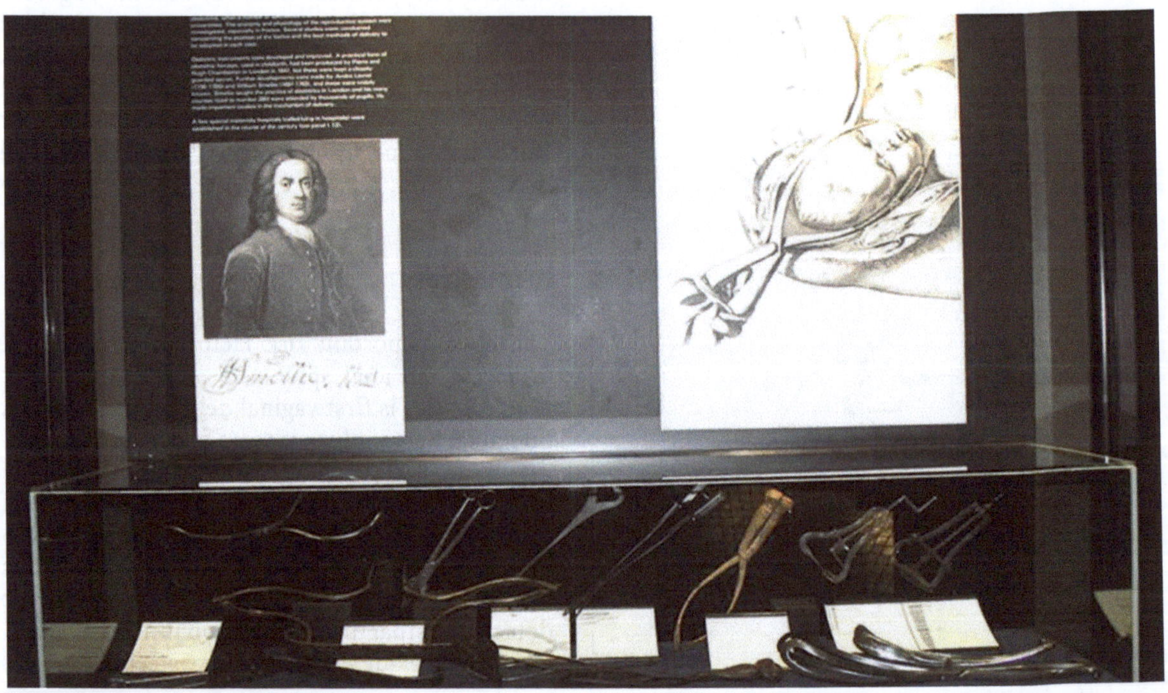

b

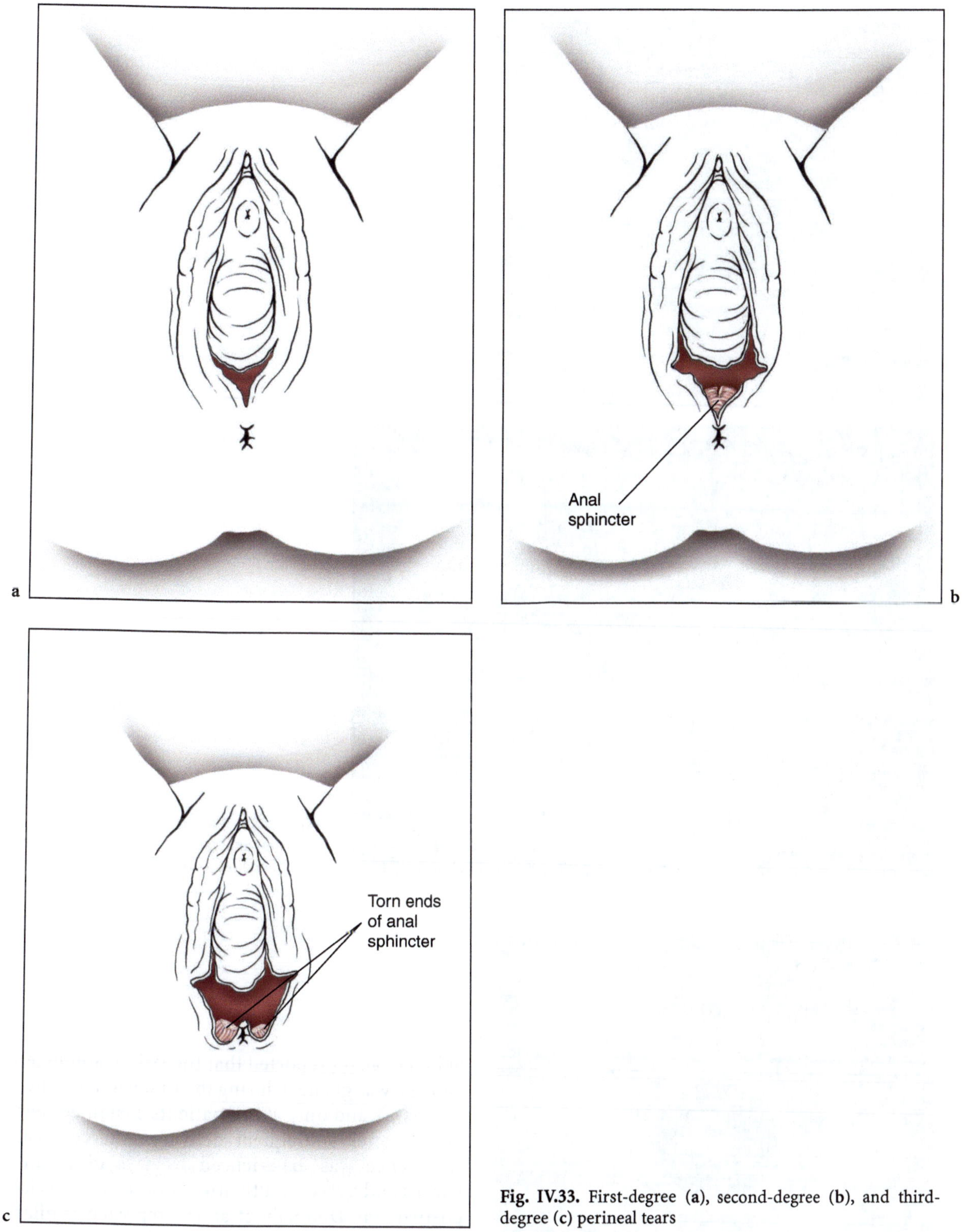

Fig. IV.33. First-degree (a), second-degree (b), and third-degree (c) perineal tears

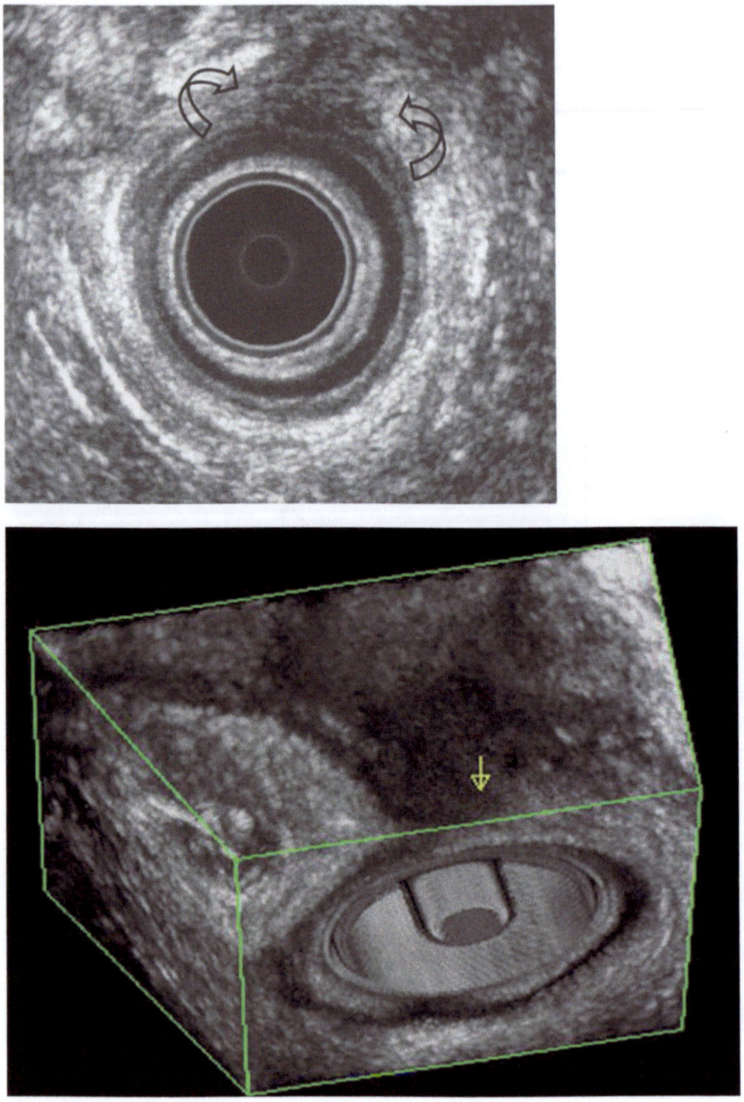

a

b

Fig. IV.34. Postpartum defect of the external anal sphincter (*open arrows*): axial plane (**a**), coronal plane (**b**)

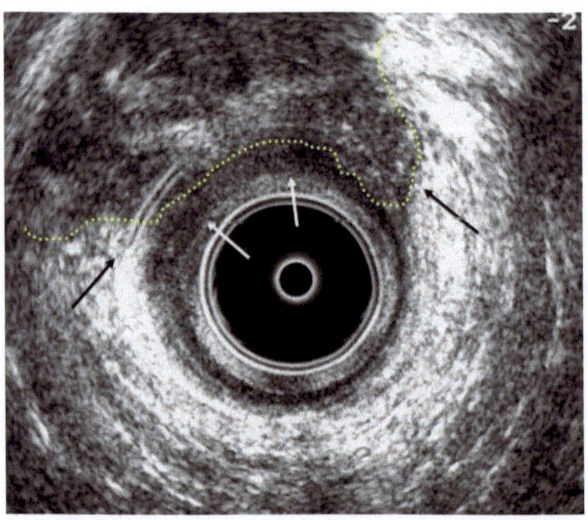

Fig. IV.35. Postpartum defect of the internal (*white arrows*) and external anal sphincters (*black arrows*), with presence of a hypoechoic area of scarring (*dots*)

Sultan et al. [5] reported that the risk of sphincter damage was greatest during the first vaginal delivery (25%), and only 4% of patients sustained new defects after subsequent delivery. Altered fecal continence was experienced by 13% of primiparous and 23% of multiparous women at 6 weeks postpartum. Donnelly et al. [6] reported similar results, with 25% of altered fecal continence 6 weeks following first vaginal delivery. In the same study, instrumental delivery and a second stage of labor prolonged beyond 60 min were associated with an 8.1-fold and 1.7-fold risk of anal sphincter

a

c

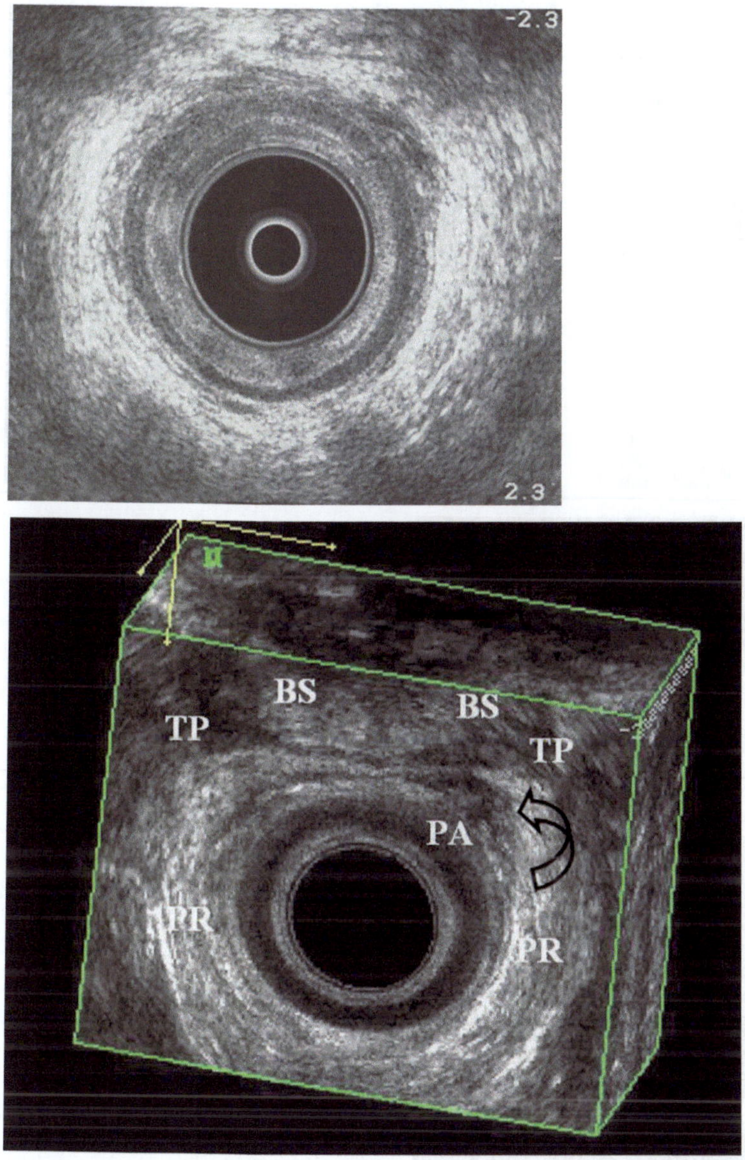

Fig. IV.36. Tear of the left puboanalis (*arrows*) (*PA*) as a scar in the medial aspect of the puborectalis (*PR*): axial plane (**a**), three-dimensional reconstruction (**b**). *TP*: transverse perineii, *BS*: bulbospongiosus muscle

injury, respectively. Handa et al. [7] also identified primiparity as the dominant risk factor of injury during childbirth. Birth weight over 4,000 g was also highly significant. Operative delivery increased the risk of sphincter laceration, with vacuum delivery presenting a greater risk than forceps delivery. Episiotomy decreased the likelihood of third-degree lacerations but increased the risk of fourth-degree lacerations. In a recent report, Abramowitz et al. [14] found that primiparae and secundiparae have the same risk factors for sphincter disruption and anal incontinence.

Endosonographic Assessment

The main indication for EAUS in patients with fecal incontinence is to detect anal sphincter defects and damage to the pelvic floor muscles (Figs. IV.34–38). There is wide variation in the incidence of clinically occult anal sphincter injuries diagnosed by ultrasonography (11–35%) after the first vaginal delivery [7, 8, 10–19]. Donnelly et al. [6] found anal sphincter injury in 35% of primiparous vaginal deliveries using EAUS. Sultan et al. [5] reviewed EAUS findings on

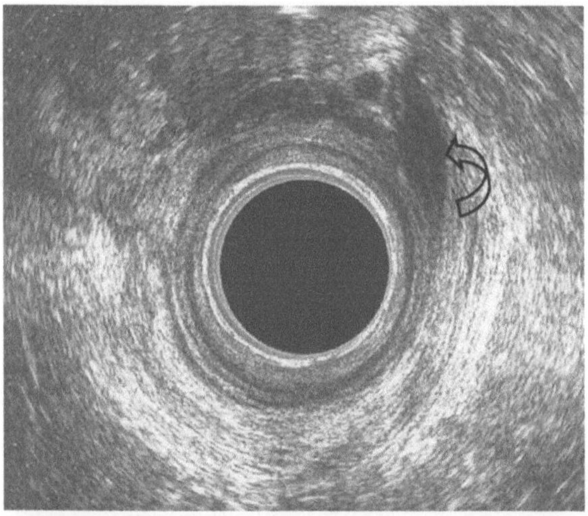
a

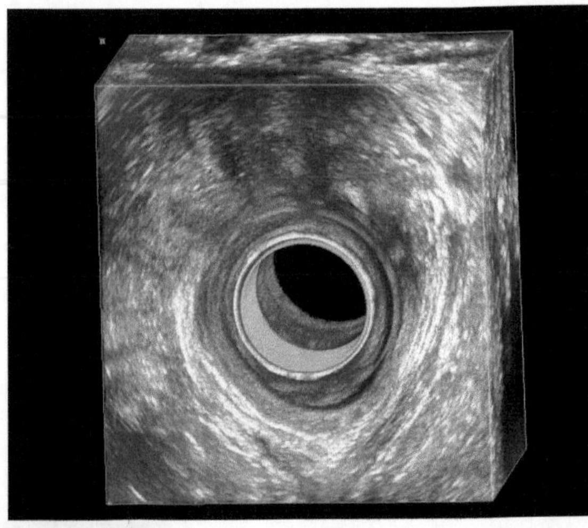
b

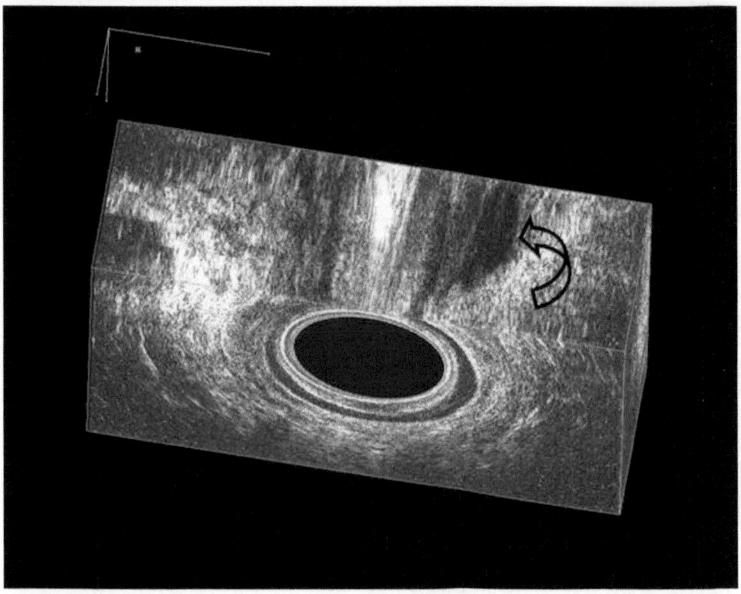
c

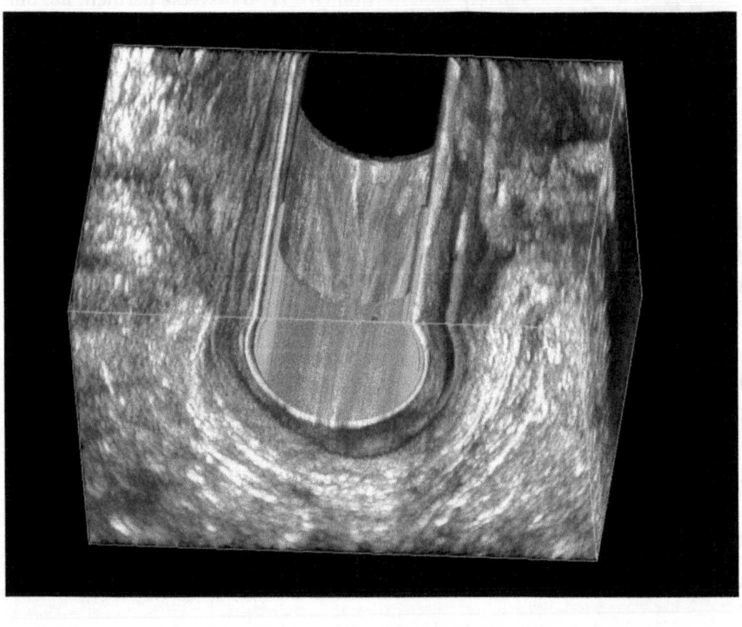
d

Fig. IV.37. Tear of the left puboanalis (*open arrows*) in the axial (**a, b**) and coronal (**c**) planes. Volume render mode (**d**)

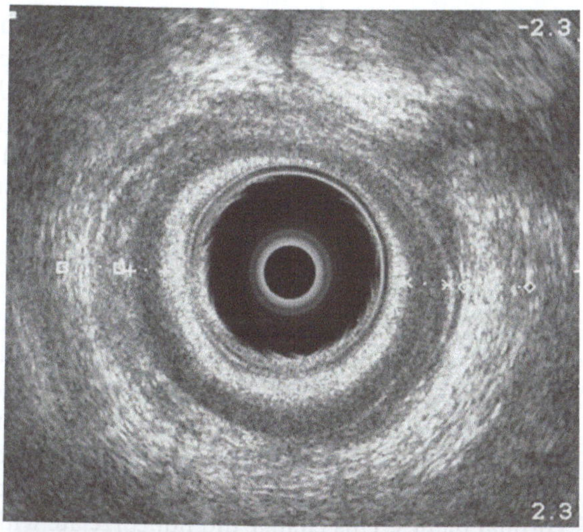

a

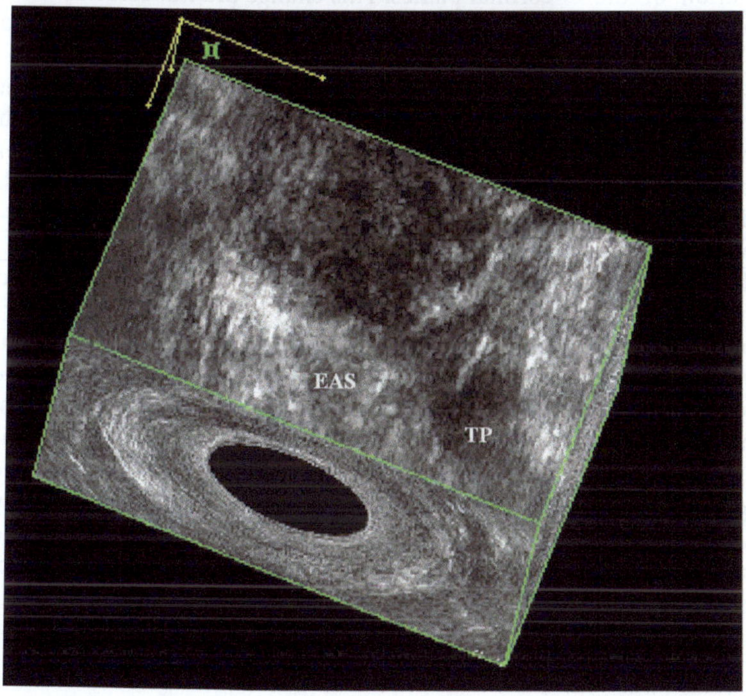

b

Fig. IV.38. Three-dimensional reconstruction in the axial (**a**) anal coronal (**b**) planes showing a tear of the left transverse perineii (*TP*) as a scar lateral to the external sphincter ring (*EAS*)

79 primiparous women before and after vaginal delivery and identified anal sphincter defects in 28 (35%), of whom nine (32%) reported altered fecal continence. Sphincter defects were not identified in those women delivered by caesarean section. Deen et al. [13] studied 46 patients with postpartum fecal incontinence symptoms and found that 87% had a recognizable anal sphincter defect on EAUS. In a prospective study, de Parades et al. [8] did not confirm previous observations that anal sphincter injury is common after forceps delivery. In a large population of 93 healthy women, anal sphincter injury was identified by ultrasonography in <13% of cases after forceps delivery, and the development of anal incontinence was not related to these defects. The only factor with significant predictive value for anal sphincter injury was perineal tear. Pinta et al. [22] analyzed possible risks factors associated with sphincter rupture during vaginal delivery. A total of 52 women with a third- or fourth-degree perineal laceration were compared with 51 primiparous women with no clinically detectable perineal laceration. EAUS found a persistent defect of

the EAS in 39 women (75%) in the rupture group compared with ten women (20%) in the control group (p<0.001). An abnormal presentation was the only risk factor for anal sphincter rupture during vaginal delivery.

Fecal incontinence related to anal sphincter defects is likely to occur even in elderly women who experienced vaginal deliveries earlier in life [15, 19]. Oberwalder et al. [23] reported that 71% of women with late-onset fecal incontinence had occult sphincter defects on EAUS results. The onset of fecal incontinence was at a median age of 61.5 years.

Obstetric trauma can be associated with damage/defects primarily to the distal part of the rectovaginal septum, as well as elongation of the length of the septum. Fecal incontinence developing after vaginal delivery can also be caused by injury to the perineal body [25]. It is the central portion of the perineum where the external anal sphincter, the bulbospongiosus, and the transverse perineal muscles meet. The perineal body has multiple and diverse functions: it anchors the anorectum, anchors the vagina, provides a physical barrier between the vagina and rectum, and maintains urinary and fecal continence.

The routine measurement of perineal body thickness (PBT) during EAUS may be valuable. Zetterstrom et al. [26] reported that 93% of incontinent women with obstetric trauma to the anal sphincter had a PBT of 10 mm or less. This result was confirmed by Fornell et al. [24] who found that PBT <10 mm was associated with incontinence for flatus and liquid stools and lower anal squeeze pressures, and also by Oberwalder et al. [27] who found that a sonographically thin (< 10 mm) perineal body was associated with anal sphincter defects in 97% of patients with fecal incontinence, a PBT of 10–12 mm was associated with sphincter defect in 36% of cases, and a PBT of 12 mm was associated with a defect in 23% of cases.

Benefits of three-dimensional (3-D) EAUS in the evaluation of fecal incontinence have been reported [15–17, 28]. Williams et al. [15] assessed changes to anal canal morphology in the absence of sphincter trauma. After delivery, there was significant shortening of the length of the anterior portion of the EAS, which could be demonstrated only with 3-D reconstructions on sagittal and coronal planes. This change did not correlate with any functional symptoms. West et al. [28] found that incontinence in parous females was not associated with loss of sphincter volume. Williams et al. [16] reported that only 68% of women with third-degree tears had 3-D EAUS evidence of sphincter damage. In another study, Williams et al. [17] determined the incidence and functional consequences of anal sphincter damage using 3-D EAUS and anal manometry in 45 women who had vaginal delivery. They found evidence of postpartum trauma in 29% of cases, involving the external sphincter in 11% of patients, the puboanalis in 11% of cases, and the transverse perineii in 7% of cases. Damage to the EAS was associated with a significant decrease in squeeze pressure and an increase in incontinence score and represented the only functionally significant component. Tears to the puboanalis or transverse perineii did not affect pressure or incontinence score.

References

1. Varma A, Gunn J, Gardiner A et al (1999) Obstetric anal sphincter injury: a prospective evaluation of incidence. Dis Colon Rectum 42:1253–1260
2. Zetterstrom JP, Mellgren A, Jensen LL et al (1999) Effect of delivery on anal sphincter morphology and function. Dis Colon Rectum 42:1253–1260
3. Nichols CM, Gill EJ, Nguyen T et al (2004) Anal sphincter injury in women with pelvic floor disorders. Obstet Gynecol 104:690–696
4. Snooks SJ, Setchell M, Swash M, Henry MM (1984) Injury to innervation of pelvic floor sphincter musculature in childbirth. Lancet 2:546–550
5. Sultan AH, Kamm MA, Hudson CN et al (1993) Anal sphincter disruption during vaginal delivery. N Engl J Med 329:1905–1911
6. Donnelly V, Fynes M, Campbell D et al (1998) Obstetric events leading to anal sphincter damage. Obstet Gynecol 92:955–961
7. Handa VL, Danielsen BH, Gilbert WM (2001) Obstetric anal sphincter lacerations. Obstet Gynecol 98:225–230
8. de Parades V, Etienney I, Thabut D et al (2004) Anal sphincter injury after forceps delivery: myth or reality? A prospective ultrasound study of 93 females. Dis Colon Rectum 47:24–34
9. Jorge JM, Wexner SD (1993) Etiology and management of fecal incontinence. Dis Colon Rectum 36:77–97

10. Lee SJ, Park JW (2000) Follow-up evaluation of the effect of vaginal delivery on the pelvic floor. Dis Colon Rectum 43:1550–1555
11. Snooks SJ, Swash M, Matthews SE, Henry MM (1990) Effect of vaginal delivery on the pelvic floor. A 5-year follow-up. Br J Surg 77:1358–1360
12. Martinez Hernandez Magro P, Villanueva Saenz E, Jaime Zavala M et al (2003) Endoanal sonography in assessment of fecal incontinence following obstetric trauma. Ultrasound Obstet Gynecol 22:616–621
13. Deen KJ, Kumar D, Williams JG et al (1993) The prevalence of anal sphincter defects in fecal incontinence. A prospective endosonic study. Gut 34:685–688
14. Abramowitz L, Sobhani I, Ganansia R et al (2000) Are sphincter defects the cause of anal incontinence after vaginal delivery? Results of a prospective study. Dis Colon Rectum 43:590–598
15. Williams AB, Bartram CI, Halligan S (2002) Alteration of anal sphincter morphology following vaginal delivery revealed by multiplanar anal endosonography. BJOG 109:942–946
16. Williams AB, Spencer JD, Bartram CI (2002) Assessment of third degree tears using three-dimensional anal endosonography with combined anal manometry: a novel technique. BJOG 109:833–835
17. Williams AB, Bartram CI, Halligan S et al (2001) Anal sphincter damage after vaginal delivery using three-dimensional anal endosonography. Obstet Gynecol 97:770–775
18. Thakar R, Sultan A (2004) Anal endosonography and its role in assessing the incontinent patient. Best Pract Res Clinic Obstet Gynaec 18:157–173
19. Sultan AH, Kamm MA, Talbot IC et al (1994) Anal endosonography for identifying external sphincter defects confirmed histologically. Br J Surg 81:463–465
20. Gold DM, Bartram CI, Halligan S et al (1999) Three-dimensional endoanal sonography in assessing anal canal injury. Br J Surg 86:365–370
21. Fitzpatrick M, Behan M, O'Connell PR, O'Herlihy C (2003) Randomized clinical trial to assess anal sphincter following forceps or vacuum assisted vaginal delivery. BJOG 110:424–429
22. Pinta TM, Kylanpaa ML, Salmi TK (2004) Primary sphincter repair: are the results of the operation good enough? Dis Colon Rectum 47:18–23
23. Oberwalder M, Dinnewitzer A, Baig MK et al (2004) The association between late-onset fecal incontinence and obstetric anal sphincter defects. Arch Surg 139:429–432
24. Fornell EU, Matthiensen L, Sjodahl R, Berg G (2005) Obstetric anal sphincter injury ten years after: subjective and objective long term effects. BJOG 112:312–316
25. Woodman PJ, Graney DO (2002) Anatomy and physiology of the female perineal body with relevance to obstetrical injury and repair. Clinical Anatomy 15:321–334
26. Zetterstrom JP, Mellgren A, Madoff RD et al (1998) Perineal body measurement improves evaluation of anterior sphincter lesions during endoanal ultrasonography. Dis Colon Rectum 41:705–713
27. Oberwalder M, Thaler K, Baig MK et al (2004) Anal ultrasound and endosonographic measurement of perineal body thickness. A new evaluation for fecal incontinence in females. Surg Endosc 18:650–654
28. West RL, Felt-Bersma RJF, Hansen BE et al (2005) Volume measurement of the anal sphincter complex in healthy controls and fecal-incontinent patients with a three-dimensional reconstruction of endoanal ultrasonography images. Dis Colon Rectum 48: 540–548

IV.4. Fecal Incontinence: Endoanal Ultrasonography and MR Imaging

M.P. Terra, J. Stoker

Introduction

To assess fecal incontinence, the physician can use different sources of information such as medical history, physical examination, a set of anorectal functional tests, and imaging techniques [1, 2]. Imaging techniques used in the diagnostic workup of patients with fecal incontinence comprise endoanal ultrasonography (EAUS), endoanal magnetic resonance (MR) imaging, external phased array MR imaging, and defecography. As this chapter focuses on demonstrating the anatomy and pathology of the anal sphincter complex, defecography will be left aside, as this technique is primarily performed in fecal incontinent patients to visualize an intussusception [3–5].

EAUS is the first imaging technique used for assessing anal sphincter pathology in patients with fecal incontinence. Before the introduction of this technique, fecal incontinence was primarily ascribed to neurogenic dysfunction, but EAUS elucidated that structural damage of the anal sphincter complex plays a crucial role in the development of fecal incontinence complaints [6–8]. EAUS is an endoluminal technique that yields images of high-contrast resolution [9]. Different layers of the anal sphincter complex can be discriminated because of tissue-dependent reflection. Some layers are low reflective (hyporeflective; darker) and other layers are high reflective (hyperreflective; brighter).

MR imaging in patients with fecal incontinence can be performed with an endoanal coil, which was introduced in the mid 1990s, or an external phased array coil [10–12]. Inherent to MR imaging are multiplanar capabilities and high contrast resolution images enabling accurate demonstration of the multilayer construction of the anal sphincter complex. Different structures can be distinguished by differences in signal intensity. Some structures produce low-intensity (hypointense) signals (e.g., external anal sphincter and other striated muscles) whereas other structures produce high-intensity (hyperintense) signals (e.g., internal anal sphincter; fat) at T2-weighted images. The use of an endoanal coil results in images of higher spatial resolution than when an external phased array coil is used although the field of view is limited. The latter is not a disadvantage in patients with fecal incontinence but might be a limitation for imaging of perianal fistulas, especially in patients with perianal Crohn's disease in which fistulas are often complex and can extend outside the field of view of endoluminal coils [13].

Techniques

Endoanal Ultrasonography

Endoanal ultrasonography is generally performed with a two-dimensional (2-D) ultrasound scanner with a 7 or 10 MHz rotating endoprobe covered by a water-filled hard sonolucent cone, providing a 360° axial view of the anal canal. No specific patient preparation is required before starting the examination. Patients can be examined in the following positions: left lateral, prone, or the lithotomy position. Performing the examination in the prone or lithotomy positions is preferable in women, as in the left lateral position, the structures at the anterior part of the anal sphincter complex are deformed, impairing accurate diagnosis. The endoprobe is covered with a condom lubricated and subsequently introduced into the anus to the level of the anorectal verge and slowly withdrawn. Images are obtained at the proximal, middle, and distal levels in the anal canal.

Besides 2-D EAUS, three-dimensional (3-D) EAUS is also available. The advantage of 3-D EAUS over 2-D EAUS is the possibility of multiplanar imaging of the anal canal, which enables demonstration of anal sphincter pathology along the length of the anal canal [14].

MR Imaging

MR imaging is generally performed at a 1.0 or 1.5 T MR unit with a dedicated endoanal coil or an external phased array coil. For MR imaging, a number of strategies can be used; here, general instructions are provided. Bowel preparation is not needed, but asking patients to fast 4 h prior the examination is necessary to reduce artifacts from bowel peristalsis. Further, asking patients to empty their bladder before starting the examination is also recommendable to prevent motion artifacts due to discomfort from a distended bladder. Bowel relaxants (one milliliter of butyl scopolamine bromide (Buscopan, 20 mg/ml; Boehringer Ingelheim, Germany) or one milligram of glucagon hydrochloride (Glucagen, Bagsvaerd, Denmark) can be injected intramuscularly just before imaging to reduce peristalsis. When an endoanal coil is used, the coil should be covered with a condom and lubricated. Lubricant produces high signal intensity nearby the coil and therefore the amount of lubricant should be limited. The endoanal coil is inserted in the anal canal in a left lateral position. After endoanal coil positioning, the patients are turned in the supine position. Supportive pads are necessary to stabilize the position of the endoanal coil. If an external phased array coil is used, the patients should be placed in the supine position with the pelvis centered at the proximal end of a posterior phased array coil in the feet-first position. An external phased array coil is placed anteriorly.

The optimal sequence for evaluating anal sphincter anatomy and pathology with endoanal or external phased array MR imaging has not been established. Generally, T2-weighted turbo spin-echo sequences can be used as basic sequence. At a 1.5 T MR unit, patients can be scanned using scan parameters within the following ranges: TR 2,500–3,500 ms, TE 70–90 ms, echo train length 10, field of view 10x10 cm (axial) and 16x16 cm (coronal), imaging matrix 256x512, 3-mm slice thickness, 0.3-mm interslice gap, and 2 excitations. Scan parameters should be optimized for the MR imaging system and endoanal coil or external phased array coil used to obtain optimal contrast resolution. Fat suppression techniques are not valuable in T2-weighted imaging in fecal incontinence. The use of T1-weighted sequences is not advisable, as its superiority above T2-weighted sequences has not been established. Phase-encoding direction should be adjusted to prevent artifacts in the anterior part of the anal sphincter complex. Axial images with slice orientation perpendicular to the anal sphincter and endoanal coil should be made. Further coronal images and, if desired, sagittal images with slice orientation parallel to the anal sphincter and endoanal coil should be obtained.

Normal Anatomy

The anal sphincter complex is comprised of different muscular layers and is enclosed by the fat-containing ischioanal space [9]. The most inner part of the anal sphincter complex is the internal anal sphincter (IAS), a smooth, circular muscle that is the terminal continuation of the circular rectal muscle. The striated external anal sphincter (EAS) is the outermost muscle of the distal anal sphincter complex and encircles the IAS. The space between the IAS and EAS, the intersphincteric space, contains fat and the longitudinal muscle. The latter is the continuation of the longitudinal muscle of the rectum. The puborectal muscle, a striated, sling-like muscle, is closely aligned to the deep part of the EAS and forms the upper outer part of the anal sphincter complex. The striated levator ani muscle is the cranial continuation of the puborectal muscle.

At EAUS, the IAS is visible as a clearly defined ring of low reflectivity (Figs. IV.39 and 40). The EAS is inseparable from the sling-like puborectal muscle and appears as an intact ring. In men, the EAS is recognizable as a ring of low reflectivity (Fig. IV.39), and in women, the EAS is mainly hyperreflective, making recognition sometimes more difficult (Fig. 40). The longitudinal muscle is a layer of variable reflectivity (Fig. IV.39).

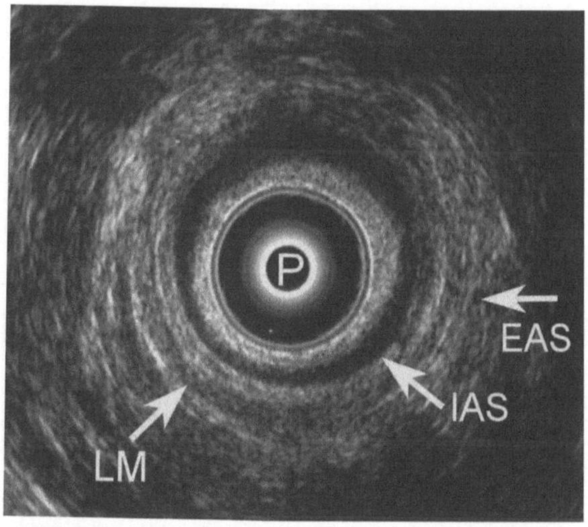

Fig. IV.39. Two-dimensional axial endoanal ultrasonography image obtained in the mid anal canal demonstrating normal male anatomy. *EAS* external anal sphincter, *IAS* internal anal sphincter, *LM* longitudinal muscle, *P* endoanal probe

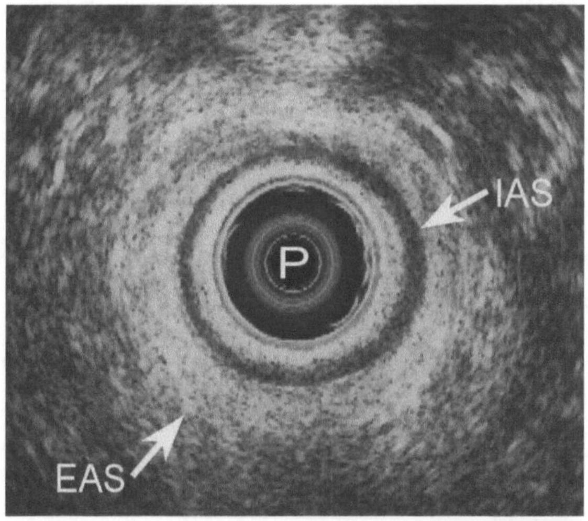

Fig. IV.40. Two-dimensional axial endoanal ultrasonography image of the mid anal canal showing normal female anatomy. The external anal sphincter is visible as a mainly hyperreflective ring (compare to Fig. IV.39). *EAS* external anal sphincter, *IAS* internal anal sphincter, *P* endoanal probe

At MR imaging on T2-weighted images, the IAS and EAS are recognizable in the axial plane as a clearly defined ring of relatively hyperintense signal intensity and relatively hypointense signal intensity, respectively (Fig. IV.41). In the coronal plane, the relation between the EAS and the puborectal muscle can be easily appreciated in contrast to the axial plane in which this is more difficult (Figs. IV.42). The hypointense longitudinal muscle often has a beaded appearance in the axial plane (Fig. IV.44). The amount of fat in the intersphincteric space is variable and may not be discernible. The puborectal muscle and levator ani have a signal intensity comparable to the EAS: relatively hypointense (Figs. IV.42 and 43).

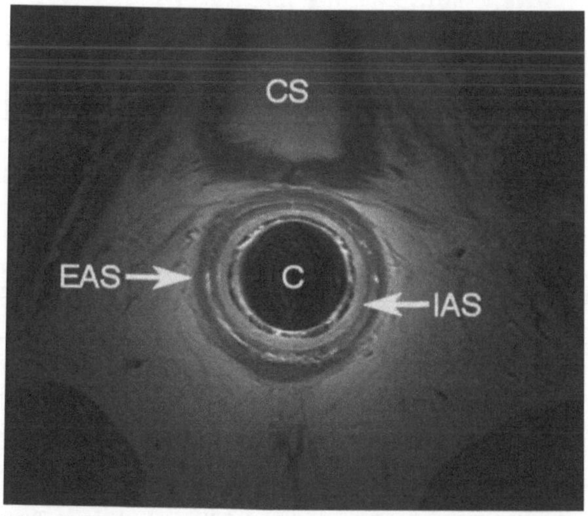

Fig. IV.41. Axial endoanal T2- weighted fast spin-echo MR image obtained in the mid anal canal visualizing normal anatomy and normal continuity of both the external and internal anal sphincter ring in a male patient. *EAS* external anal sphincter, *IAS* internal anal sphincter, *CS* corpus spongiosum, *C* endoanal coil

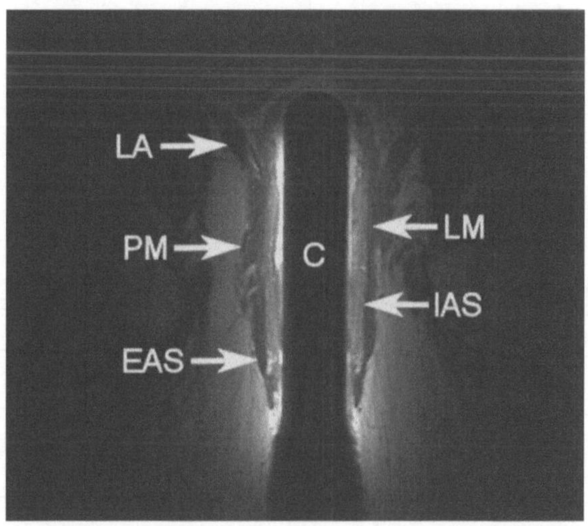

Fig. IV.42. Endoanal T2- weighted fast spin-echo MR image demonstrating normal anatomy in the coronal plane in a 68-year-old man. *EAS* external anal sphincter, *IAS* internal anal sphincter, *LM* longitudinal muscle, *PM* puborectal muscle, *LA* levator ani, *C* endoanal coil

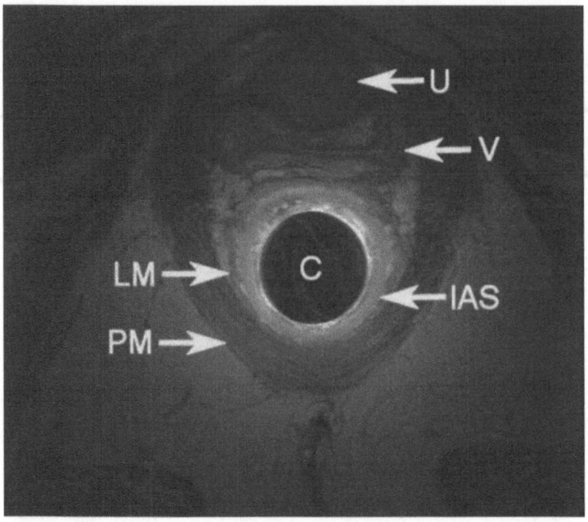

Fig. IV.43. Axial endoanal T2- weighted fast spin-echo MR image obtained through the upper part of the anal sphincter complex showing the normal sling-like configuration of the puborectal muscle in a female patient. *IAS* internal anal sphincter, *LM* longitudinal muscle, *PM* puborectal muscle, *V* vagina, *U* urethra, *C* endoanal coil

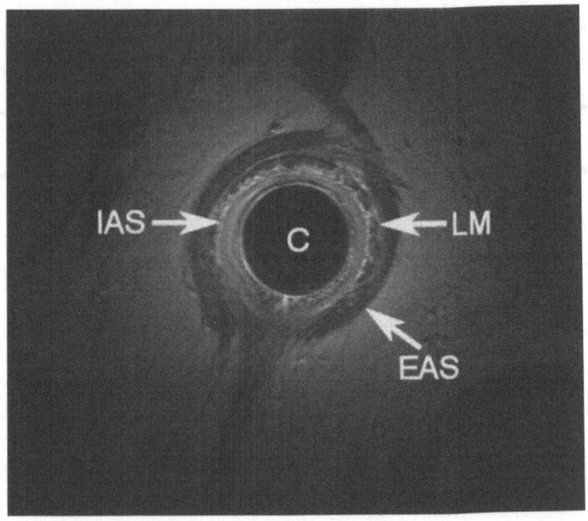

Fig. IV.44. Endoanal T2- weighted fast spin-echo MR image demonstrating the beaded appearance of the longitudinal muscle in the axial plane at the lower edge of the anal sphincter complex in a male patient. *EAS* external anal sphincter, *IAS* internal anal sphincter, *LM* longitudinal muscle, *C* endoanal coil

Anal Sphincter Complex Lesions

In fecal incontinent patients, EAUS and MR imaging focus mainly on visualizing the IAS and EAS, as damage of these two muscles proved to be a major cause of fecal incontinence [7, 8, 15–19]. IAS and EAS lesions are comprised of defects, scar tissue, and muscle volume anomalies.

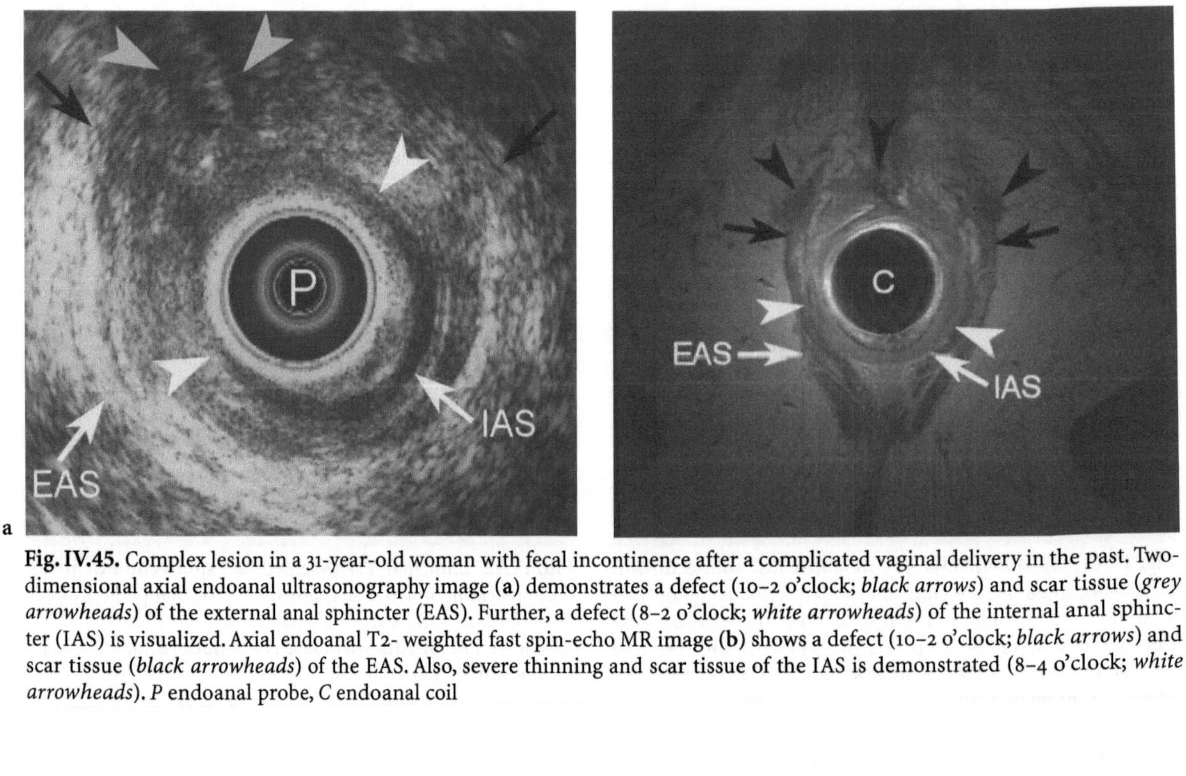

Fig. IV.45. Complex lesion in a 31-year-old woman with fecal incontinence after a complicated vaginal delivery in the past. Two-dimensional axial endoanal ultrasonography image (**a**) demonstrates a defect (10–2 o'clock; *black arrows*) and scar tissue (*grey arrowheads*) of the external anal sphincter (EAS). Further, a defect (8–2 o'clock; *white arrowheads*) of the internal anal sphincter (IAS) is visualized. Axial endoanal T2- weighted fast spin-echo MR image (**b**) shows a defect (10–2 o'clock; *black arrows*) and scar tissue (*black arrowheads*) of the EAS. Also, severe thinning and scar tissue of the IAS is demonstrated (8–4 o'clock; *white arrowheads*). *P* endoanal probe, *C* endoanal coil

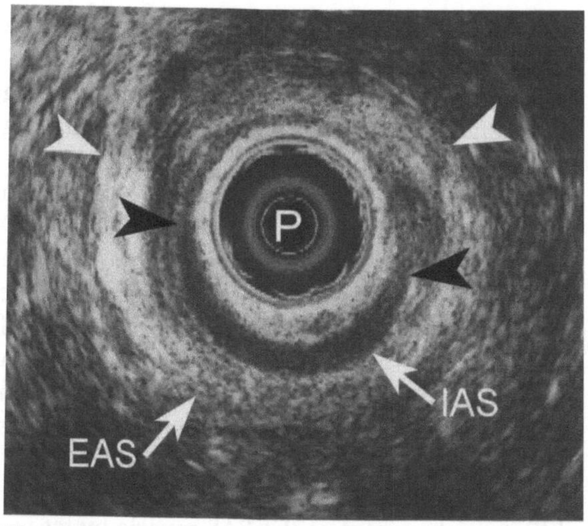

Fig. IV.46. Two-dimensional endoanal ultrasonographic image showing a defect of the internal (9–3 o'clock; *black arrowheads*) and external anal sphincter (10–2 o'clock; *white arrowheads*) at the anterior part of the anal sphincter complex in a 35-year-old woman with fecal incontinence complaints and a complicated vaginal delivery in the past. *EAS* external anal sphincter, *IAS* internal anal sphincter, *P* endoanal probe

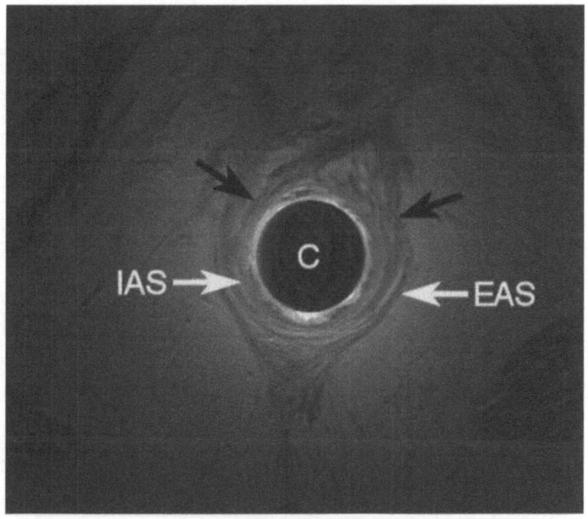

Fig. IV.47. Scar tissue and a defect of the internal (IAS) and external anal sphincter (EAS) (10–2 o'clock; *black arrows*) and diffuse thinning of the IAS and EAS ring at axial endoanal T2-weighted fast spin-echo MR imaging in a 67-year-old woman with fecal incontinence and a complicated vaginal delivery in the past. *C* endoanal coil

Defects and Scar Tissue

Defects of the IAS and EAS are defined at EAUS as an interruption of the fibrillar echotexture (Figs. IV.45a and 46) and at MR imaging as a discontinuity of the muscle ring (Figs. IV.45b and 47) [9, 10, 20]. Defects of the IAS and EAS can be isolated or may be accompanied by each other. Isolated IAS defects are mostly due to prior anorectal surgery whereas isolated EAS defects and combined IAS and EAS defects have generally an obstetric origin. Defects following obstetric trauma are frequently located at the anterior part of the anal sphincter complex (Figs. IV.45, 46, and 47) [7, 16, 19]. Healing of defects is accompanied by the formation of granulation tissue, which leads to scar tissue. Scar tissue is recognized at EAUS by loss of the normal architecture, with an area of amorphous texture that usually has low reflectiveness (Fig. IV.45a) [9, 20]. At MR imaging, scar tissue is visible as a hypointense deformation of the normal pattern of the muscle layer due to replacement of muscle cells by fibrous tissue (Figs. IV.45b and 47) [10].

To describe the extent of defects and/or scar tissue in the axial plane, we advocate reading in hours from a clock face or reporting of regions (e.g., right anterolateral, left posterior). In both cases, the physician should refer to the patient in the classic lithotomy position. The longitudinal extent can be indicated by the level of the anal canal (EAUS: proximal, middle, and distal) or in millimeter distance from the lower edge of the EAS (MR imaging).

Muscle Volume Anomalies

IAS thickness increases and EAS thickness decreases with age [21, 22]. These age-related effects should be differentiated from pathological thinning or thickening of both anal sphincter muscles. Thickness of the IAS can be defined accurately in millimeters at both EAUS and MR imaging, as the boundaries of the IAS are clearly visualized, resulting in an accurate delineation (Figs. IV.39–41). Generally, IAS thickness in adults is considered to be normal when it ranges from 2 to 4 mm, irrespective of patient age. Abnormal thickening (>4 mm) of the IAS can be found in patients with solitary rectal ulcer syndrome, and abnormal thinning (<2 mm) in patients with idiopathic degeneration [23, 24]. The above-mentioned range for normal IAS thickness and cutoff values for pathological thickening or thinning of the IAS apply only for endoluminal imaging, as

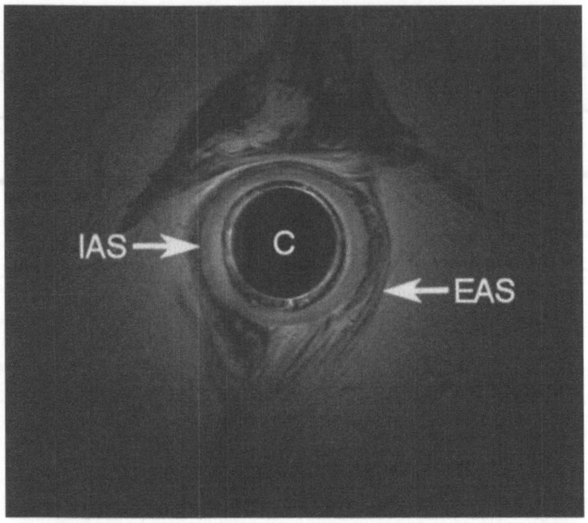

Fig. IV.48. Axial endoanal T2- weighted fast spin-echo MR image showing mild thinning of the external anal sphincter (EAS) muscle and diffuse replacement of EAS muscle by fat in a 68-year-old woman with fecal incontinence and diabetic mellitus. *IAS* internal anal sphincter, *C* endoanal coil

they have not yet been established at external phased array MR imaging.

Measuring the thickness of the EAS is difficult at 2-D EAUS, as the boundaries of the EAS are heterogeneous and therefore more complicated to define. EAS thickness can more easily be determined at MR imaging, as the demarcation of the EAS to the surrounding tissues is clearer. In healthy subjects, the average thickness of the EAS at endoanal MR imaging is approximately 4 mm [22]. Beets-Tan et al. reported that sphincter measurement with external phased array MR imaging is as reliable as that with endoanal MR imaging [25]. A previous study in four men and five nulliparous women showed an excellent correlation between EAS thickness measurements at 3-D EAUS and endoanal MR imaging [26]. Although EAS thickness measurements can accurately be made at 3-D EAUS and MR imaging, the role of these linear measurements is limited [27]. A recent study showed no significant difference in EAS thickness measurements between patients with and without EAS atrophy [28].

EAS atrophy, thinning of the EAS muscle, or diffuse replacement of the EAS muscle by fat is a common pathological muscle volume anomaly in patients with fecal incontinence [10, 28–30]. Atrophy of the EAS results from damage of the pudendal nerve, the principal nerve innervating the anorectum [31]. Demonstration of EAS atrophy is difficult at 2-D EAUS as firstly, fatty infiltration cannot be distinguished from normal muscle tissue; and secondly, the boundaries of the EAS are hard to determine (Figs. IV.39 and 40). EAS atrophy can easily be defined at MR imaging, as the delineation of the greater part of the EAS to the surrounding tissues is clear, and fat results in a hyperintense signal and is therefore easily recognized within the hypointense EAS [10] (Figs. IV.48 and 49). Important risk factors for pudendal

a 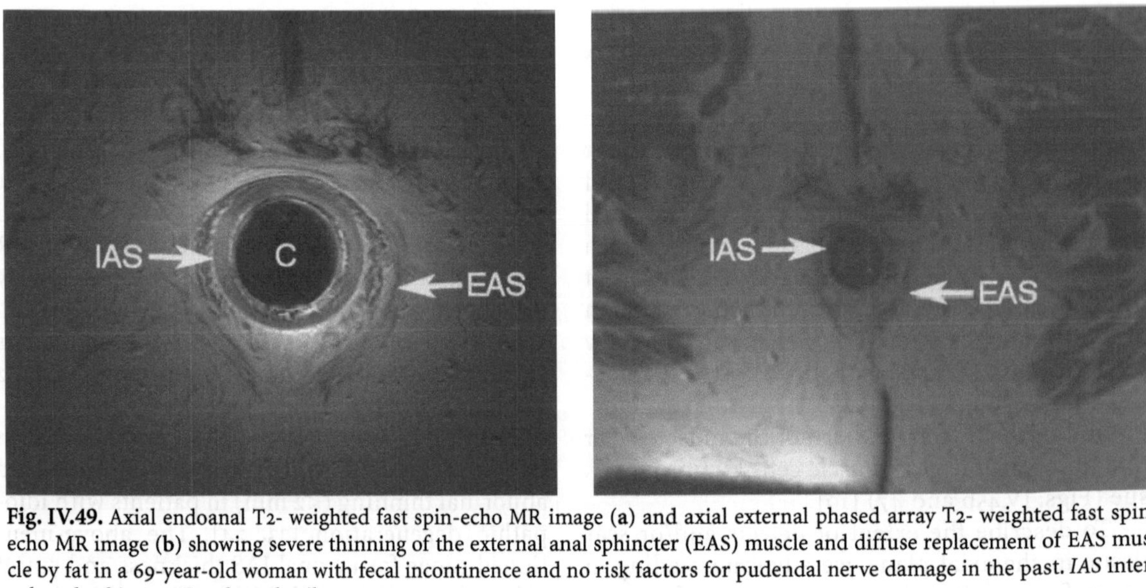 b

Fig. IV.49. Axial endoanal T2- weighted fast spin-echo MR image (**a**) and axial external phased array T2- weighted fast spin-echo MR image (**b**) showing severe thinning of the external anal sphincter (EAS) muscle and diffuse replacement of EAS muscle by fat in a 69-year-old woman with fecal incontinence and no risk factors for pudendal nerve damage in the past. *IAS* internal anal sphincter, *C* endoanal coil nerve damage comprise obstetric details in women (i.e., high-birth-weight infant, a long second stage of labor, forceps delivery), neurological disorders (cerebral, spinal, local disorder), straining for chronic constipation, diabetes mellitus, or simply the neuropathy of aging [31]. Depicting EAS atrophy is of importance in patients with fecal incontinence, as a previous study demonstrated – as did some physiological studies [32–34] – that atrophy of the EAS due to pudendal nerve damage is a negative predictor for the outcome of surgery of an EAS defect (anterior anal sphincter repair) [35]. The authors of that study have shown that outcome of anterior anal sphincter repair was significantly better in patients without EAS atrophy compared with those patients with EAS atrophy.

In contrast to EAS atrophy, pathological thickening of the EAS is seldom discussed in the literature, and its clinical value is not well established.

Comparative and Reproducibility Studies

Endoanal Ultrasonography versus Endoanal MR Imaging

Several studies investigated the diagnostic accuracy of 2-D EAUS and endoanal MR imaging in assessing anal sphincter integrity. Both EAUS and endoanal MR imaging have been validated physiologically, histologically, and intraoperatively as accurate tools in mapping internal and EAS defects [36–42]. Some studies compared these competitive techniques for demonstrating IAS and EAS pathology. Malouf and colleagues evaluated prospectively 2-D EAUS and endoanal MR imaging in 52 patients with fecal incontinence and reported that both techniques are comparable in diagnosing EAS defects [43]. Further, they suggested the inferiority of endoanal MR imaging in demonstrating IAS defects. Another study compared retrospectively 2-D EAUS and endoanal MR imaging to surgery in 22 patients with fecal incontinence and found MR imaging to be the most accurate technique for depicting IAS and EAS defects [20]. The reported results of those studies vary. Some of the variability can be attributed to differences in study design, patient population, and level of experience of readers. The current consensus is that both techniques can be used for demonstrating defects of the anal sphincter complex [30].

As explained before, depiction of EAS atrophy at 2-D EAUS is difficult. By contrast, the diagnostic accuracy of endoanal MR imaging for the diagnosis of EAS atrophy has been thoroughly investigated, and all studies reported that EAS atrophy can be accurately demonstrated with endoanal MR imaging [20, 27, 35, 44–47]. Rociu and colleagues compared 2-D EAUS and endoanal MR imaging for the depiction of EAS atrophy and found that EAS atrophy can only be accurately depicted at endoanal MR imaging and not at EAUS [20]. These findings are in concordance with another study evaluating both techniques in 20 women with fecal incontinence due to obstetric trauma [35]. Williams et al. found that patients with a thin IAS (<2 mm) and/or a poorly defined EAS at EAUS were more likely to have EAS atrophy and endoanal MR imaging should be considered to determine whether the sphincter is grossly atrophic [47]. Accurate assessment of EAS atrophy at endoanal MR imaging can be made by quantitative measurements of the area of remaining EAS and of the percentage of fat content of the EAS [35, 44, 47]. A recent study in 18 female patients with fecal incontinence evaluated whether 3-D EAUS measurements could be used to detect EAS atrophy [48]. The authors reported that despite the multiplanar capability, 3-D EAUS was not able to demonstrate EAS atrophy. In clinical practice, there are no "hard" criteria available for the visual diagnosis of EAS atrophy at MR imaging, but a recent study showed a relation between EAS squeeze function parameters obtained at anal manometry and the qualitative assessment of EAS atrophy by radiologists at endoanal MR imaging [28]. We suggest using the following qualitative grading system to assess atrophy at MR imaging: no atrophy (no thinning and no replacement of sphincter muscle by fat) (Fig. IV.41), mild atrophy (<50% thinning and/or replacement of sphincter muscle by fat) (Fig. IV.48), or severe atrophy (≥50% thinning and/or replacement of sphincter muscle by fat) (Fig. IV.49a, b). Although the clinical value of grading EAS atrophy has not been established yet, it might be that grading atrophy has an impact on the outcome of anterior anal sphincter repair. The hypothesis that patients with mild atrophy will fare better after anterior anal sphincter repair than patients with severe EAS atrophy should be analyzed in future studies.

Endoanal MR Imaging versus External Phased Array MR Imaging

Both 2-D EAUS and endoanal MR imaging have been shown, as described above, to be useful in detecting defects of the anal sphincter complex. Nevertheless, both techniques have the drawback that they can mainly be performed only at specialized centers, as a dedicated endoluminal probe or coil is necessary. Additionally, the introduction of the endoluminal device is uncomfortable. These two disadvantages of EAUS and endoanal MR imaging could be overcome with the use of external phased array coils. MR imaging with external phased array coils has already taken a central place in visualizing perineal disease and rectal tumors [49–51]. Previous studies show that external phased array MR imaging is also of great worth for demonstrating anal anatomy [52]. Until recently, the diagnostic value of this MR imaging technique in detecting EAS and IAS defects, as well as demonstrating EAS atrophy in patients with fecal incontinence, has not been established. A recent study in 30 patients with fecal incontinence due to mixed etiologies compared external phased array MR imaging to endoanal MR imaging for the depiction of IAS and EAS defects [12]. The study reported that both techniques did not significantly differ for the depiction of IAS and EAS defects. As endoanal MR imaging showed its superiority over EAUS for demonstrating EAS atrophy, atrophy of the EAS could till recently only be accurately demonstrated at the first technique. However, another recent study reported that external phased array MR imaging and endoanal MR imaging did not significantly differ in their ability to depict EAS atrophy, with good agreement [11].

Reproducibility Studies

Error and variation in image interpretation has been described as radiology's "Achilles' heel," and each imaging method must be reasonably reproducible between observers [53]. Gold et al. determined the interobserver agreement of 2-D EAUS for assessing anal sphincter disruption in 51 patients who were referred for EAUS to assess possible sphincter abnormalities [54]. They found very good agreement between observers for detecting IAS and EAS defects. A previous study evaluated the interobserver agreement of endoanal MR imaging and found that interobserver agreement was less than reported for EAUS [55]. The authors of that study found a moderate overall interobserver agreement for the assessment of sphincter integrity and reported that agreement was strongest if the anal sphincters were either both disrupted or both intact. Similar to that study, a weak interobserver agreement of endoanal MR imaging was described for the detection of anal sphincter defects in another reproducibility study of MR imaging [12]. This study evaluated the interobserver agreement of external phased array MR imaging as well, which was poor to fair between different observers. The latter study assessed, besides the between-observers variation, the variation between observations of a single observer for assessing the integrity of the anal sphincter complex, as apparent disagreement between observers may be due to both intra- and interobserver variation. The intraobserver agreement ranged from fair to very good for endoanal MR imaging and external phased array MR imaging, with a stronger intraobserver agreement for each observer familiar with his/her own specific MR imaging technique.

Reported results about the reproducibility of imaging techniques for demonstrating EAS atrophy are sparse in the literature. To our knowledge, only one study evaluated observer reproducibility in assessing EAS atrophy with endoanal MR imaging and external phased array MR imaging [11]. In line with reported results of interobserver agreement for the detection of EAS defects [12, 55], this study found a moderate interobserver agreement of endoanal MR imaging for the detection of EAS atrophy. The reproducibility between observers was moderate to good for external phased array MR imaging. The intraobserver agreement was moderate to very good for endoanal MR imaging and fair to very good for external phased array MR imaging. Also in that study, the reproducibility of observations of a single observer seemed to be related to the experience level of an observer with endoanal MR imaging and external phased array MR imaging, respectively.

The fact that results among radiologists vary considerably for depicting anal sphincter defects and EAS atrophy at MR imaging can be explained by the relatively limited number of manuscripts discussing anal sphincter pathology at MR imaging. This may lead to a higher contribution of personal experience in reading. The latter might also be a consequence of the fact that there are no "hard" criteria available for the visual diagnosis of

EAS atrophy. Training radiologists in interpreting the changes in sphincter morphology that are demonstrated in patients with defects or atrophy of the anal sphincter complex might improve reader performance for both MR imaging techniques.

Role of Imaging Techniques in the Diagnostic Workup

EAUS, endoanal MR imaging, and external phased array MR imaging are competitive techniques in the diagnostic workup of fecal incontinence. They have a central position in assessing pathology of the EAS and IAS muscles, as physical examination is not reliable in detecting EAS and IAS defects [56]. Electromyography is a painful test and precludes an assessment of the structural and functional integrity of the entire sphincter complex [57, 58], and anal manometry is not able to differentiate between sphincter dysfunction due to structural sphincter injury or pudendal nerve damage [59]. Further, pudendal nerve latency testing is not 100% conclusive for demonstrating pudendal nerve damage, as this technique measures only the conduction time of the fastest muscle fibers, and latencies may be normal even in the presence of EAS atrophy [1].

Patients with fecal incontinence are initially treated conservatively, including with dietary measures (fibers, avoidance of foods that cause diarrhea or urgency), medical treatment (antidiarrheal medications, bulking agents), and pelvic floor rehabilitation (electrical stimulation and biofeedback) [1]. If these treatment options have failed, patients with structural damage of the EAS may be considered for surgery (anterior anal sphincter repair). Previous studies report that some patients with an initially good response to anterior anal sphincter repair have shown deterioration of function in the long term due to the coexistence of atrophy of the EAS [60]. No surgical option is available for patients with an isolated disruption of the IAS.

An overview of the literature concerning imaging techniques in patients with fecal incontinence shows that EAUS, endoanal MR imaging, and external phased array MR imaging are all valuable tools in the diagnostic workup of patients with fecal incontinence but that local expertise is the major factor for decisions about the preferred technique. As EAUS is, in contrast to MR imaging, a relatively simple, fast, and inexpensive technique, the present consensus is that EAUS can be used as the primary technique and MR imaging as the second-line technique, depending on availability and observer's experience level. The major advantage of MR imaging above EAUS is the accurate demonstration of EAS atrophy. As described above, EAS atrophy proved to be an indicator for poor outcome of anterior anal sphincter repair. Therefore, to select patients to benefit from anterior anal sphincter repair, besides demonstrating the presence and extent of an EAS defect, the detection of EAS atrophy is also of importance. In these situations, MR imaging is mandatory as a complementary technique to EAUS in the diagnostic workup of fecal incontinence.

References

1. Madoff RD, Parker SC, Varma MG, Lowry AC (2004) Faecal incontinence in adults. Lancet 364:621–632
2. Bharucha AE (2003) Fecal incontinence. Gastroenterology 124:1672–1685
3. Fuchsjager MH, Maier AG (2003) Imaging fecal incontinence Eur J Radiol 47:108–116
4. Jorge JM, Habr-Gama A, Wexner SD (2001) Clinical applications and techniques of cinedefecography. Am J Surg 182:93–101
5. Wiersma TG, Mulder CJ, Reeders JW (1997) Dynamic rectal examination: its significant clinical value. Endoscopy 29:462–471
6. Parks AG, Swash M, Urich H (1977) Sphincter denervation in anorectal incontinence and rectal prolapse. Gut 18:656–665
7. Sultan AH, Kamm MA, Hudson CN et al (1993) Anal-sphincter disruption during vaginal delivery. N Engl J Med 329:1905–1911
8. Sultan AH, Johanson RB, Carter JE (1998) Occult anal sphincter trauma following randomized forceps and vacuum delivery. Int J Gynaecol Obstet 61:113–119
9. Bartram CI (2003) Ultrasound. In: Bartram CI, DeLancey JO, Halligan S et al (eds) Imaging pelvic floor disorders. Springer, Berlin Heidelberg New York
10. Rociu E, Stoker J, Zwamborn AW, Lameris JS (1999) Endoanal MR imaging of the anal sphincter in fecal incontinence. Radiographics 19:S171–S177
11. Terra MP, Beets-Tan RG, van der Hulst VPM et al

(2005) MR imaging in evaluating atrophy of the external anal sphincter in patients with fecal incontinence. AJR Am J Roentgenol (*in press*)
12. Terra MP, Beets-Tan RG, van der Hulst VPM et al (2005) Anal sphincter defects in patients with fecal incontinence: endoanal versus external phased-array MR imaging. Radiology 236:886–895
13. Horsthuis K, Stoker J (2004) MRI of perianal Crohn's disease. AJR Am J Roentgenol 183:1309–1315
14. Gold DM, Bartram CI, Halligan S et al (1999) Three-dimensional endoanal sonography in assessing anal canal injury. Br J Surg 86:365–370
15. Abbasakoor F, Nelson M, Beynon J et al (1998) Anal endosonography in patients with anorectal symptoms after haemorrhoidectomy. Br J Surg 85:1522–1524
16. Kamm MA (1994) Obstetric damage and faecal incontinence. Lancet 344:730–733
17. Snooks S, Henry MM, Swash M (1984) Faecal incontinence after anal dilatation. Br J Surg 71:617–618
18. Speakman CT, Burnett SJ, Kamm MA, Bartram CI (1991) Sphincter injury after anal dilatation demonstrated by anal endosonography. Br J Surg 78:1429–1430
19. Sultan AH, Kamm MA, Hudson CN, Bartram CI (1994) Third degree obstetric anal sphincter tears: risk factors and outcome of primary repair. BMJ 308:887–891
20. Rociu E, Stoker J, Eijkemans MJ et al (1999) Fecal incontinence: endoanal US versus endoanal MR imaging. Radiology 212:453–458
21. Frudinger A, Halligan S, Bartram CI et al (2002) Female anal sphincter: Age-related differences in asymptomatic volunteers with high-frequency endoanal US. Radiology 224:417–423
22. Rociu E, Stoker J, Eijkemans MJC, Lameris JS (2000) Normal anal sphincter anatomy and age. and sex-related variations at high-spatial-resolution endoanal MR imaging. Radiology 217:395–401
23. Halligan S, Sultan A, Rottenberg G, Bartram CI (1995) Endosonography of the anal sphincters in solitary rectal ulcer syndrome. Int J Colorectal Dis 10:79–82
24. Vaizey CJ, Kamm MA, Bartram CI (1997) Primary degeneration of the internal anal sphincter as a cause of passive faecal incontinence. Lancet 349:612–615
25. Beets-Tan RG, Morren GL, Beets GL et al (2001) Measurement of anal sphincter muscles: endoanal US, endoanal MR imaging, or phased-array MR imaging? A study with healthy volunteers. Radiology 220:81–89
26. Williams AB, Bartram CI, Halligan S et al (2002) Endosonographic anatomy of the normal anal canal compared with endocoil magnetic resonance imaging. Dis Colon Rectum 45:176–183
27. Williams AB, Malouf AJ, Bartram CI et al (2001) Assessment of external anal sphincter morphology in idiopathic fecal incontinence with endocoil magnetic resonance imaging. Dig Dis Sci 46:1466–1471
28. Terra MP, Deutekom M, Beets-Tan RG et al (2006) Relation between external anal sphincter atrophy at endoanal magnetic resonance imaging and clinical, functional, and anatomic characteristics in patients with fecal incontinence. Dis Colon Rectum (*in press*)
29. Stoker J, Halligan S, Bartram CI (2001) Pelvic floor imaging. Radiology 218:621–641
30. Stoker J, Bartram CI, Halligan S (2002) Imaging of the posterior pelvic floor. Eur Radiol 12:779–788
31. Rao SS (2004) Pathophysiology of adult fecal incontinence. Gastroenterology 126:S14–S22
32. Gilliland R, Altomare DF, Moreira H Jr. et al (1998) Pudendal neuropathy is predictive of failure following anterior overlapping sphincteroplasty. Dis Colon Rectum 41:1516–1522
33. Jacobs PP, Scheuer M, Kuijpers JH, Vingerhoets MH (1990) Obstetric fecal incontinence. Role of pelvic floor denervation and results of delayed sphincter repair. Dis Colon Rectum 33:494–497
34. Londono-Schimmer EE, Garcia-Duperly R, Nicholls RJ (1994) Overlapping anal sphincter repair for faecal incontinence due to sphincter trauma: five year follow-up functional results. Int J Colorectal Dis 9:110–113
35. Briel JW, Stoker J, Rociu E et al (1999) External anal sphincter atrophy on endoanal magnetic resonance imaging adversely affects continence after sphincteroplasty. Br J Surg 86:1322–1327
36. Cuesta MA, Meijer S, Derksen EJ et al (1992) Anal sphincter imaging in fecal incontinence using endosonography. Dis Colon Rectum 35:59–63
37. Deen KI, Kumar D, Williams JG et al (1993) Anal sphincter defects. Correlation between endoanal ultrasound and surgery. Ann Surg 218:201–205
38. DeSouza NM, Puni R, Gilderdale DJ, Bydder GM (1995) Magnetic resonance imaging of the anal sphincter using an internal coil. Magn Reson Q 11:45–56
39. DeSouza NM, Hall AS, Puni R et al (1996) High resolution magnetic resonance imaging of the anal sphincter using a dedicated endoanal coil. Comparison of magnetic resonance imaging with surgical findings. Dis Colon Rectum 39:926–934
40. Law PJ, Kamm MA, Bartram CI (1991) Anal endosonography in the investigation of faecal incontinence. Br J Surg 78:312–314
41. Meyenberger C, Bertschinger P, Zala GF, Buchmann P (1996) Anal sphincter defects in fecal incontinence: Correlation between endosonography and surgery. Endoscopy 28:217–224
42. Nielsen MB, Hauge C, Pedersen JF, Christiansen J (1993) Endosonographic evaluation of patients with

anal incontinence: findings and influence on surgical management. AJR Am J Roentgenol 160:771–775
43. Malouf AJ, Williams AB, Halligan S et al (2000) Prospective assessment of accuracy of endoanal MR imaging and endosonography in patients with fecal incontinence. AJR Am J Roentgenol 175:741–745
44. Briel JW, Zimmerman DD, Stoker J et al (2000) Relationship between sphincter morphology on endoanal MRI and histopathological aspects of the external anal sphincter. Int J Colorectal Dis 15:87–90
45. DeSouza NM, Puni R, Zbar A (1996) MR imaging of the anal sphincter in multiparous women using an endoanal coil: Correlation with in vitro anatomy and appearances in fecal incontinence. Am J Roentgenol 167:1465–1471
46. Fletcher JG, Busse RF, Riederer SJ et al (2003) Magnetic resonance imaging of anatomic and dynamic defects of the pelvic floor in defecatory disorders. Am J Gastroenterol 98:399–411
47. Williams AB, Bartram CI, Modhwadia D et al (2001) Endocoil magnetic resonance imaging quantification of external anal sphincter atrophy. Br J Surg 88:853–859
48. West RL, Dwarkasing S, Briel JW et al (2005) Can three-dimensional endoanal ultrasonography detect external anal sphincter atrophy? A comparison with endoanal magnetic resonance imaging. Int J Colorectal Dis 20: 328–333
49. Beets-Tan RG, Beets GL, van der Hoop AG et al (2001) Preoperative MR imaging of anal fistulas: Does it really help the surgeon? Radiology 218:75–84
50. Beets-Tan RG, Beets GL, Vliegen RF et al (2001) Accuracy of magnetic resonance imaging in prediction of tumour-free resection margin in rectal cancer surgery. Lancet 357:497–504
51. DeSouza NM, Gilderdale DJ, Coutts GA et al (1998) MRI of fistula-in-ano: a comparison of endoanal coil with external phased array coil techniques. J Comput Assist Tomogr 22:357–363
52. Morren GL, Beets-Tan RG, van Engelshoven JM (2001) Anatomy of the anal canal and perianal structures as defined by phased-array magnetic resonance imaging. Br J Surg 88:1506–1512
53. Robinson PJ (1997) Radiology's Achilles' heel: error and variation in the interpretation of the Rontgen image. Br J Radiol 70:1085–1098
54. Gold DM, Halligan S, Kmiot WA, Bartram CI (1999) Intraobserver and interobserver agreement in anal endosonography. Br J Surg 86:371–375
55. Malouf AJ, Halligan S, Williams AB et al (2001) Prospective assessment of interobserver agreement for endoanal MRI in fecal incontinence. Abdom Imaging 26:76–78
56. Keating JP, Stewart PJ, Eyers AA et al (1997) Are special investigations of value in the management of patients with fecal incontinence? Dis Colon Rectum 40:896–901
57. Enck P, von Giesen HJ, Schafer A et al (1996) Comparison of anal sonography with conventional needle electromyography in the evaluation of anal sphincter defects. Am J Gastroenterol 91:2539–2543
58. Tjandra JJ, Milsom JW, Schroeder T, Fazio VW (1993) Endoluminal ultrasound is preferable to electromyography in mapping anal sphincteric defects. Dis Colon Rectum 36:689–692
59. Sultan AH, Kamm MA, Talbot IC et al (1994) Anal endosonography for identifying external sphincter defects confirmed histologically. Br J Surg 81: 463–465
60. Malouf AJ, Norton CS, Engel AF et al (2000) Long-term results of overlapping anterior anal-sphincter repair for obstetric trauma. Lancet 355:260–265

Invited Commentary

J.J. Tjandra

Endoanal ultrasound is an important adjunct in the assessment of patients with fecal incontinence [1, 2]. A thorough clinical history of the bowel function, including dietary, pharmacologic, surgical, and social history, together with a detailed anorectal examination, remain the most important basis in patient management. A careful anorectal examination with attention to perineal scars and digital rectal examination would yield much information and guidance to patient management.

Many of the specialized investigations such as anorectal physiology and endoanal ultrasound serve to confirm the clinical impression. The main function of endoanal ultrasound is to define the presence and extent of sphincter defect(s) and scarring and whether the process involves either or both anal sphincters [3]. In our center, sonographic thickness of either the internal or external anal sphincters has not been found to correlate with anal sphincter pressures or Wexner's continence score [4]. Neither did they predict the outcome of a sphincter repair.

In addition, prolonged pudendal nerve conduction is not related with sonographic thickness of the external anal sphincter [5]. In a review of 51 women with bilaterally prolonged pudendal nerve terminal motor latency, the sonographic thickness of the external sphincter was similar to that of normal female controls with normal continence and normal pudendal nerve terminal motor latency.

While magnetic resonance imaging (MRI) might show features suggestive of sphincter atrophy such as fat replacement, these MR appearances have not been correlated with histology. Some atrophy presumably occurs with all muscles, including anal sphincters, with aging; however, more work is required to quantify this concept of sphincter atrophy for this to be scientifically valid. Atrophy can also occur in a patchy fashion within the anal sphincters, which further complicates its assessment. MRI is costly and not readily accessible. These are factors which will impede its role in the management of fecal incontinence.

A direct back-to-back examination with both two-dimensional (2-D) and three-dimensional (3-D) endoanal ultrasound was performed in 102 patients by a single examiner in our center. The 2-D endoanal ultrasound was performed and reported first, followed by the 3-D endoanal ultrasound. No additional information was obtained with the 3-D examination. Instead, the 3-D examination yielded confusing findings in 11 patients, especially with reference to the length of the sphincter defect. Hence, with experienced operators, 3-D endoanal ultrasound does not provide any further benefit than the standard 2-D examination.

Endoanal ultrasound provides good images of the anatomy of the pelvic floor and anal sphincters. This has largely replaced the need for the painful needle electromyography [6]. However, functional assessment with anorectal physiology remains important [7–9]. A low-resting anal canal pressure in the presence of an intact internal sphincter suggests internal sphincter dysfunction, especially if the patient complains of passive fecal incontinence. The presence of poor resting and squeeze anal pressures in the presence of sonographically intact anal sphincters would suggest stretched anal injuries, especially if there is diffuse hypoechogenicity within the external sphincter. By contrast, presence of prolonged pudendal nerve terminal motor latency would be an additional contributing factor to fecal incontinence.

Endoanal ultrasound aids decision making in the management of fecal incontinence. Presence of an isolated defect of the external anal sphincter on endoanal ultrasound would be an indication for sphincter repair if the defect exceeds 25% of the circumference and the patient is significantly symptomatic [10]. A coexisting defect of the internal anal sphincter is a poor prognostic factor to successful sphincter repair, and patients should be appropriately counseled; an injectable therapy with a bulking agent, such as silicone biomaterial (PTQ) might be necessary at a later stage.

Following maximal conservative therapy with dietary management and pelvic floor physiotherapy, an injectable bulking agent [11] would be the preferred initial treatment in patients with internal sphincter dysfunction presenting with passive fecal incontinence and reduced resting anal pressure. On the other hand, if there are multiple deficits, such as concomitant pudendal neuropathy, internal sphincter dysfunction, and multiple defects of the external sphincter, then sacral neuromodulation [12] is more likely to be effective.

Endoanal ultrasound does have some limitations. Even with 3-D sonography, anal canal length is best established physiologically using anorectal manometry rather than by endoanal ultrasound [13]. In addition, the inexperienced physician might confuse the normal deficiency of the perineal body in the upper anal canal in women with a sphincter defect. Presence of a large rectocele could also make interpretation of an anterior sphincter defect difficult.

Despite such limitations, endoanal ultrasound is a useful adjunct to the clinical assessment of fecal incontinence. It is portable and easy to perform, and should be part of the armamentarium of any colorectal surgeon interested in the pelvic floor.

References

1. Tjandra JJ, Milsom JW, Stolfi VM et al (1992) Endoluminal ultrasound defines anatomy of the anal canal and pelvic floor. Dis Colon Rectum 35:465–470
2. Rieger N, Tjandra JJ, Solomon M (2004) Endoanal and endorectal ultrasound: applications in colorectal surgery. Aust NZ J Surg 74(8):671–675
3. Tjandra JJ, Ooi BS, Tang CL (2001) Faecal incontinence after lateral sphincterotomy is often associated with other occult sphincter defects: a study using endoanal sonography. Aust NZ J Surg 71:598–602
4. Jorge JM, Wexner SD (1993) Etiology and management of fecal incontinence. Dis Colon Rectum 36: 77–97
5. Tjandra JJ, Han WR, Carey M et al (2000) Prolonged pudendal nerve conduction is not associated with sonographic thickness of the external anal sphincter. Aust NZ J Surg 70 [Suppl]:A66
6. Tjandra JJ, Milsom JW, Schroeder T, Fazio VW (1993) Endoluminal ultrasound is preferable to needle EMG in the assessment of anal sphincteric defect. Dis Colon Rectum 36:689–692
7. Ooi BS, Tjandra JJ (1999) Fecal seepage in males with paradoxically high resting anal tone may be associated with anismus. Dis Colon Rectum 42:824–825
8. Ooi BS, Tjandra JJ, Tang CL et al (2000) Anorectal physiological testing before and after a successful sphincter repair: a prospective study. Colorectal Dis 2000; 2:220–228
9. Tjandra JJ, Ooi BS, Han WR (2000) Anorectal physiological testing for bowel dysfunction in patients with spinal cord lesions. Dis Colon Rectum 2000; 43:927–931
10. Tjandra JJ, Han WR, Goh J et al (2003) Direct repair vs overlapping sphincter repair: A randomized controlled trial. Dis Colon Rectum 46:937–943
11. Tjandra JJ, Lim JF, Hiscock R, Rajendra P (2004) Injectable silicone biomaterial for fecal incontinence due to internal anal sphincter dysfunction is effective. Dis Colon Rectum 47:2138–146
12. Tjandra JJ, Lim JF, Matzel K (2004) Sacral nerve stimulation – an emerging treatment for faecal incontinence. Aust NZ J Surg 74:1098–1106
13. Tjandra JJ, Han WR (2003) Measurement of anal sphincter length with endoanal ultrasound is functionally unhelpful. Dis Colon Rectum 46:A39

Section V

Endoanal Ultrasonography in the Evaluation of Perianal Sepsis and Fistula-in-ano

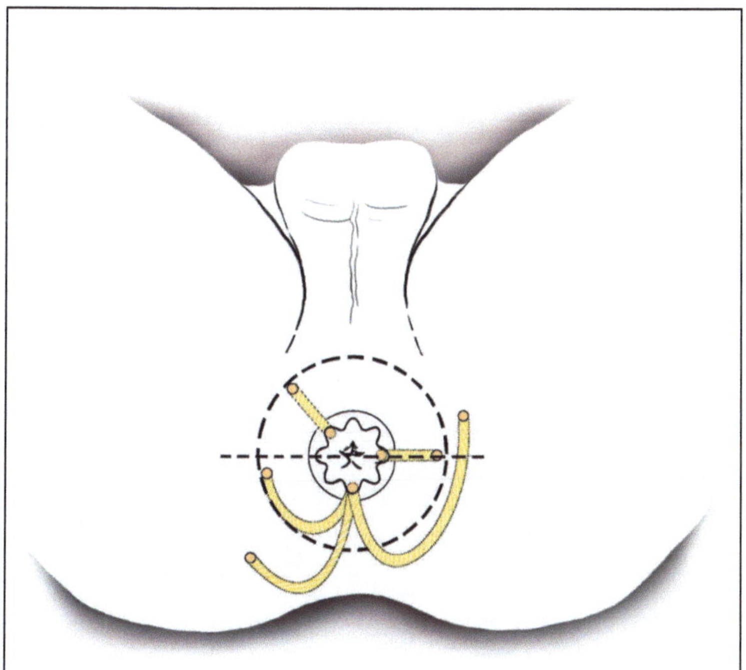

V.1. Introduction

G.A. Santoro, G. Di Falco

The pathogenesis of anorectal abscesses and fistulas is generally attributed to an infection of the anal glands of Herrmann and Desfosses (cryptoglandular hypothesis) [1]. These glands, numbering about six, are usually located in the subepithelial position, in the intersphincteric space, or in the external sphincter, with ducts that enter at the base of the anal crypts of Morgagni at the dentate line level. Occasionally, the glands may be situated cephalad or caudal to the dentate line. Infection of the glands can result in an abscess, which can spread in a number of directions, usually along the path of least resistance, and can lead to the subsequent development of an anal fistula (Fig. V.1). Shafik proposed that all anorectal abscesses or fistulas originate as a central space infection, which spreads to the other perianal spaces along the central septa [2, 3].

Classification

Five presentations of anorectal abscess have been described (Fig. V.2) [1]:

1. Submucosal abscess, which arises from an infected crypt in the anal canal and is located under the mucosa. Rectal examination may reveal a tender submucosal mass, which may not be readily apparent by anoscopy
2. Intersphincteric abscess, which represents between 2% and 5% of perirectal abscesses. In this condition, the infection dissects in the intersphincteric plane and can spread cephalad (high type) or caudal (low type)
3. Perianal abscess, which is the most common type, occurs in 40–45% of cases and is identified as a superficial, tender mass outside the

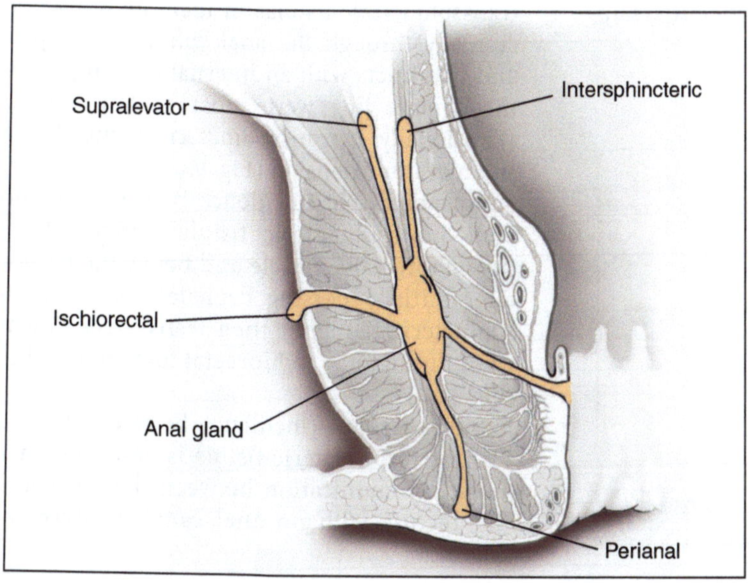

Fig. V.1. Infection of the anal gland in the intersphincteric plane can spread to a number of different locations

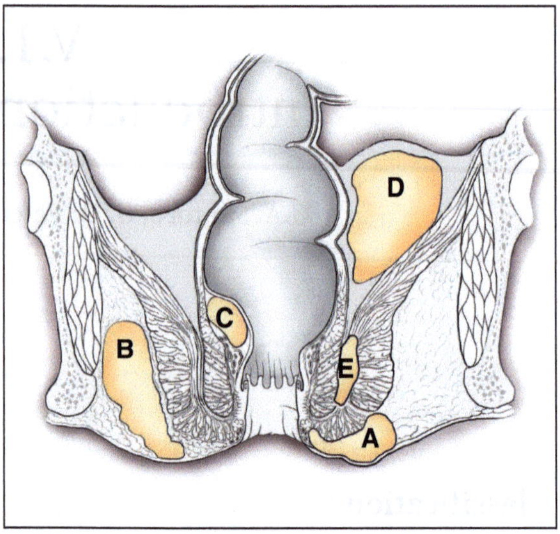

Fig. V.2. Types of anorectal abscesses: *A* perianal, *B* ischiorectal, *C* submucosal, *D* supralevator, *E* intersphincteric

anal verge. Physical examination reveals an area of erythema, induration, or fluctuance, and anoscopic examination can demonstrate pus exuding at the base of a crypt (Fig. V.3)

4. Ischiorectal abscess, which is seen in 20–25% of patients, may present as a large, erythematous, indurated, tender mass on the buttock or may be virtually inapparent. The patient complains only of severe pain or is febrile
5. Supralevator abscess, which is relatively rare, comprises less than 2.5% of perirectal abscesses. It may occur as a cephalad extension of an intersphincteric or transsphincteric abscess or may be associated with a pelvic inflammatory condition (Crohn's disease, diverticulitis, salpingitis) or pelvic surgery.

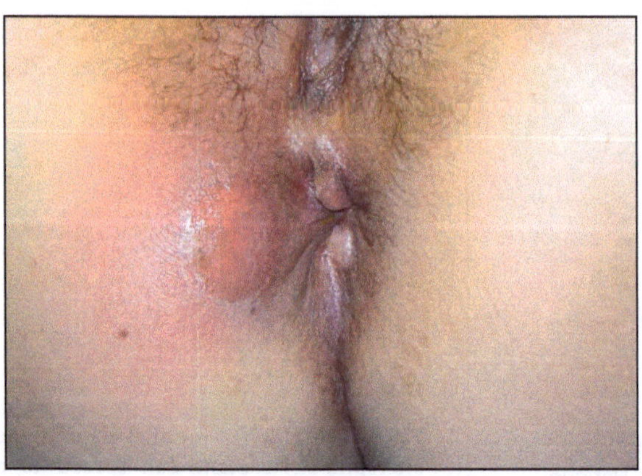

Fig. V.3. Perianal abscess

Sepsis can spread through the different perianal spaces and become a horseshoe infection (Fig. V.4).

Anorectal fistula represents a communication between two epithelial surfaces: the perianal skin and the anal canal or rectal mucosa [1]. Any fistula is characterized by an internal opening, a primary tract, and an external or perineal opening (Fig. V.5). Occasionally, the primary tract can present a secondary extension or a fistula can be without a perineal opening. Parks et al. [4] classified the main tract of the fistula in relationship to the sphincters into four types:

1. Intersphincteric (incidence between 55% and 70%): An intersphincteric fistula passes through the internal sphincter and through the intersphincteric plane to the skin (Fig. V.6). Only the most superficial portions of the tract pass through the subcutaneous external sphincter. Secondary extension may be observed to proceed cephalad in the intersphincteric plane (high blind tract)
2. Transsphincteric (incidence between 55% and 70%): Transsphincteric fistula passes through both the internal and external sphincters into the ischiorectal fossa and to the skin (Fig. V.7). The level of the tract determines one of three types of transsphincteric fistula: high (traversing the upper two thirds of the external sphincter), mid, or low (Fig. V.8). It has been suggested that the height of the internal opening does not always reflect the level at which a transsphincteric fistula crosses the external anal sphincter. Buchanan et al. [5] suggested that half of the transsphincteric fistulas in their study tracked cranially through the anal sphincter complex and that tracts with an internal opening above the dentate line were most acutely angled. Occasionally, a transsphincteric fistula has a supralevator extension (Fig. V.9)
3. Suprasphincteric (incidence between 1% and 3%): Suprasphincteric fistula courses above the puborectalis muscle and below the levator after initially passing cephalad as an intersphincteric fistula. It then transverses downward through the ischiorectal fossa to the skin (Fig. V.10)
4. Extrasphincteric (incidence between 2% and 3%): Extrasphincteric fistula is described by a direct communication between the perineum and rectum with no anal canal involvement (Fig. V.11).

a

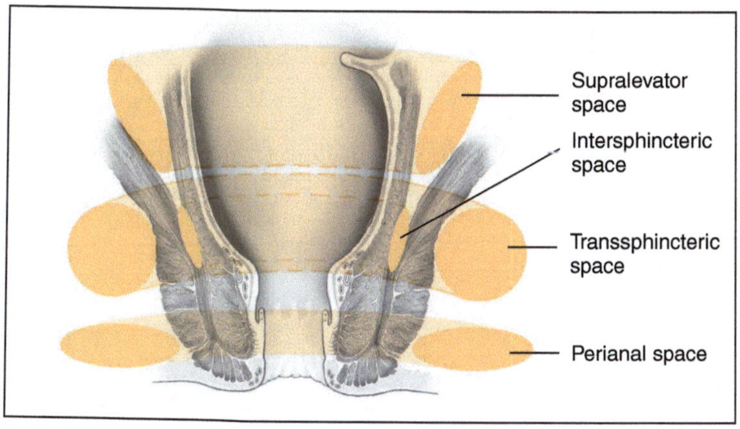

b

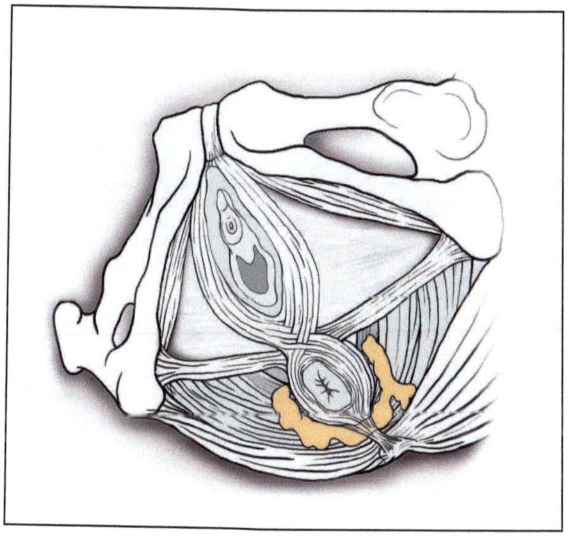

Fig. V.4. Schematic representation of horseshoe extension of anal sepsis in the different perianal spaces (**a**, **b**)

Submucous fistulas are those in which the tract is subsphincteric and does not involve or pass the sphincter complex. Anovaginal fistulas have an extension toward the vaginal introitus. Secondary tracts may develop in any part of the anal canal or may extend circumferentially in the intersphincteric, ischioanal, or supralevator spaces (horseshoe extensions). Fazio [6] classified fistulas as *simple* or *complex*. Superficial, intersphincteric, or low transsphincteric fistulas not complicated by abscesses or secondary tracts are considered *simple* fistulas. High transsphincteric, suprasphincteric, or extrasphincteric fistulas, presence of multiple secondary tracts or large abscesses, internal openings high in the anal canal, anterior fistulas in women, recurrent or persistent fistulas after previous operations, and fistulas in Crohn's disease are considered *complex* fistulas [7].

Identification of Fistula Tract

Accurate evaluation of patients with perianal sepsis is crucial for the treatment plan. Intersphincteric tracts usually open externally very close to the anal verge, and transsphincteric and other more complicated tracts will open further away, as they will have to traverse the external anal sphincter first. Physical examination may reveal the thickened tract proceeding into the anal canal if the fistula has a relatively superficial position, and anoscopic examination may demonstrate purulent material exuding from the base of the crypt. According to Goodsall's rule [8], when the external opening lies anterior to the transverse plane, the internal opening tends to be located radially and in the same position as is the external opening. Conversely, when the external opening lies posterior to this plane, the internal

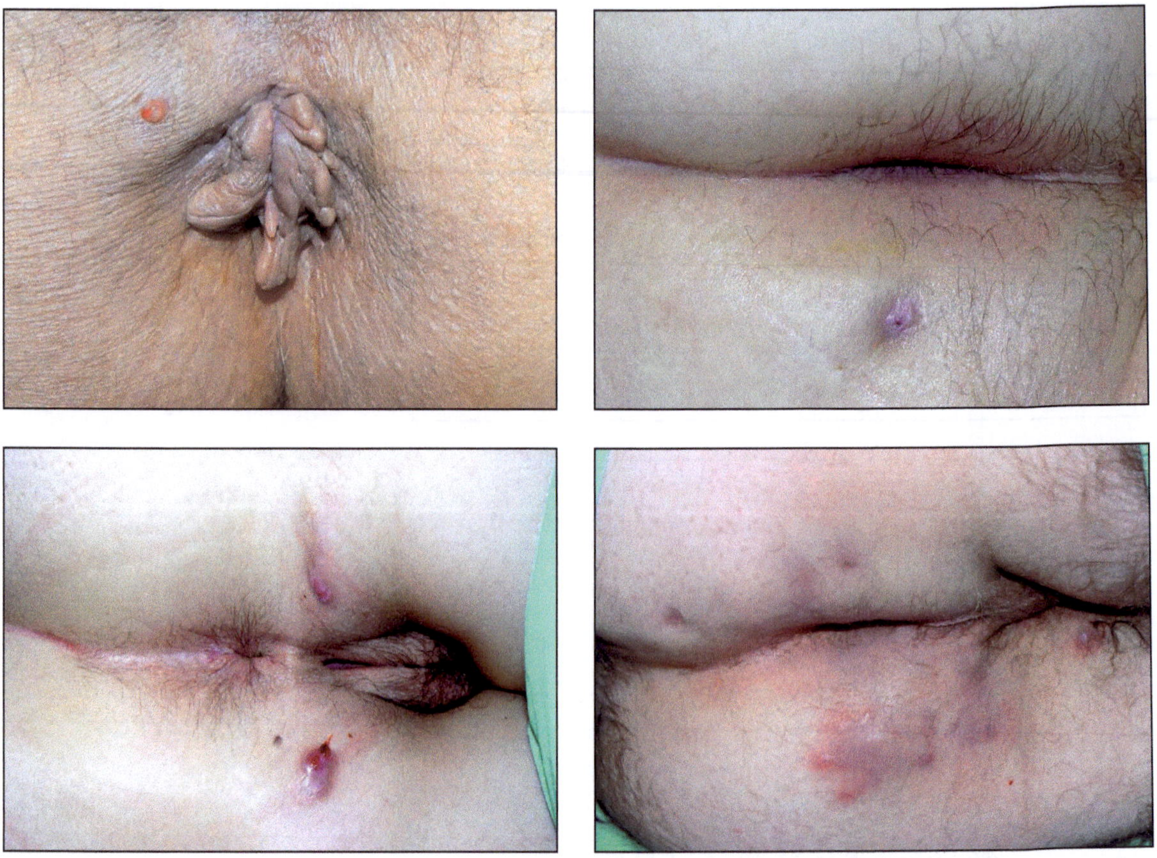

a b c d

Fig. V.5. Different types of external orifices (**a–d**)

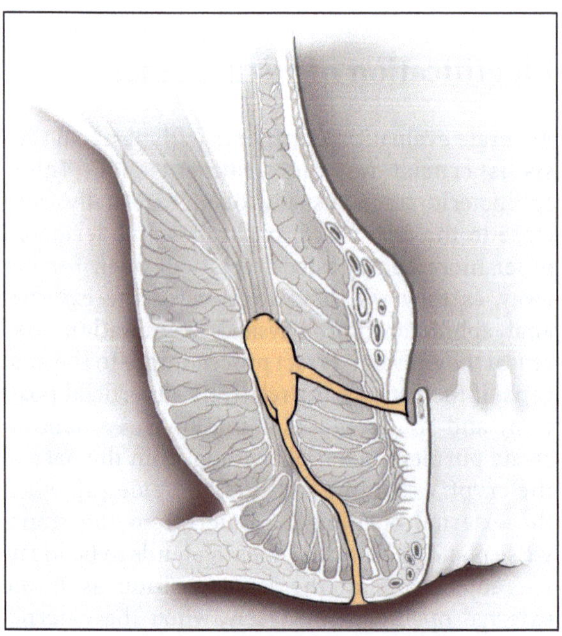

Fig. V.6. Schematic drawing of intersphincteric fistula

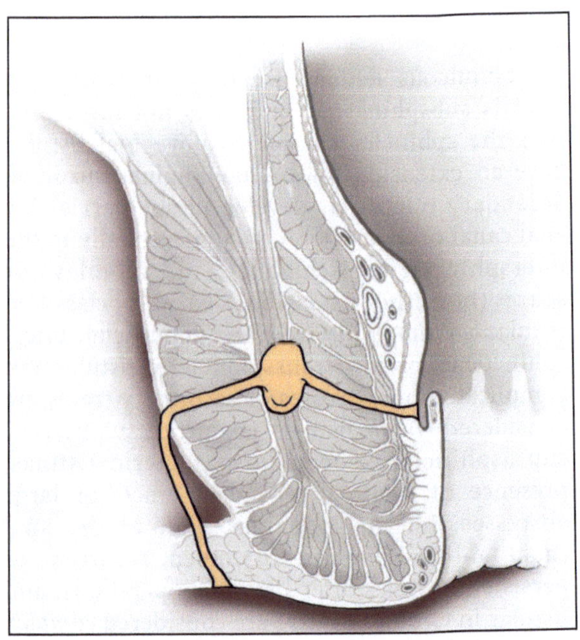

Fig. V.7. Schematic drawing of transsphincteric fistula

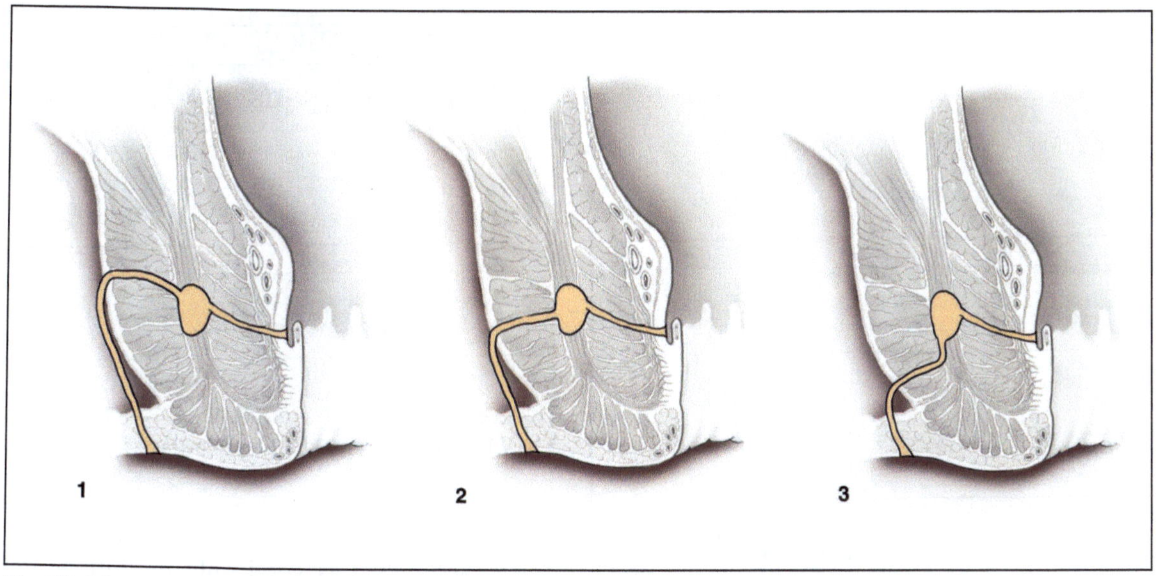

Fig. V.8. Schematic drawing of different types of transsphincteric fistula: *1* high, *2* mid, *3* low

opening is usually located in the posterior midline, irrespective of the site of the external opening (Fig. V.12). In the literature [9], a positive predictive value has been reported of 59% for primary fistulas (anterior fistulas: 72%, posterior fistulas: 41%) and 41% for recurrent fistulas (anterior fistulas: 67%, posterior fistulas: 12.5%) and, consequently, the use of Goodsall's rule alone in decision making before surgical intervention is not recommended.

Passage of a probe from both the external and the internal openings may confirm the course of the tract (Fig. V.13). However, a stenotic or sharply angulated tract may preclude complete passage from either end. Furthermore, this method is potentially dangerous because a false tract can be

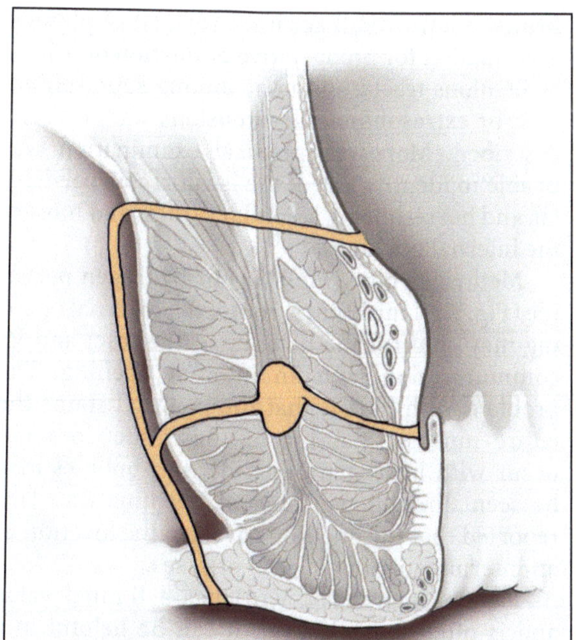

Fig. V.9. Schematic drawing of transsphincteric fistula with supralevator extension

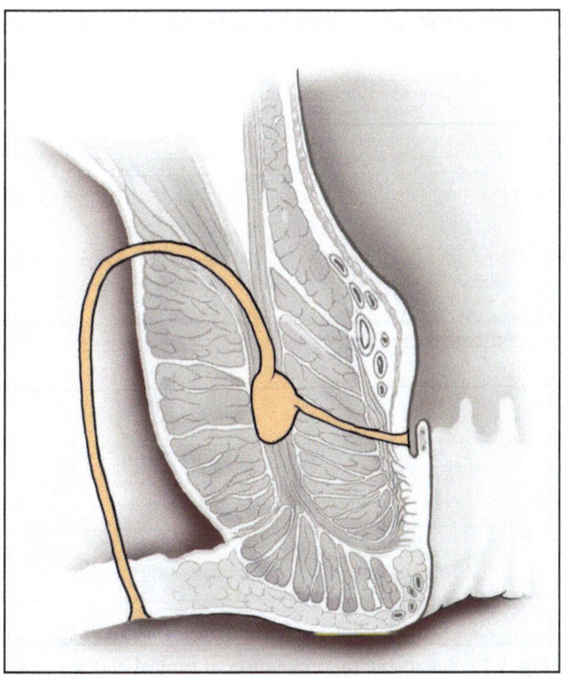

Fig. V.10. Schematic drawing of suprasphincteric fistula

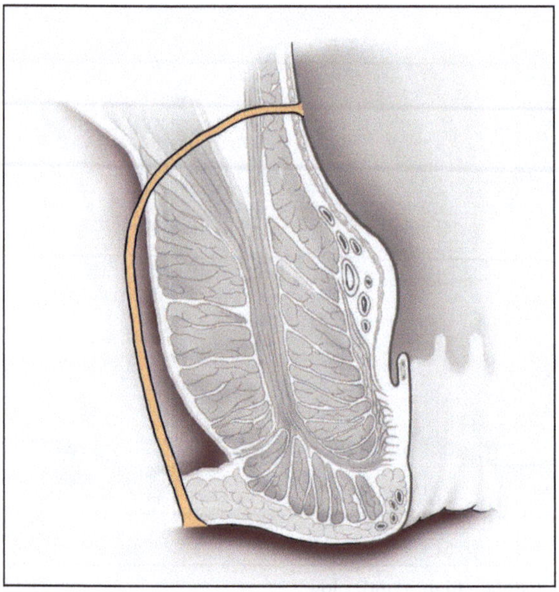

Fig. V.11. Schematic drawing of extrasphincteric fistula

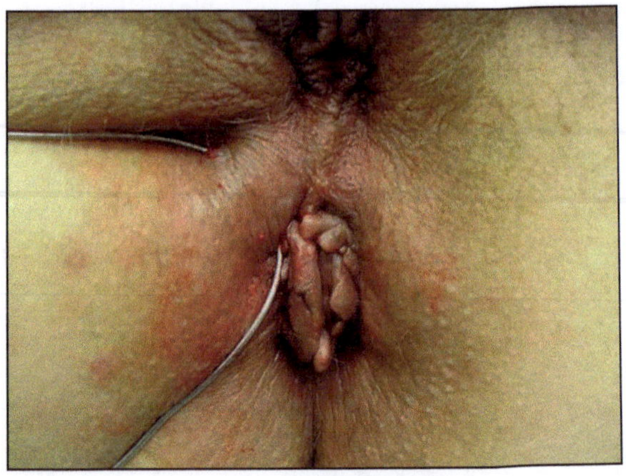

Fig. V.13. A probe is passed through the tract

made by an inexperienced surgeon. Seow-Choen et al. [10] reported results obtained by evaluating 38 patients. Physical examination was performed by a consultant and a research fellow, and the best accuracy rates were 85.3%, 71.4%, and 78.8% for primary and secondary tracts and the internal openings, respectively. Among primary tracts, physical examination could reach a very good accuracy in identifying superficial (100%) and transsphincteric (100%) tracts. As for secondary tracts, accuracy was good only for infralevator tracts (100%) but was inadequate for both supralevator (63.6%) and intersphincteric (33.3%) tracts. Deen et al. [11] evaluated 18 patients by physical examination and were able to identified only 50% of the internal openings and 27.3% of the horseshoe tracts. Poen at al. [12] studied 21 patients with fistulas. In their study, physical examination allowed a correct diagnosis of primary tracts in 38% of patients (less accurate in intersphincteric than transsphincteric fistulas) whereas 62% of patients were unclassified. The internal openings and secondary tracts were identified in 71% and 60% of patients, respectively. Ratto et al. [13] confirmed a low overall accuracy (65.4%) of physical examination for preoperative evaluation of primary fistulous tracts, and none among suprasphincteric or extrasphincteric extensions was correctly described. Moreover, physical examination was unable to identify any of the ischiorectal, pelvirectal, and horseshoeing secondary tracts and most of the internal openings.

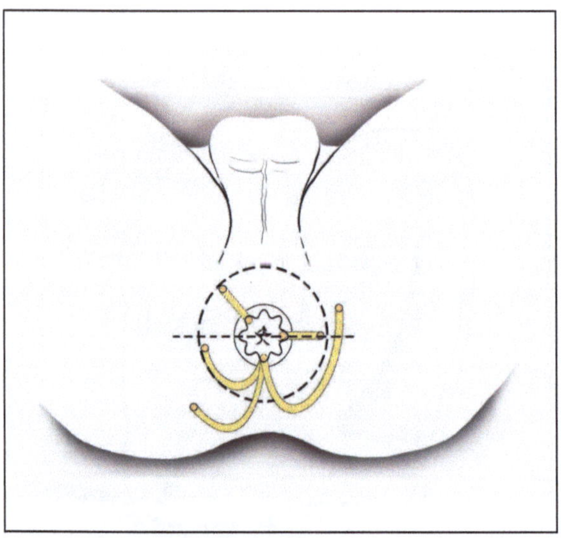

Fig. V.12. Schematic representation of typical courses of fistula tracts according to Goodsall's rule

Methylene blue (Fig. V.14) or hydrogen peroxide (Fig. V.15) injection through the external opening may confirm the patency of the tract and its communication with an internal opening. The problem with blue is that the material stains the entire mucosa. Staining of the tissue does not occur with hydrogen peroxide, and bubbles may be seen through the internal opening. Cho [14] reported that this method revealed the location of an internal opening in 76% of cases.

Fistulography (Fig. V.16) has a limited value and is often not tolerated. It can be helpful in a chronic fistula with an external opening distant from the anus. However, it can offer only indirect

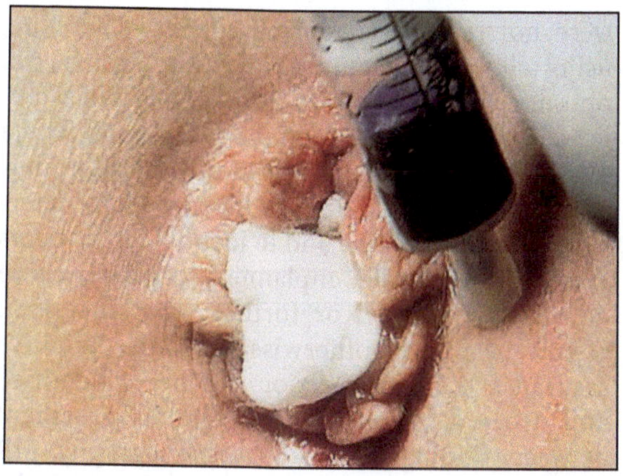

Fig. V.14. Methylene blue injection through the external orifice

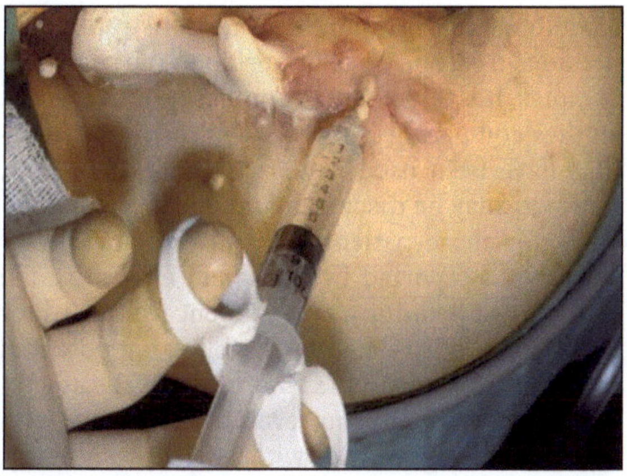

Fig. V.15. Hydrogen peroxide injection through the external orifice

and not very reliable information on the involvement of anal sphincters. Weisman et al. [15] found fistulography a useful diagnostic procedure in 26 of 27 (96.3%) patients studied and were able to alter surgical management in 48% of patients. Kuijpers and Schulpen [16] examined 25 patients with anal fistula and found that the fistulograms were correct in only 16%, and the internal orifice was identified in only 24% of patients. They considered fistulography an inaccurate and unreliable procedure and did not recommend it in the diagnosis of fistula-in-ano.

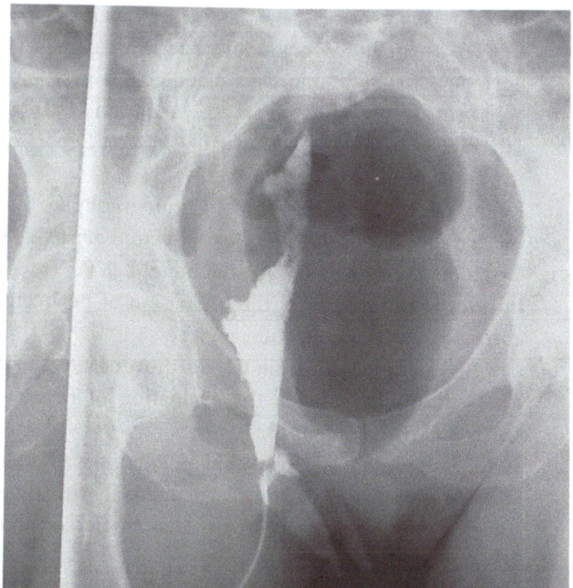

Fig. V.16. Fistulogram demonstrates the course of an extrasphincteric fistula

The importance of endoanal ultrasound (EAUS) in evaluating patients with perianal sepsis has been confirmed in numerous studies [10–13, 17–22]. The ultrasonographic images of the fistulous tract are well correlated with the operative findings [17, 18]. EAUS has better diagnostic specificity and sensitivity for the topography of the fistula and for the relationship between the sphincter and the fistula when compared with digital examination and computerized tomography [10].

Magnetic resonance imaging (MRI) has been suggested as a better diagnostic procedure [23–26]. However, differences in definition of fistulous tract have been described in relation to the technique used. Endoanal coil has been used for a long time; however, it has low definition of fistulas outside of the sphincter and, recently, a phased array technique has been preferred [27, 28]. Considering technical characteristics, time consumption, costs, and availability of the instruments in hospitals, in our opinion, MRI should be used in cases of complex fistula secondary to Crohn's disease, which is often associated with large abscesses and multiple tracts outside of the sphincter or in recurrent fistula, to distinguish fibrosis from active sepsis when EAUS is unable to give reliable information [29]. Buchanan et al. [30] have shown that surgery guided by MRI can reduce further recurrence by about 75% in recurrent fistula-in-ano.

In the following chapters, accuracy and reliability of endoanal ultrasonography in the evaluation of perianal abscesses and fistulas will be discussed. Endoanal ultrasonography and endoanal MRI will then be compared to determine which technique is more accurate for demonstration of a fistulous tract and its relationship to the sphincter complex. It is important to emphasize that in most studies comparing EAUS and MRI, surgical findings have been used as the gold standard. This, however, may be discussed and questioned, especially for those patients who did not heal after surgery. As reported by Buchanan et al. [21], the difficulty of defining a true reference standard for fistula-in-ano is related to the following potential source of bias: operators who perform the assessments can have differing levels of experience with anal endosonography or with MRI and, similarly, surgeons who perform the operations have different levels of experience. Barker et al. [31] showed that 9% of all fistulas do not heal, because fistulous tracts that were identified by endoanal MRI were not recognized during surgery. Therefore, using clinical outcome as the final arbiter can minimize potential biases. Because it is well established that the most common cause of fistula recurrence is infection missed at surgical examination, patients should be followed up to determine clinical outcome and to identify any patients who require further unplanned surgery because of a failure to heal or further recurrence [21]. Fistula healing is, otherwise, the only definitive assurance that all infection has been identified and treated. Thus, if there is disagreement between findings at anal endosonography, MR imaging, and surgical examination, it should be assumed to be correct the findings associated to fistula healing. This is defined as the outcome-derived reference standard [21].

References

1. Corman ML (1993) Anorectal abscess and fistula. In: Corman ML (ed) Colon and rectal surgery, 3rd edn. Lippincott, Philadelphia, pp. 133–187
2. Shafik A (1979) A new concept of the anatomy of the anal sphincter mechanism and the physiology of defecation. VI. The central abscess: a new clinicopathologic entity in the genesis of anorectal suppuration. Dis Colon Rectum 22:336–351
3. Shafik A (1979) A new concept of the anatomy of the anal sphincter mechanism and the physiology of defecation. VII. Anal fistula: a simplified classification. Dis Colon Rectum 22:408–414
4. Parks AG, Gordon PH, Hardcastle JD (1976) A classification of fistula-in-ano. Br J Surg 63:1–12
5. Buchanan GN, Williams AB, Bartram CI et al (2003) Potential clinical implications of direction of a trans-sphincteric anal fistula track. Br J Surg 90:1250–1255
6. Fazio VW (1987) Complex anal fistulae. Gastroenterol Clin North Am 16:93–114
7. Saller M, Fuchs KH, Kraemer M, Thiede A (1998) Stepwise concept for treatment of complex anal fistulas. Zentralb Chir 123:840–845
8. Goodsall DH (1900) Anorectal fistula. In: Goodsall DH, Miles WE (eds) Diseases of the anus and rectum, part I. Longmans, Green, London, pp. 92
9. Gunawardhana PA, Deen KI (2001) Comparison of hydrogen peroxide instillation with Goodsall's rule for fistula-in-ano. Aust NZ J Surg 71:472–474
10. Seow-Choen F, Burnett S, Bartram CI, Nicholls RJ (1991) Comparison between anal endosonography and digital examination in the evaluation of anal fistulae. Br J Surg 78:445–447
11. Deen KI, Williams JG, Hutchinson R et al (1994) Fistulas in ano: endoanal ultrasonographic assessment assists decision making for surgery. Gut 35:391–394
12. Poen AC, Felt-Bersma RJF, Eijsbouts QA et al (1998) Hydrogen peroxide-enhanced transanal ultrasound in the assessment of fistula-in-ano. Dis Colon Rectum 41:1147–1152
13. Ratto C, Gentile E, Merico M et al (2000) How can the assessment of fistula-in-ano be improved? Dis Colon Rectum 43:1375–1382
14. Cho DY (1999) Endosonographic criteria for an internal opening of fistula-in-ano. Dis Colon Rectum 42:515–518
15. Weisman RI, Orsay CP, Pearl RK, Abcarian H (1991) The role of fistulography in fistula-in-ano. Report of five cases. Dis Colon Rectum 34:181–184
16. Kuijpers HC, Schulpen T (1985) Fistulography for fistula-in-ano: is it useful? Dis Colon Rectum 28:103–104
17. Cataldo PA, Senagore A, Luchtefeld MA (1993) Intrarectal ultrasound in the evaluation of perirectal abscesses. Dis Colon Rectum 36:554–558
18. Law PJ, Talbot RW, Bartram CI, Northover JMA (1989) Anal endosonography in the evaluation of perianal sepsis and fistula in ano. Br J Surg 76:752–755
19. Sudol-Szopinska I, Szczepkowski M, Panorska AK et al (2004) Comparison of contrast-enhanced with non-contrast endosonography in the diagnostics of anal fistulas. Eur Radiol 14:2236–2241
20. Lindsey I, Humphreys MM, George BD, Mortensen NJ (2002) The role of anal ultrasound in the management of anal fistulas. Colorectal Dis 4:118–122

21. Buchanan GN, Halligan S, Bartram CI et al (2004) Clinical examination, endosonography and MR imaging in preoperative assessment of fistula in ano: comparison with outcome-based reference standard. Radiology 233:674–681
22. Bartram C, Buchanan G (2003) Imaging anal fistula. Radiol Clin N Am 41:443–457
23. Halligan S, Healy JC, Bartram CI (1998) Magnetic resonance imaging of fistula-in-ano: STIR or SPIR? Br J Radiol 71:141–145
24. Buchanan G, Halligan S, Taylor S et al (2004) MRI of fistula in ano: inter and intraobserver agreement and effects of directed education. AJR Am J Roentgenol 183:135–140
25. Beets-Tan RGH, Beets GL, Gerritsen van der Hoop A et al (2001) Preoperative MR imaging of anal fistula: does it really help the surgeon? Radiology 218:75–84
26. Maier AG, Funovics MA, Kreuzer SH et al (2001) Evaluation of perianal sepsis: comparison of anal endosonography and magnetic resonance imaging. J Magnet Reson Imaging 14:254–260
27. DeSouza NM, Gilderdale DJ, Coutts GA et al (1998) MRI of fistula-in-ano: a comparison of endoanal coil with external phased array coil techniques. J Comput Assist Tomogr 22:357–363
28. Hussain SM, Stoker J, Schouten WR et al (1996) Fistula-in-ano: endoanal sonography versus endoanal MR imaging in classification. Radiology 200:475–481
29. Gustafsson UM, Kahvecioglu B, Astrom G et al (2001) Endoanal ultrasound or magnetic resonance imaging for preoperative assessment of anal fistula: a comparative study. Colorectal Dis 3:189–197
30. Buchanan G, Halligan S, Williams A et al (2002) Effect of MRI on clinical outcome of recurrent fistula-in-ano. Lancet 360:1661–1662
31. Barker PG, Lunniss PJ, Armstrong P et al (1994) Magnetic resonance imaging of fistula in ano: technique, interpretation and accuracy. Clin Radiol 49:7–13

V.2.
Accuracy and Reliability of Endoanal Ultrasonography in the Evaluation of Perianal Abscesses and Fistula-in-ano

G.A. Santoro, C. Ratto

The configuration of perianal sepsis and the relationship of abscesses or fistulas with internal and external sphincters are most important factors influencing the results of surgical management [1]. Preoperative identification of all loculate purulent areas and definition of the anatomy of the primary fistulous tract, secondary extensions, and the internal opening plays an important role in adequate planning of the operative approach in order to ensure complete drainage of abscesses, to prevent early recurrence after surgical treatment, and to minimize iatrogenic damage of sphincters and the risk of minor or major degrees of incontinence. It has been suggested that detailed knowledge of fistula characteristics may allow a reduction in the occurrence of both these adverse events [2]. Clinical evaluation, including fistula probing, has severe limitations on account of poor reliability in detecting the location of the internal opening and the possible existence of secondary tracts [3–7]. On the other hand, fistulography, traditionally adopted in the diagnostic workup, has been shown to be of poor accuracy in correlating the tract route with the local anatomic musculature and spaces [2–3, 8–9].

Over the last two decades, endoanal ultrasonography (EAUS) has been demonstrated to be a very helpful diagnostic tool, showing interesting features in accurately assessing all fistula or abscess characteristics [4–6, 9–13]. EAUS can be easily repeated while following patients with perianal sepsis to choose the optimal timing and modality of surgical treatment, to evaluate integrity or damage of sphincters after operation, and to identify fistula recurrence. EAUS still has some limitations and requires experience, but it is a rapid, simple, and well-tolerated technique. It also gives information about the state of the anal sphincters, which is valuable in performing successful fistula surgery. A fistula tract affecting minimal muscle can be safely excised, but where the bulk of external sphincter muscle is affected, it is best treated by seton drainage or mucosal advancement flap [1]. However, EAUS does not provide an adequate deep and global display of all adjacent pelvic and perineal spaces that may be involved.

The addition of hydrogen peroxide injection through the external opening of the fistula appears to improve the diagnostic accuracy of standard EAUS; where it is injected, hydrogen peroxide produces a significant increase in the echogenicity of the fistulous tract, which then appears as hyperechoic instead of hypoechoic. This method of hydrogen-peroxide-enhanced ultrasonography (HPUS) can thus be helpful in identifying tracts that had not been observed at the standard EAUS examination or the presence of which had not been definitively established [14, 15]. It can be also particularly useful when an active fistulous tract needs to be distinguished from postsurgical or posttrauma scar tissue that can cause tissue alterations that are difficult to analyze [15]. Moreover, HPUS has proven superior to conventional EAUS in the assessment and classification of fistula-in-ano in patients with Crohn's disease [16].

A new technique is three-dimensional (3-D) EAUS, which enables reconstruction of transversal images of the anal canal in the coronal and sagittal planes. The use of 3-D EAUS might be very helpful in tracing the pathway of a tract and should be able to provide a significant contribution by increasing accuracy. *Volume render mode* is a special feature that successfully can be applied to high-resolution 3-D data volumes. Imaging processing includes maximum intensity, minimum intensity, and summed voxel projections, combined with positional or intensity weighting. This technique changes the depth information of 3-D data volume so information inside the cube to some extent is reconstructed.

Endoanal Ultrasonography Findings

The ultrasound examination is generally started using 10 MHz, changing to 7 or 5 MHz to optimize visualization of the deeper structures external to the anal sphincters. The puborectalis muscle and external, longitudinal, and internal sphincters should always be identified and used as referents for the spatial orientation of the fistula or abscess.

An anal abscess appears as a hypoechoic dishomogeneous area, sometimes with hyperechoic spots within it, possibly in connection with a fistulous tract directed through the anal canal lumen. Infection can spread in a number of directions, usually along the path of least resistance (Fig. V.17). Abscesses are classified as superficial (Fig. V.18), intersphincteric (Fig. V.19), ischiorectal (Fig. V.20), supralevator (Fig. V.21), pelvirectal (Fig. V.22), and horseshoe (Fig.V.23).

An anal fistula appears as a hypoechoic tract, which is followed along its crossing of the subepithelium, internal or external sphincters, and through the perianal spaces. With regard to the anal sphincters, according to the classification by Parks et al. [3], the fistulous primary tract can be classified into four types:

1. Intersphincteric tract, which is presented as a band of poor reflectivity within the longitudinal layer, causing widening and distortion of an otherwise narrow intersphincteric plane (Figs. V.24 and 25). The tract goes through the intersphincteric space without traversing the external sphincter fibers
2. Transsphincteric tract, in which the extension through the external sphincter is clearly shown by a poorly reflective tract running out through the external sphincter and disrupting its normal architecture (Fig. V.26). The point at which the main tract of the fistula traverses the sphincters defines the fistula level. The transsphincteric fistulas are divided into high, medium, or low, corresponding to the ultrasound level of the anal canal. The low

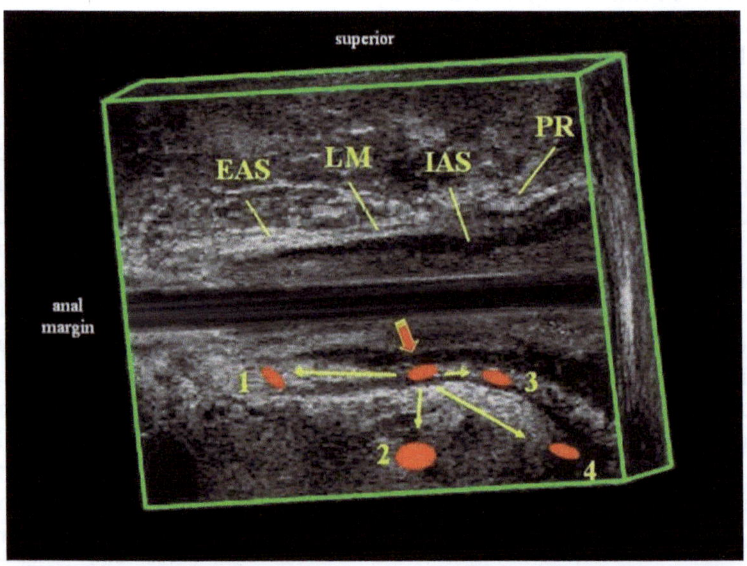

Fig. V.17. Sagittal view from a three-dimensional data set. Infection of the anal gland at the level of the dentate line (*arrow*) can spread superficially (*1*) or in the ischioanal (*2*), intersphincteric (*3*), or suprasphincteric (*4*) spaces. *EAS* external anal sphincter, *LM* longitudinal muscle, *IAS* internal anal sphincter, *PR* puborectalis muscle

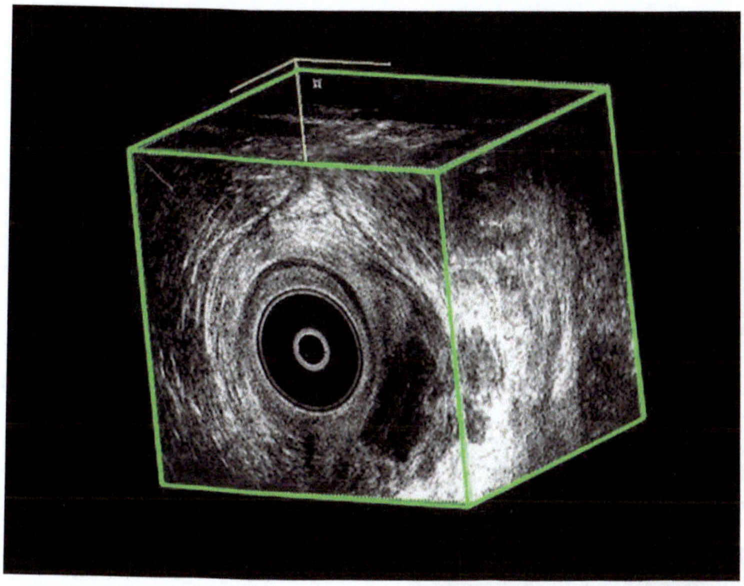

Fig. V.18. Acute superficial abscess presenting as an area of low reflectivity in the left side of the anal canal below the level of the internal sphincter

transsphincteric tract traverses only the distal third of the external sphincter at the lower portion of the medium anal canal (Fig. V.27). The medium transsphincteric tract traverses both sphincters, external and internal, in the middle part of the medium anal canal (Fig. V.28). The high transsphincteric tract traverses both sphincters in the higher part of the medium anal canal in the space below the puborectalis muscle (Fig. V.29)

3. Suprasphincteric tract, which goes above or through the puborectalis level (Fig. V.30). To detect supralevator extension, it is often necessary to fit the rectal balloon system to make contact with the distal rectal wall
4. Extrasphincteric tract, which may be seen close to but more laterally placed around the external sphincter (Fig. V.31).

Differentiation between granulated tracts and scars is sometimes difficult. Straight tracts are easily identified, but smaller and oblique tracts are more difficult to image. Secondary tracts, when present, are related to the main one and are

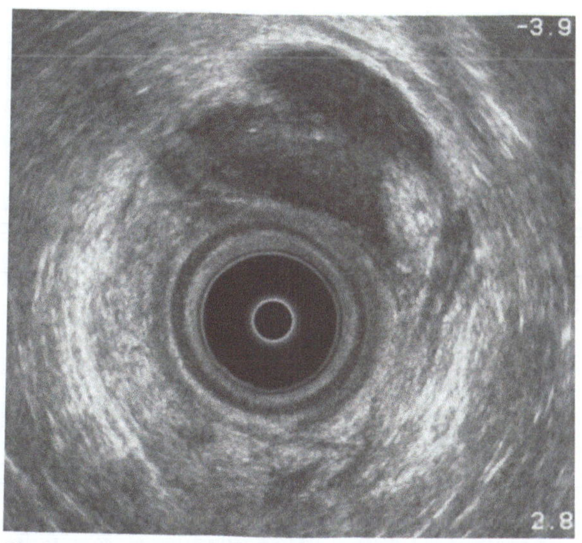

Fig. V.19. Acute intersphincteric abscess presenting as an area of low reflectivity in the anterior intersphincteric space

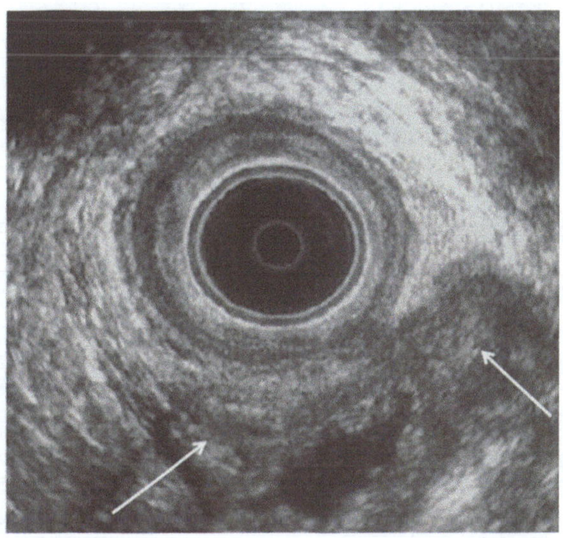

Fig. V.20. Acute abscess in the deep posterior ischioanal space (*arrows*)

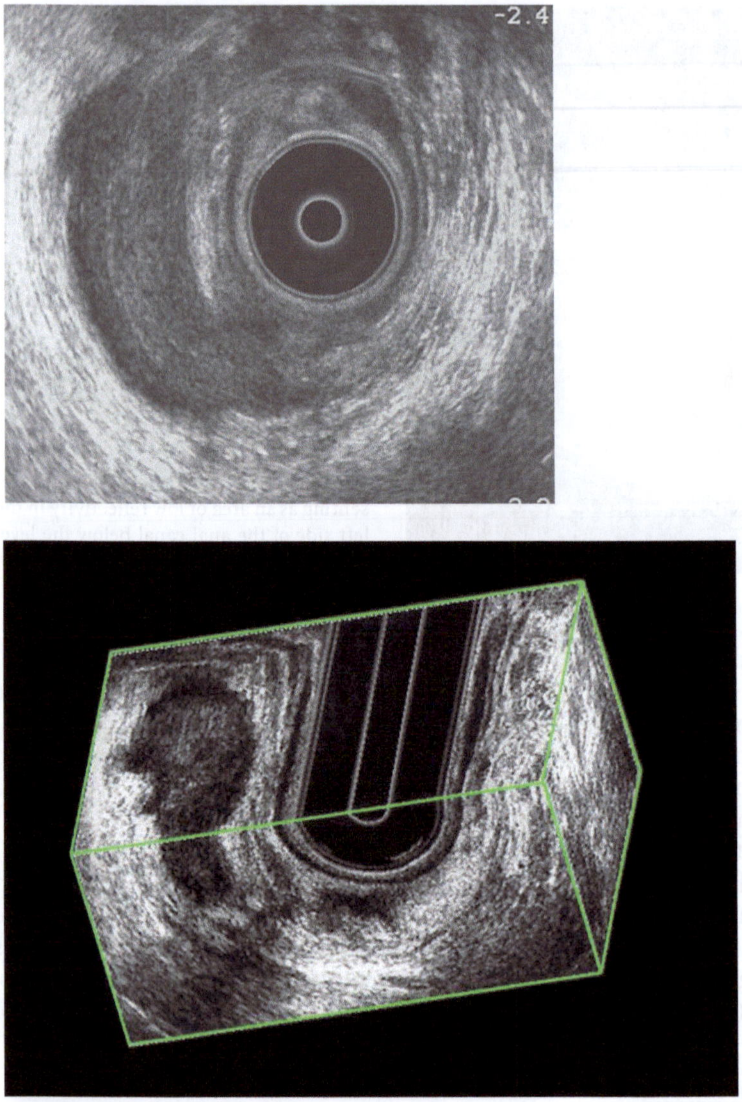

a

b

Fig. V.21. Acute supralevator abscess presenting as an area of low reflectivity in the right side of the anal canal deep beyond the puborectalis muscle (a). Coronal view from a three-dimensional data set (b). The longitudinal extension of the collection is more easily appreciated

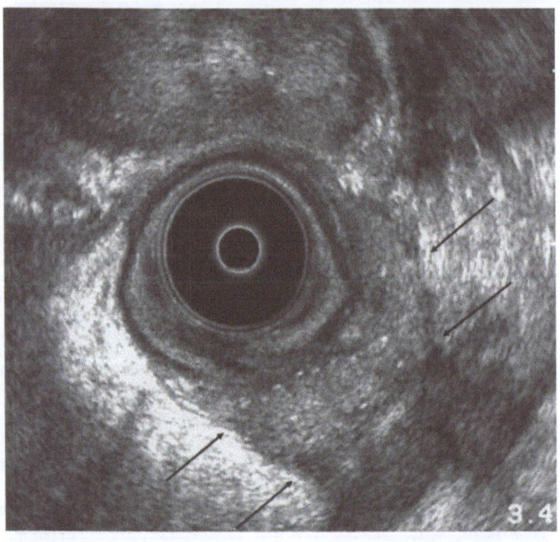

Fig. V.22. Pelvirectal abscess (*arrows*) at the prostate level, developed for a dehiscence of a colorectal anastomosis for rectal cancer

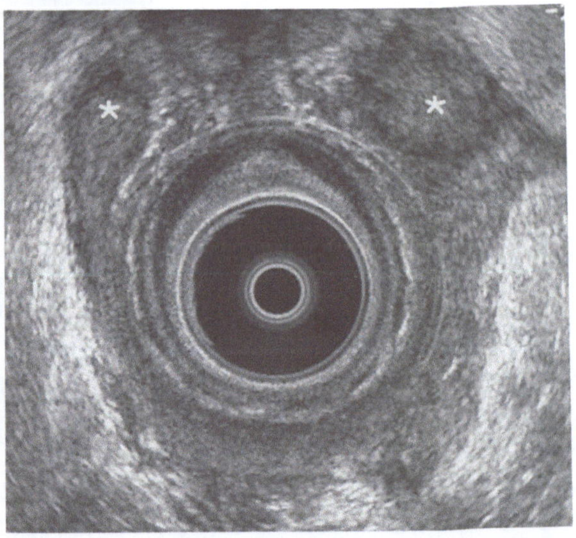

Fig. V.23. Horseshoe collection in the supralevator space

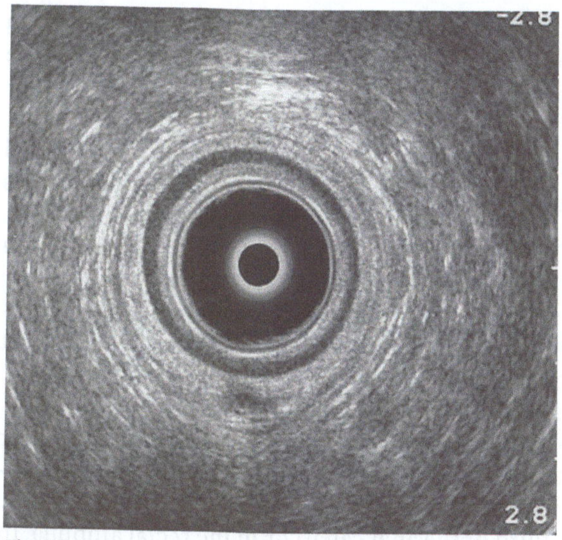

Fig. V.24. Posterior intersphincteric fistula at 6 o'clock

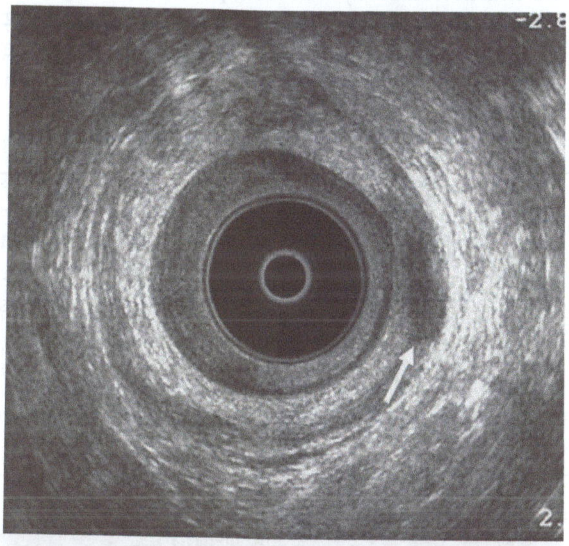

a

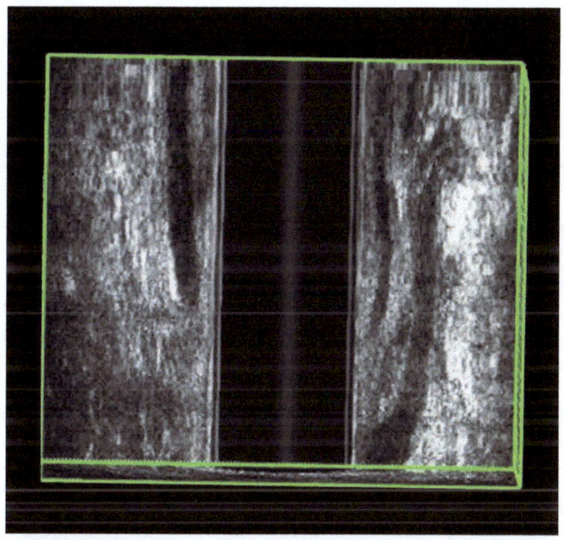

b

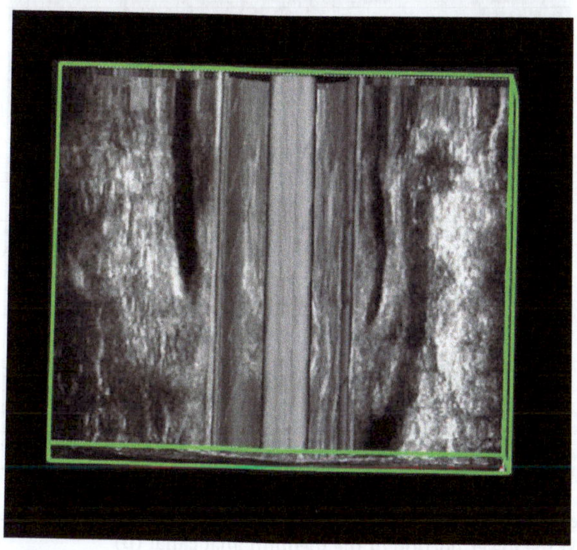

c

Fig. V.25. Axial endosonographic image of mid anal canal level. A hypoechoic area in the intersphincteric space is present at 3 o'clock (*arrow*) (**a**). Three-dimensional reconstruction in the coronal plane confirms an intersphincteric tract, appearing as a band of poor reflectivity within the plane, causing widening and distortion of an otherwise narrow plane. The tract extends through the intersphincteric space without traversing the external sphincter fibers (**b**). Volume render mode of the same image as in b (**c**)

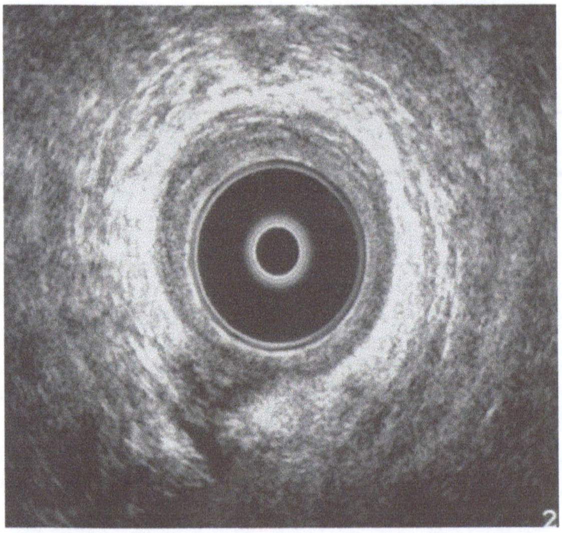

Fig. V.26. Posterior transsphincteric tract extending through the external sphincter

classified as intersphincteric, transsphincteric, suprasphincteric, or extrasphincteric (Fig. V.32). Similarly, horseshoe tracts, when identified, are categorized as intersphincteric, suprasphincteric, or extrasphincteric (Fig. V.33).

The dentate line is not visible as an anatomical structure but is assumed to be just below the midpoint of the internal sphincter. For this reason, the internal opening of an anal fistula is seldom clearly defined.

Endosonographic criteria for the site of an internal opening, according to Cho [17], are the following:

1. An appearance of a root-like budding formed by the intersphincteric tract, which contacts the internal anal sphincter (IAS) (Fig. V.34)
2. An appearance of a root-like budding with an IAS defect (Fig. V.35)
3. A subepithelial breach connecting to the intersphincteric tract through an IAS defect (Fig. V.36).

The site is categorized as being above, at, or below the dentate line (in relation to the presumed location of the dentate line at the middle third of the anal canal) or in the rectal ampulla. In addition, the site of the internal opening can also be characterized by the clock position, being classified from 1 to 12 o'clock. The internal opening can be identified as hypoechoic (when acute inflammation is present) or hyperechoic (when chronically inflamed).

After standard EAUS examination, in patients in whom the external fistula opening is patent, 1.0–2.0 ml of 3% hydrogen peroxide can be injected very slowly using an 18-gauge plastic cannula via this opening while ultrasonic scanning of the anal canal is performed [18]. When no obvious external opening is present, a focal, elevated, erythematous region immediately adjacent to the

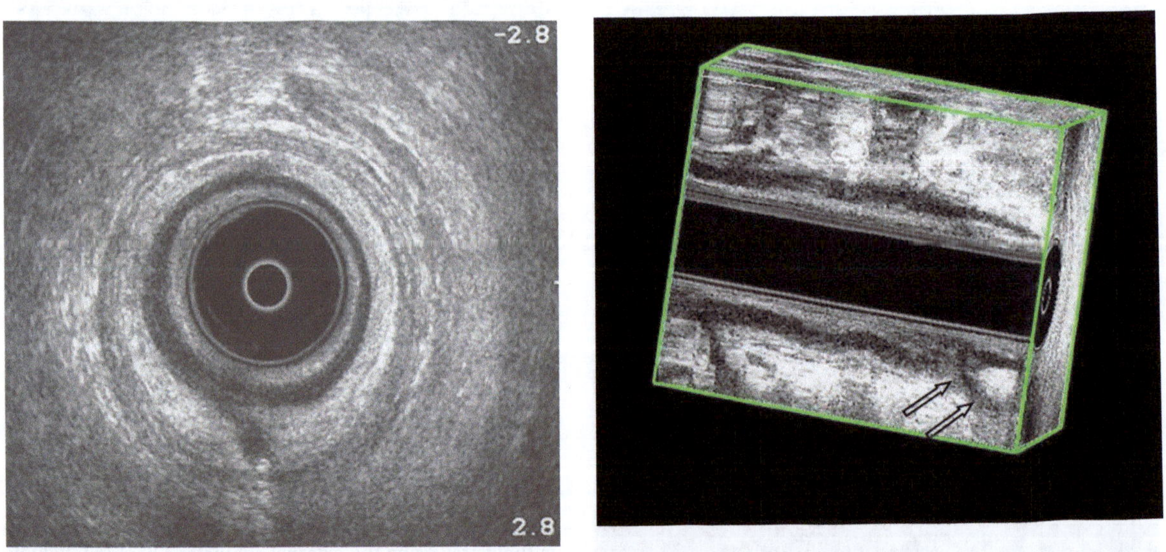

Fig. V.27. Low transsphincteric fistula at 6 o'clock (**a**). Sagittal view from a three-dimensional data set confirming that the tract (*arrows*) traverses only the distal third of the external sphincter at the lower portion of the medium anal canal (**b**)

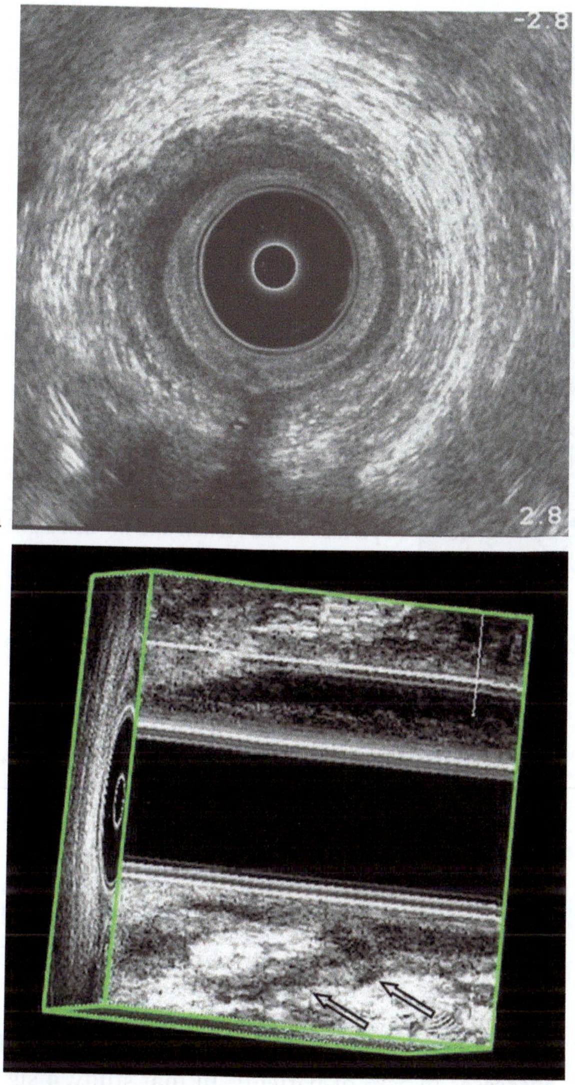

a

b

Fig. V.28. Medium transsphincteric fistula at 6 o'clock (**a**). Sagittal view from a three-dimensional data set confirming that the tract (*arrows*) traverses the middle part of the external sphincter (**b**)

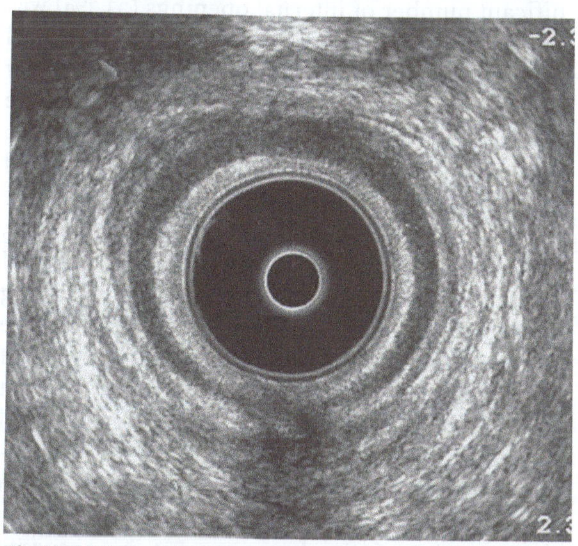

Fig. V.29. High transsphincteric tract traversing both sphincters in the higher part of the medium anal canal in the space below the puborectalis

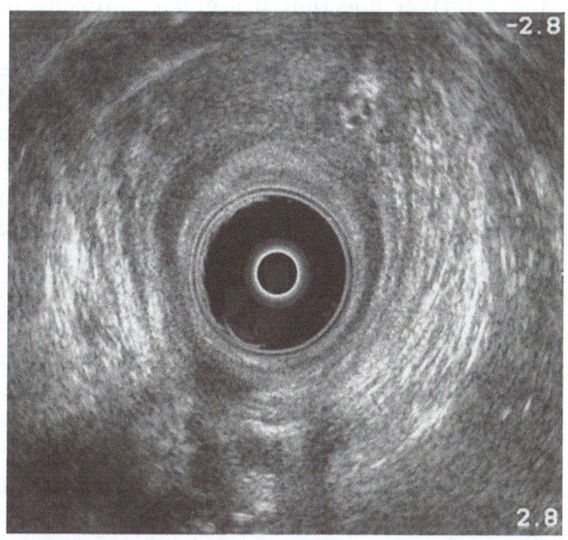

Fig. V.30. Suprasphincteric tract extending through the puborectalis muscle

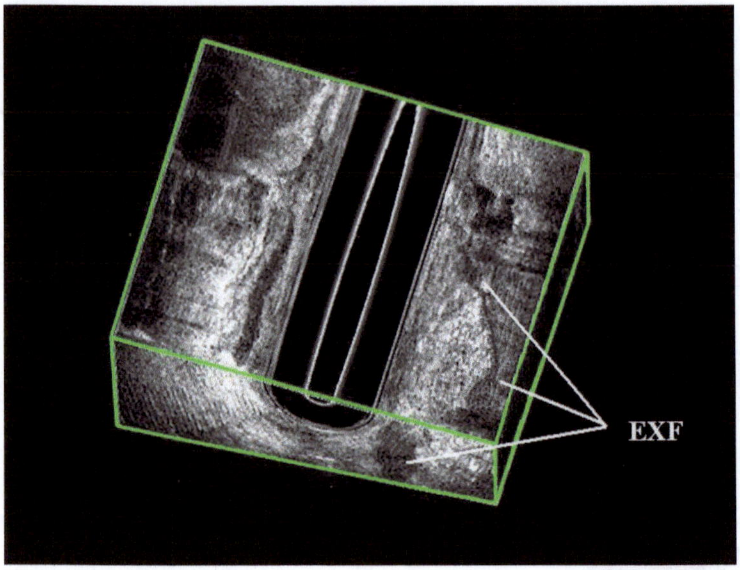

Fig. V.31. Extrasphincteric fistula (*EXF*) with direct communication between the perineum and rectum and no anal canal involvement

anal orifice is frequently identified. The soft catheter tip should be firmly pressed onto or probed into the center of this region, where the skin is easily broken, and the external opening located. Gas is a strong ultrasound reflector, and after injection fistula tracks become hyperechoic, and the internal opening is identified as an echogenic breach at the submucosa (Fig. V.37). According to Navarro-Luna et al. [19], injection should be performed in two phases: an initial injection of a small amount of hydrogen peroxide and a further injection at a greater pressure to determine whether there are secondary tracts that initially might be undetected [19]. During this technique, however, the operator must be careful because the injected hydrogen peroxide often results in bubbling into the anal canal, which then acts as a barrier to the ultrasound wave. Another disadvantage inherent to hydrogen peroxide injection is the very strong reflection that occurs at a gas/tissue interface, which blanks out any detail deep beyond this interface. The bubbles produced by hydrogen peroxide induce acoustic shadowing deep beyond the tract, so all information deep beyond the inner surface of the tract is lost (Fig. V.38). To reduce this potential pitfall of imaging, a volume-rendered 3-D data set can facilitate the following of a tortuous fistula tract due to the transparency and depth information (Fig. V.39).

Accuracy and Reliability

EAUS is able to identify the echo structure of the anal sphincters and allow the accurate identification of perianal sepsis. An early report [10] from St. Mark's Hospital, London, described the good tolerability of this procedure and its accuracy for the selective identification of fistula and abscess configurations. Primary tracts were correctly detected in 91.7% of patients and perianal abscesses in 75% of patients. In that study, a significant number of internal openings (33.3%) was not identified by use of a break in the mucosal layer as endosonographic criterion, possibly because of the proximity of the mucosa to the probe so that it was not within focal range. Subsequently, Seow-Choen et al. [5] underlined the high accuracy of EAUS in detecting a large proportion of internal openings, intersphincteric, and transsphincteric tracts. They described revised ultrasonographic criteria for identifying an internal opening, which included one or more of the following features: a hypoechoic breach of the subepithelial layer of the anorectum, a defect in the circular muscles of the internal anal sphincter, and a hypoechoic lesion of the normally hyperechoic longitudinal muscle abutting on the normally hypoechoic circular smooth muscle. In spite of the improvement in accuracy (73%), their results revealed no significant differ-

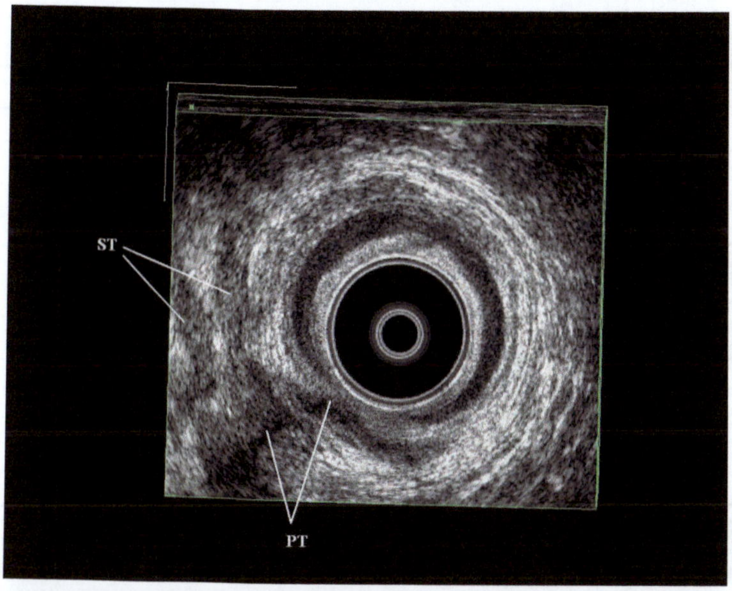

a

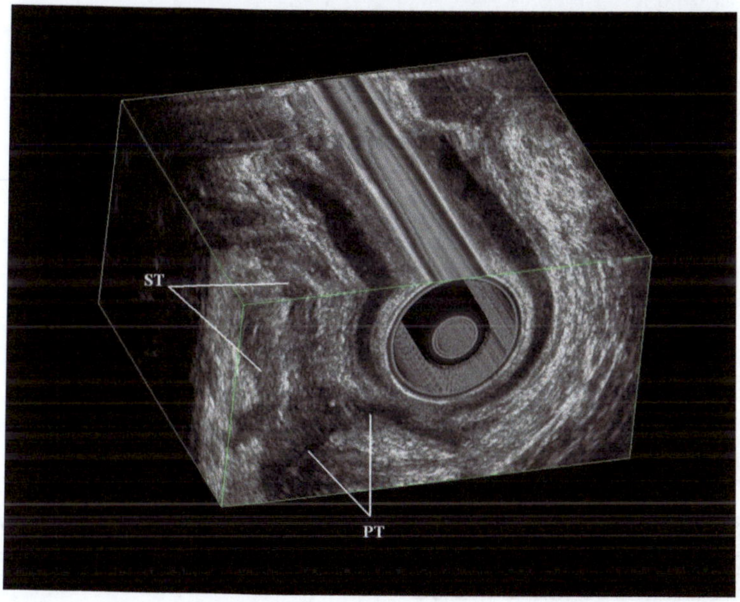

b

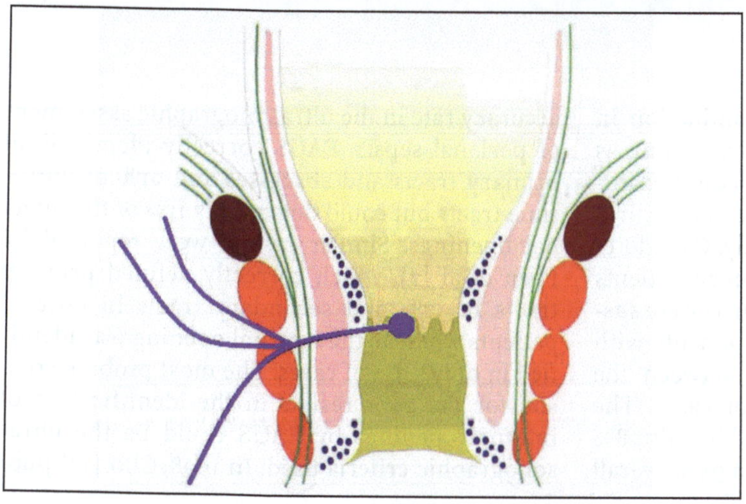

c

Fig. V.32. Posterior transsphincteric fistula (**a**) (*PT* primary tract) with two secondary transsphincteric tracts (*ST* secondary tracts) extending through the ischioanal space. Three-dimensional reconstruction (**b**). Schematic representation (**c**)

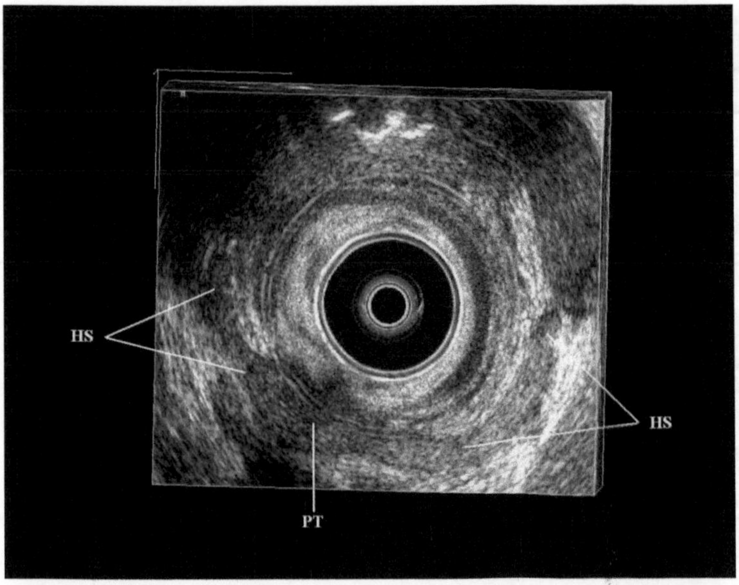

a

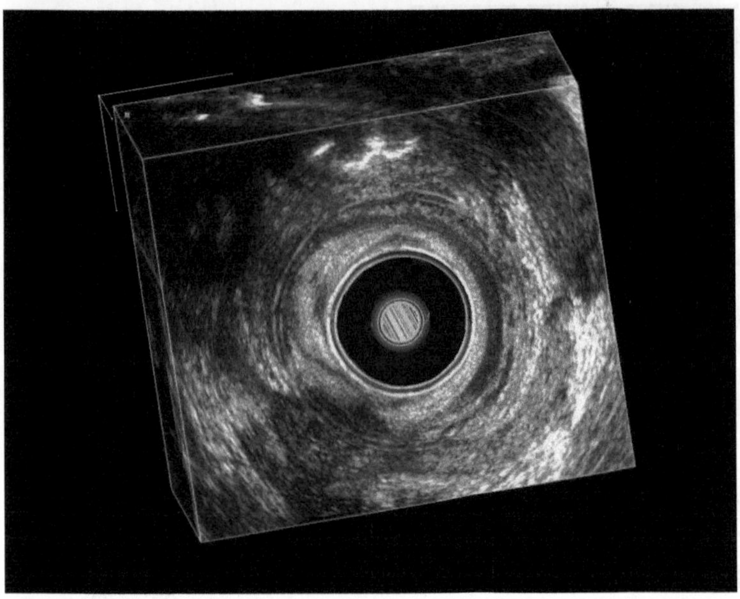

b

Fig. V.33. Posterior transsphincteric fistula (**a**) (*PT* primary tract) with horseshoe (*HS*) secondary extension through the intersphincteric space. Volume render mode (**b**)

ence between EAUS and digital examination in the assessment of internal openings. Among 35 patients with fistulas and 34 with abscesses examined by Kuntz et al. [12], EAUS showed an accuracy rate of 77.1 and 100%, respectively. Cataldo et al. [11] used EAUS intraoperatively in 24 patients in whom perianal abscesses and fistulas were suspected and correctly identified all patients with abscess, defining the relationship between the abscesses and sphincters in 63% of cases. The internal opening, however, was found in only 28% of patients. Deen et al. [6] obtained a 94% overall accuracy rate in the ultrasonographic assessment of perianal sepsis. EAUS correctly identified all primary tracts and abscesses and 91% of horseshoe tracts but could detect only 11% of the internal openings. Similar results were reported by Poen et al [7], which correctly defined primary tracts in 57% and secondary tracts in 60% of patients whereas the internal opening was identified in only 5.3% of cases. The most probable reason for the poor results in the identification of internal openings by EAUS could be the ultrasonographic criteria used. In 1998, Cho [17] pub-

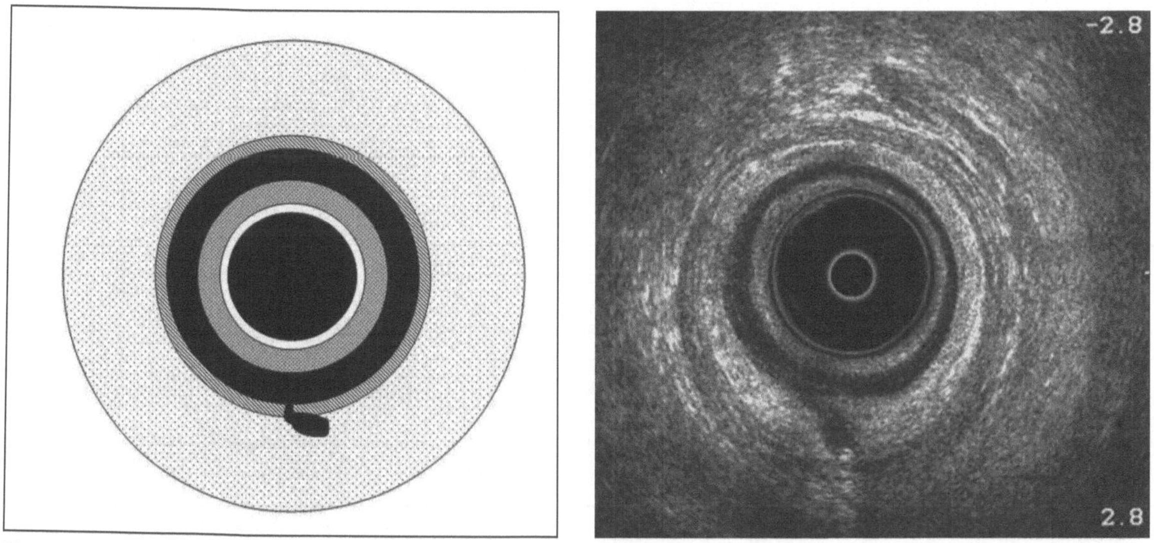

a b

Fig. V.34. First endosonographic criteria for the site of an internal opening according to Cho [17]: an appearance of a root-like budding formed by the intersphincteric tract, which contacts the internal sphincter (**a, b**)

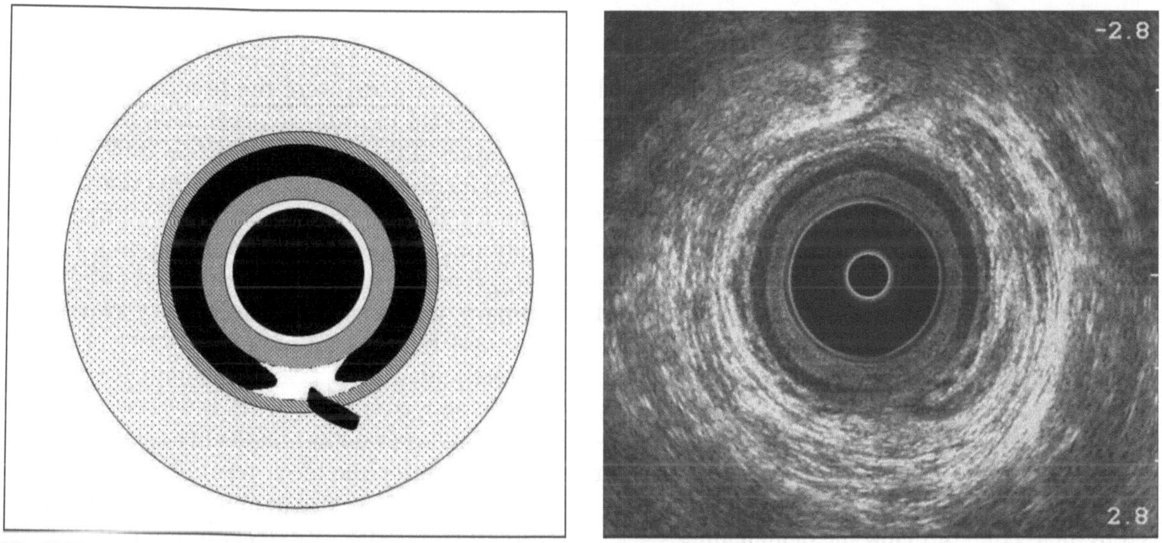

a b

Fig. V.35. Second endosonographic criteria for the site of an internal opening according to Cho [17]: a root-like budding with an appearance of internal sphincter defect due to inflammatory changes within the sphincter increasing its reflectivity locally (**a, b**)

lished new criteria for diagnosing internal opening. Using a combination of his three endosonographic criteria, the sensitivity of EAUS was 94%, specificity 87%, positive predictive value 81%, and negative predictive value 96%. Ratto et al. [14] showed that although EAUS improves definition of fistula anatomy compared with clinical evaluation alone, it is not accurate in defining primary tracts in approximately one half of patients. EAUS was more accurate in transsphincteric fistulas than intersphincteric tracts but could not correctly identify suprasphincteric or extrasphincteric tracts.

The major problems while investigating primary tracts with EAUS occur because of the structure alterations of the anal canal and perianal muscles and tissues, which can overstage the fistula, or poor definition of the tract when filled with inflammatory tissue, which can downstage the fistula. The disappointing results of EAUS in diagnosing extrasphincteric fistulas could be due to the echogenicity of the fistula, especially those

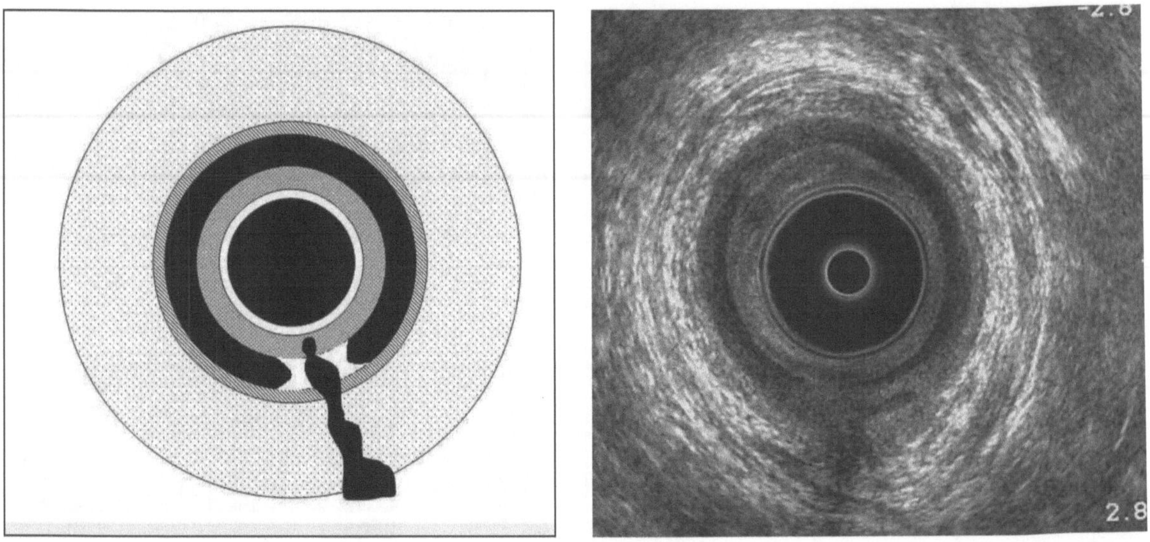

a b

Fig. V.36. Third endosonographic criteria for the site of an internal opening according to Cho [17]: a subepithelial breach connecting to the intersphincteric tract through an internal sphincter defect (**a, b**)

with narrow lumen, which is practically identical to the fat tissue in the ischiorectal fossa and to the short focal length of the transducer and thus prevents imaging fistula from running a large distance from the anal canal. Concerning secondary tracts, approximately two thirds of all patients were accurately identified, and false findings occurred mostly because of overstaging. EAUS did not adequately identify any secondary ischiorectal, pelvirectal, or horseshoe tracts. In comparison with clinical assessment, EAUS significantly improved accuracy in finding the internal openings, but it could not categorize it in 15–20% of patients, particularly when the opening was located in the rectum or below the dentate line.

The reported diagnostic accuracy of HPUS ranges from 71 to 95% for primary tracts and from 63 to 96.1% for secondary tracts while that of standard EAUS ranges from 50 to 91.7% for the primary tract and from 60 to 68% for secondary tracts (Table V.1). The highest concordance is usually reported for primary transsphincteric fistulas while the major of diagnostic difficulty is still the adequate identification of primary supra- and extrasphincteric fistulas. HPUS also can contribute to a more accurate identification of the internal opening. In comparison to results reported using standard EAUS with an accuracy ranging from 5.3 to 93.5%, the reported accuracy of HPUS is higher, ranging from 48 to 96.6%. Cheong et al. [26] were the first to describe the use of HPUS in order to accentuate tissue interface layers at the level of the fistula tract and suggested its usefulness particularly in recurrent and complex fistulas. Subsequently, in a prospective study of 21 patients with fistula-in-ano, Poen et al. [7] reported an HPUS accuracy rate of 95% for primary tracts, 71% for secondary extensions, and 48% for internal openings. Ratto et al. [14] correctly identified 75% of primary tracts using HPUS, and compared with EAUS, this method was more accurate in identifying transsphincteric and intersphincteric tracts. However, both EAUS and HPUS were unable to identify suprasphincteric and extrasphincteric tracts. Approximately 85% of secondary tracts were correctly staged with HPUS, with an accuracy of nearly 90% for intersphincteric and ischiorectal tracts. HPUS failed, however, to improve the ability of EAUS to identify the internal openings, particularly when located below the dentate line or in the rectal ampulla. In this regard, Moscowitz et al. [27] reported a 61.1% correlation between HPUS and surgical findings of the internal opening, with a positive predictive value of 84%. Poor results were reported by Ortiz et al. [28], who correctly identified an internal opening endosonographically in 62.5% of patients (32% with intersphincteric fistulas, 77% with transsphincteric fistulas, and 17% with suprasphincteric fistulas).

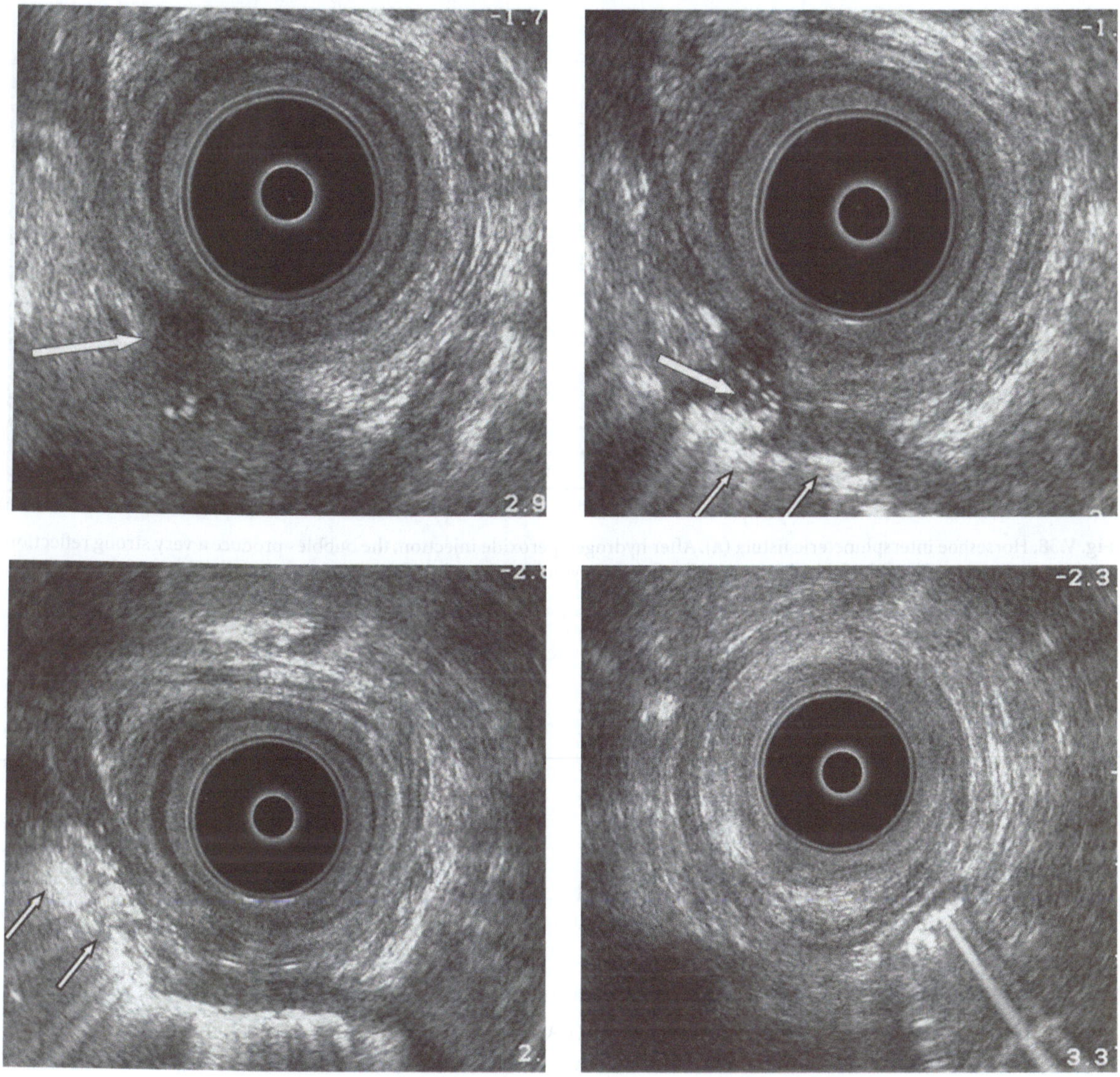

a b c d

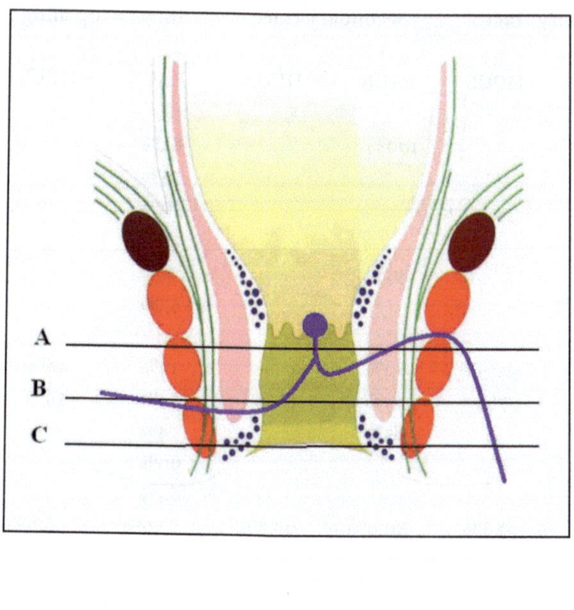

e

Fig. V.37. Posterior transsphincteric tract extending through the external sphincter (*arrow*). No secondary extensions are clearly visible. Higher part of the anal canal (level A) (**a**). After hydrogen peroxide, fistula tract becomes hyperechoic (*large arrow*), and a secondary hyperchoic horseshoe extension through the left and right ischioanal spaces (*small arrows*) becomes evident. Middle part of the anal canal (level B) (**b, c**). Lower part of the anal canal (level C) subcutaneous echogenic area at 5 o'clock (external opening) (**d**). Schematic representation of the fistulous tract at the three different levels (**e**)

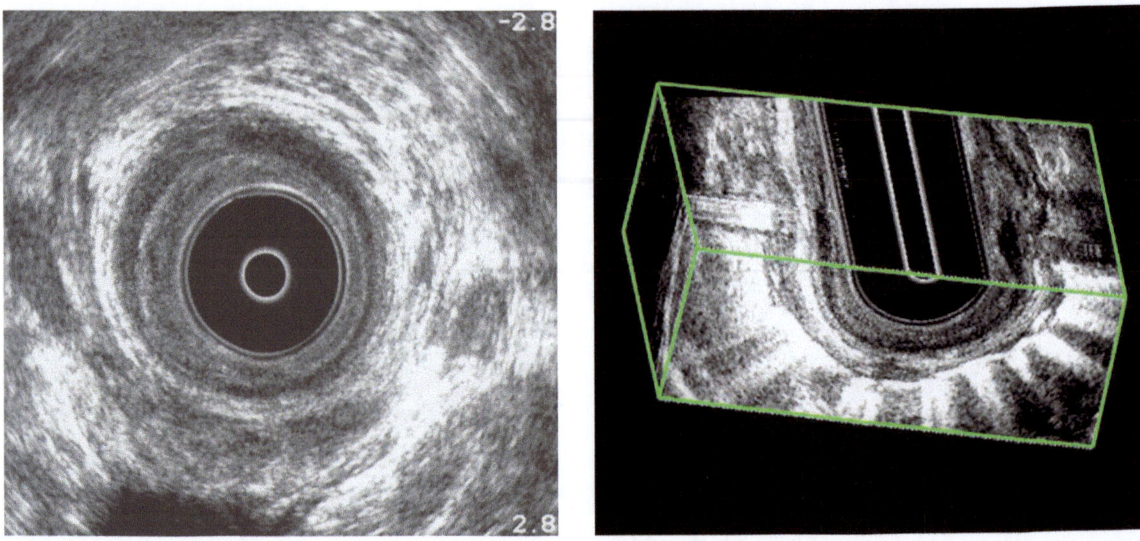

a b

Fig. V.38. Horseshoe intersphincteric fistula (**a**). After hydrogen peroxide injection, the bubbles produce a very strong reflection at the gas/tissue interface, which blanks out any detail deep beyond this interface (**b**). All information deep beyond the inner surface of the tract is lost

There were no statistically significant differences in the identification of an internal opening by EAUS between recurrent fistula (67%) and non-recurrent fistula (62%). They concluded that the accuracy of HPUS for the identification of internal openings is still insufficient to justify preoperative endosonography as a diagnostic method for routine use in patients with fistula-in-ano.

Navarro et al. [19] reported excellent results with hydrogen peroxide enhancement. HPUS was able to identify the internal opening in 94% of cases and whether the tract was linear or curvilinear in 95% of cases. The ultrasound level coincided with surgical findings in 85% of patients, and chronic fistula cavities were confirmed by surgery in 75% of patients. These results were confirmed by

Table V.1. Comparison of endoanal ultrasonography (EAUS) and hydrogen-peroxide-enhanced transanal ultrasound (HPUS) in the evaluation of fistula-in-ano. Review of the literature

Authors	Patients (no.)	EAUS probe	Primary tract		Secondary tract		Internal opening	
			EAUS	HPUS	EAUS	HPUS	EAUS	HPUS
Law et al. [10]	22	7 MHz	95%		100%		82%	
Seow-Choen et al. [5]	36	7 MHz	75%				75%	
Lunniss et al. [20]	20	7 MHz	70%				70%	
Cataldo et al. [11]	24	7 MHz	63%				28%	
Deen et al. [6]	18	7 MHz	100%		91%		11%	
Hussain et al. [21]	28	7 MHz	36%				57%	
Kuntz et al. [12]	35	7 MHz	77%					
Poen et al. [7]	21	7 MHz	62%	95%	60%	71%	14%	48%
Ratto et al. [14]	26	10 MHz	50%	77%	65%	88%	54%	54%
Gustafsson et al. [22]	23	10 MHz	61%		65%		74%	
Navarro et al. [23]	55	10 MHz	85%				96%	
Joo et al. [24]	25	10 MHz	76%				64%	
Ratto et al. [25]	89	10 MHz	84.3%	97.8%	80.9%	98.8%	87.6%	96.6%

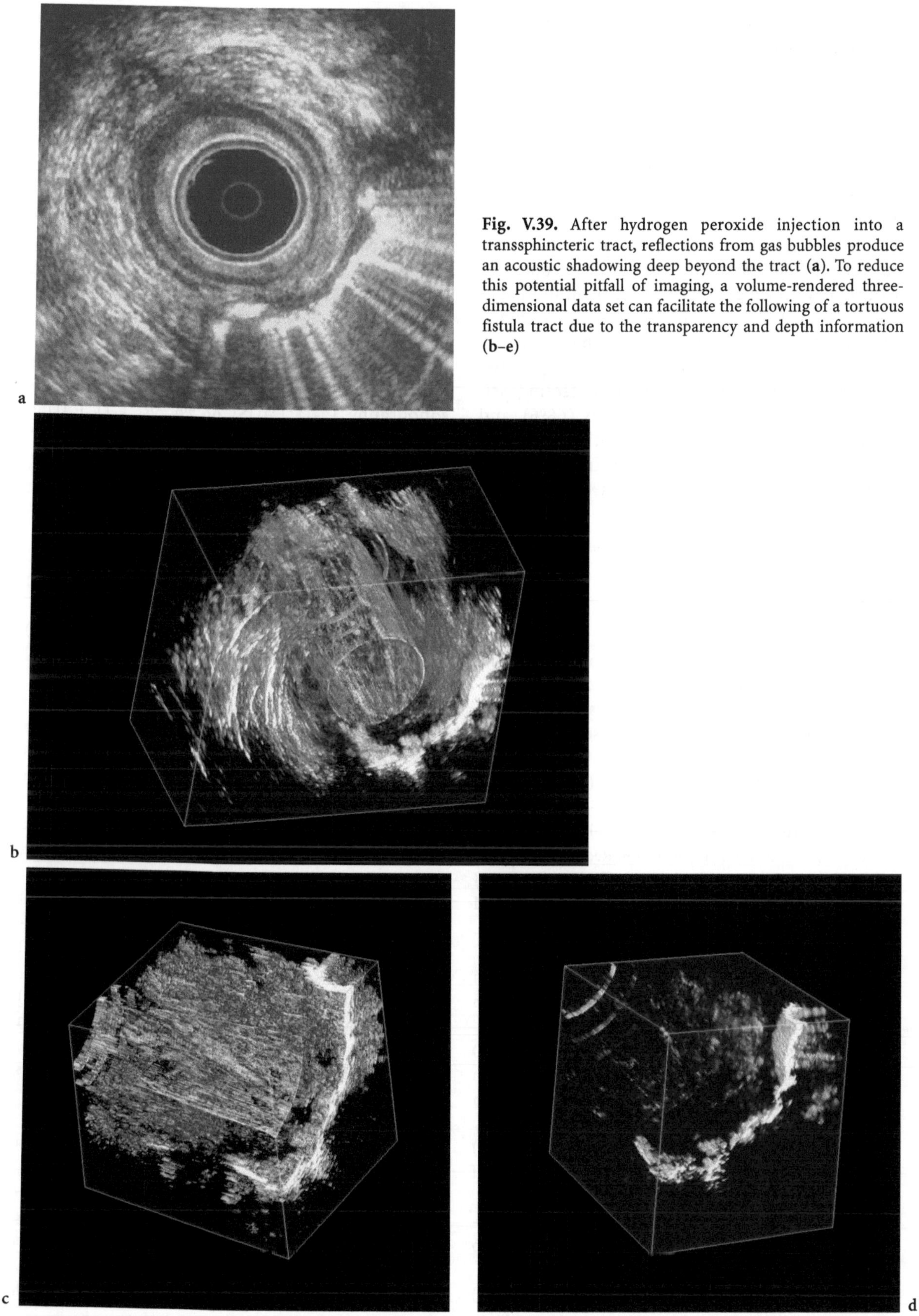

Fig. V.39. After hydrogen peroxide injection into a transsphincteric tract, reflections from gas bubbles produce an acoustic shadowing deep beyond the tract (**a**). To reduce this potential pitfall of imaging, a volume-rendered three-dimensional data set can facilitate the following of a tortuous fistula tract due to the transparency and depth information (**b–e**)

Sudol-Szopinska et al. [15], who found HPUS significantly increased the accuracy of standard noncontrast EAUS in identifying internal opening (89% vs. 65%, respectively) and in differentiating simple from complex tracts (92% vs.75%, respectively; $p<0.00001$).

More recently, the availability of the 3-D imaging system has provided another very useful tool for accurate assessment of endoanal and endorectal ultrasound examination. With regard to anal fistulas, with this method, the operator can review the entire series of ultrasound images reconstructed along all planes desired (coronal, sagittal, transverse, oblique). Buchanan et al. [29], in 19 patients with recurrent or complex fistulas, reported accurate results in detecting primary tracts (81%), secondary tracts (68%), and internal openings (90%). The addition of hydrogen peroxide (3-D HPUS) did not improve these features (accuracies of 71%, 63%, and 86%, respectively). West et al. [30] reported that 3-D HPUS and endoanal MRI are equally adequate for the evaluation of perianal fistulas. The methods agreed in 88% of cases for the primary fistula tract, in 90% for the location of the internal opening, in 78% for secondary tracts, and in 88% for fluid collections. Using 3-D imaging, Ratto et al. [25] reported an accuracy of 98.5% for primary tracts, 98.5% for secondary tracts, and 96.4% for internal openings compared with 89.4%, 83.3%, and 87.9%, respectively, when the two-dimensional (2-D) system was used. Our experience [31] with 57 patients with perianal fistulas confirms that 3-D reconstructions improves the accuracy of EAUS in the identification of the internal opening compared with standard ultrasonography (2-D EAUS: 66.7% vs. 3-D EAUS: 89.5%; $P=0.0033$). Primary tracts, secondary tracts, and abscesses were correctly evaluated by both procedures.

References

1. Joy HA, Williams JG (2002) The outcome of surgery for complex anal fistula. Colorectal Dis 4:254–261
2. Corman ML (1993) Anorectal abscess and fistula. In: Corman ML (ed) Colon and rectal surgery, 3rd edn. Lippincott, Philadelphia, pp 133–187
3. Parks AG, Gordon PH, Hardcastle JD (1976) A classification of fistula-in-ano. Br J Surg 63:1–12
4. Kuijpers HC, Schulpen T (1985) Fistulography for fistula-in-ano: is it useful? Dis Colon Rectum 28:103–104
5. Seow-Choen F, Burnett S, Bartram CI, Nicholls RJ (1991) Comparison between anal endosonography and digital examination in the evaluation of anal fistulae. Br J Surg 78:445–447
6. Deen KI, Williams JG, Hutchinson R (1994) Fistulas in ano: endoanal ultrasonographic assessment assists decision making for surgery. Gut 35:391–394
7. Poen AC, Felt-Bersma RJF, Eijsbouts QA et al (1998) Hydrogen peroxide-enhanced transanal ultrasound in the assessment of fistula-in-ano. Dis Colon Rectum 41:1147–1152
8. Weisman RI, Orsay CP, Pearl RK, Abcarian H (1991) The role of fistulography in fistula-in-ano. Report of five cases. Dis Colon Rectum 34:181–184
9. Shouler PJ, Grimley RP, Keighley MR, Alexander-Wiliams J (1986) Fistula-in-ano is usually simple to manage surgically. Int J Colorectal Dis 1:113–115
10. Law PJ, Talbot RW, Bartram CI, Northover JMA (1989) Anal endosonography in the evaluation of perianal sepsis and fistula in ano. Br J Surg 76:752–755
11. Cataldo PA, Senagore A, Luchtefeld MA (1993) Intrarectal ultrasound in the evaluation of perirectal abscesses. Dis Colon Rectum 36:554–558
12. Kuntz C, Glaser F, Buhr HJ, Herfarth C (1994) Endoanal ultrasound. Indications and results. Chirurg 65:352–357
13. Lindsey I, Humphreys MM, George BD, Mortensen NJ (2002) The role of anal ultrasound in the management of anal fistulas. Colorectal Dis 4:118–122
14. Ratto C, Gentile E, Merico M et al (2000) How can the assessment of fistula-in-ano be improved? Dis Colon Rectum 43:1375–1382
15. Sudol-Szopinska I, Szczepkowski M, Panorska AK et al (2004) Comparison of contrast-enhanced with non-contrast endosonography in the diagnostics of anal fistulas. Eur Radiol 14:2236–2241
16. Sloots CEJ, Felt-Bersma RJF, Poen AC et al (2001) Assessement and classification of fistula-in-ano in patients with Crohn's disease by hydrogen peroxide enhanced transanal ultrasound. Int J Colorectal Dis 16:292–297
17. Cho DY (1999) Endosonographic criteria for an internal opening of fistula-in-ano. Dis Colon Rectum 42:515–518
18. Kruskal JB, Kane RA, Morrin MM (2001) Peroxide-enhanced anal endosonography: technique, image interpretation and clinical applications. Radiographics 21:S173–S189
19. Navarro-Luna A, Garcia-Domingo MI, Rius-Macias J,

Marco-Molina C (2004) Ultrasound study of anal fistulas with hydrogen peroxide enhancement. Dis Colon Rectum 47:108–114

20. Lunniss PJ, Kamm MA, Phillips RKS (1994) Factors affecting continence after surgery for anal fistula. Br J Surg 81:1382–1385
21. Hussain SM, Stoker J, Schouten WR et al (1996) Fistula-in-ano: endoanal sonography versus endoanal MR imaging in classification. Radiology 200:475–481
22. Gustafsson UM, Kahvecioglu B, Astrom G et al (2001) Endoanal ultrasound or magnetic resonance imaging for preoperative assessment of anal fistula: a comparative study. Colorectal Dis 3:189–197
23. Navarro A, Rius J, Collera P et al (1998) Anal fistulas: results of ultrasonographic studies. Dis Colon Rectum 41:A57
24. Joo JS, Son KS, Lee HS, Lee SK (1998) Preoperative evaluation of anal fistula by endorectal ultrasonography. Dis Colon Rectum 41:A46–47
25. Ratto C, Grillo E, Parello A et al (2005) Endoanal ultrasound-guided surgery for anal fistula. Endoscopy 37:1–7
26. Cheong DM, Nogueras JJ, Wexner SD, Jagelman DG (1993) Anal endonography for recurrent anal fistulas: image enhancement with hydrogen peroxide. Dis Colon Rectum 36:1158–1160
27. Moscowitz I, Baig MK, Noguearas JJ et al (2003) Accuracy of hydrogen peroxide enhanced endoanal ultrasonography in assessment of the internal opening of an anal fistula complex. Tech Coloproctol 7:133–137
28. Ortiz H, Marzo J, Jemenez G, DeMiguel M (2001) Accuracy of hydrogen peroxide-enhanced ultrasound in the identification of internal openings of anal fistulas. Colorectal Dis 4:280–283
29. Buchanan GN, Halligan S, Bartram CI et al (2004) Clinical examination, endosonography and MR imaging in preoperative assessment of fistula in ano: comparison with outcome-based reference standard. Radiology 233:674–681
30. West RL, Dwarkasing S, Felt-Bersma RJF et al (2004) Hydrogen peroxide-enhanced three-dimensional endoanal ultrasonography and endoanal magnetic resonance imaging in evaluating perianal fistulas: agreement and patient preference. Eur J Gastroenterol Hepat 16:1319–1324
31. Santoro GA, Ratto C, Di Falco G (2004) Three-dimensional reconstructions improve the accuracy of endoanal ultrasonography in the identification of internal openings of anal fistulas. Colorectal Dis 6 [Suppl 2]:P214

Clinical Cases

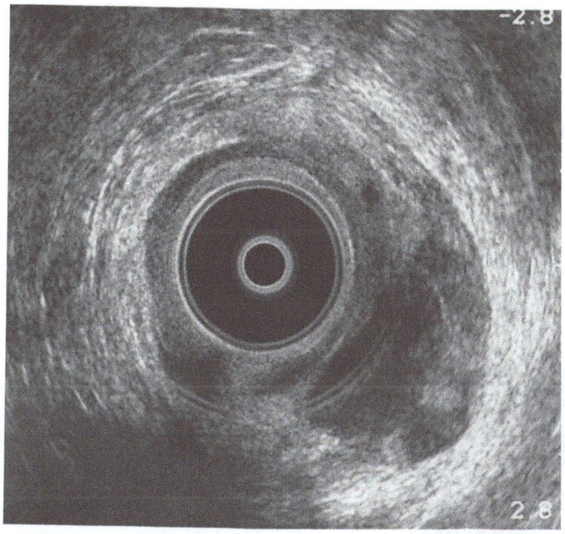

a

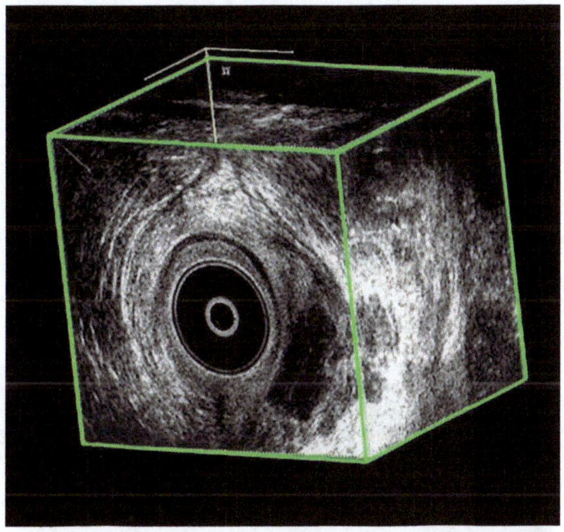

b

Case V.1. A 23-year-old man complaining of perianal pain. Physical examination reveals a left lateral, superficial, tender mass outside the anal verge. Axial endosonographic image of lower anal canal level reveals a large hypoechoic area (**a**). Three-dimensional endoanal ultrasonography confirms the presence of an acute superficial abscess (**b**). The patient underwent immediate incision and drainage

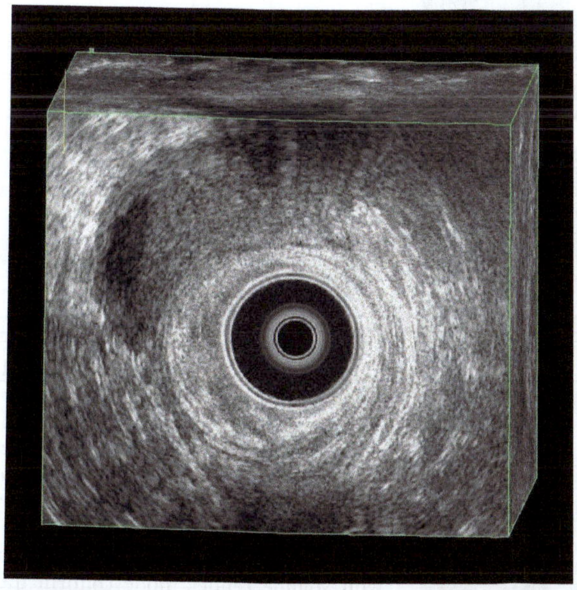

a

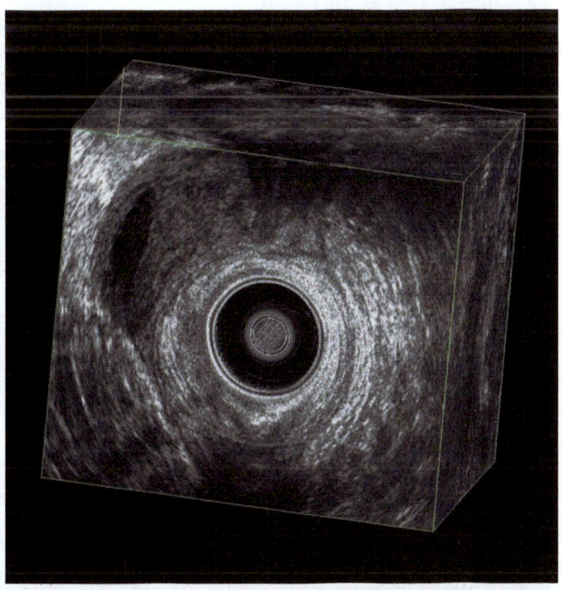

b

Case V.2. A 47-year-old man complaining of fever and perianal pain. Physical examination reveals an anterior, superficial, tender mass outside the anal verge. Three-dimensional reconstruction in the axial plane reveals a large hypoechoic area (**a**). Volume render mode confirms the presence of an acute superficial abscess (**b**). The patient underwent immediate incision and drainage

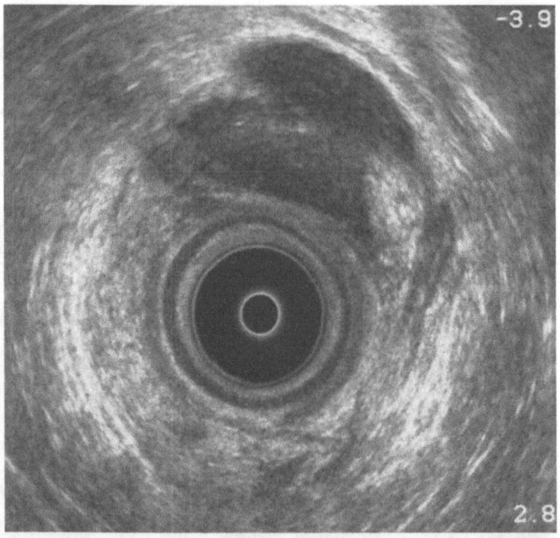

a

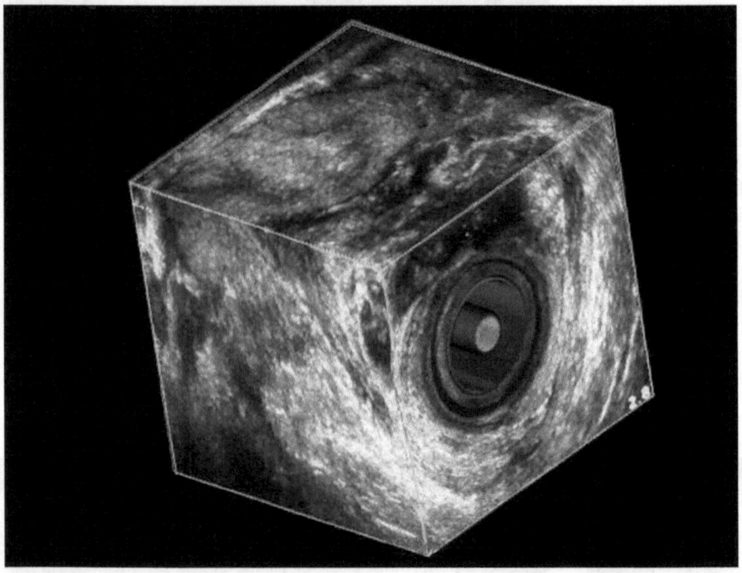

b

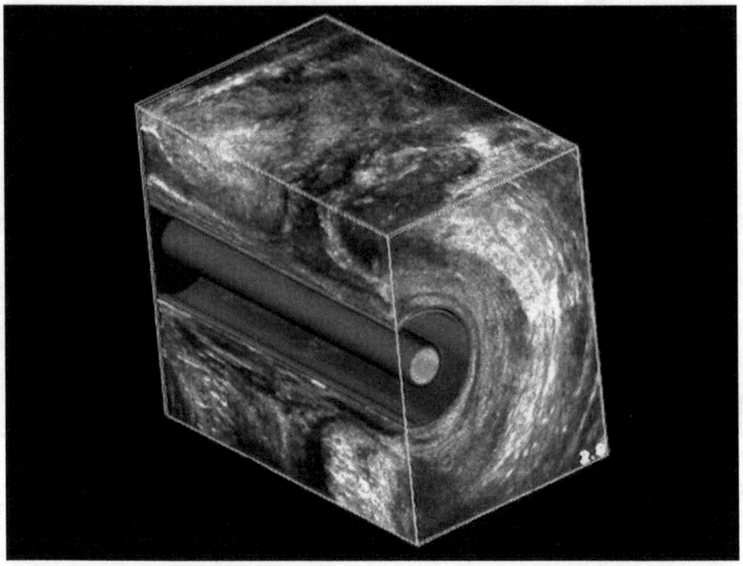

c

Case V.3. A 63-year-old man complaining of fever and perirectal pain. Digital rectal examination reveals an anterior, tender mass at the dentate line level 2 cm from the anal verge. Axial endosonographic image of mid anal canal level reveals a large hypoechoic area in the anterior intersphincteric zone (**a**). Three-dimensional endoanal ultrasonography scans with volume render mode confirm the presence of an acute anterior intersphincteric abscess (**b, c**). The patient underwent immediate drainage through the intersphincteric space

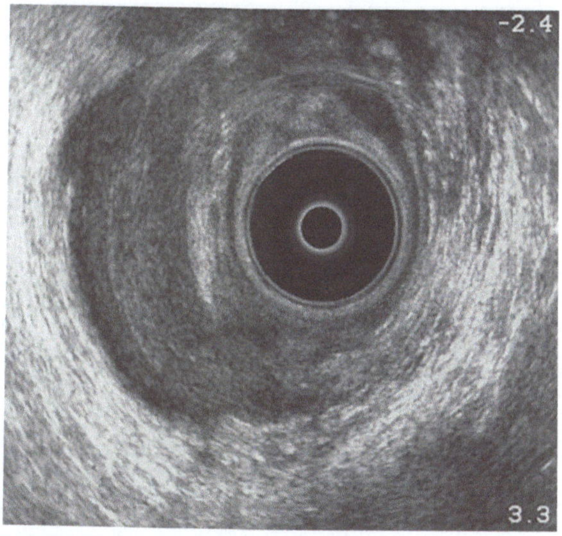

a

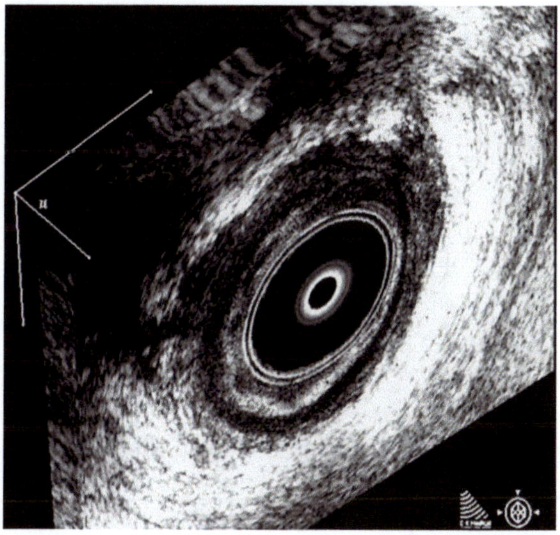

b

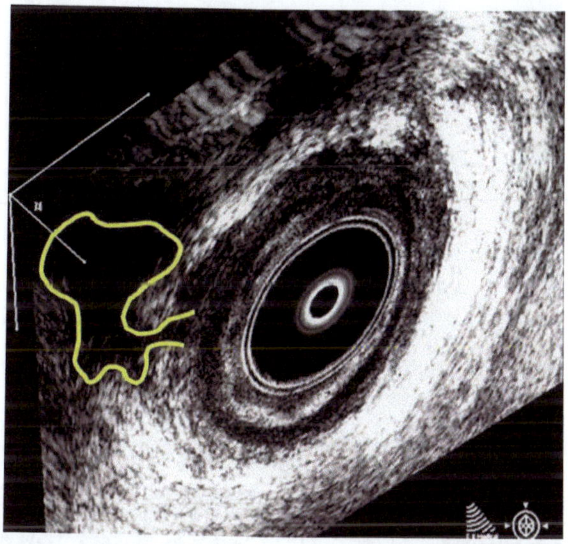

c

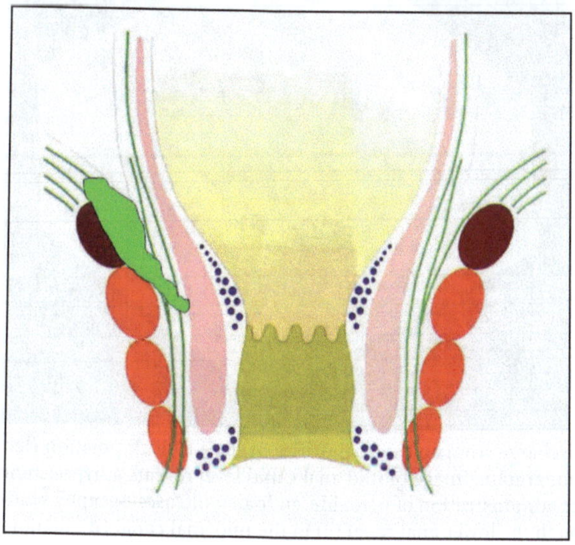

d

Case V.4. A 45-year-old woman complaining of fever and perirectal pain. Digital rectal examination reveals a right lateral, supralevator, tender mass at 4 cm from the anal verge. Axial endosonographic image of the upper anal canal level reveals a large hypoechoic dishomogeneous area in the right lateral supralevator space (**a**). Three-dimensional endoanal ultrasonography reconstruction confirms the presence of an acute supralevator abscess (**b, c**). Drawing in the coronal plane (**d**)

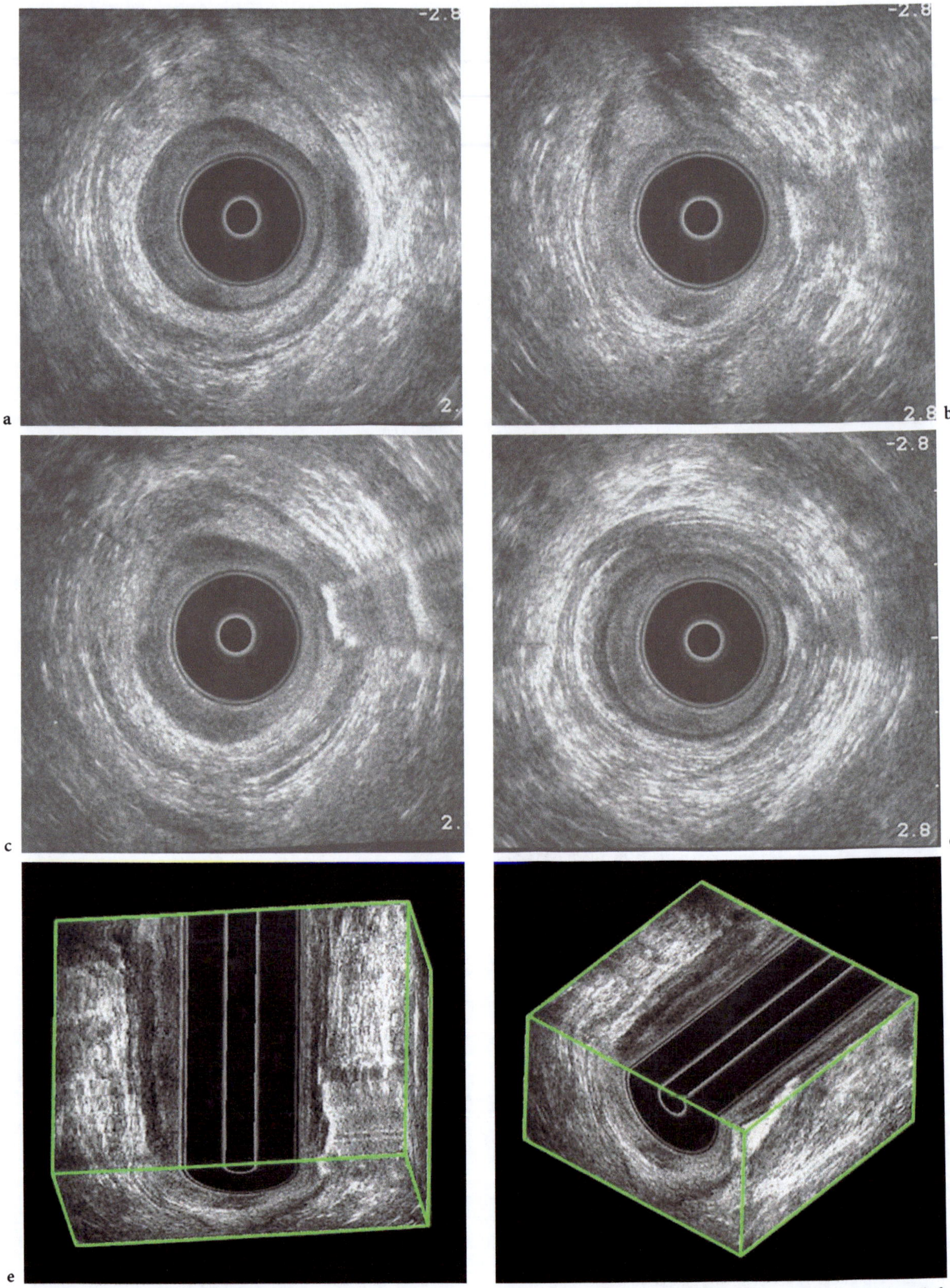

Case V.5. A 57-year-old man complaining of perianal purulent discharge from an external orifice at the 3 o'clock position (left lateral side) immediately adjacent to the anal canal. Axial endosonographic image of mid anal canal level reveals a hypoechoic area in the intersphincteric zone at the 3 o'clock position (**a**). After administration of peroxide, endoanal ultrasonography scans show a direct communication that extends from the skin (**b**) through the lower anal canal (**c**) to the mid anal canal (**d**), demonstrating a simple intersphincteric fistula. Three-dimensional hydrogen-peroxide-enhanced ultrasonography confirms the presence of left lateral intersphincteric fistula (**e, f**)

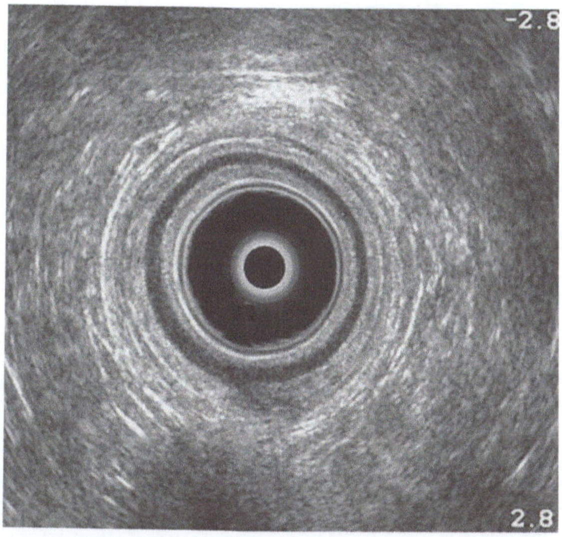

a

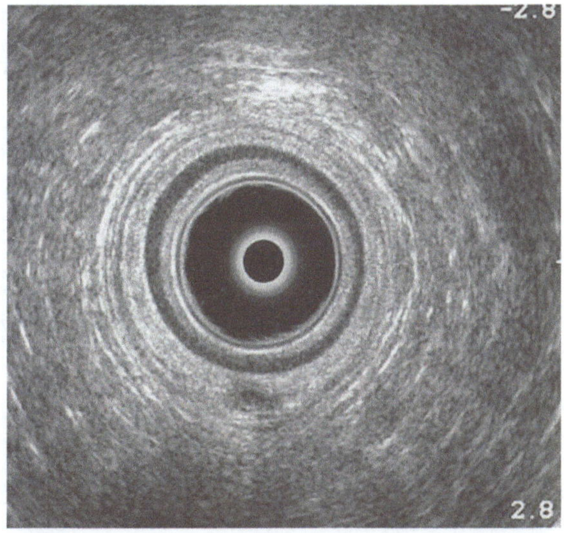

b

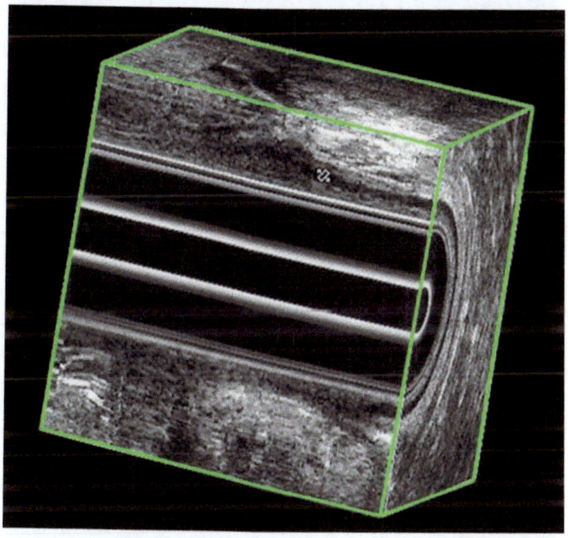

c

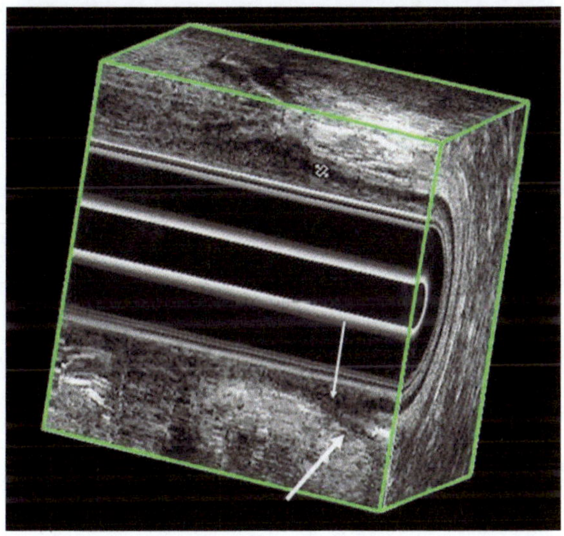

d

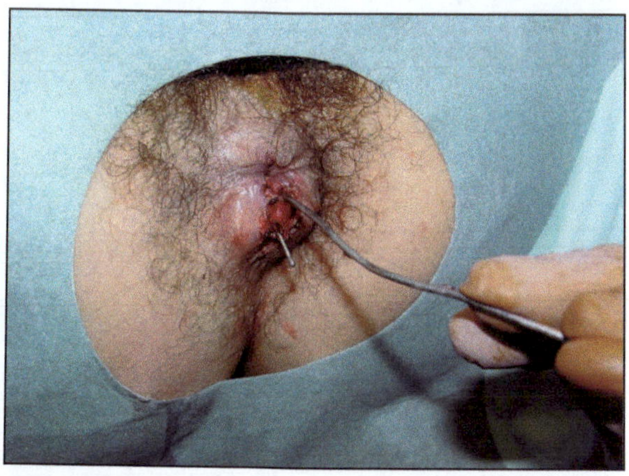

e

Case V.6. A 28-year-old woman complaining of purulent discharge from the anus. Axial endosonographic images of mid anal canal level reveal a hypoechoic area in the posterior intersphincteric zone (**a, b**). Three-dimensional reconstruction in the sagittal plane confirms an intersphincteric fistula, appearing as a band of poor reflectivity within the intersphincteric plane (*large arrow*), communicating with the anal canal (internal orifice; *small arrow*) (**c, d**). The patient underwent an unroofing procedure (**e**)

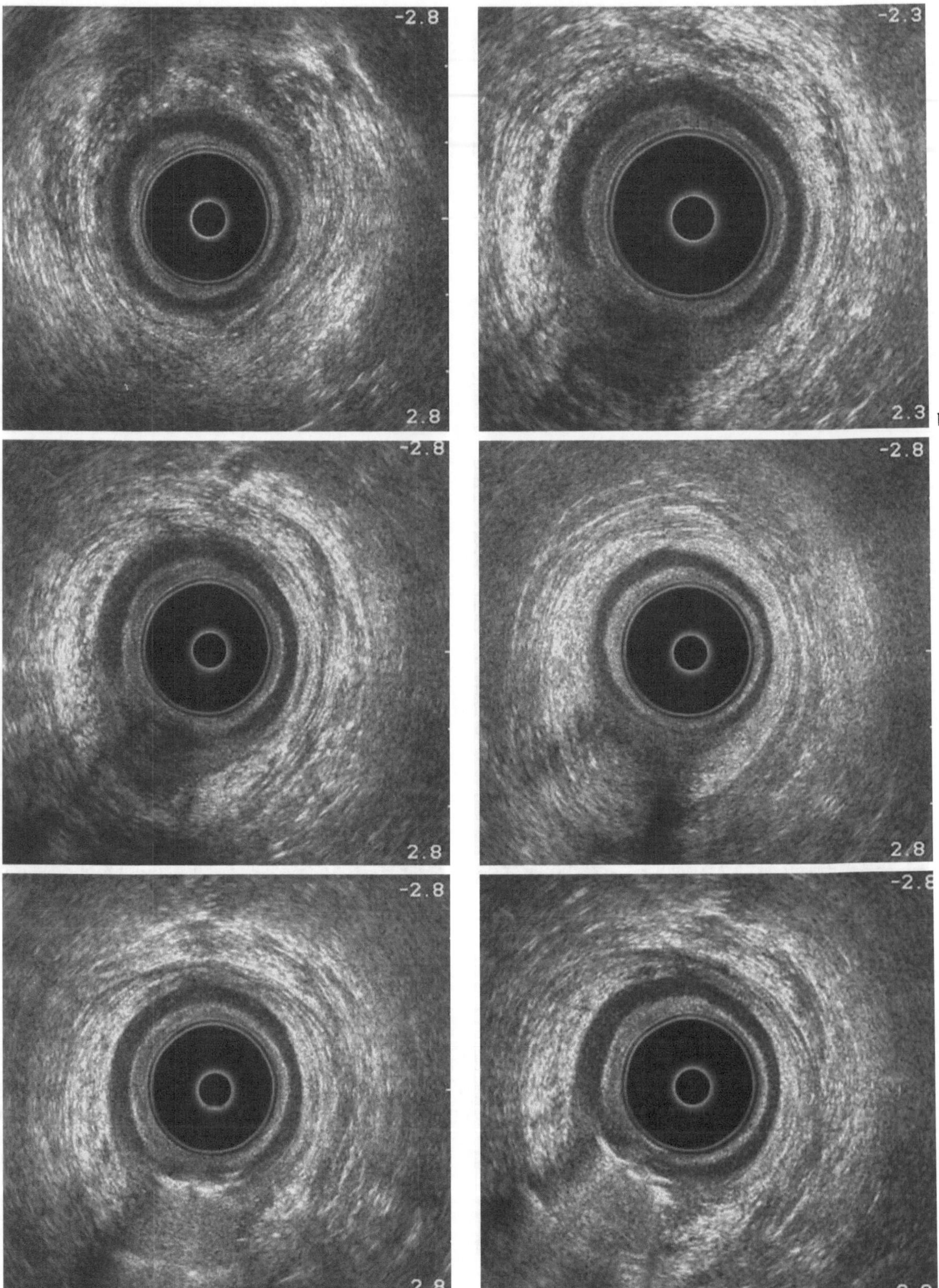
-2.8
2.8
a
-2.3
2.3
b
-2.8
2.8
c
-2.8
2.8
d
-2.8
2.8
e
-2.8
2.8
f

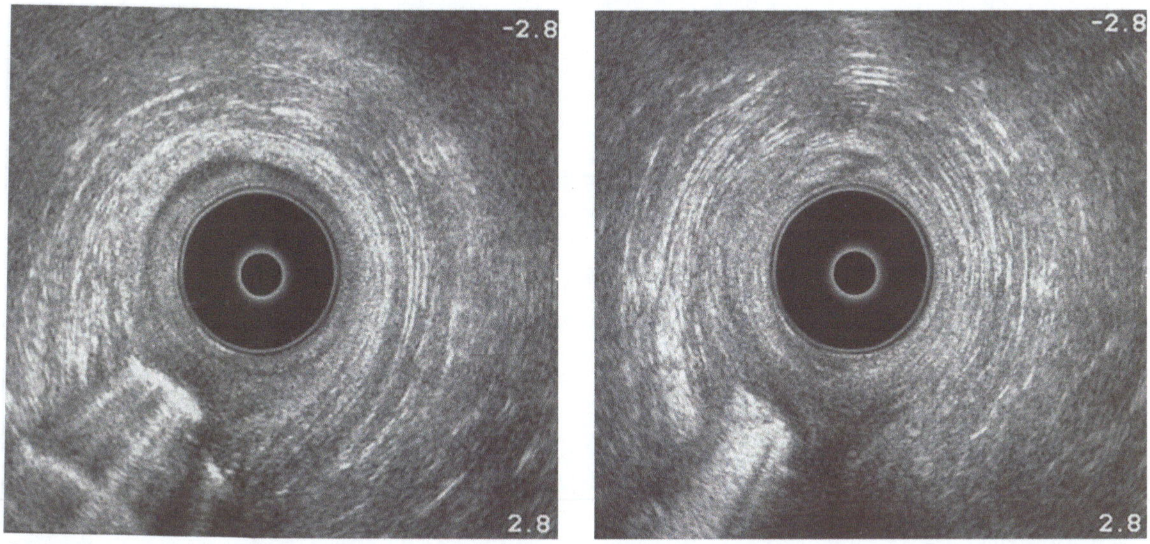

g h

Case V.7. A 53-year-old man complaining of recurrent perianal purulent discharge. Physical examination reveals a cutaneous opening at the 6 o'clock position. Axial endosonographic image at the upper anal canal level shows a normal anatomy (**a**). At mid anal canal level, endoanal ultrasonography (EAUS) scans reveal a posterior hypoechoic tract extending through the external sphincter, with an appearance of internal sphincter defect at the 6 o'clock position (**b, c**) (second endosonographic criteria for the site of an internal opening according to Cho [17]). The fistula also tracks downward at the lower anal canal level (**d**). After peroxide injection, the EAUS scans confirm immediate communication with the anal canal (**e, f**) with the transsphincteric fistula extending caudally (**g, h**)

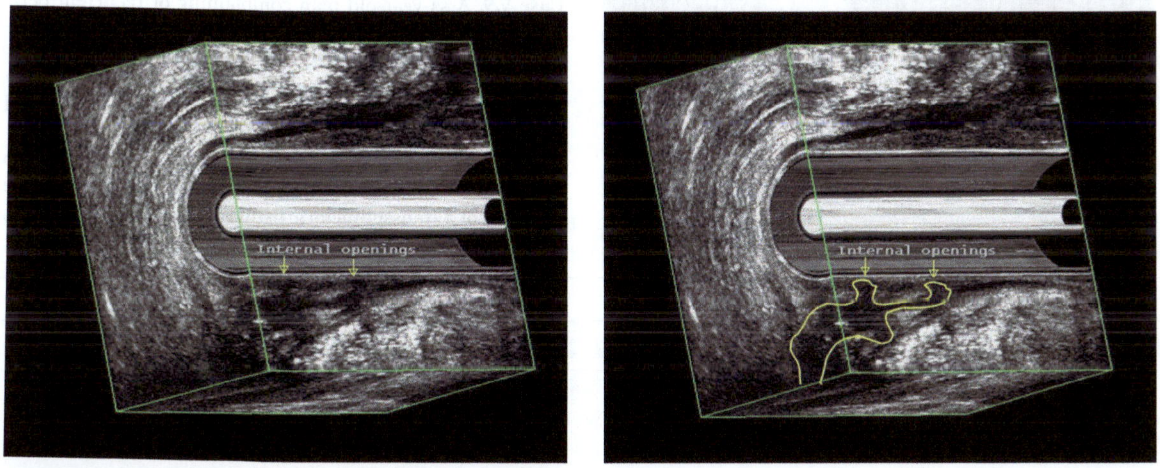

a b

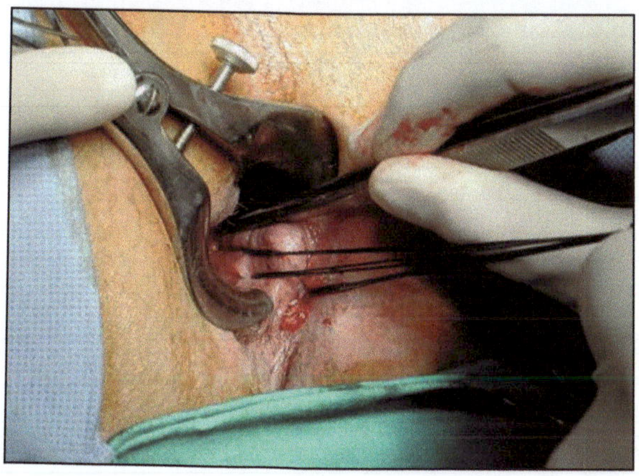

c

Case V.8. A 43-year-old woman complaining of anal pain and perianal purulent discharge from an external orifice at the 6 o'clock position. Sagittal view from a three-dimensional data set shows a transsphincteric tract with two internal openings that traverses the middle part of the external sphincter (**a, b**). At surgery, the presence of two internal openings was confirmed, and two cutting setons were inserted through this complex fistulous tract (**c**)

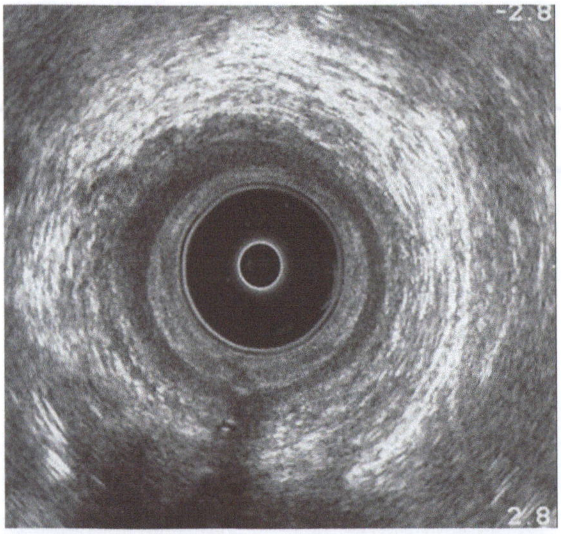

a

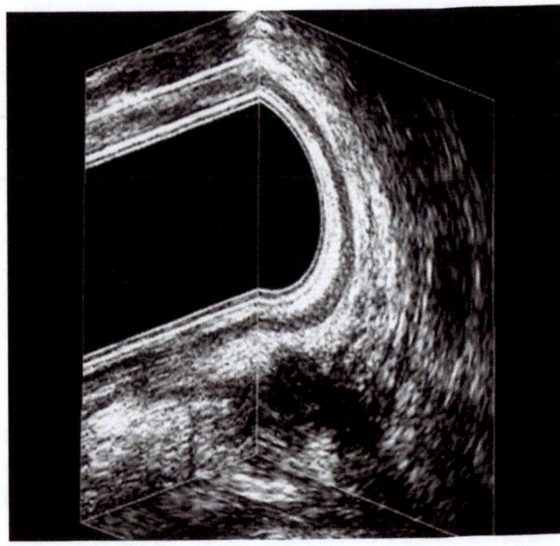
b

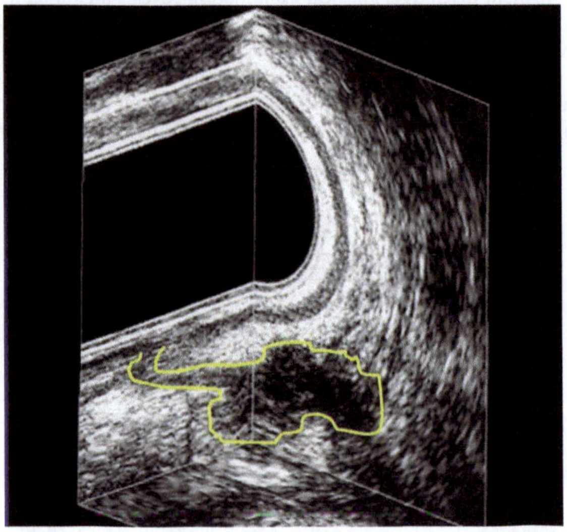
c

Case V.9. A 53-year-old man complaining of recurrent perianal purulent discharge. Physical examination reveals a cutaneous opening at the 6 o'clock position. Axial endosonographic image at mid anal canal level shows a posterior hypoechoic tract extending through the internal and external sphincters at the 6 o'clock position (**a**) (third endosonographic criteria for the site of an internal opening according to Cho [17]). Three-dimensional ultrasonography scan confirms the presence of a transsphincteric fistula at the 6 o'clock position, traversing the middle part of the external sphincter and communicating with a small perianal abscess (**b, c**)

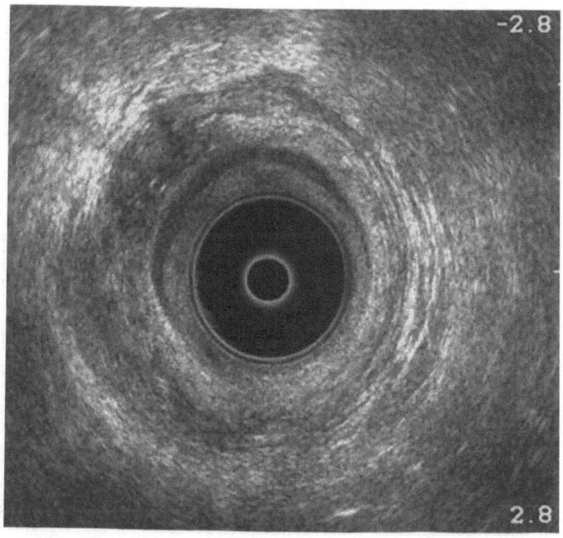

a

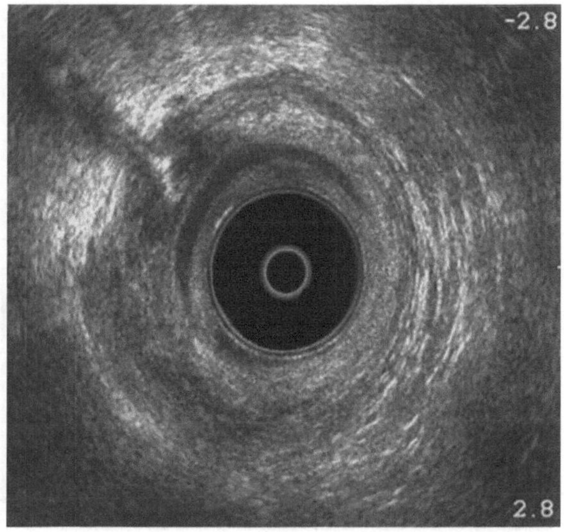

b

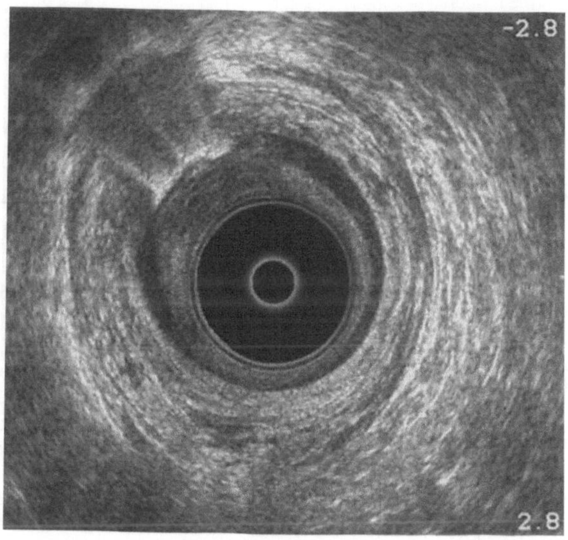

c

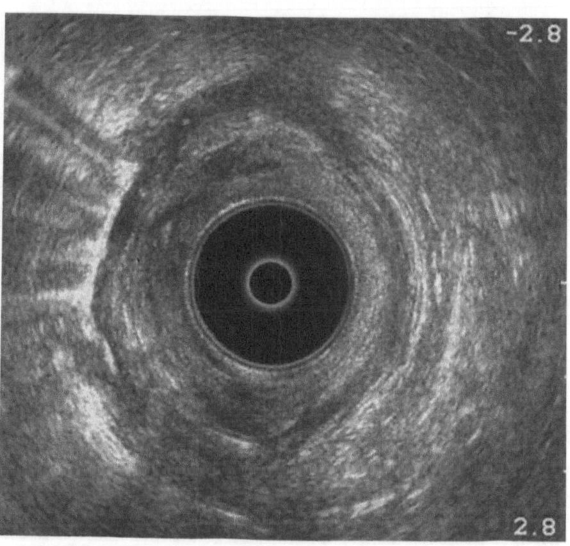

d

Case V.10. A 55-year-old man complaining of rectal pain and perianal purulent discharge from an external orifice at the 11 o'clock position. Preliminary endoanal ultrasonography (EAUS) scan at mid anal canal level reveals irregular thickening in the right lateral intersphincteric plane with a hypoechoic area containing air (hyperechoic spet) at the 11 o'clock position (**a**). After peroxide injection, the EAUS scan shows immediate communication with the area at the 11 o'clock position and through the internal anal sphincter with the anal lumen (**b**). Fistula extends anteriorly (**c**) and posteriorly (**d**) into the intersphincteric plane (horseshoe intersphincteric fistula)

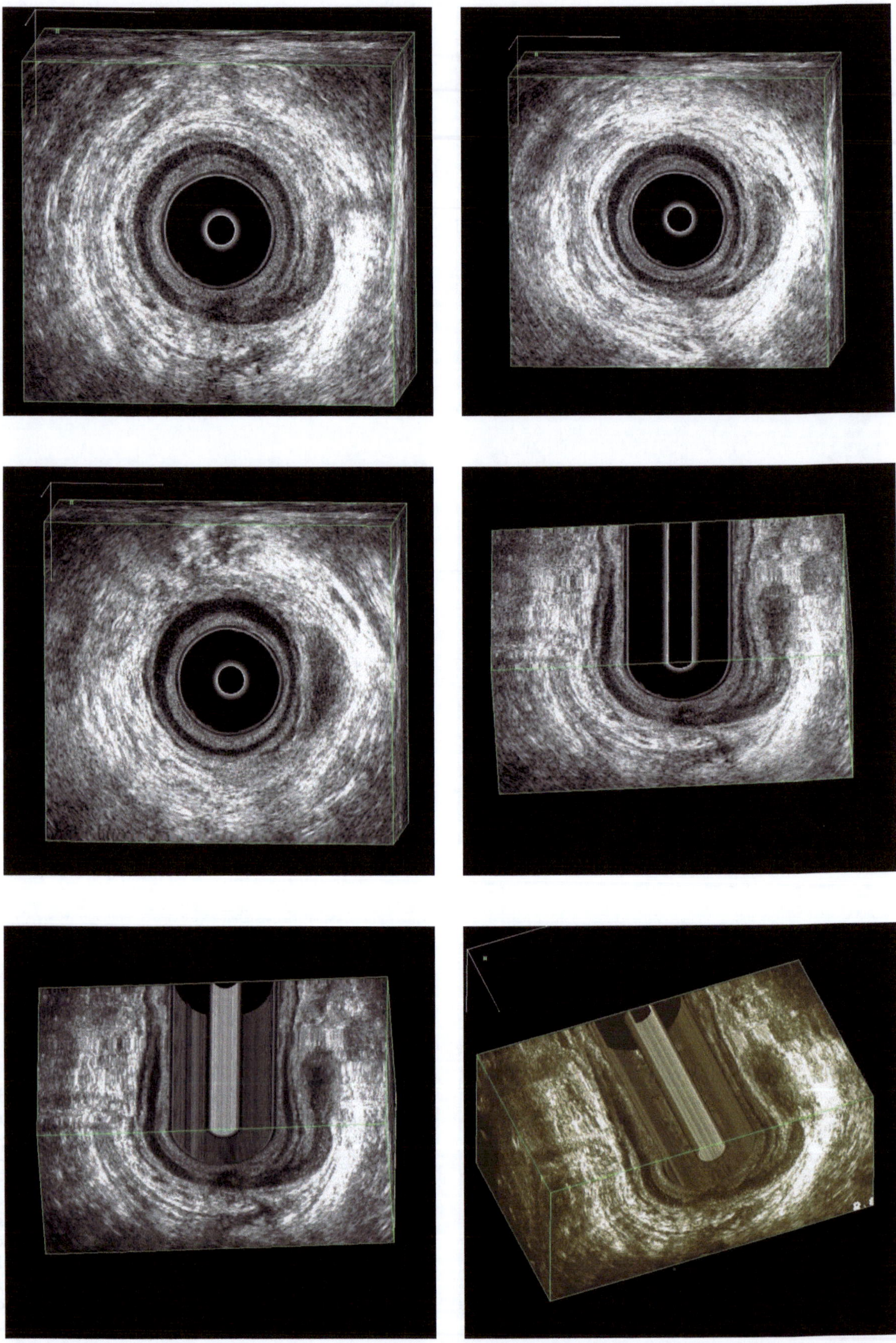

a b c d e f

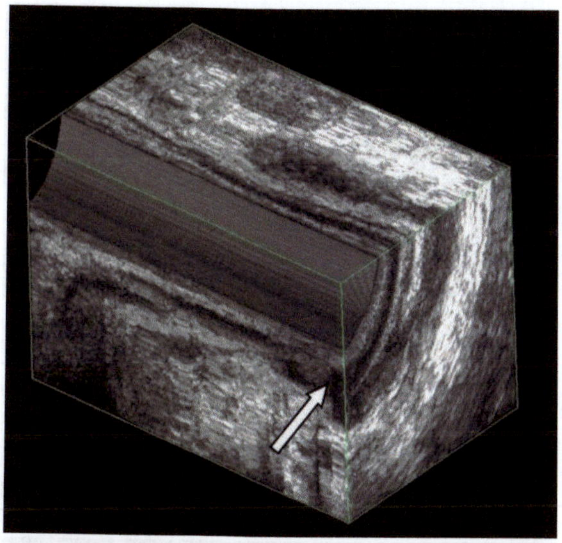
g

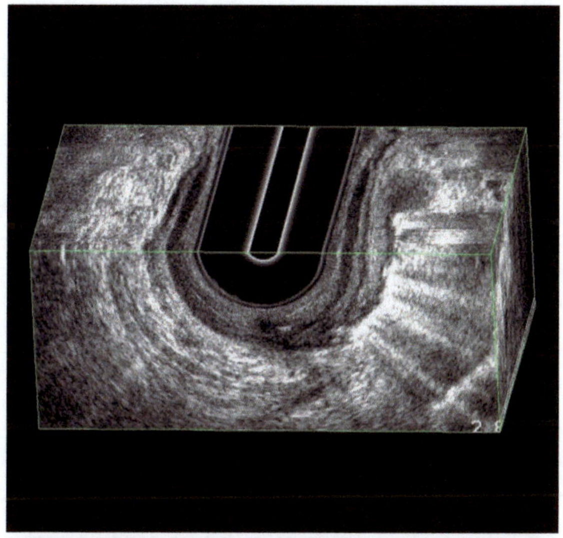
h

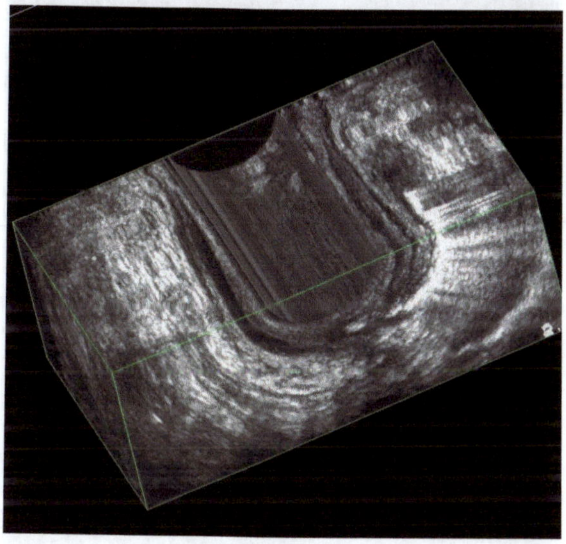
i

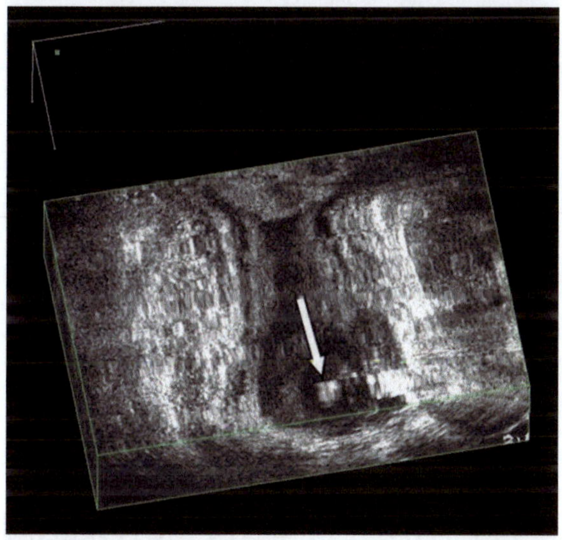
l

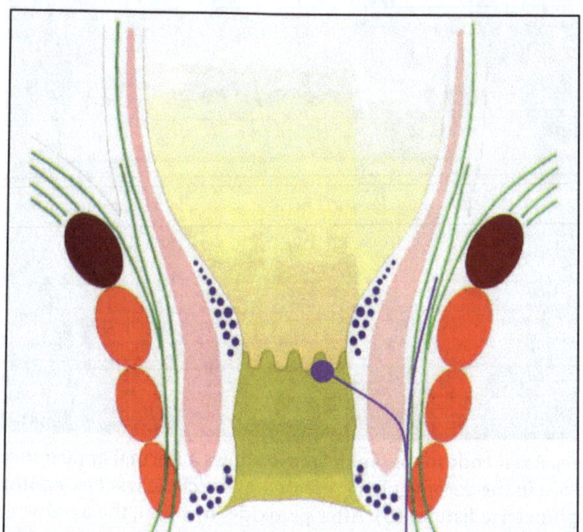
m

Case V.11. A 34-year-old woman complaining of recurrent perianal purulent discharge. Physical examination reveals a cutaneous opening at the 6 o'clock position. At mid anal canal level, three-dimensional reconstruction in the axial plane reveals a hypoechoic intersphincteric tract with an appearance of internal sphincter defect at the 6 o'clock position (**a**) (second endosonographic criteria for the site of an internal opening according to Cho [17]). The fistula also tracks upward and laterally into the intersphincteric plane (**b**, **c**). Reconstruction in the coronal plane confirms an intersphincteric fistula, with the internal opening at the 6 o'clock position, extending upward and laterally within the longitudinal layer (**d**). The tract causes widening and distortion of the intersphincteric plane without traversing the external sphincter. Volume render mode (**e**, **f**). Reconstruction in the sagittal plane confirms the presence of the internal opening at the 6 o'clock position (*arrow*) (**g**). After administration of peroxide, endoanal ultrasonography scan shows immediate communication with the anal lumen below the level of the internal anal sphincter and the extent of the intersphincteric fistula (**h**). Volume render mode (**i**). Internal orifice (*arrow*) (**l**). Drawing in the axial plane shows extent of the intersphincteric fistula (**m**)

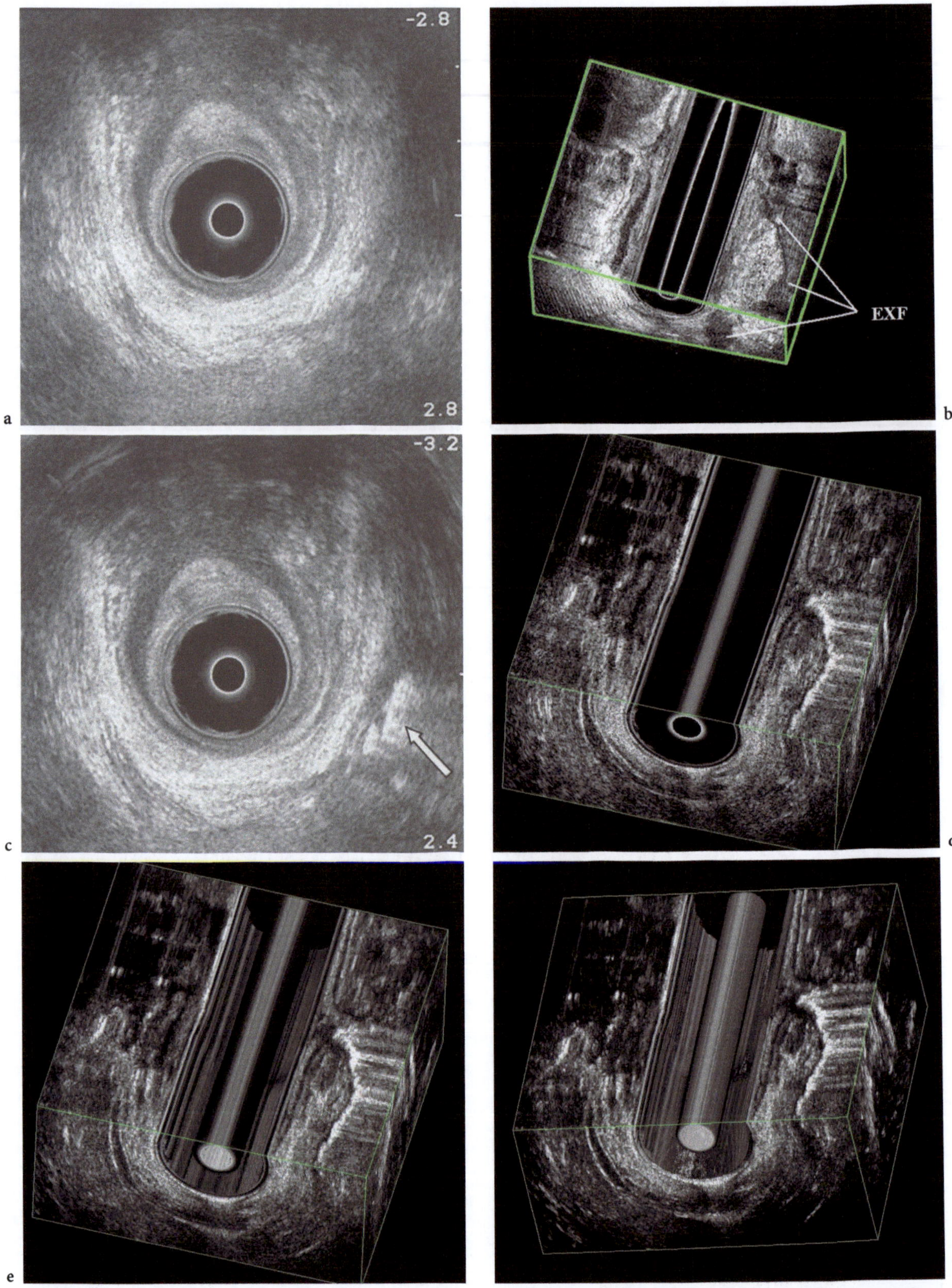

Case V.12. A 29-year-old man referred for recurrent perianal fistula. Axial endosonographic image shows a normal appearance of upper anal canal level (**a**). Three-dimensional (3-D) reconstruction in the coronal plane reveals a hypoechoic tract extending upward outside the internal and external sphincters (*EXF*, extrasphincteric fistula) (**b**). After peroxide injection, the axial scan shows the presence of bright echoes (*arrows*) at the 4 o'clock position at the upper anal canal level (**c**). 3-D hydrogen-peroxide-enhanced ultrasonography confirms an extrasphincteric fistula communicating with the rectal ampulla (**d**). Volume render mode (**e, f**)

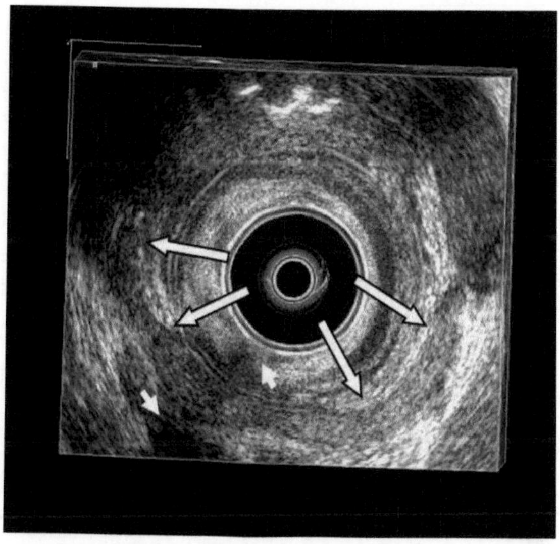

a

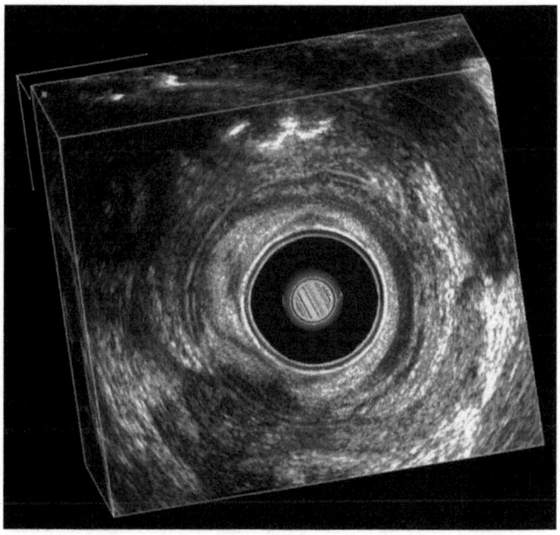

b

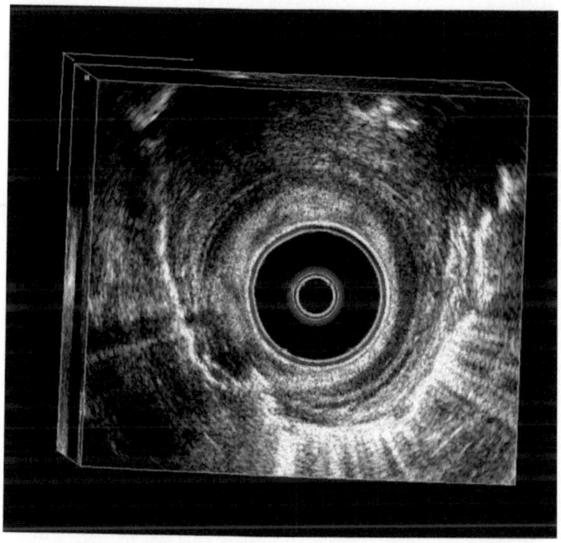

c

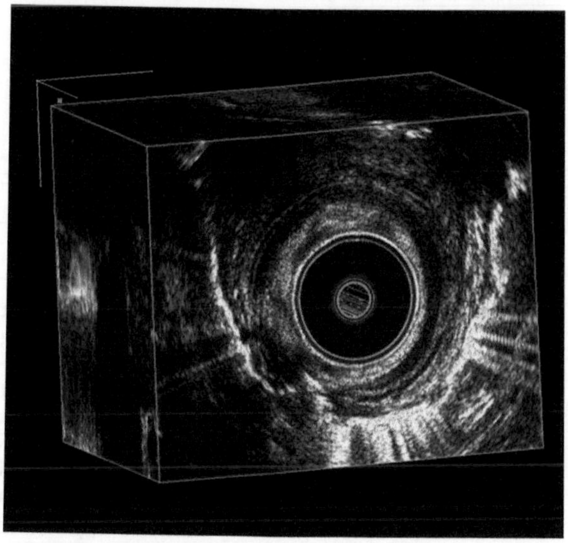

d

Case V.13. A 33-year-old man complaining of recurrent perianal fistula and purulent discharge from an external orifice at the 7 o'clock position. Three-dimensional endoanal ultrasonography (EAUS) scan at mid anal canal level shows a posterior hypoechoic tract extending through the internal and external sphincters (*small arrows*) and an irregular thickening in the right and left lateral intersphincteric plane (*large arrows*) (**a**). Volume render mode (**b**). After peroxide injection, the EAUS scan shows immediate communication through the internal sphincter into the anal lumen, with horseshoe extension into the intersphincteric plane (**c**). Volume render mode confirms the presence of a posterior transsphincteric fistula, with internal opening at the 7 o'clock position and secondary horseshoe intersphincteric extension (**d**)

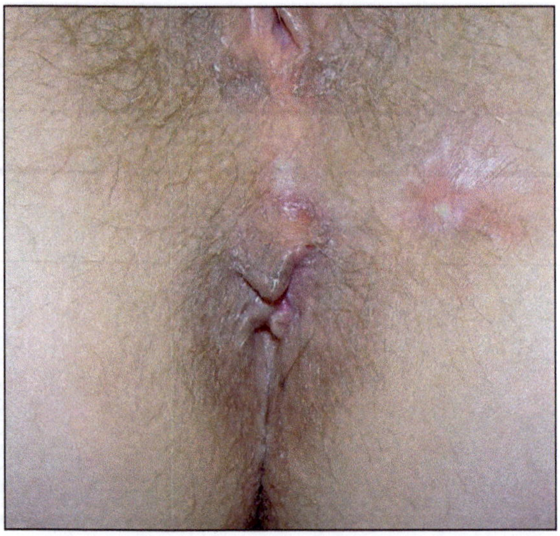

a

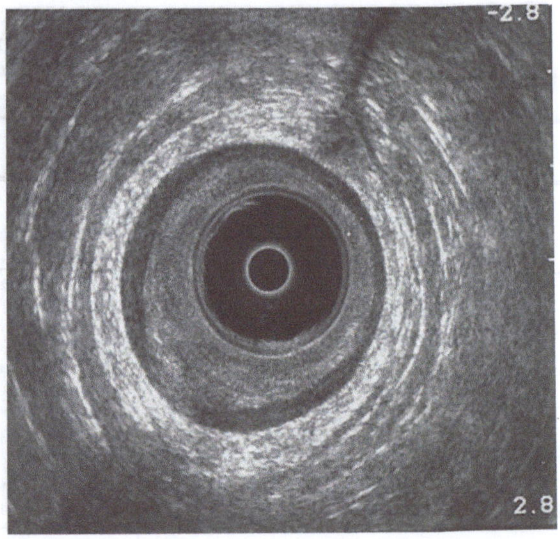

b

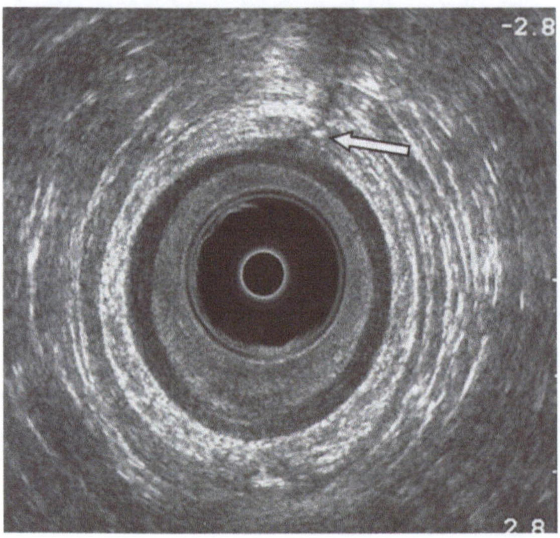

c

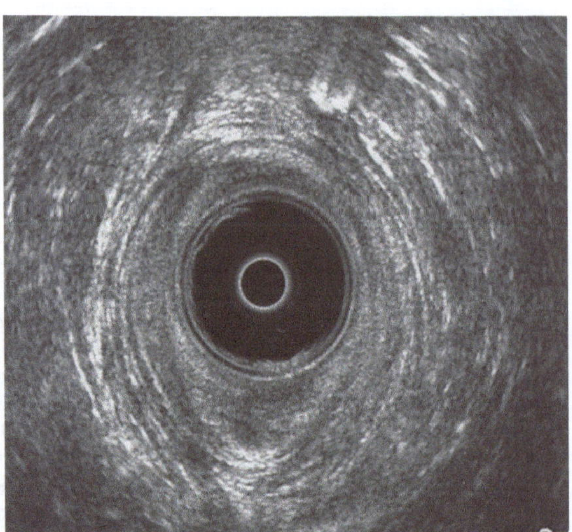

d

Case V.14. A 27-year-old woman referred for recurrent perianal fistula. Physical examination reveals a cutaneous scar at the 2 o'clock position where the external fistulous opening was previously located (**a**). Preliminary endoanal ultrasonography (EAUS) scan shows an anterior hypoechoic tract extending through the internal and external sphincters (**b**). After probing into the center of the cutaneous scar, the skin is easily broken and the peroxide injected into the external opening. The EAUS scans show immediate communication with the transsphincteric tract (**c, d**)

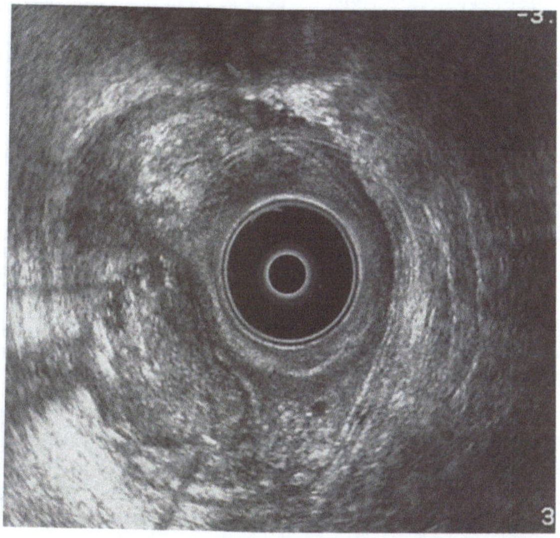
a

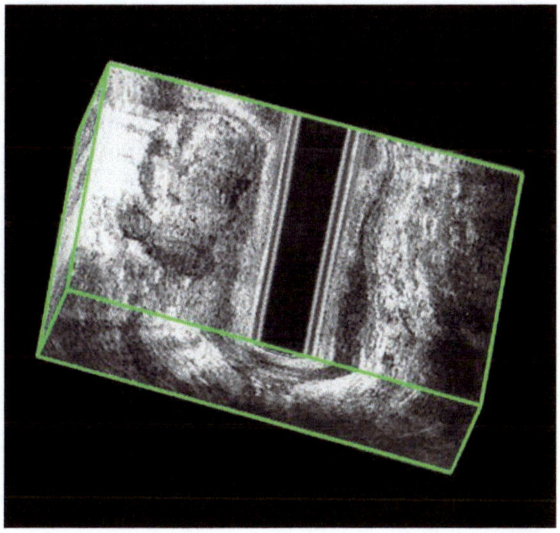
b

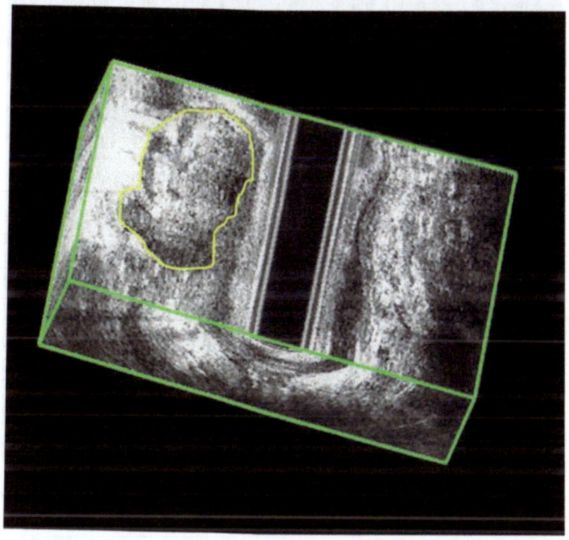
c

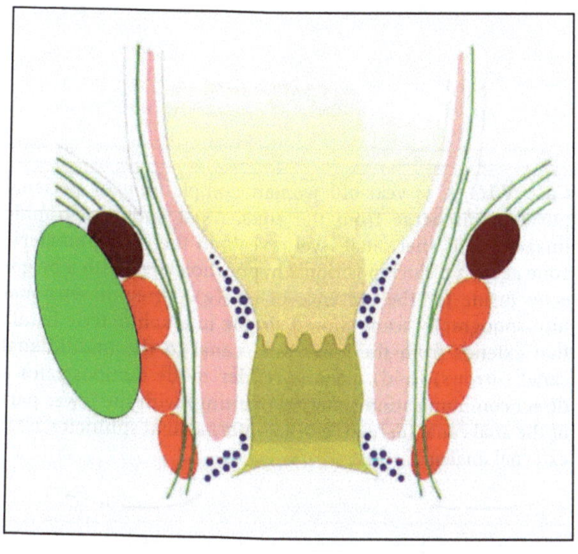
d

Case V.15. A 35-year-old man complaining of perirectal pain. Digital rectal examination reveals a right lateral tender mass at 2 cm from the anal verge. Axial endosonographic image of mid anal canal level reveals a large dishomogeneous area in the right lateral ischioanal space (**a**). Three-dimensional reconstruction in the coronal plane confirms the presence of a chronic ischioanal abscess (**b, c**). Drawing in the axial plane (**d**). The patient underwent drainage through the ischioanal space

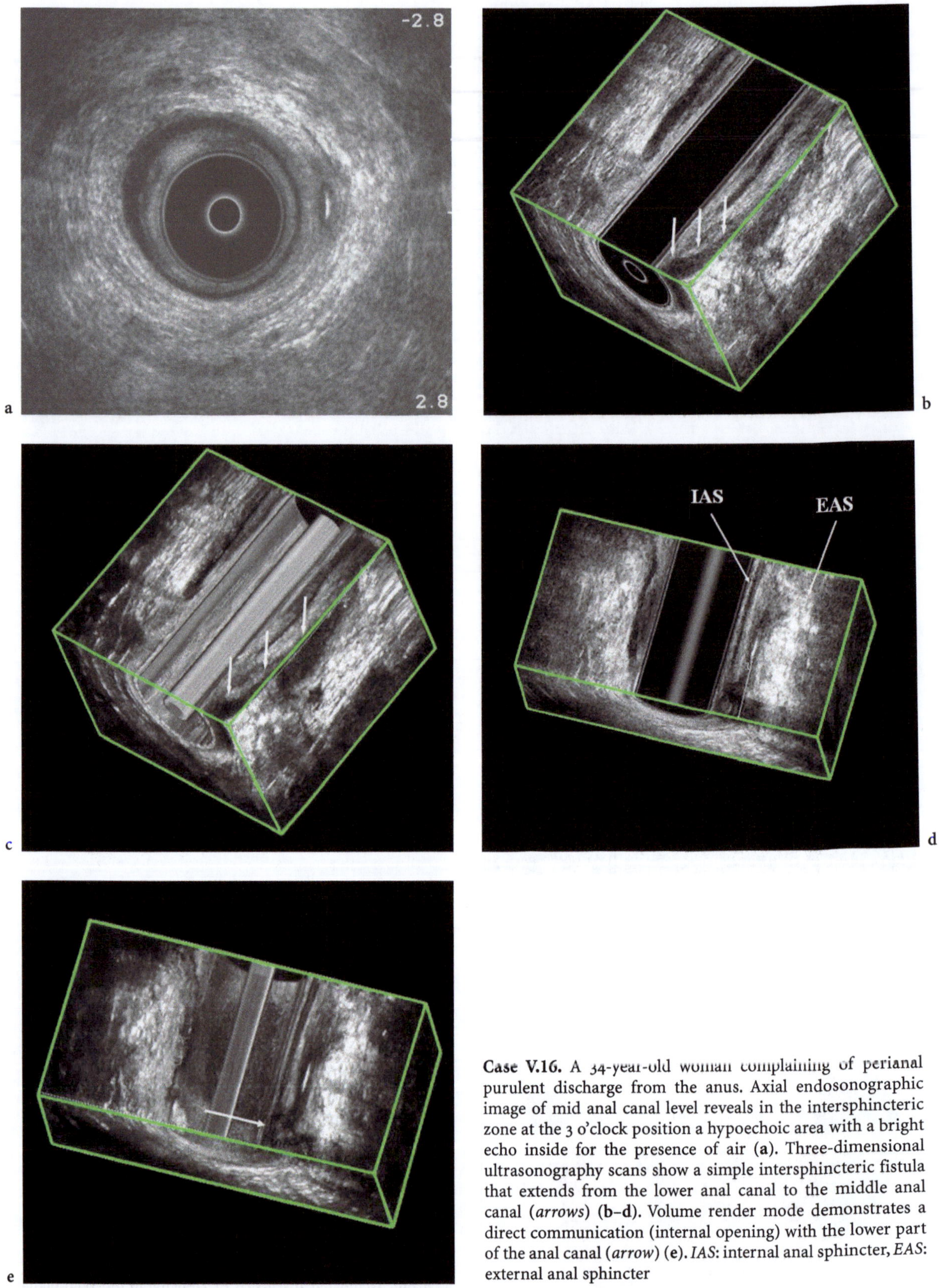

Case V.16. A 34-year-old woman complaining of perianal purulent discharge from the anus. Axial endosonographic image of mid anal canal level reveals in the intersphincteric zone at the 3 o'clock position a hypoechoic area with a bright echo inside for the presence of air (**a**). Three-dimensional ultrasonography scans show a simple intersphincteric fistula that extends from the lower anal canal to the middle anal canal (*arrows*) (**b–d**). Volume render mode demonstrates a direct communication (internal opening) with the lower part of the anal canal (*arrow*) (**e**). *IAS*: internal anal sphincter, *EAS*: external anal sphincter

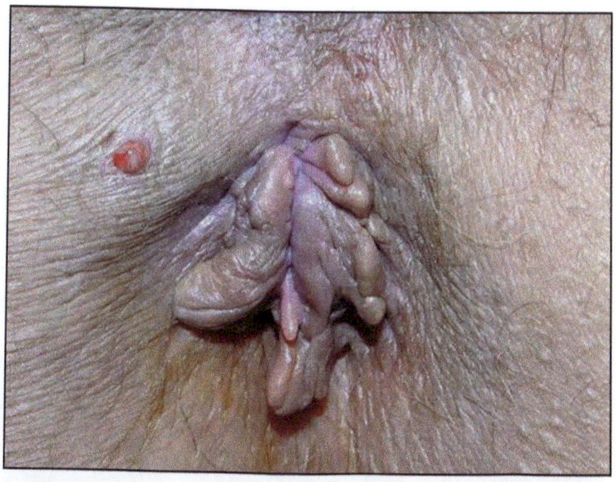

a

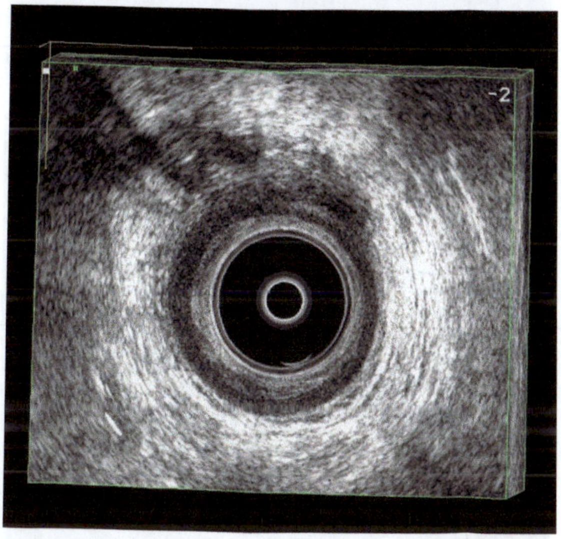

b

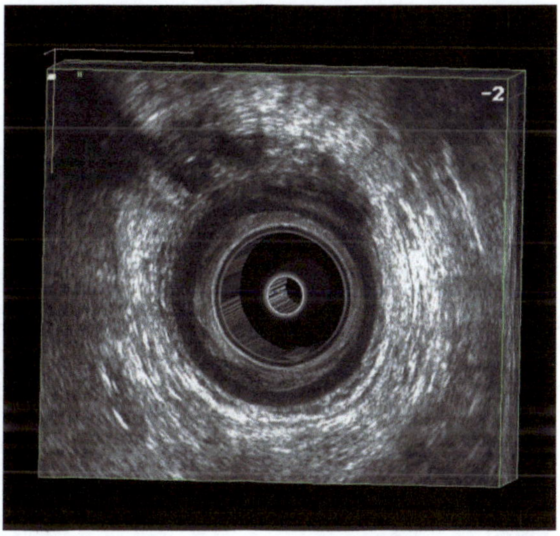

c

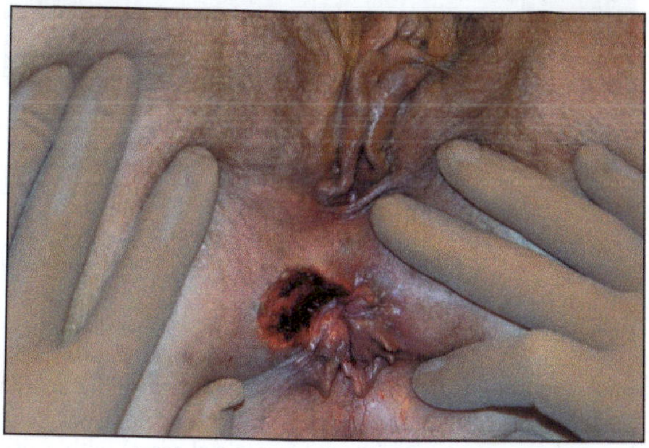

d

Case V.17. A 36-year-old woman complaining of perianal purulent discharge. Physical examination reveals a cutaneous opening at the 11 o'clock position (**a**). Axial endosonographic image at mid anal canal level shows an anterior hypoechoic tract extending through the external sphincter, which contacts the internal sphincter at the 12 o'clock position (transsphincteric fistula) (**b**). Volume render mode (**c**). The patient underwent a laid-open procedure (**d**)

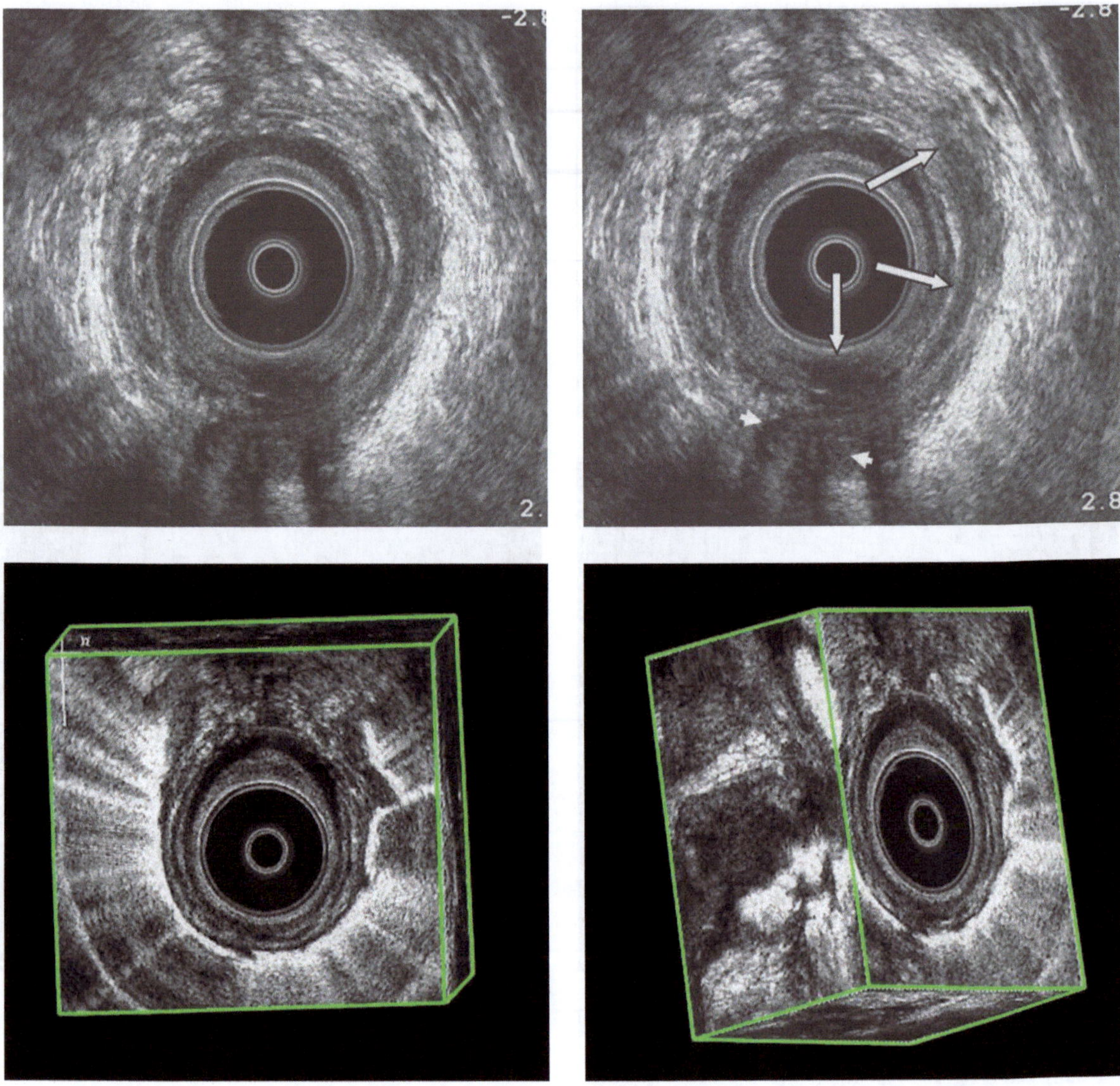

a b c d

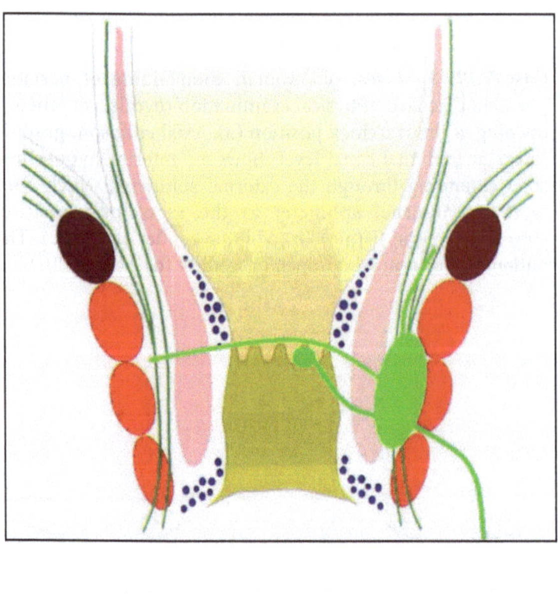

e

Case V.18. A 53-year-old man complaining of fever and purulent discharge from an external orifice at the 6 o'clock position. Axial endoanal ultrasonography (EAUS) scans at mid anal canal level show a posterior, large, intersphincteric hypoechoic area (acute intersphincteric abscess) with a primary tract (*small arrows*) extending from this area through the external sphincter (transsphincteric fistula) and a secondary tract extending through the left side of the intersphincteric plane (*large arrows*) (**a**, **b**). After peroxide injection, the EAUS scan reveals an horseshoe extension into the intersphincteric plane (**c**). Three-dimensional reconstruction on the sagittal plane shows upward extension of the horseshoe secondary tract (**d**). Drawing in the axial plane shows extent of the abscess and fistulas (**e**)

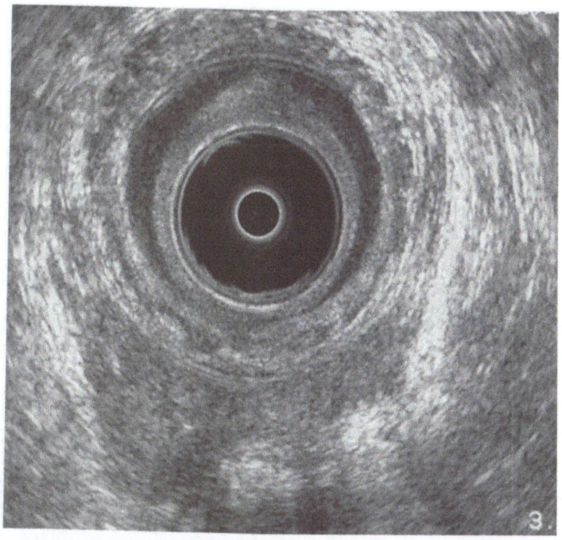

a

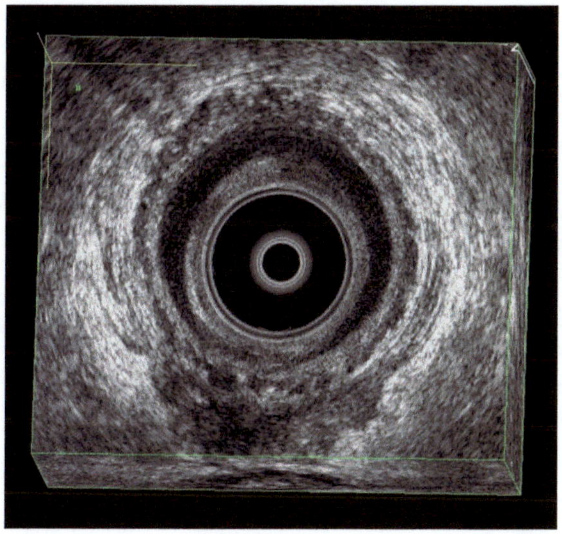

b

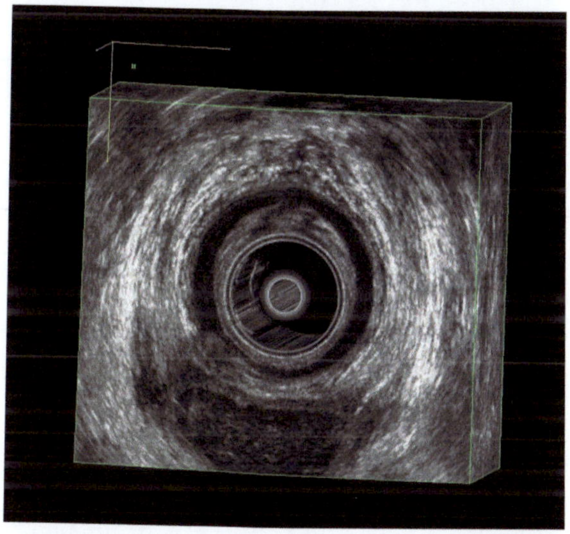

c

Case V.19. A 58-year-old man complaining of fever and perirectal pain. Digital rectal examination reveals a posterior tender mass at the dentate line level 2 cm from the anal verge. Axial endosonographic image of mid anal canal level reveals a large hypoechoic area in the posterior intersphincteric zone (**a**). Three-dimensional endoanal ultrasonography scan confirms the presence of an acute posterior intersphincteric abscess (**b**). Volume render mode (**c**)

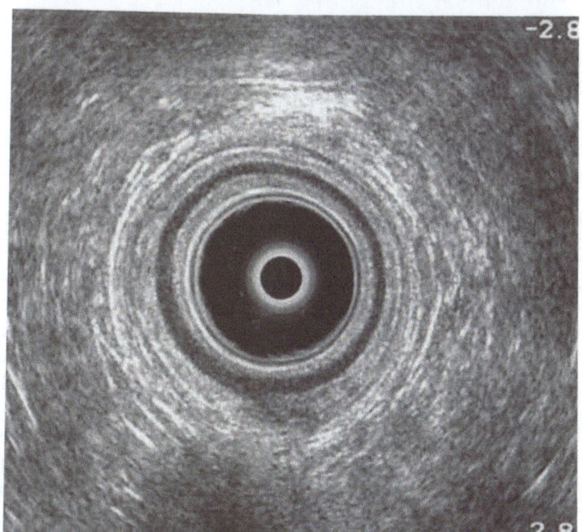

a

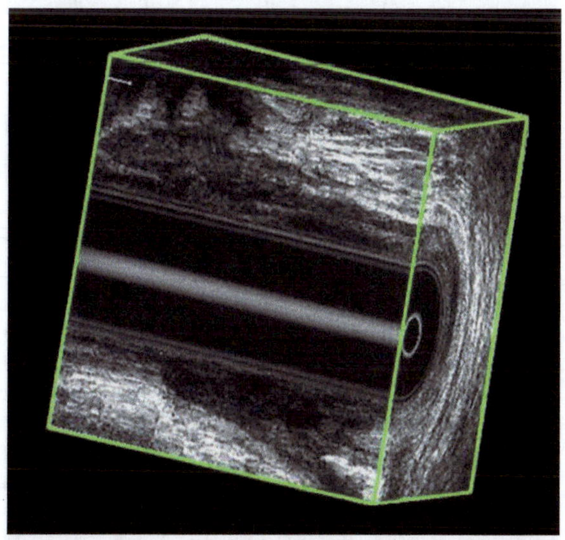

b

Case V.20. A 37-year-old woman complaining of perianal pain. Axial endosonographic image of mid anal canal level reveals a hypoechoic area in the intersphincteric zone at the 6 o'clock position (**a**). Sagittal view from a three-dimensional data set shows a low intersphincteric tract (**b**). The patient underwent a laid-open procedure

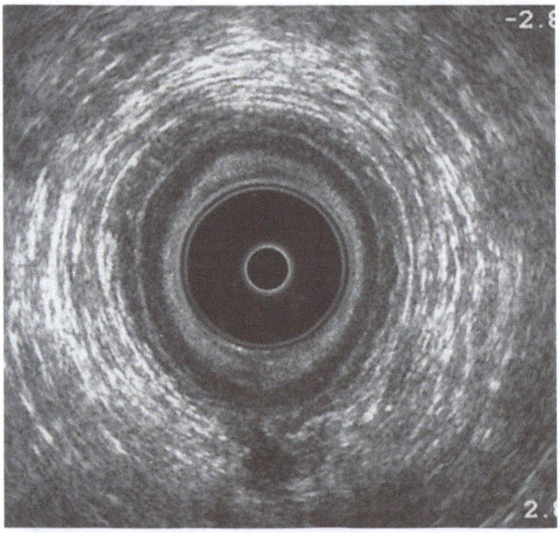
a

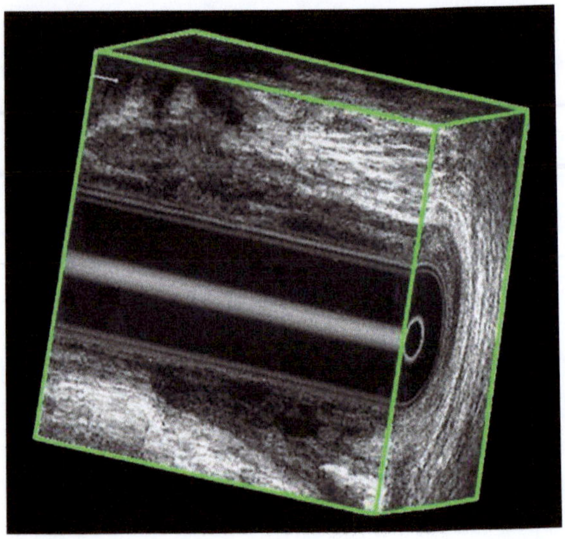
b

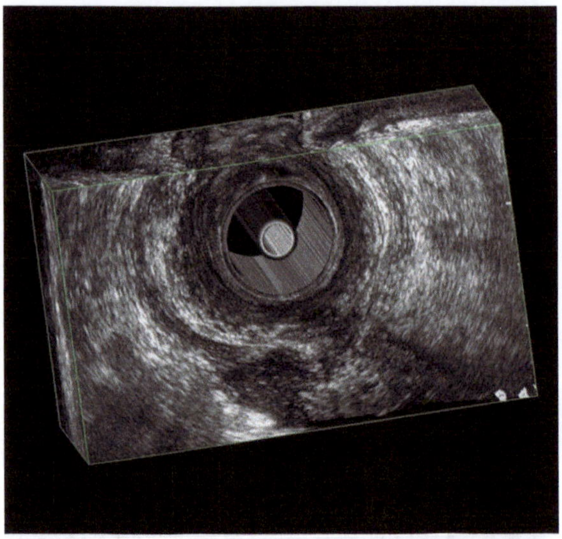
c

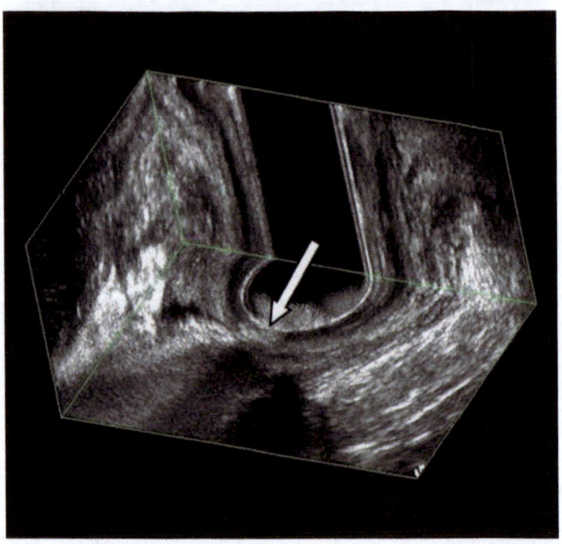
d

Case V.21. A 43-year-old man complaining of recurrent perianal purulent discharge. Physical examination reveals a cutaneous opening at the 6 o'clock position. Axial endosonographic image at mid anal canal level shows a posterior hypoechoic tract extending through the external sphincter, which contacts the internal sphincter at the 6 o'clock position (third endosonographic criteria for the site of an internal opening according to Cho [17]) (**a**). Sagittal view from a three-dimensional data set confirming the presence of a low transsphincteric fistula that traverses only the distal third of the external sphincter (**b**). Volume render mode (**c, d**). The internal opening is located at the 6 o'clock position (*arrow*). After demonstration of the limited involvement of the external sphincter, the patient underwent a fistulotomy, with no loss of continence

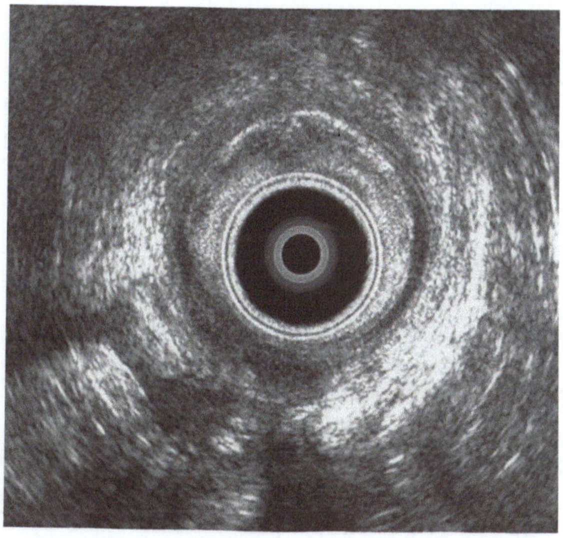

a

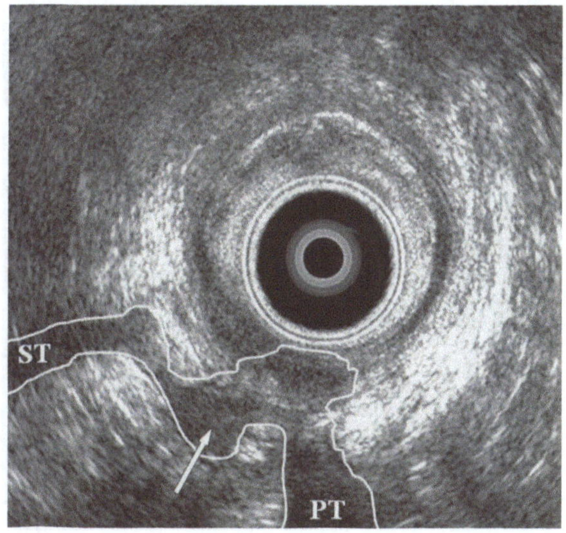

b

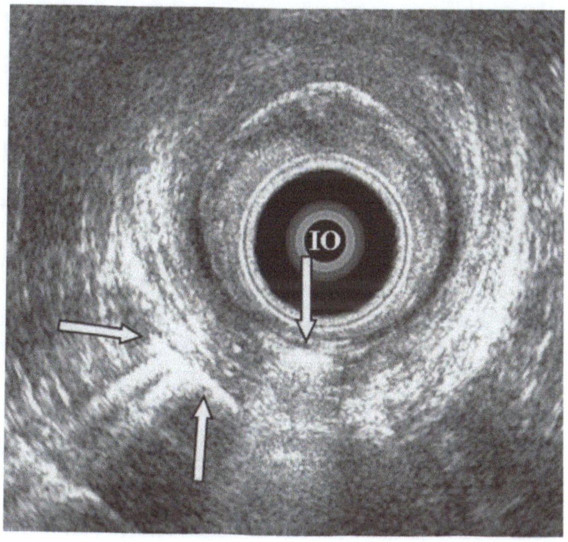

c

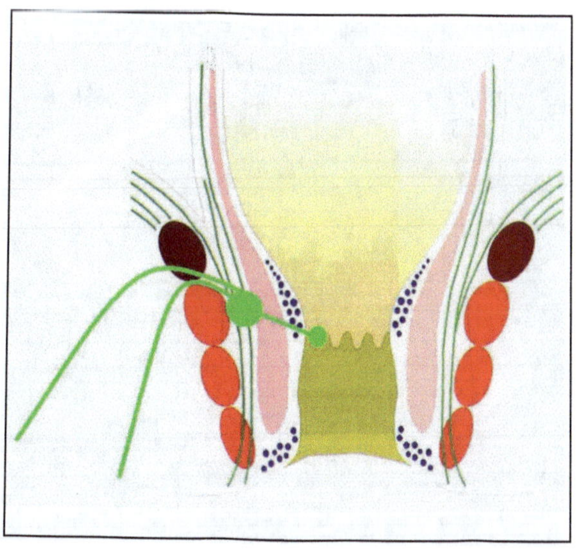

d

Case V.22. A 28-year-old woman referred for recurrent perianal fistulas. Physical examination reveals two external openings at the 6 and 9 o'clock positions, respectively. Axial endoanal ultrasonography (EAUS) scan shows an intersphincteric hypoechoic area (acute intersphincteric abscess) at the 6 o'clock position (*arrow*), with a primary tract (*PT*) extending posteriorly from this area through the puborectal muscle (suprasphincteric fistula) and a secondary tract (*ST*) extending in the right side and traversing the puborectal muscle at the 9 o'clock position (**a**, **b**). After injection of peroxide from the external opening at the 6 o'clock position, the EAUS scan reveals an immediate communication with the anal lumen (*IO* internal opening) (**c**). Drawing in the axial plane shows extent of the abscess and fistulas (**d**)

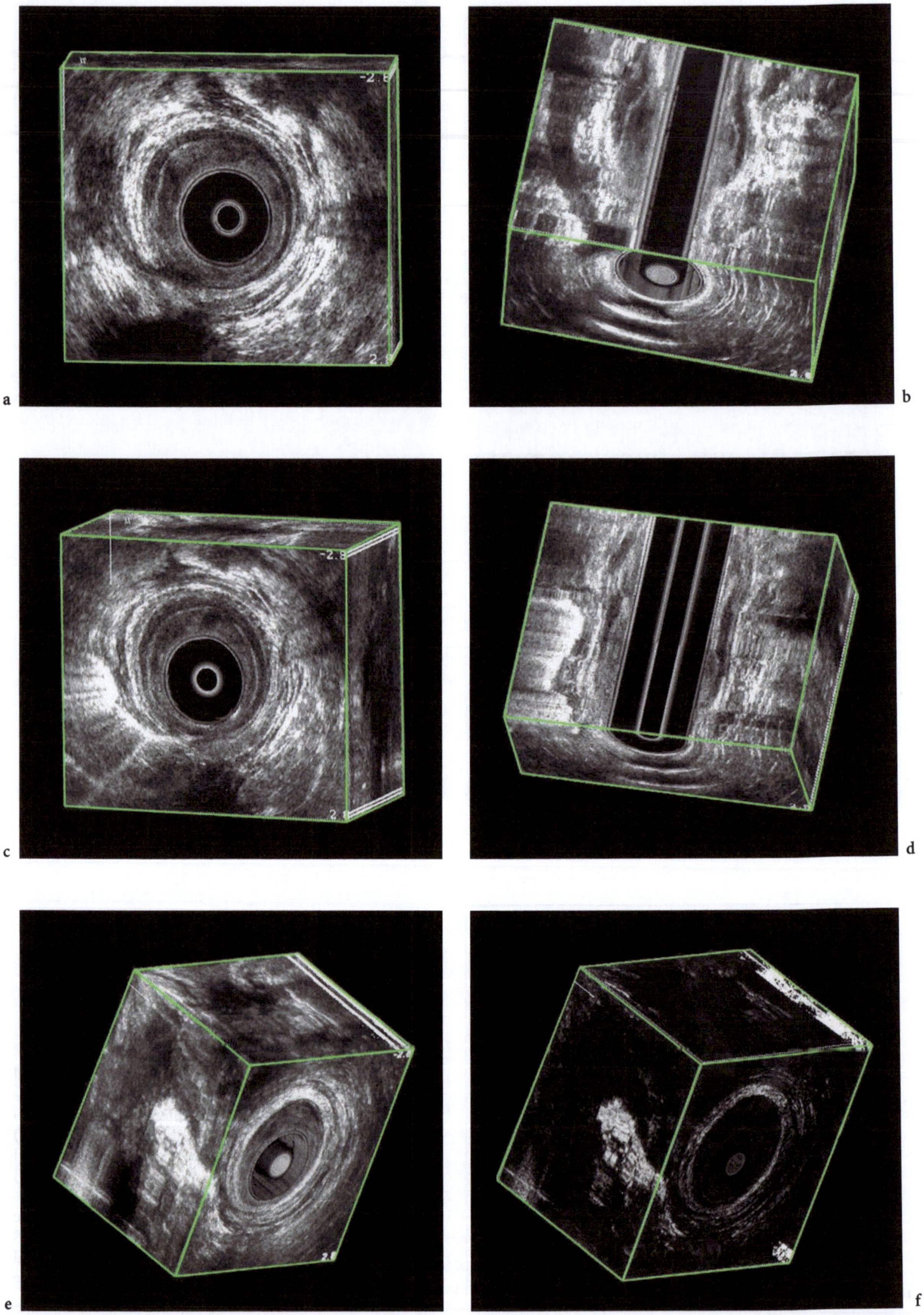
a
b
c
d
e
f

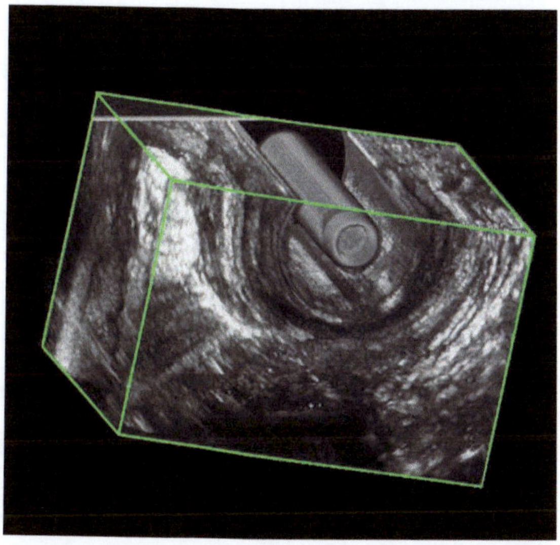
g

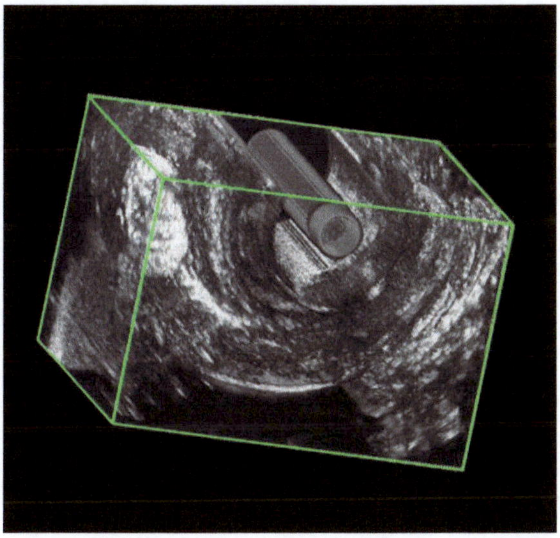
h

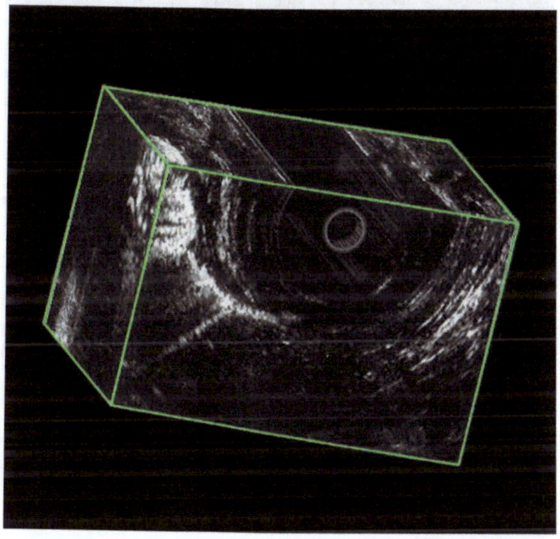
i

Case V.23. A 26-year-old man with recurrent perianal Crohn's disease. Axial endosonographic image of mid anal canal level reveals a hypoechoic area into the right ischiorectal fossa (acute abscess) with a primary tract extending from this area and traversing the external and internal sphincter at the 6 o'clock position (transsphincteric fistula) (**a**). Three-dimensional reconstruction on the coronal plane shows upward extension of the ischiorectal abscess (**b**). After peroxide injection through a cutaneous orifice at the 9 o'clock position (right lateral side) endoanal ultrasonography scans with volume render mode confirm the presence of an acute ischiorectal abscess (**c-f**) with a transsphincteric fistula (**g-i**)

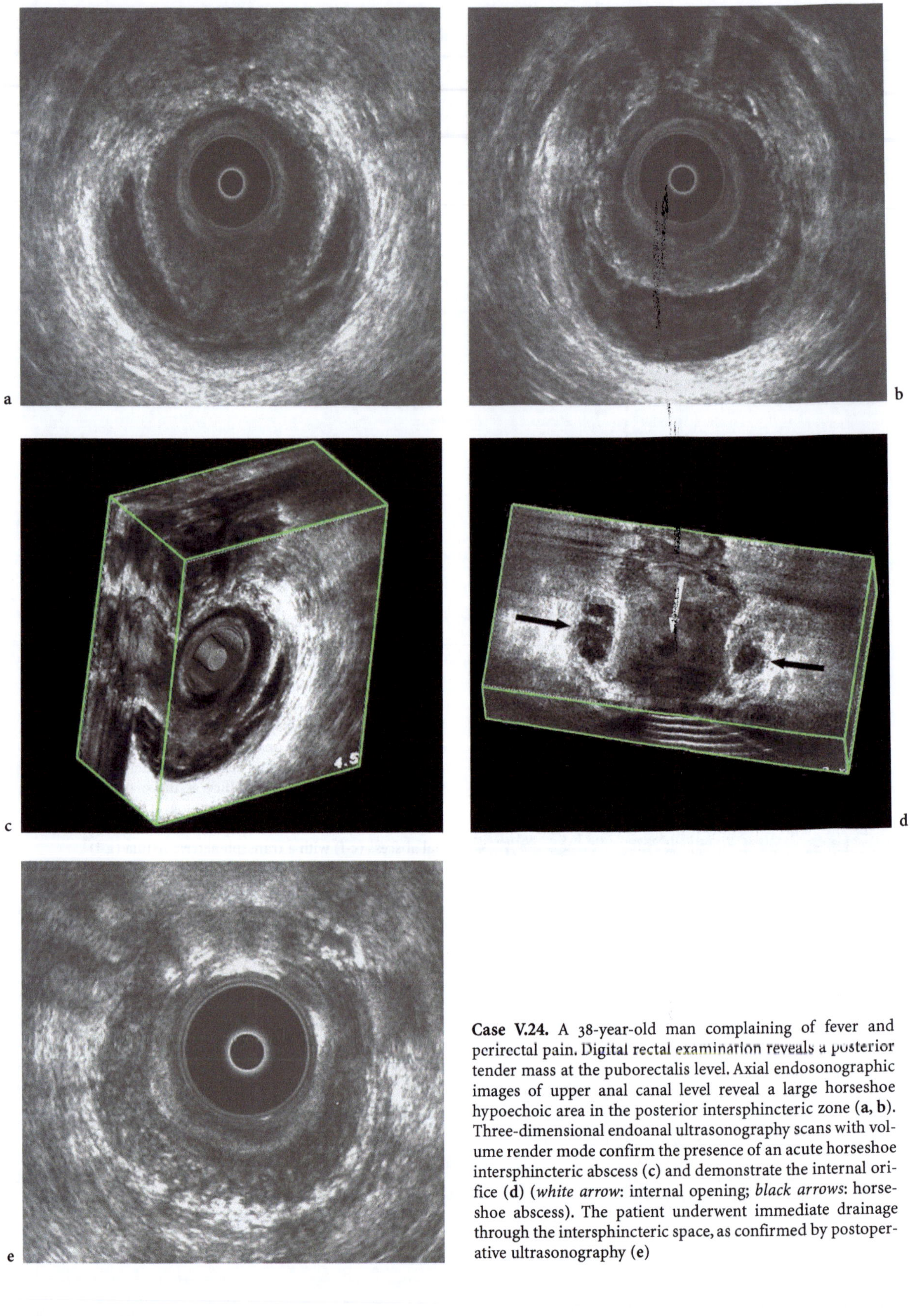

Case V.24. A 38-year-old man complaining of fever and perirectal pain. Digital rectal examination reveals a posterior tender mass at the puborectalis level. Axial endosonographic images of upper anal canal level reveal a large horseshoe hypoechoic area in the posterior intersphincteric zone (**a**, **b**). Three-dimensional endoanal ultrasonography scans with volume render mode confirm the presence of an acute horseshoe intersphincteric abscess (**c**) and demonstrate the internal orifice (**d**) (*white arrow*: internal opening; *black arrows*: horseshoe abscess). The patient underwent immediate drainage through the intersphincteric space, as confirmed by postoperative ultrasonography (**e**)

V.3. Imaging Perianal Sepsis: Anal Endosonography or MR Imaging?

S. Halligan

A variety of imaging techniques have been used to evaluate fistula-in-ano and perianal sepsis over the years. Some these are more useful than others, and practitioners experienced in this field tend to agree that fistulography and computed tomography (CT) scanning, even in the era of multidetector-row scanning, are not very helpful [1]. This is because in order be of any significant clinical use, an imaging test has to bring something to the surgeon's table that is additional to the information provided at his or her examination under anesthetic (EUA). The surgeon is primarily concerned with the relationship of the fistula tract to the sphincter complex – i.e., the fistula classification [2]. This allows the surgical approach to be planned carefully and appropriately. Fistula-in-ano has a tendency to recur despite seemingly adequate surgery, and recurrence is usually due to infection that has escaped surgical detection at EUA and thus gone untreated. Identification of sepsis that would otherwise have been missed is unquestionably the prime role for preoperative imaging in these patients, and there is now little doubt, if any, that magnetic resonance imaging (MRI) is best-suited to this task. However, there are other aspects of assessment that sometimes cause the surgeon considerable trouble. Identifying the radial site and level of the internal opening is one example, and is a well-recognized problem at EUA in some patients – patients in whom an internal opening is not detected have a high chance of relapse. Imaging may be used to direct the surgeon to the enteric communication when this is not immediately apparent at EUA, and anal endosonography (AES) is particularly adept in this setting. It should also be borne in mind that although radiologists (and surgeons) are constantly searching for the "one best test," most investigations provide complementary and additive information, and there are no disadvantages to performing both MRI and AES in the same patient where local circumstances, availability, and economics allow.

Anal Endosonography

AES has already been discussed in the context of perianal sepsis in Chapter 2 of this Section. When considering the comparison between AES and MRI, it is worthwhile focussing on exactly what it is that sonography does well. It is well-established that ultrasound generally best images structures that are close to the transducer surface, and the higher the frequency of the transducer, the more this condition will apply. AES is most used for assessment of anal sphincter injury in the context of fecal incontinence [3] because the anal sphincters, lying close to the transducer, are imaged with high spatial resolution. It follows then, that in the context of fistula-in-ano, those aspects of the fistula that lie close to or within the sphincter complex will be imaged with most precision. In particular, using modern 10 -MHz transducers [4], endosonography is particularly well suited to identification of the internal opening because it usually lies right at the probe surface. When considering identification of the internal opening, it is important to realize that a tract extending right up to the anal mucosal surface is rarely seen. Although a breach in the subepithelial layer of the anal canal is occasionally present, it is more com-

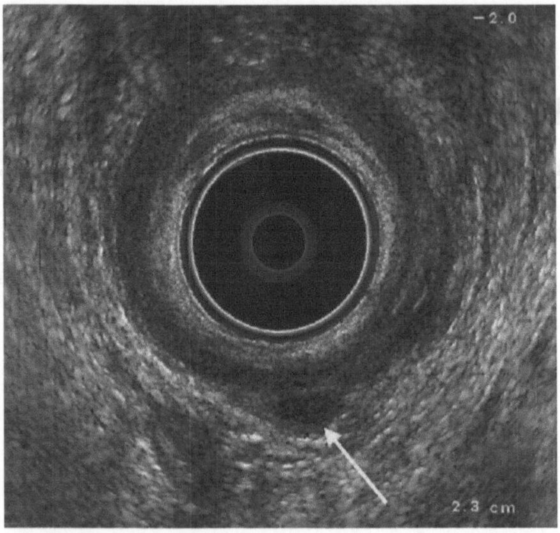

Fig. V.40. Anal endosonography reveals a focus of intersphincteric sepsis posteriorly at 6 o'clock at dentate line level (*arrow*). This was the site of the internal opening - note that the tract cannot be traced right to the anal canal lumen

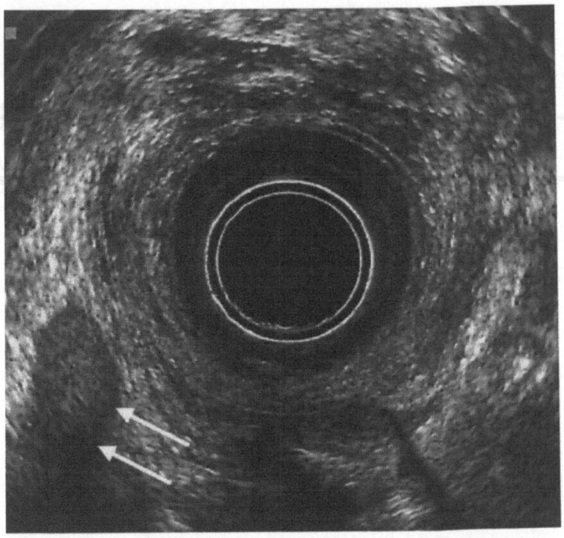

Fig. V.42. Anal endosonography shows a collection in the right posterior quadrant of the ischioanal fossa (*arrows*). Loss of peripheral signal makes it difficult to trace this in its entirety (see Fig. V.49)

mon for the position of the internal opening to be revealed by a hypoechoic focus in the intersphincteric space that abuts the internal sphincter (Fig. V.40), often with a small corresponding defect in the internal sphincter. Because intersphincteric fistulas never stray beyond the intersphincteric space, they are usually well visualized by AES (Fig. V.41).

It also follows that isolated intersphincteric abscesses are also well seen using AES. In the

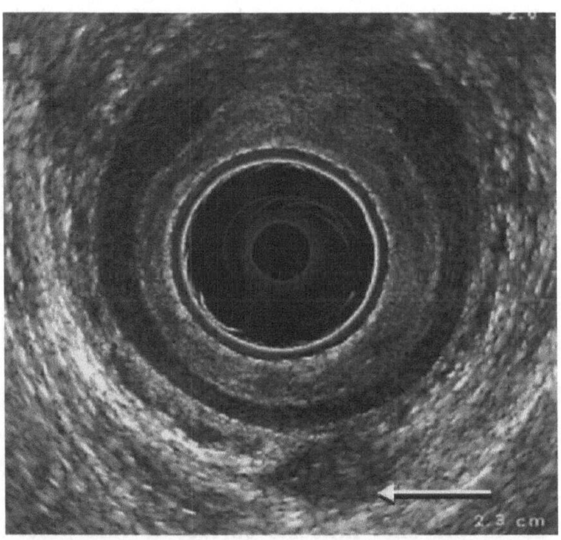

Fig. V.41. Anal endosonography shows an intersphincteric fistula (*arrow*). Note that the fistula is medial to the external sphincter

author's practice, the technique has considerable utility in patients known to have had a fistula previously and who have new symptoms suggesting that they are developing further sepsis but in whom digital anal examination is normal. AES facilitates quick and easy diagnosis of intersphincteric abscesses in this situation, many of which are small and impalpable but which are well seen on ultrasound because of the high spatial resolution of the technique.

Transsphincteric fistulas are revealed by tracts that cross the external sphincter to reach the ischioanal (ischiorectal) fossa. As would be expected, extensions are revealed as hypoechoic fluid collections, but it is here that AES starts to lag behind MRI. The further the extensions are from the anal canal, the less well they are visualized by AES (Fig. V.42). This is because the depth of penetration of the ultrasound beam is limited, especially at higher frequencies. It should also be noted that endoanal MRI suffers from similar limitations [5]. Also, AES cannot reliably distinguish infection from fibrosis since both appear hypoechoic [6]. This causes particular difficulties in patients with recurrent disease since infected tracts and fibrotic scars are frequently combined. Attempts have been made to clarify the course of tracts by injecting hydrogen peroxide or ultrasound contrast agents into the external opening during examination [7, 8]. However, gas formed within the tract as a result may cause acoustic

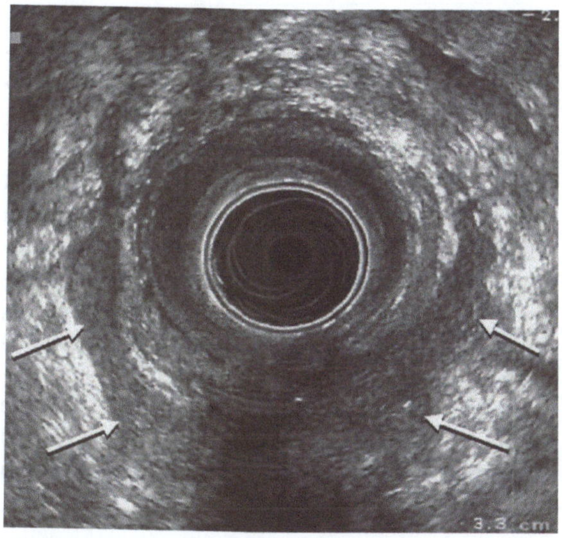

Fig. V.43. Anal endosonography showing an obvious large extension (*arrows*). The surrounding anatomy is distorted, and it is difficult to be sure whether the extension is infralevator, supralevator, or includes elements of both

shadowing that mimics an extension. Indeed, this phenomenon potentially occurs with any tract that contains air. For example, intersphincteric fistulas may be inadvertently classified as transsphincteric as a result.

The levator plate (pelvic floor) is a crucial landmark for surgeons since the treatment options for patients with supralevator and infralevator sepsis may differ significantly. Notably, the levator plate forms a relative barrier to surgical drainage, and supralevator sepsis usually means

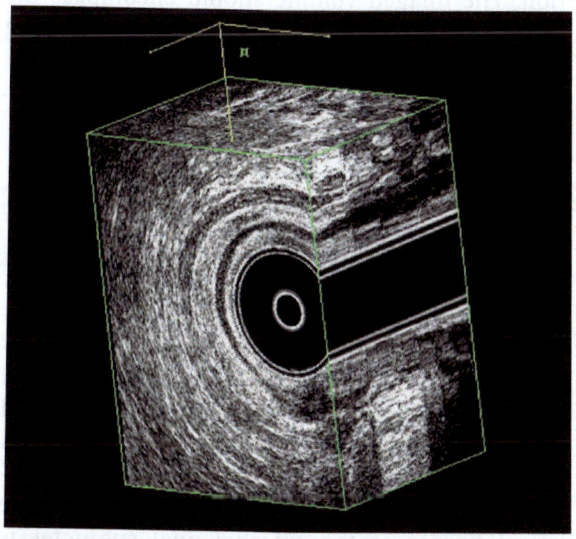

Fig. V.44. Three-dimensional anal endosonography

extensive surgical incision if adequate drainage is to be achieved. AES has great difficulty visualizing the precise position of the levator plates because they lie in the same plane as the ultrasound beam and, moreover, they are poorly differentiated from surrounding structures (unlike their appearance on MRI). The result is that it can be very difficult to determine if a collection is supra- or infralevator (Fig. V.43). Some workers have attempted to overcome this disadvantage by employing three-dimensional (3-D) acquisition [9] (Fig. V.44), but this remains largely experimental.

It was initially hoped that AES would revolutionize preoperative fistula classification, a view supported by early studies [10]. However, subsequent work has been inconclusive. For example, some investigators have found the technique useful [11, 12] while others have found it no better than digital examination [6].

MR Imaging

In recent years, MRI has emerged as the leading contender for preoperative classification of fistula-in-ano. It not only classifies tracts accurately, but also identifies diseases that would otherwise have been missed – an area where it excels more than any other technique, including EUA. MRI has had a palpable effect on surgical treatment and, ultimately, patient outcome.

Coils

The technique for MRI is extremely simple and can be achieved with most equipment. For example, field strength does not appear to be a critical factor for good results [13]. Initial reports of MRI necessarily used the body coil [14–18], and the introduction of external phased array surface coils further increased signal-to-noise ratio (SNR) and spatial resolution [19, 20]. The best spatial resolution is achieved by using dedicated endoluminal anal coils [21]. It should be noted that these endoluminal coils are not the same as rectal coils, being smaller and designed for location in the anus. Their availability remains relatively restricted. Endoluminal coils are susceptible to motion artefact, but this can be reduced by careful patient preparation. For example, patients should be asked to try to relax the sphincter and pelvic floor as much as possible, and due attention should be paid to comfort, including supporting the coil and patient with pads [22]. Spasmolytics may help to reduce motion-induced artefacts – either 20 mg hyoscine butylbromide (Buscopan) or 1 mg glucagon intramuscularly.

The exact choice of coil depends on personal preference, availability, the patient group studied, and the clinical question in each particular patient. A study of ten patients with cryptoglandular fistulas found an endoluminal coil superior to a surface coil [23] whereas a subsequent study of 30 patients found a body coil superior overall because the limited field of view inevitable with endoluminal imaging meant that distant extensions were missed [5]. A third study compared endoluminal and phased array coils in 20 patients and found that while the endoluminal coil was superior for classification of the primary track, extensions were better imaged using the superior field-of-view of the external coil [24]. These results suggest clearly that a large field-of-view is necessary whenever extensions are suspected, for example, in patients with recurrent fistula or Crohn's disease. The high spatial resolution of endoluminal coils makes them ideal for demonstrating precisely the location and height of the internal opening, rather like AES, and they may have a special role for demonstrating ano- or rectovaginal fistulas, which are notoriously difficult to image [25]. They are also valuable when simultaneous information on the degree of any sphincter disruption is needed, which may be the case in patients who have had previous surgery. Endoluminal coils are sometimes difficult to place due to anal stenosis or local pain as a result of extensive infection. The author found that an endoluminal coil could not be sited in 17% of his patients [5], but Stoker and colleagues failed in only 3% [22], possibly reflecting differing patient populations.

Where circumstances allow, it is likely that optimal examination will be achieved using a combination of both external and endoluminal coils. However, it should be borne in mind that accuracy with external coils alone remains high [5, 16–20], and lack of an endoluminal coil alone is insufficient reason to avoid preoperative MRI of fistula-in-ano.

Sequences

Various investigators have adopted different strategies with respect to the sequences used to image fistula-in-ano, but all agree that anatomic precision is needed in combination with some method by which infection is highlighted. Many investigators employ the rapid and convenient fast-spin-echo, T2-weighted sequence, which provides good contrast between hyperintense fluid within the tract and its hypointense fibrous wall while simultaneously enabling good discrimination between the several layers of the anal sphincter. Others have used T1-weighted sequences, which must be combined with intravenous contrast for the fistula to be highlighted. Fat suppression techniques are also widely used, and the author favors short T1 inversion recovery (STIR) imaging, which combines fat suppression with high conspicuity of active tracts.

Imaging Planes

It is vital that imaging planes are aligned with respect to the anal canal. Because the anal canal is tilted forward from the vertical by approximately 45°, straight axial and coronal images are unsatisfactory. Instead, oblique axial and coronal planes orientated orthogonal and parallel to the anal sphincter are required and are planned easily from a midline sagittal image. It is important that the imaged volume extends several centimeters above the levators and also includes the whole presacral space, both of which are common sites for extensions. The entire perineum should also be included. Occasionally, tracts may extend for several centimeters, and any tract visible on the standard volume must be followed to its termination. The imaged volume should encompass the whole sensitive region of the coil when using endoanal receivers.

Interpretation

The success of MRI for preoperative classification of fistula-in-ano is a direct result of its sensitivity for tracts and abscesses combined with high anatomic precision and ability to image in surgically relevant planes. Accurate preoperative classification is achieved by correctly relating the imaged fistula to the anal sphincter. Active tracks are filled with pus and granulation tissue and thus appear as hyperintense longitudinal structures on T2-weighted or STIR sequences. Unlike ultrasound, the lateral border of the external anal sphincter is

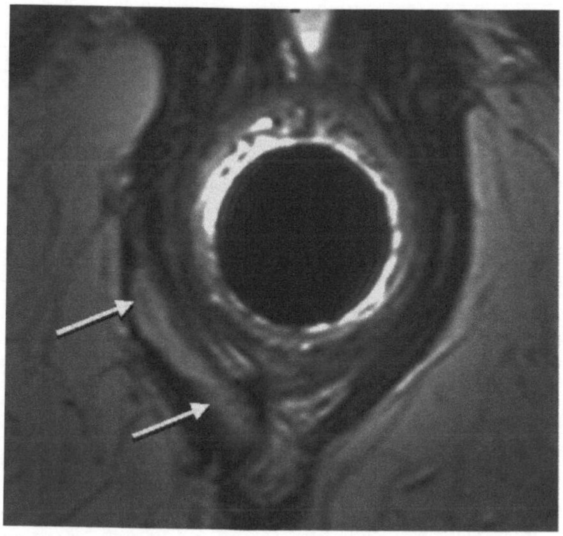

Fig. V.45. Endoanal magnetic resonance image of an extensive intersphincteric fistula (*arrows*). Note that there in no sepsis in the ischioanal fossa (compare with Fig. V.46)

clearly visualized in most patients using MRI. This makes it relatively easy to determine whether a fistula is contained by the external sphincter or has extended beyond it. If a fistula remains contained by the external sphincter throughout its course, then it is highly likely to be intersphincteric (Fig. V.45). In contrast, any evidence of a tract in the ischioanal fossa effectively excludes an intersphincteric fistula. However, transsphincteric, suprasphincteric, and extrasphincteric fistulas all share the common feature of a tract lying beyond the confines of the external sphincter.

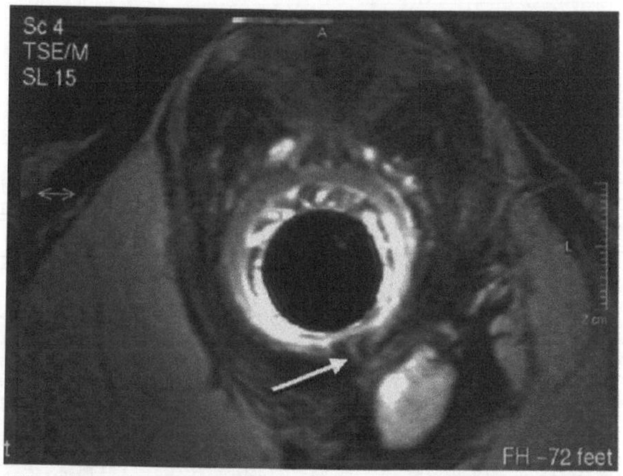

Fig. V.46. Endoanal magnetic resonance image of a transsphincteric fistula. There is a primary track in the left posterior aspect of the ischioanal fossa. The internal opening is well demonstrated (*arrow*)

While a transsphincteric fistula will be the commonest cause of a tract in the ischioanal fossa (Fig. V.46), differentiation between these three fistulas is only possible by locating the internal opening and determining the course between this and the primary tract. The exact location of the internal opening can be difficult to define. Two questions need to be answered: what is the radial site of the internal opening and what is its level? The vast majority of anal fistulas open into the anal canal at the level of the dentate line commensurate with the cryptoglandular hypothesis of fistula pathogenesis. Furthermore, most fistulas enter posteriorly at 6 o'clock. Unfortunately, the dentate line cannot be identified as a discrete anatomical entity either on AES or MRI, even when using endoanal receiver coils, but its general location can be estimated with sufficient precision for imaging to be worthwhile. The dentate line lies at approximately midanal canal level, which is midway between the superior border of the puborectalis muscle and the most caudal extent of the subcutaneous external sphincter. These landmarks define the "surgical" anal canal (as distinct from the "anatomical" anal canal, which is shorter and defined as the canal caudal to the anal valves). Dentate level is probably appreciated best using coronal views, but with experience, its location can be estimated from axial views with reasonable precision. Any tract that penetrates the pelvic floor above the level of the puborectalis muscle is potentially a suprasphincteric or extrasphincteric fistula. The level of the internal opening distinguishes between these, being anal in the former and rectal in the latter (Fig. V.47).

The radial site of the internal opening is simple to identify if the fistula can be traced into the anal lumen. However, like endosonography, it is frequently impossible to trace a tract right up to the anal mucosa. In such cases, an intelligent deduction must be made as to where the internal opening is likely to be, which is best done by looking to where there is maximal intersphincteric sepsis. The intersphincteric space and longitudinal layer is often seen as a low-intensity ring lying between the internal and external sphincter. The internal sphincter is hyperintense on both T2-weighted fast-spin-echo and STIR sequences.

The major advantage of MRI over AES is the facility with which it can image extensions. Like fistula tracts, extensions are revealed as hyperintense regions on T2-weighted and STIR imaging. The commonest type of extension is one that arises from the apex of a transsphincteric tract and

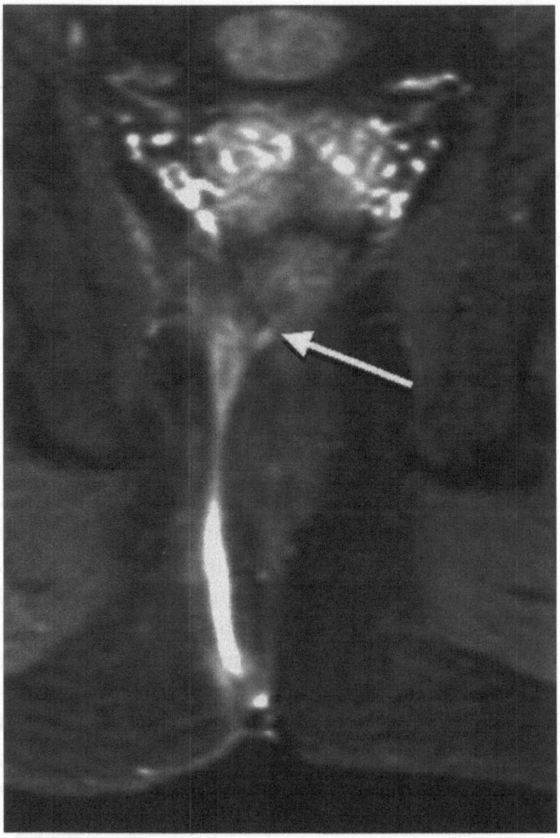

Fig. V.47. Coronal image from a body-coil magnetic resonance examination showing a right-sided ischioanal tract with an enteric communication (*arrow*) above the puborectalis, diagnosing an extrasphincteric fistula

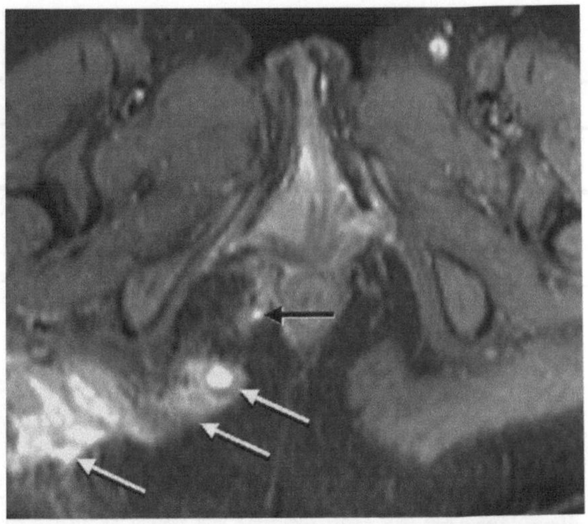

Fig. V.49. Same patient as Fig. V.42. The distant extension into the buttock (*white arrows*) is much better appreciated on magnetic resonance imaging than on anal endosonography. Note that the extension is well away from the primary tract (*black arrow*)

extends into the roof of the ischioanal fossa (Fig. V.48). The major benefit of MRI is that it can alert the surgeon to extensions that would otherwise be missed since they can travel several centimeters from the primary tract (Fig. V.49), which makes them difficult to detect by clinical examination or EUA. It is especially important to search for supralevator extensions (Fig. V.50) since these are not only difficult to detect but pose specific difficulties with treatment. Complex extensions are especially common in patients with recurrent fistula-in-ano or those who have Crohn's disease [19, 20].

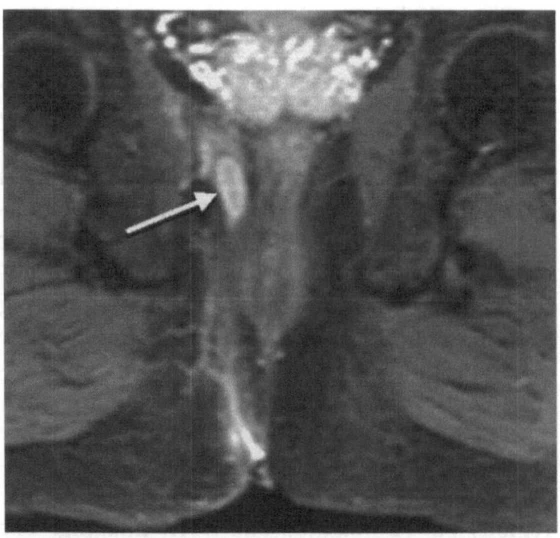

Fig. V.48. Surface coil magnetic resonance imaging clearly demonstrates an extension (*arrow*) into the roof of the right ischioanal fossa

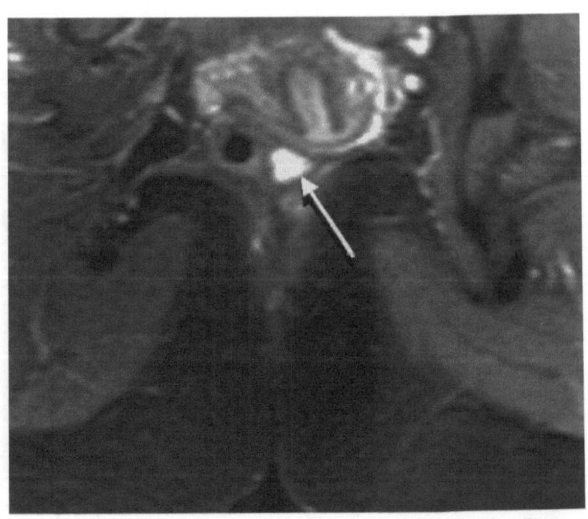

Fig. V.50. Coronal image from a body-coil magnetic resonance examination showing a supralevator abscess (*arrow*)

Comparisons between MR Imaging and Anal Endosonography

A variety of investigators have directly compared AES with MRI, both with and without an endoanal coil, and these comparisons have found endosonography variously superior [26], equivalent [27, 28], or inferior [7, 8]. On the face of it, these comparisons are confusing and unhelpful. In the author's opinion, much of this uncertainty stems from relative unfamiliarity with one of the techniques under evaluation, both of which are highly dependent (like all imaging tests) on expert interpretation.

The true potential of MRI was not fully appreciated until the study by Lunniss and coworkers [16], who imaged 16 patients with cryptoglandular fistula-in-ano and compared the MR classification with that obtained at subsequent EUA. MRI proved correct in 14 of the 16 cases (88%), immediately suggesting that it was the most accurate preoperative assessment yet available. However, the remaining two patients, in whom MR suggested disease but EUA had been normal, re-presented some months later with disease at the site initially indicated by MRI. This led the authors to conclude "MRI is the most accurate method for determining the presence and course of anal fistulae" [16]. This work was confirmed rapidly by others and subsequently elaborated on. Spencer and colleagues independently classified 37 patients into those with simple or complex fistulas on the basis of MRI and EUA and found that imaging was the better predictor of outcome, with positive and negative predictive values of 73% versus 57% and 87% versus 64% for MR and surgery, respectively [29]. This study implied clearly that MRI and outcome were closely related and again raised the possibility that preoperative MRI could help identify features that underpinned postoperative recurrence. Beets-Tan and colleagues extended this hypothesis by investigating the therapeutic impact of preoperative MRI; the MRI findings in 56 patients were revealed to the operating surgeon after they had completed an initial EUA [19]. MRI provided important additional information that precipitated further surgery in 12 of the 56 patients (21%), predominantly in those with recurrent fistulas or Crohn's disease [19].

Buchanan and coworkers hypothesized that the therapeutic impact and thus beneficial effect of preoperative MRI would be greatest in patients with recurrent fistulas since these had the most chance of harboring occult infection while also being the most difficult to evaluate clinically [20]. After an initial EUA, they revealed the findings of preoperative MRI in 71 patients with recurrent fistulas and left any further surgery to the discretion of the operating surgeon. They found that postoperative recurrence was only 16% for surgeons who always acted if MRI suggested they had missed areas of infection whereas recurrence was 57% for surgeons who instead chose always to ignore imaging [20]. The authors were thus able to demonstrate that correct use of MRI could ultimately affect clinical outcome, something that has not been achieved for AES. Furthermore, of the 16 patients who needed further unplanned surgery, MRI initially correctly predicted the site of this disease in all cases [20]. Using a similar approach, the same research group also investigated the effect of preoperative MRI on clinical outcome in patients presenting with primary fistula-in-ano, finding that the scheduled surgical approach changed in 10% as a result [30].

Ever since Lunniss's work suggested that EUA might be an imperfect reference standard with which to judge MRI [16], comparative studies have been plagued by the lack of a genuine reference standard. It is now well recognized that surgical findings at EUA are often incorrect. In particular, there are frequent false negatives. In a recent comparative study of endosonography, MRI, and EUA in 34 patients with fistulas due to Crohn's disease, Schwartz and coworkers found that a combination of results of at least two modalities was necessary in order to arrive at a correct classification [27]. Indeed, it is well established that many surgical false negatives only reveal themselves during long-term clinical follow-up and, at this point in time, comparative studies that ignore clinical outcome are likely to be seriously flawed at best. In what the author believes is the best comparison to date, Buchanan and coworkers classified 108 primary tracts using clinical examination in the clinic, AES, and MRI and compared the findings to a reference standard that was based on ultimate clinical outcome [31]. Digital evaluation correctly classified 61% of primary tracts in comparison to 81% for AES and 90% for MRI [31]. While MRI was superior in every comparison made by the authors, AES was particularly adept at correctly predicting the site of the internal opening, achieving this in 91% compared with 97% for MRI [31]. However, there was little doubt that MRI was a superior technique overall.

Conclusion

In the author's opinion, if imaging has to be restricted to one test, then MRI is the clear favorite. However, as stated already, AES and MRI may provide complementary information, and no harm comes from performing both. AES does have some clear advantages although these are related to the fact that it is relatively cheap and simple to perform rather than its technical performance. It is rapid and well tolerated by patients and, unlike MRI, can be performed easily in the outpatient clinic or even on the ward since machines are easily portable. It should also be borne in mind that AES is vastly superior to digital examination in the clinic and is therefore well worth performing, especially if MRI is unavailable or if there is no specific expertise in its interpretation. Also, a major role of AES in fistula disease is to assess the degree of sphincter disruption in those patients who become anally incontinent following surgery.

References

1. Halligan S, Stoker J (2006) Imaging fistula-in-ano: State-of-the-art. Radiology (*in press*)
2. Parks AG, Gordon PH, Hardcastle JD (1976) A classification of fisula-in-ano. Br J Surg 63:1–12
3. Sultan AH, Kamm MA, Hudson CN et al (1993) Anal sphincter disruption during vaginal delivery. N Engl J Med 329:1905–1911
4. Frudinger A, Halligan S, Bartram CI et al (2002) Female anal sphincter: Age-related differences in asymptomatic volunteers with high frequency endoanal US. Radiology 224:417–423
5. Halligan S, Bartram CI (1998) MR imaging of fistula in ano: are endoanal coils the gold standard? AJR Am J Roentgenol 171:407–412
6. Choen S, Burnett S, Bartram CI, Nicholls RJ (1991) Comparison between anal endosonography and digital examination in the evaluation of anal fistulae. Br J Surg 78:445–447
7. Kruskal JB, Kane RA, Morrin MM (2001) Peroxide-enhanced anal endosonography: technique, image interpretation, and clinical applications. Radiographics 21:173–189
8. Chew SS, Yang JL, Newstead GL, Douglas PR (2003) Anal fistula: Levovist-enhanced endoanal ultrasound: a pilot study. Dis Colon Rectum 46: 377–384
9. Buchanan GN, Bartram CI, Williams AB et al (2005) Value of hydrogen peroxide enhancement of three-dimensional endoanal ultrasound in fistula-in-ano. Dis Colon Rectum 48:141–147
10. Law PJ, Talbot RW, Bartram CI et al (1989) Anal endosonography in the evaluation of perianal sepsis and fistula-in-ano. Br J Surg 76:752–755
11. Deen KI, Williams JG, Hutchinson R et al (1994) Fistula in ano: endoanal ultrasonographic assessment assists decision making for surgery. Gut 35:391–394
12. Lindsey I, Humphreys MM, George BD, Mortensen NMJ (2002) The role of anal ultrasound in the management of anal fistulas. Colorectal Dis 4:118–122
13. Madsen SM, Myschetzky PS, Heldmann U et al (1999) Fistula in ano: evaluation with low-field magnetic resonance imaging (0.1 T). Scand J Gastroenterol 34:1253–1256
14. Fishman-Javitt MC, Lovecchio JL, Javors B et al (1987) The value of MRI in evaluating perirectal and pelvic disease. Magn Reson Imaging 5:371–380
15. Koelbel G, Schmiedl U, Majer MC et al (1989) Diagnosis of fistulae and sinus tracts in patients with Crohn disease: value of MR imaging. AJR Am J Roentgenol 152:999–1003
16. Lunniss PJ, Armstrong P, Barker PG et al (1992) Magnetic resonance imaging of anal fistulae. Lancet 340:394–396
17. Barker PG, Lunniss PJ, Armstrong P et al (1992) Magnetic resonance imaging of fistula-in-ano: technique, interpretation and accuracy. Clin Radiol 49:7–13
18. Spencer JA, Ward J, Beckingham IJ et al (1996) Dynamic contrast enhanced MR imaging of perianal fistulas. AJR Am J Roentgenol 167:735–741
19. Beets-Tan RG, Beets GL, van der Hoop AG et al (2001) Preoperative MR imaging of anal fistulas: Does it really help the surgeon? Radiology 218:75–84
20. Buchanan G, Halligan S, Williams A et al (2002) Effect of MRI on clinical outcome of recurrent fistula-in-ano. Lancet 360:1661–1662
21. Hussain SM, Stoker J, Schouten WR et al (1996) Fistula in ano: endoanal sonography versus endoanal MR imaging in classification. Radiology 200:475–481

22. Stoker J, Rociu E, Zwamborn AW et al (1999) Endoluminal MR imaging of the rectum and anus: technique, applications, and pitfalls. Radiographics 19:383–398
23. Stoker J, Hussain SM, van Kempen D et al (1996) Endoanal coil in MR imaging of anal fistulas. AJR Am J Roentgenol 166:360–362
24. DeSouza NM, Gilderdale DJ, Coutts GA et al (1998) MRI of fistula-in-ano: a comparison of endoanal coil with external phased array coil techniques. J Comput Assist Tomogr 22:357–363
25. Stoker J, Rociu E, Schouten WR, Laméris JS (2002) Anovaginal and rectovaginal fistulas: endoluminal sonography versus endoluminal MR imaging. AJR Am J Roentgenol 178:737–741
26. Orsoni P, Barthet M, Portier F et al (1999) Prospective comparison of endosonography, magnetic resonance imaging and surgical findings in anorectal fistula and abscess complicating Crohn's disease. Br J Surg 86:360–364
27. Schwartz DA, Wiersema MJ, Dudiak KM et al (2001) A comparison of endoscopic ultrasound, magnetic resonance imaging, and exam under anesthesia for evaluation of Crohn's perianal fistulas. Gastroenterology 121:1064–1072
28. Gustafsson UM, Kahvecioglu B, Astrom G, Graf W (2001) Endoanal ultrasound or magnetic resonance imaging for preoperative assessment of anal fistula: a comparative study. Colorectal Dis 3:189–197
29. Spencer JA, Chapple K, Wilson D et al (1998) Outcome after surgery for perianal fistula: predictive value of MR imaging. AJR Am J Roentgenol 171:403–406
30. Buchanan GN, Halligan S, Williams AB et al (2003) Magnetic resonance imaging for primary fistula in ano. Br J Surg 90:877–881
31. Buchanan GN, Halligan S, Bartram CI et al (2004) Clinical examination, endosonography, and magnetic resonance imaging for preoperative assessment of fistula-in-ano: Comparison to an outcome based reference standard. Radiology 233:674–681

V.4. Fistula-in-ano: Endoanal Ultrasonography versus Endoanal MR Imaging – A Gastroenterologist Perspective

R.J.F. Felt-Bersma

Introduction

Accurate preoperative assessment of perianal fistulas is necessary for planning the most suitable surgical procedure and avoiding complications or recurrences. Currently, the main techniques are endoanal ultrasonography (EAUS) and magnetic resonance imaging (MRI). EAUS has proved to be very valuable in delineating perianal fistulas, especially when hydrogen peroxide is used as a contrast medium [hydrogen-peroxide-enhanced ultrasonography (HPUS)]. Visualization is improved, and an accurate preoperative assessment of fistulas is obtained [1–9]. Three-dimensional (3-D) EAUS enables axial images of the anal canal to be reconstructed in the coronal and sagittal planes. The use of 3-D images provides more information on the anatomy of anorectal disorders [10]. MRI is also very effective in preoperative assessment of perianal fistulas [11–16].

EAUS Compared with MRI

Several studies have compared EAUS with MRI (Figs. V.51 and 52), with different conclusions [17–25]. One study determined agreement between 3-D HPUS and endoanal MRI in preoperative assessment of perianal fistulas and compared these results with surgical findings [17]. Twenty-one patients (aged 26–71 years) with clinical symptoms of a cryptoglandular perianal fistula and a visible external opening underwent preoperative 3-D HPUS, endoanal MRI, and surgical exploration. Experienced observers blinded for each other's findings assessed the results separately. A description of each fistula was made and the following characteristics were recorded: classification of the primary fistula tract according to Parks (intersphincteric, transsphincteric, extrasphincteric, suprasphincteric [26], horseshoe or not classified, presence of secondary tracts (circular or linear), and location of an internal opening.

The median time between 3-D HPUS and endoanal MRI was 66 days, and the median time between the last study (3-D HPUS or endoanal MRI) and surgery was 154 days. Agreement for the primary fistula tract was 81% for 3-D HPUS and surgery, 90% for endoanal MRI and surgery as well as for 3-D HPUS and endoanal MRI. For secondary tracts, agreement for circular tracts was 67% for 3-D HPUS and surgery, 57% for endoanal MRI and surgery, and 71% for 3-D HPUS and endoanal MRI. For linear tracts, agreement was 76% for 3-D HPUS and surgery, 81% for endoanal MRI and surgery, and 71% for 3-D HPUS and endoanal MRI. Agreement for the location of an internal opening was 86% for 3-D HPUS and surgery as well as for endoanal MRI and surgery and 90% for 3-D HPUS and endoanal MRI. It was concluded that 3-D HPUS and endoanal MRI have a good agreement, especially for classification of the primary fistula tract and location of an internal opening and show good agreement when compared with surgical findings. Both 3-D HPUS and endoanal MRI can be used as a reliable method for preoperative evaluation of perianal fistulas.

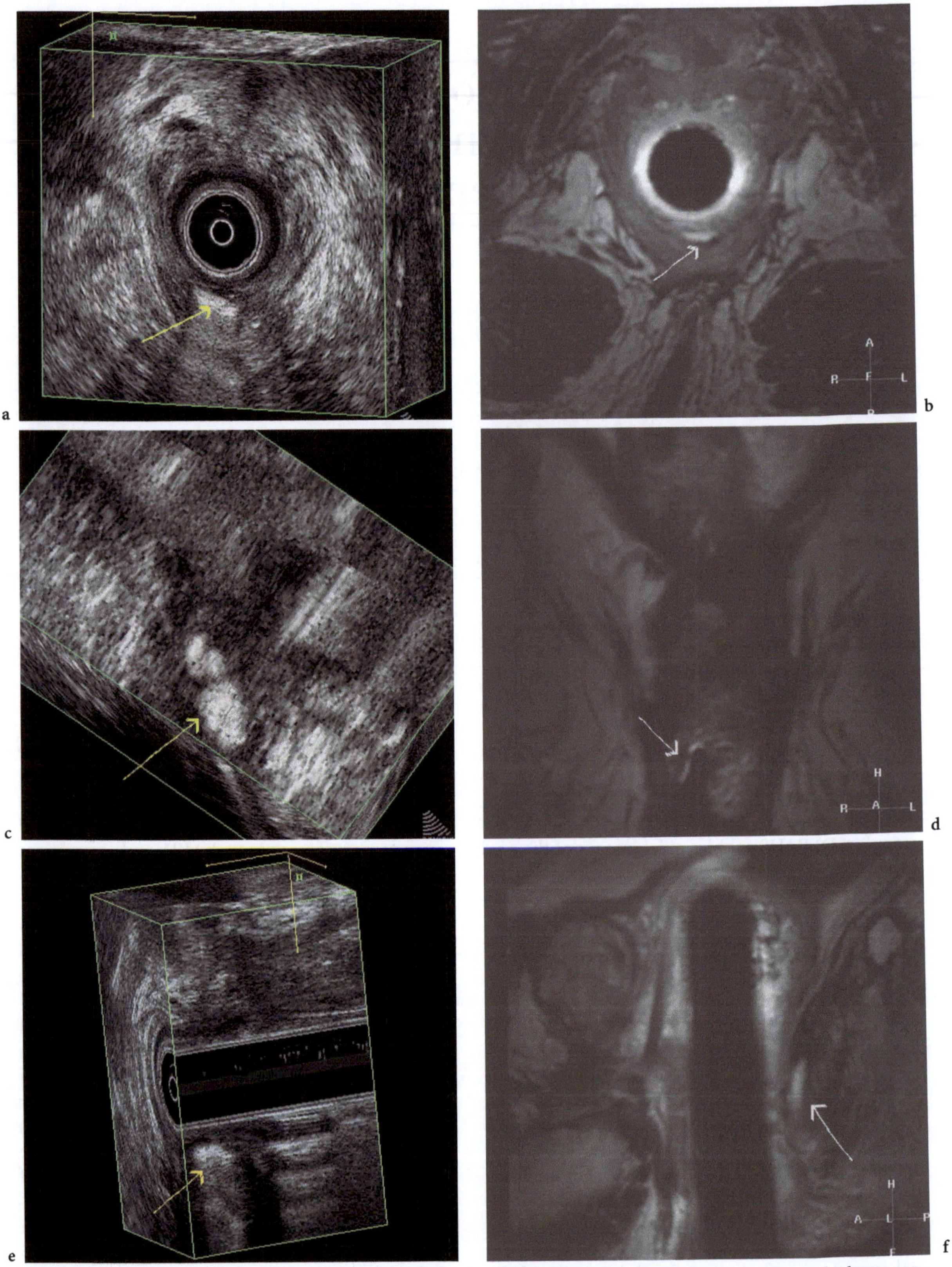

Fig. V.51. Transsphincteric fistula and internal opening (*arrow*): transversal image with three-dimensional (3-D) hydrogen-peroxide-enhanced ultrasonography (HPUS) (**a**) and endoanal (T2) magnetic resonance imaging (MRI) (**b**), frontal image with 3-D HPUS (**c**) and endoanal (T2) MRI (**d**), and lateral image with 3-D HPUS (**e**) and endoanal (T2) MRI (**f**)

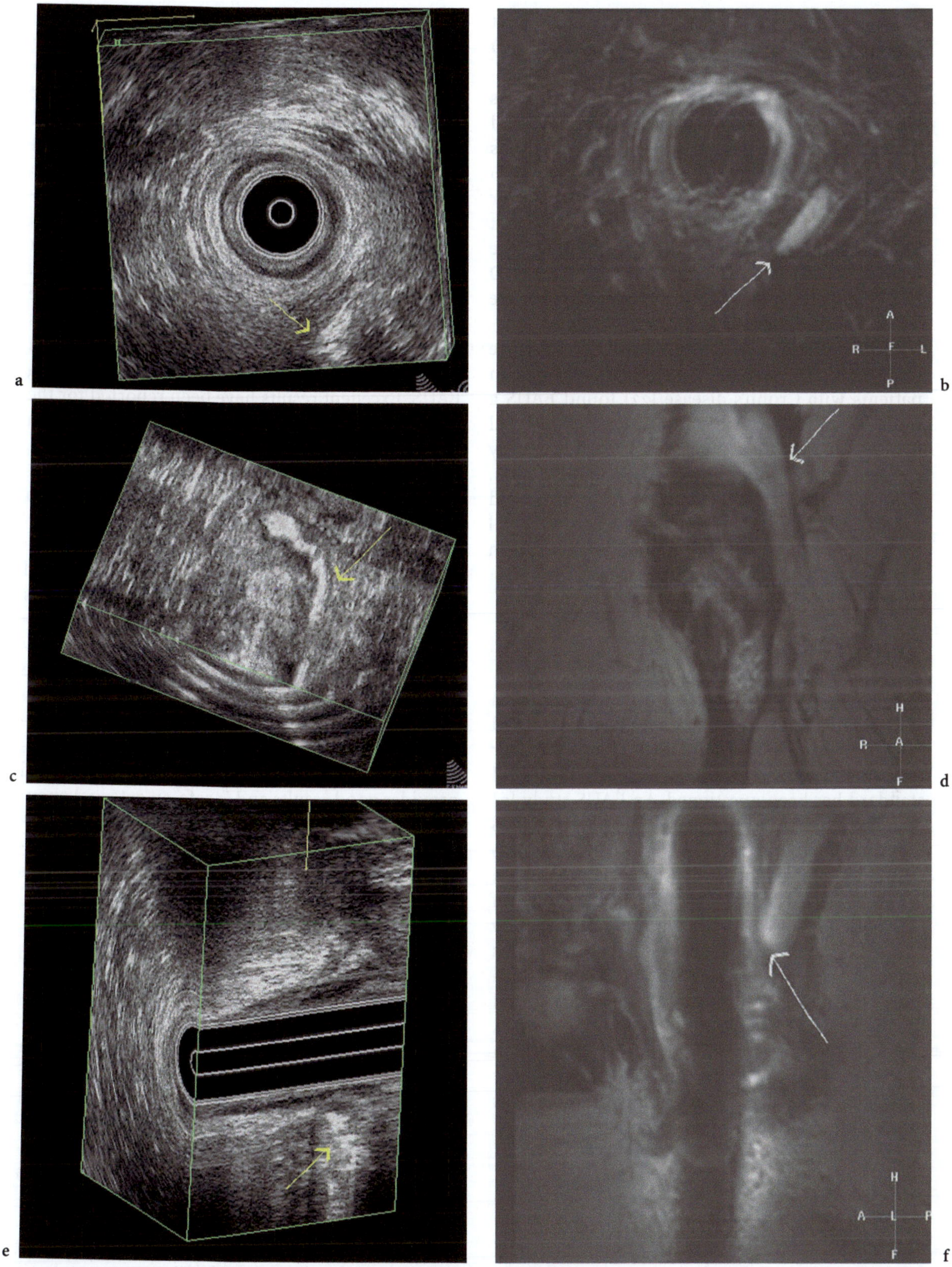

Fig. V.52. Horseshoe fistula (*arrow*): transversal image with anal three-dimensional (3-D) hydrogen-peroxide-enhanced ultrasonography (HPUS) (**a**) and endoanal (T2) magnetic resonance imaging (MRI) (**b**), frontal image with 3-D HPUS (**c**) and endoanal (T2) MRI (**d**), and lateral image with 3-D HPUS (**e**) and endoanal (T2) MRI (**f**)

Another study in 40 patients who were not yet operated were compared concerning their 3-D HPUS and endoanal MRI findings [18]. The interval between 3-D HPUS and endoanal MRI was only 14 days. Comparison of both techniques and patient preference was assessed. The methods agreed in 88% for the primary fistula tract, 90% for the location of the internal opening, 78% for secondary tracts, and 88% for fluid collection. There was no significant difference between the amount of discomfort experienced during 3-D HPUS and endoanal MRI or in patient preference for one procedure over the other.

Three studies [19–21] found MRI to be more accurate than EAUS not using HPUS. A study in patients with Crohn's disease [22] found EAUS a more sensitive modality for imaging perianal Crohn's disease than pelvic MRI; another study concluded the same with body coil MRI [23]. Others [24, 25] concluded that EAUS, MRI, and examination under general anesthesia were all accurate tests for determining fistula anatomy in patients with perianal Crohn's disease.

Gold Standard

In most studies mentioned, surgery was used as a gold standard [17, 19–21, 23] although EAUS and MRI are both well-established techniques for assessing fistulas. The use of surgery as a gold standard has been questioned. An EAUS study [2] demonstrated two secondary tracts with HPUS that were not found during surgery. These patients developed a recurrent fistula, suggesting that these branches were actually present at the time of HPUS. In a follow-up study with 37 patients, body coil MRI was shown to make better predictions regarding patient outcome than were surgical findings [15]. Another study [23] with 23 patients found that in two patients who did not heal after surgery, EAUS showed an extension and/or abscess, which was not identified at the time of operation. For body coil MRI, the corresponding number was three. In the same study, no internal opening was found during surgery in three patients.

Techniques Used in EAUS and MRI

The results in the studies mentioned above [17–25] differ, and different techniques for MRI and EAUS were used. One reasons for the different results found could be the use of different probes for EAUS. Better results were found when a linear probe or biplane probe [22, 24] was used; 3-D EAUS may also improve imaging [17, 18]. Most studies mentioned had earlier used a body coil [19, 21–24]. Body-coil MRI may give additional information on structures further away from the anal canal, but it can be difficult to make a distinction between fistula tracts and vessels [22]. With an endocoil, more precise information can be obtained from the anal sphincter [17, 18, 20, 25].

An important issue is that hydrogen peroxide was not used in many of the comparative studies mentioned above [20–25]. This could be a reason for some of the disappointing results found using EAUS. Excellent results have been reported for the assessment of perianal fistulas when hydrogen peroxide is used as a contrast medium [1–9, 17, 18]. The accuracy for determining the Parks classification can rise by 30% with HPUS [2]. A problem encountered by conventional EAUS is that it is difficult to distinguish between scar tissue and active fistulas. When hydrogen peroxide is introduced into the external opening, a fistula tract appears as hyperechoic. This way, it is easier to identify a fistula tract as well as the internal opening or any secondary tracts. The use of hydrogen peroxide has proved to be a safe method. In our center, no complications have occurred due to the introduction of hydrogen peroxide nor are any documented in the studies mentioned. Although this method provides good results and is safe, an external opening must be visible to introduce hydrogen peroxide. EAUS can be performed in patients with claustrophobia, extreme obesity, and metallic implants (pacemaker) where MRI cannot be used.

Conclusion

Anal endosonography and MRI are both excellent techniques in imaging perianal fistulas. In anal endosonography, enhancement with HPUS improves diagnostic yield; however, an external fistula opening has to be present. Three-dimensional EAUS will possibly also increase visibility. With MRI, an endoanal coil probably has advantages although several enhancement techniques with a body coil are also very accurate. EAUS can be used in cases where MRI is not possible, such as claustrophobia, extreme obesity, and metallic implants. Also, EAUS is less expensive than MRI.

References

1. Cheong DMO, Nogueras JJ, Wexner SD, Jagelman DG (1993) Anal endosonography for recurrent anal fistulas: image enhancement with hydrogen peroxide. Dis Colon Rectum 36:1158–1160
2. Poen AC, Felt-Bersma RJF, Eijsbouts QAJ, et al (1998) Hydrogen peroxide-enhanced transanal ultrasound in the assessment of fistula-in-ano. Dis Colon Rectum 41:1147–1152
3. Ratto C, Gentile E, Merico M et al (2000) How can the assessment of fistula-in-ano be improved? Dis Colon Rectum 43:1375–1382
4. Sloots CEJ, Felt-Bersma RJF, Poen AC, Cuesta MA (2001) Assessment and classification of never operated and recurrent cryptoglandular fistulas-in-ano using hydrogen peroxide enhanced transanal ultrasound. Colorectal Dis 3:422–426
5. Sloots CEJ, Felt-Bersma RJF, Poen AC et al (2001) Assessment and classification of fistula-in-ano in patients with Crohn's disease by hydrogen peroxide enhanced transanal ultrasound. Int J Colorectal Dis 16:292–297
6. Sudol-Szopinska I, Jakubowski W, Szczepkowski M (2002) Contrast-enhanced endosonography for the diagnosis of anal and anovaginal fistulas. J Clin Ultrasound 30:145–150
7. Sudol-Szopinska I, Gesla J, Jakubowski W et al (2002) Reliability of endosonography in evaluation of anal fistulae and abscesses. Acta Radiol 43:599–602
8. Navarro-Luna A, Garcia-Domingo MI, Rius-Macias J, Marco-Molina C (2004) Ultrasound study of anal fistulas with hydrogen peroxide enhancement. Dis Colon Rectum 47:108–114
9. Buchanan GN, Bartram CI, Williams AB et al (2005) Value of hydrogen peroxide enhancement of three dimensional fistula-in-ano. Dis Colon Rectum 48:141–147
10. Christensen AF, Nyhuus B, Nielsen MB, Christensen H (2005) Three-dimensional anal endosonography may improve diagnostic confidence of detecting damage to the anal sphincter complex. Br J Radiol 78: 308–311
11. Szyszko TA, Bush J, Gishen P et al (2005)Endoanal magnetic resonance imaging of fistula-in-ano: a comparison of STIR with gadolinium-enhanced techniques. Acta Radiol 46:3–8
12. Maccioni F, Colaiacomo MC, Stasolla A et al (2002) Value of MRI performed with phased-array coil in the diagnosis and pre-operative classification of perianal and anal fistulas. Radiol Med 104:58–67
13. Morris J, Spencer JA, Ambrose NS (2000) MR imaging classification of perianal fistulas and its implications for patient management. Radiographics 20:623–637.
14. Stoker J, Fa VE, Eijkemans MJ et al (1998) Endoanal MRI of perianal fistulas: the optimal imaging planes. Eur Radiol 8:1212–1216
15. Spencer JA, Chapple K, Wilson D et al (1998) Outcome after surgery for perianal fistula: predictive value of MR imaging. AJR Am J Roentgenol 171:403–406
16. DeSouza NM, Gilderdale DJ, Coutts GA et al (1998) MRI of fistula-in-ano: a comparison of endoanal coil with external phased array coil techniques. J Comput Assist Tomogr 22:357–363
17. West RL, Zimmerman DD, Dwarkasing S et al (2003) Prospective comparison of hydrogen peroxide-enhanced three-dimensional endoanal ultrasonography and endoanal magnetic resonance imaging of perianal fistulas. Dis Colon Rectum 46: 1407–1415
18. West RL, Dwarskasing S, Felt-Bersma RJF et al (2004) Hydrogen peroxide-enhanced three-dimensional endoanal ultrasonography and endoanal magnetic resonance imaging in evaluating perianal fistulas: agreement and patient preference. Gastroenterol Hepatol 16:1319–1324
19. Buchanan GN, Halligan S, Bartram CI et al (2004) Clinical examination, endosonography, and MRI imaging in preoperative assessment of fistula-in-ano: comparison with outcome-based reference standard. Radiology 233:674–681
20. Hussain SM, Stoker J, Schouten WR et al (1996) Fistula in ano: endoanal sonography versus endoanal MR imaging in classification. Radiology 200:475–481
21. Lunniss PJ, Barker PG, Sultan AH et al (1994) Magnetic Resonance imaging of fistula-in-ano. Dis Colon Rectum 37:708–718
22. Orsoni P, Barthet M, Portier F et al (1999) Prospective comparison of endosonography, magnetic resonance imaging and surgical findings in anorectal fistula and abscess complicating Crohn's disease. Br J Surg 86:360–364
23. Gustafsson UM, Kahvecioglu B, Astrom G et al (2001) Endoanal ultrasound or magnetic resonance imaging for preoperative assessment of anal fistula: a comparative study. Colorectal Dis 3:189–197
24. Schwartz DA, Wiersema MJ, Dudiak KM et al (2001) A comparison of endoscopic ultrasound, magnetic resonance imaging and exam under anesthesia for evaluation of Crohn's perianal fistulas. Gastroenterology 121:1064–1072
25. Stoker J, Rociu E, Schouten WR, Lameris JS (2002) Anovaginal and rectovaginal fistulas: endoluminal sonography versus endoluminal MR imaging. Am J Roentgenol 178:737–741
26. Parks AG, Gordon PH, Hardcastle JD (1976) A classification of fistula-in-ano. Br J Surg 63:1-12

Invited Commentary

T.L. Hull

Anorectal sepsis can be categorized as either anal abscesses or the resultant anal fistula. Most anorectal sepsis is uncomplicated and can be managed with straightforward evaluation, exam, and surgical intervention.

Anal Abscesses

All anal abscesses need adequate drainage. Many drainage procedures can be performed in the emergency room or the office with local anesthesia. When this is not possible or the diagnosis is in doubt, drainage with general or regional anesthesia in the operating room (OR) is indicated. Usually, the abscess can be delineated with careful, deliberate palpation. The surgeon feels a definite island of thickening when the remainder of the anal canal is soft and relaxed due to operative anesthesia. When an abscess is suspected and none can be found, further modalities may be helpful to elucidate the etiology. A full proctologic exam will rule out mucosal lesions (such as acute herpes of the rectum), which can mimic an acute anal abscess. Additionally, patients may present with a partially drained abscess with a tiny external opening and induration. This type of presentation requires further drainage to adequately drain the cavity.

This section deals with the consideration of imaging modalities to further evaluate the area of the anorectum at the pelvic diaphragm in situations of suspected sepsis. Anal endosonography has proven to be a useful tool when abscess is suspected but not found at operative exam. Even sonographers with limited experience can see the hypoechoic area. Two drawbacks are pain, which can be severe with probe insertion, and identifying abscesses that are located extended distances from the anal canal (i.e., they may be outside the focal length of the probe). If the anal endosonography can be performed in the operative suite, pain would not be a factor. We have found the most productive use for endosonography to be imaging intersphincteric abscesses, which are small, especially in a scarred anal canal. Additionally, in neutropenic patients who make limited purulent fluid and the surgeon wishes to submit them to the least amount of anal canal manipulation, anal endosonography may be quite helpful to image the anal region. Magnetic resonance imaging (MRI) may provide more information when the endosonography cannot be performed in the OR or the abscess is felt to be outside the focal length of the probe. In some situations, computed tomography (CT) may also be helpful, particularly if an abscess is suspected from a supralevator component. Diseases such as Crohn's disease or perforated diverticulitis are examples of these types of circumstances. The CT can give additional information about the bowel wall of the offending area that cannot be obtained from endosonography. The possibility of using several modalities together for complex cases, such as complicated perianal Crohn's disease with abscess formation, should be considered. MRI and endosonography can show paths of abscess tracking, which may not be as complete with either study alone.

About 10% of patients will develop a recurrent abscess [1, 2]. Etiology of recurrence in one study was insufficient prior treatment, incorrect diagnosis, or missed components [3]. For patients with recurrence, repeat drainage is mandatory with emphasis on complete drainage. The diagnosis must be verified, and for those with suspected missed components, further imaging may be helpful.

In summary, the majority of anal abscesses do not require specialized testing. Full drainage of pus through a large incision making the external opening as close to the sphincter mechanism as possible will be sufficient. Packing should be avoided, and the edges of the wound should be sufficiently opened so that closure over a partially drained cavity does not occur. Alternately, insertion of a catheter with a mushroom-shaped head will also provide drainage while allowing the cavity to collapse around the catheter. Then the patient can return to the office in about 3 weeks and the catheter injected with peroxide. If there is no extravasation into the anal canal, the catheter is removed. Likewise, if there is communication with the anal canal or there continues to be drainage from the external opening, a fistula is suspected. Approximately 37% of patients will form a fistula [1, 2]

Anal Fistula

Fistulas can be organized into simple and complex forms. Most are simple, and no preoperative planning is required [4]. For these patients, simple fistulotomy will be the preferred operative treatment. In the minority, where no internal opening can be found or recurrent anal sepsis and a fistula develop, further imaging may be helpful.

With this in mind, the real question is: What is the best imaging modality to evaluate fistulas that are not straightforward? Most literature does not really address this dilemma. The ideal study would be a prospective, blinded, randomized trial to see if there are differences when examined before and after looking at cure *and incontinence rates* when comparing preoperative endosonography [two-dimensional (2-D) vs. three-dimensional (3-D)] and MRI. The CT scan currently does not seem to offer sufficient sphincter delineation to be a choice. Additionally, cost would need to be a studied variable, as the MRI is more expensive than the endosonography. Since this study does not exist, the current literature should be evaluated always while reflecting on the ideal study and how current studies compare.

With current knowledge, it appears that the internal opening is equally poorly seen with the endosonography and MRI. However, if the internal opening cannot be detected in the OR, further imaging burns no bridges and may provide valuable information. In practice, this is ideally how imaging would be used, and current studies do not provide information on how often the internal opening is revealed when it cannot be demonstrated at operative exam. Studies compare the number of times MRI or endosonography correctly identify and agree with either each other or the OR exam at elucidating the internal opening. While this is useful, it does not fully guide how imaging should be used for discovering the internal opening that the surgeon cannot find in the everyday practice setting.

The frustration of examining a patient in the OR without finding the internal opening (even with a noted external opening) is the clinical situation that requires assistance from further imaging. Three-dimensional endosonography may have an advantage – over 2-D imaging, especially – as it allows the ability to go back and examine the surrounding tissue after the exam is completed and to look for tracts and amount of muscle enveloped in the fistula. Certainly, if there is concern regarding dividing muscle and possible postoperative fecal incontinence, a 3-D image that visualizes exactly the amount of sphincter distal to the fistula would be helpful in planning surgical treatment strategy.

An interesting finding not highlighted in Chap. V.4, titled “Fistula-In-Ano: Endoanal Ultrasonography versus Endoanal MR Imaging – A Gastroenterologist Perspective” was the finding in the paper by West et al. [5] on the number of times secondary tracts were missed by the surgeon. When examining the results, the agreement for discovering primary tracts was 81% 3-D (with hydrogen peroxide enhancement) and surgery, 90% MRI and surgery, and 90% 3-D and MRI. However, when looking at secondary circular tracts, agreement was 67% for 3-D and surgery, 57% for MRI and surgery, but 71% for 3-D and MRI. This is again noted in that chapter where the authors question surgery as the gold standard and rightfully point out that another study using hydrogen-peroxide-enhanced endosonography found two missed secondary tracts after surgery [6]. These important finding may be a clue regarding recurrence after treatment of fistula, i.e., that the surgeon does not always discover secondary tracts, and this could be a source of continued or persistent sepsis. Therefore, when treatment does not heal, further imaging from these modalities may be of value with the intention of looking for secondary tracts.

Many anterior fistulas in women are straightforward and traverse into the perineal body or the vagina. They are classified as complex because simple fistulotomy is usually avoided to decrease the chances of fecal leakage after the procedure.

When planning the operative treatment of these fistulas, anal endosonography is strongly considered. The poor closure record with mucosal advancement flaps may be related to a sphincter defect, which may be difficult to detect. Anal endosonography can demonstrate an anterior defect and clearly change the operative approach. For this reason, I prefer anal endosonography prior to planning the surgical approach for anterior fistulas in women.

In summary, hydrogen-peroxide-enhanced endosonography seems to improve detection of tracts and separation of scar from the tract. When reviewing the studies cited in these chapters, it is not always clear if the participants were blinded about other findings. Also, there are different ways of performing endosonography (i.e., probe size or use of hydrogen peroxide), which also is not clearly stated. Likewise, MRI can be done with different techniques, and comparison of today's machines with those even 5 years ago may not accurately reflect the advancement in technology. Perhaps the most interesting thing gleaned from these reviews is that surgeons miss secondary tracts in the OR. This is proved with the additional imaging techniques. The summary statement from the "Introduction," which states that when judging results we should use the outcome-derived reference standard – namely, fistula healing – is true. After all, this is the result we should be most interested in obtaining.

Conclusion

Most anal sepsis can be managed without further imaging. Treatment of recurrent disease and sepsis with an unusual presentation may be augmented with further imaging. This also includes complex perianal Crohn's disease and supralevator sepsis. Exactly which imaging modality is preferable remains unclear in the current literature. Focused studies with the clear endpoint of sepsis that has healed/been eradicated, along with clear study designs free from bias, are needed. Also, current imaging technology must be fairly matched (i.e., modern MRI, 3-D endosonography, etc.) in order to obtain an impartial comparison.

References

1. Hamalainen KP, Sainio AP (1998) Incidence of fistulas after drainage of acute anorectal abscesses. Dis Colon Rectum 41:1357–1361
2. Vasilevsky CA, Gordon PH (1984) The incidence of recurrent abscesses or fistula-in-ano following anorectal suppuration. Dis Colon Rectum 27: 126–130
3. Chrabot CM, Prasad ML, Abcarian H (1983) Recurrent anorectal abscesses. Dis Colon Rectum 26:105–108
4. Fazio VW (1987) Complex anal fistulae. Gastroenterol Clin North Am 16:93–114
5. West RL, Zimmermann DD, Dwarkasing S et al (2003) Prospective comparison of hydrogen peroxide-enhanced three-dimensional endoanal ultrasonography and endoanal magnetic resonance imaging of perianal fistulas. Dis Colon Rectum 46:1407–1415
6. Poen AC, Felt-Bersma RJF, Eijsbouts QAJ et al (1998) Hydrogen peroxide-enhanced transanal ultrasound in the assessment of fistula-in-ano. Dis Colon Rectum 41:1147–1152

Section VI

Update in the Evaluation of Outlet Obstruction

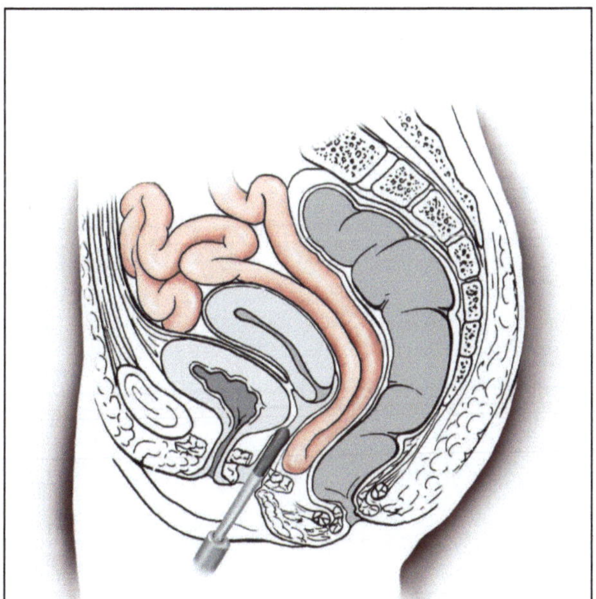

VI.1. Introduction

G.A. Santoro, A. Stuto

Anorectal outlet obstruction, also known as obstruction defecation syndrome (ODS), is a pathological condition due to a variety of causes and is characterized by an impaired expulsion of the bolus after calling to defecate. Patients complain of different symptoms, including incomplete evacuation with or without painful effort, unsuccessful attempts with long periods spent in bathroom, return visit to the toilette, use of perineal support, manual assistance (insertion of finger into the vagina or anal canal), extreme straining to defecate, dependence on enema and/or laxatives, hemorrhoidal prolapse, perineal pain/discomfort when standing, fragmented defecation and fecal incontinence. These symptoms often lead to a poor quality of life.

Prevalence of the entire spectrum of constipation, of which ODS is part, accounts for 14.7% in the US adult population [1] while the true prevalence of ODS among the population is not known even if the feeling is that it is underestimated. The causes and the pathway to developing a morbid condition in ODS is schematically represented in Fig.VI.1. After ruling out pelvic and rectal tumor, the main distinction in the pathogenesis of ODS is between functional and mechanical causes (Table VI.1). Failure to release the anal sphincters or paradoxical contraction of the puborectalis muscle are considered the main and most frequent functional causes of ODS [2]. In these patients, biofeedback can achieve reactivation of the inhibitory capacity of all pelvic floor muscles involved in defecation, with an improvement in symptoms of 50% [3–4].

The most relevant mechanical causes of ODS are rectocele, rectal intussusception, enterocele, genital prolapse, and descending perineum. It is fundamental to distinguish between rectal causes (rectocele and intussusception) and extrarectal causes (enterocele, genital prolapse, and descending perineum).

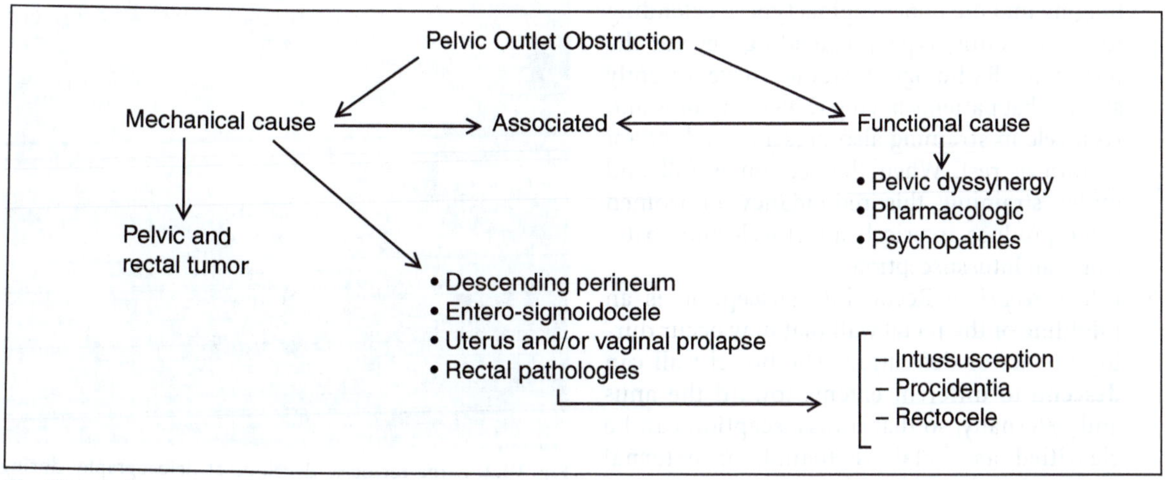

Fig. VI.1. Pathogenesis of obstructed defecation syndrome

Table VI.1. Pathophysiology of obstructed defecation syndrome

Mechanism	Common causes
Mechanical outlet obstruction	Rectal intussusception External prolapse Enterocele
Dissipation of force vector	Rectocele Descending perineum syndrome Total rectal prolapse
Functional outlet obstruction	Inefficient inhibition of internal anal sphincter: • Hirschsprung, Chagas, hereditary internal sphincter myopathy Inefficient relaxation of striated pelvic floor muscles: • paradoxical puborectalis contraction, spinal cord lesion, multiple sclerosis
Defective rectal filling sensation	Idiopathic megarectum Rectal hyposensitivity (blunted rectum)

Pathologic Clinical Conditions

1. *Rectocele*: Rectocele is classically defined as a herniation of the rectal wall through a defect in the posterior rectovaginal septum in the direction of the vagina. This abnormal condition is documented either under straining or during defecation at the proctogram (Fig. VI.2) or during rectal examination (Fig. VI.3). Rectoceles may be classified according to their position (low, middle, high), size (small <2 cm, medium 2–4 cm, large >4 cm) and degree (type 1: with bulging into the upper vagina; type 2: extending to the introitus; type 3: extending beyond the introitus). Radiological studies have recently shown that patients having ODS symptoms and rectocele in straining also present a redundant rectum at rest. When the rectum is full and under straining, this redundancy in women could produce anteriorly a rectocele and posteriorly an intussusception
2. *Intussusception*: Rectal intussusception is an infolding of the rectal wall that may occur during the act of defecation. The bowel wall can descend to different extents toward the anus and externally, so that intussusception can be classified as rectal, rectoanal, or external (external prolapse)
3. *Rectal mucosal prolapse*: This is an intussusception with involvement of the rectal mucosa only (Fig. VI.4)
4. *Enterocele*: It is a herniation of the small bowel or sigmoid colon (sigmoidocele) into a deep pouch of Douglas, which protrudes into the

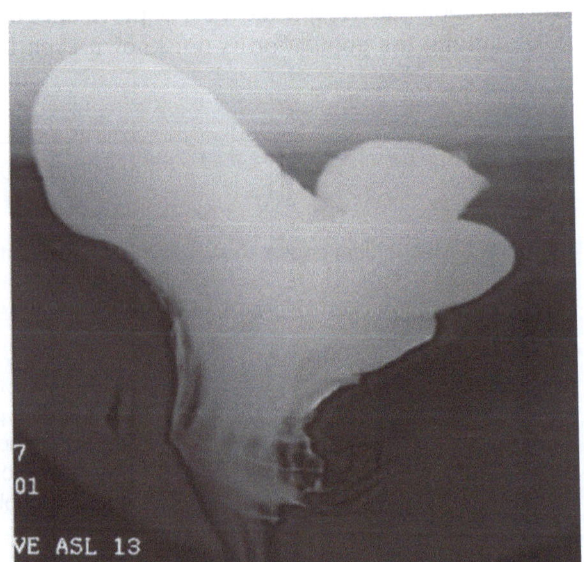

Fig. VI.2. Large rectocele develops at defecography during straining a 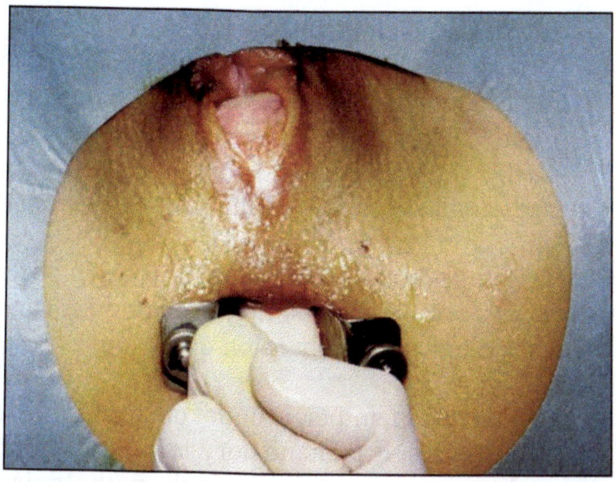 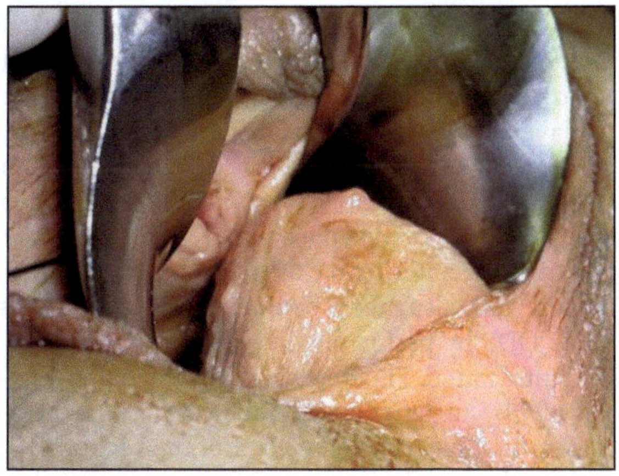 b

Fig. VI.3. Small (a) and large (b) rectocele at clinical examination

vagina or rectum (Fig. VI.5). Enteroceles occur almost exclusively in women, and most of them succeed vaginal or abdominal hysterectomy.

The presence of these anatomic deformities must not be considered a pathologic condition per se but must always be correlated to the symptoms and patient's quality of life. A small rectocele (<2 cm) is a common finding in healthy women at defecography [5]. Freimanis et. al. [6] demonstrated the presence of a rectocele, intussusception, pelvic descent, or puborectalis spasm in 67% of asymptomatic volunteers studied by standard defecography. On the other hand, it is well established that rectal intussusception, mucosal rectal prolapse, rectocele, and enterocele are common findings in the defecogram of patients suffering from defecation disorders [7].

In patients with ODS symptoms, mechanical obstruction is nearly always associated to a combination of scenarios of the different pathological conditions mentioned above. For this reason, we strongly believe that symptomatic rectocele is a syndrome in which rectocele is only the easiest anatomical defect detectable. The pathogenesis of ODS is still matter of debate and controversy, and currently, two main causes are recognized as leading factors. Excessive straining during defecation leads to a traction neuropathy with subsequent weakened pelvic floor and perineal descent [8–9]. Traction neuropathy during childbirth has been considered as a main factor causing ODS. More recently, a novel theory has been proposed to explain ODS and the related symptoms (Longo A, XIV Colorectal Symposium, Ft. Lauderdale, FL USA, 2003). This theory starts from the observa-

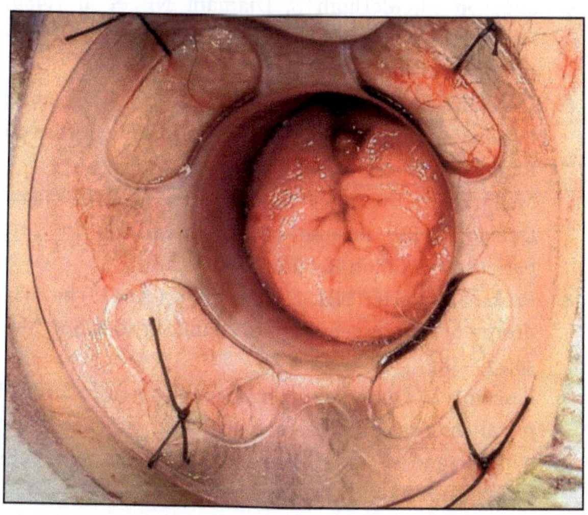

Fig. VI.4. Circumferential mucosal rectal prolapse

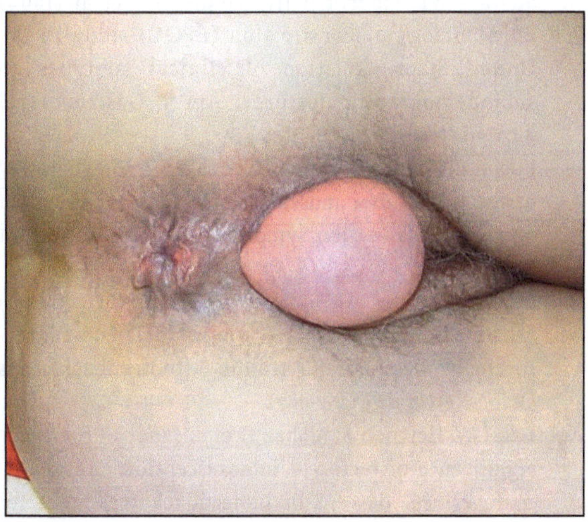

Fig. VI.5. Descending perineum in a patient with enterocele tion of comparative anatomic and histological studies conducted on cadavers with and without evidence of rectocele and intussusception. In cadavers with rectocele and/or intussusception, two main pictures could be demonstrated: an increased overall capacity of the rectal ampulla and thinning or disappearance of the muscular layer of the anterior rectal wall. The latter observation has also been demonstrated in patients with ODS by performing transanal or transvaginal ultrasound. This theory places the pathogenesis of ODS in patients with rectocele and/or intussusception in a primary defect of the rectum.

Further study is needed for a better understanding of this common condition, but nevertheless, in recent years, the scientific community agrees on several aspect of ODS:

1. Rectocele is not the unique pathological finding in ODS. It is very frequent in healthy asymptomatic women and it should not be considered a pathological condition only because it is evident at clinical examination or at the defecography
2. In ODS, anatomical findings must always be matched with patients' complaints and quality of life
3. ODS could be due to rectal causes, such as rectocele and intussusception, as well as secondary to extrarectal causes, such as genital prolapse, enterocele, and sigmoidocele
4. In ODS, mechanical obstruction is nearly always associated to a combination scenario of different pathological conditions: according to this, in ODS patients, an accurate diagnostic workup is mandatory to rule out all pathological conditions that can be responsible
5. It is important to use diagnostic tools in order to achieve a more complete anatomical and physiologic comprehension of the scenario.

In conclusion, in pelvic outlet obstruction due to rectal causes, it is mandatory to keep in mind the relevance of possible occult pathologies, equating symptoms with clinical findings and imaging, balancing potential outcomes with surgical risks, and analyzing the different surgical techniques available.

The purpose of this section is to put into perspective the numerous procedures that have been described for the diagnosis of this condition. Accuracy and reliability of endoanal, endorectal, dynamic anorectal, transvaginal, and transperineal dynamic ultrasonography in the evaluation of outlet obstruction will be discussed. Defecographic study of rectal evacuation in constipated patients will be discussed in detail. Finally, the role of the new technique of dynamic magnetic resonance imaging in patients with pelvic organ prolapse will be evaluated.

References

1. Stewart WF, Liberman JN, Sandler RS et al (1999) Epidemiology of constipation (EPOC) study in the United States: relation of clinical subtypes to sociodemographic features. Am J Gastroenterol 94:3530–3540
2. Fucini C, Ronchi O, Elbetti C (2001) Electromyography of the pelvic floor musculature in the assessment of obstructed defecation symptoms. Dis Colon Rectum 44:1168–1175
3. Mimura T, Roy AJ, Storrie JB, Kamm MA (2000) Treatment of impaired defecation associated with rectocele by behavioral retraining (biofeedback). Dis Colon Rectum 43:1267–1272
4. Lau CW, Heymen S, Alabaz O et al (2000) Prognostic significance of rectocele, intussusception and abnormal perineal descent in biofeedback treatment for constipated patients with paradoxical puborectalis contraction. Dis Colon Rectum 43:478–482
5. Shorvon PJ, McHugh S, Diamant NE et al (1989) Defecography in normal volunteers: results and implications. Gut 30:1737–1749
6. Freimanis MG, Wald A, Caruana B, Bauman DH (1991) Evacuation proctography in normal volunteers. Invest Radiol 26:581–585
7. Mellgren A, Bremmer S, Johansson C et al (1994) Defecography. Results of investigations in 2816 patients. Dis Colon Rectum 37:1133–1141
8. Parks AG, Porter NH, Hardcastle J (1966) The syndrome of the descending perineum. Proc R Soc Med 59:477–482
9. Pescatori M, Quondamcarlo C (1999) A new grading of rectal internal mucosal prolapse and its correlation with diagnosis and treatment. Int J Colorectal Dis 14:245–249

VI.2. Accuracy and Reliability of Endoanal, Endorectal, Dynamic Anorectal, and Transvaginal Ultrasonography in the Evaluation of Outlet Obstruction

G.A. Santoro, G. Di Falco

Standard diagnostic proctologic procedures in the assessment of patients with obstructed defecation include clinical evaluation, endoscopy, manometry [1], electromyography [2], and radiologic techniques such as evacuation proctography [3], colpocystodefecography and dynamic magnetic resonance imaging (DMRI) [4]. Several reports have described the sonographic evaluation of female pelvic floor dysfunction [5–20]. Ultrasonography may provide several data on anal sphincter integrity and morphology, rectovaginal septum, and integrity of the rectal wall and may also have a role in diagnosing enterocele, rectocele, rectal intussusception, and mucosal prolapse and in evaluating pelvic floor dyssynergy. Most abnormalities, however, require evacuation for diagnosis, and the role of ultrasound in the evaluation of patients with outlet obstruction remains to be defined.

Technical Issues

In the study of outlet obstruction, different ultrasonographic techniques can be used: (1) endoanal (EAUS) and endorectal (ERUS) ultrasonography [5–11], (2) dynamic anorectal endosonography (DAE) [12–14], (3) transvaginal ultrasonography (TVUS) [15, 16], and (4) dynamic transperineal ultrasonography (DTP-US) [17, 18]. Technical aspects of EAUS and ERUS have already been reported in Section II, and the technique of dynamic transperineal ultrasonography will be described in detail in another chapter of this section. We will focus on the other two procedures: dynamic anorectal ultrasonography and transvaginal ultrasonography.

Dynamic Anorectal Endosonography

Anorectal ultrasonography is performed using a biplane, high-frequency, rigid linear transducer (B-K Medical 8658 probe) (Fig. VI.6). For the examination, the patient is placed in the left lateral position. After conventional inspection of the rectal wall and the anal canal, the probe is introduced and directed to the ventral rectal wall. To achieve an optimal

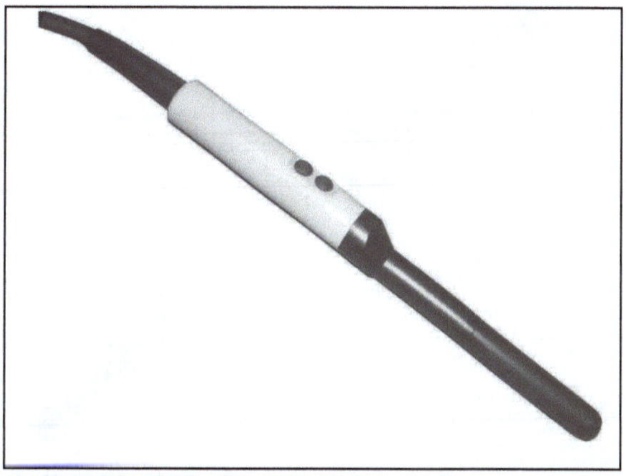

Fig. VI.6. Biplane, high-frequency, anorectal transducer (B-K Medical 8658 probe)

acoustic contact, the rectum should be filled with 50 ml of water or, alternatively, can a water-filled balloon mounted on the probe. The minimal distance between the peritoneal cavity and the inner anal verge [peritoneal-anal distance (PAD)] is determined during rest. The patient is then asked to strain maximally, and the PAD is determined again. The difference between PAD at rest and during maximal strain can be calculated [12, 13]. Other variables examined are the length and thickness of the anal sphincter and puborectalis muscles at rest, during voluntary contraction (squeezing), and during a defecation movement (straining) [14]. Healthy individuals show a decrease in length and an increase in thickness of the anal sphincter during voluntary contraction. During straining, the anal sphincter increases in length and decreases in thickness. The puborectalis muscle also relaxes, resulting in an increased length and decreased thickness.

A source of conflict may derive from the sonographic methodology used. It has been suggested that the left lateral decubitus position of patients during examination is not physiologically. However, the relative dynamics of intrapelvic organs may be unaffected by the change in gravity. Some authors [12] ask the patient to produce a defecation effort, leaving the ultrasound probe in the same position. There is, however, a tendency for the probe to be expelled when the patient strains forcefully. Indeed, it is possible to resist probe expulsion and thereby splinting the rectum during the evacuation, but this may inhibit enterocele formation. Other authors [11] have found these problems can be overcome by moving the probe in tandem with the perineum.

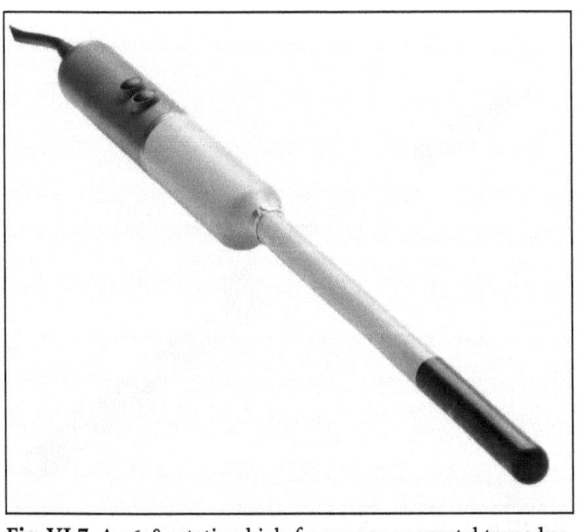

Fig. VI.7. A 360° rotating high-frequency anorectal transducer (B-K Medical 2050 probe)

Transvaginal Ultrasonography

TVUS involves placing the probe inside the vagina. For this application, two different types of high-frequency ultrasound transducers can be used. For evaluation of transaxial projections, a high-frequency (up to 16 MHz) 360° transducer with a built-in automatic three-dimensional (3-D) acquisition system is used (B-K Medical 2050 probe) (Fig. VI.7). The image plane of this transducer is 90° to the longitudinal axis. The 2050 has a completely cylindrical probe finger so that the vaginal wall does not have to adapt to various diameters of the probe. For sagittal and conventional transverse imaging of the pelvic floor, including color Doppler, a biplane, high-frequency transducer with a long linear and transverse array is used (B-K Medical 8658 probe) (Fig. VI.6). Both arrays are placed at 90° to each other and at 90° to the longitudinal axis. The transducer can be placed resting on the posterior vaginal wall. With the patient lying on her back on a table or in a gynecological chair, the anterior vaginal wall will softly contact the surface of the ultrasound transducer without disturbing the functional anatomy (Fig. VI.8).

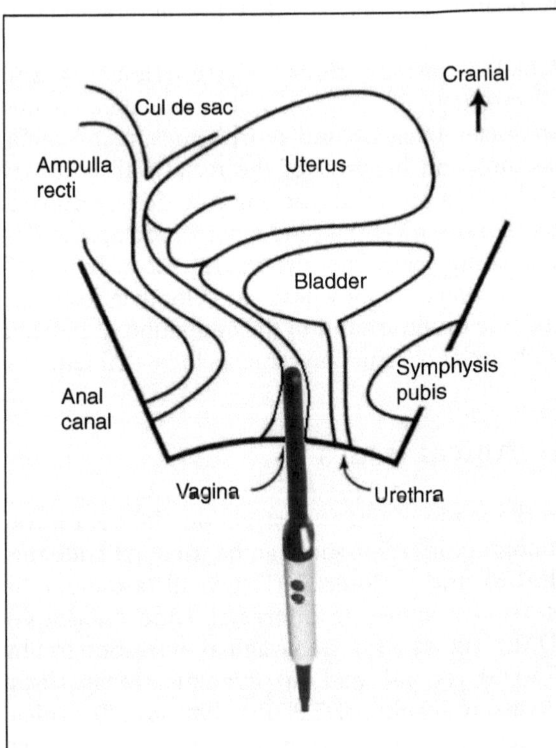

Fig. VI.8. Schematic representation of transvaginal ultrasonography

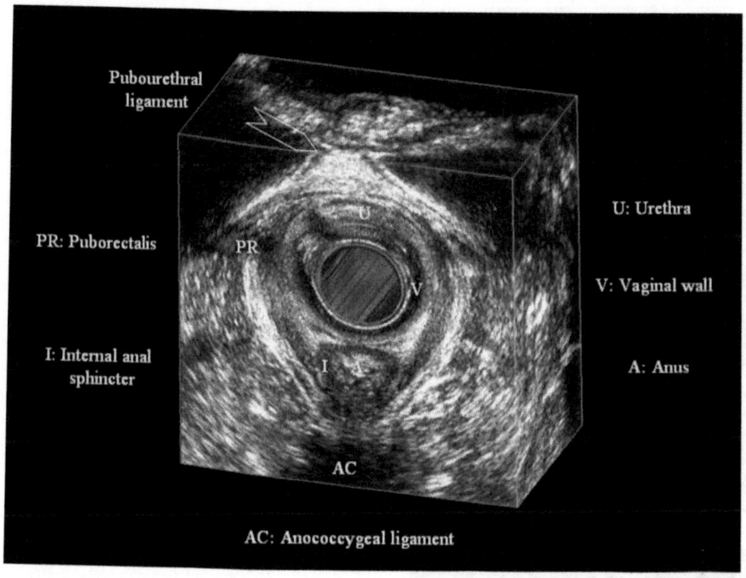

Fig. VI.9. Transvaginal ultrasonography. The urethra is seen anterior to the vagina with the anal canal dorsal to the vagina. The puborectalis is demonstrated as an almost ellipsoidal structure encircling the anal canal, the vagina, and the urethra

TVUS allows evaluation of a complex set of anatomical structures of the pelvic floor (Fig. VI.9). At the level of the external urethral meatus, the anal canal will be seen posteriorly in the image, together with the external anal sphincter (EAS), the internal anal sphincter (IAS), and often the superficial transverse perineal muscles within the perineal body in nullipara women. Introducing the transducer further in the cephalad direction (proximal) will image the ischiopubic rami, the symphysis pubis, the urethra, and the pubourethral ligament (Fig. VI.9). The puborectalis muscle will be seen inferior and lateral to the anal canal, depicting a soft curve up anterior and lateral to the vagina, forming almost an ellipsoidal structure before attaching itself to the inferior side of the symphysis pubis (Fig. VI.9). Posteriorly to the anal canal, the anococcygeal ligament can be identified as a black triangle in the ultrasound image (Fig. VI.9).

Ultrasonographic Abnormal Findings and Correlation to Clinical Conditions

Anal Sphincter

Patients with obstructed defecation may have clinically asymptomatic, unsuspected sphincter damage following vaginal delivery, anal surgery, or trauma [5, 6]. Woods et al. [6] reported that 71% of patients with rectal prolapse and incontinence had an abnormality in the anal sphincter complex on EAUS. In 19% of patients, the defects were isolated to the IAS, in 14% of patients the defects were isolated to the EAS, and in 38% of patients the defects were found in both the IAS and EAS. Anal sphincter tears are likely to contribute to symptoms of incontinence following surgical correction of obstructed defecation. Therefore, it is mandatory to identify preoperatively any sphincteric lesions in order to plan an adequate management.

Nielsen et al. [7] suggested that EAUS should be considered in patients with obstructed defecation to identify patients with internal sphincter hypertrophy. Halligan et al. [8] examined 21 patients with histologically proven solitary rectal ulcer syndrome (SRUS), a condition linked pathophysiologically with rectal prolapse, in order to determine the frequency of any ultrasound abnormality. The submucosa was inhomogeneous, and thickness increased in patients with SRUS compared with control asymptomatic subjects (median 4.0 mm vs. 2.0 mm; $P<0.0001$). IAS diameter was increased (median 3.8 mm vs. 2.0 mm; $P<0.0001$), as was the cross-sectional area (median 241 sq mm vs. 112 sq mm; $P<0.0001$). EAS diameter was also increased (median 8.5 mm vs. 7.0 mm; $P=0.0173$). The authors suggested that apparent muscle hypertrophy on ultrasound may diagnose those

a

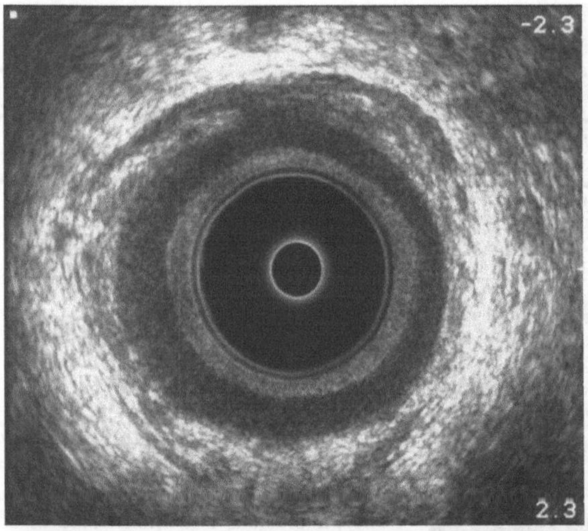

b

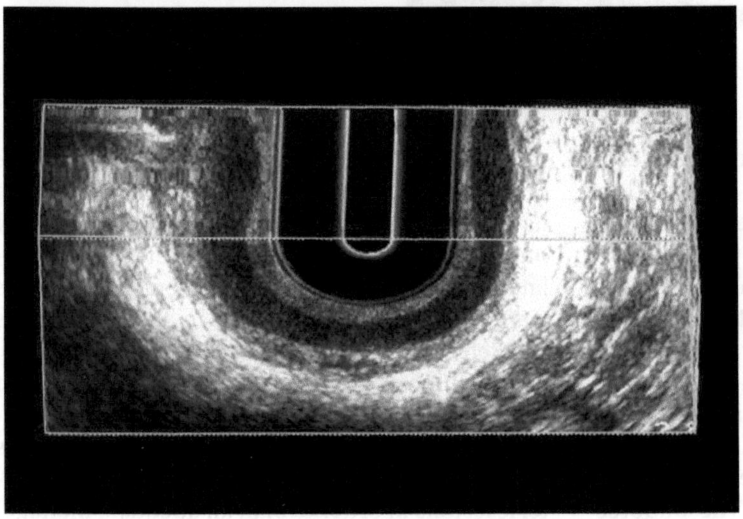

Fig. VI.10. Internal anal sphincter hypertrophy in a patient with solitary rectal ulcer syndrome (**a**). Three-dimensional reconstruction on coronal plane (**b**)

patients with SRUS in whom defecatory difficulty is a predominant symptom (Fig. VI.10). Poen et al. [9] showed asymmetry and thickening of the IAS and submucosa in 12 patients with complete rectal prolapse. After laparoscopic rectopexy, the maximum IAS thickness decreased from 3.0 mm to 2.6 mm (P=0.02). In a study from Dvorkin et al. [10], the EAUS scans of 18 patients with full-thickness rectal prolapse were compared with those of 23 asymptomatic controls. Patients with rectal prolapse showed a characteristic elliptical morphology in the anal canal, with anterior/posterior submucosal distortion (Fig. VI.11). IAS and submucosa thickness and area were greater in all quadrants of the anal canal (especially upper) in patients with rectal prolapse. There was statistical evidence of a relationship between increases in all measured variables and the finding of rectal prolapse. The authors suggested that the cause of sphincter distortion and increased thickness is the result of mechanical stress placed on the sphincter from the prolapse and compensatory hypertrophy. After surgical correction of the prolapse, the IAS decreased in thickness. An irregular and asymmetrical aspect of the anal sphincter on EAUS and TVUS was also revealed by Damon et al. [11] in 23 patients with full-thickness rectal prolapse or rectoanal intussusception. Interestingly, in this group of patients, the anal sphincter asymmetry index, identified by anal

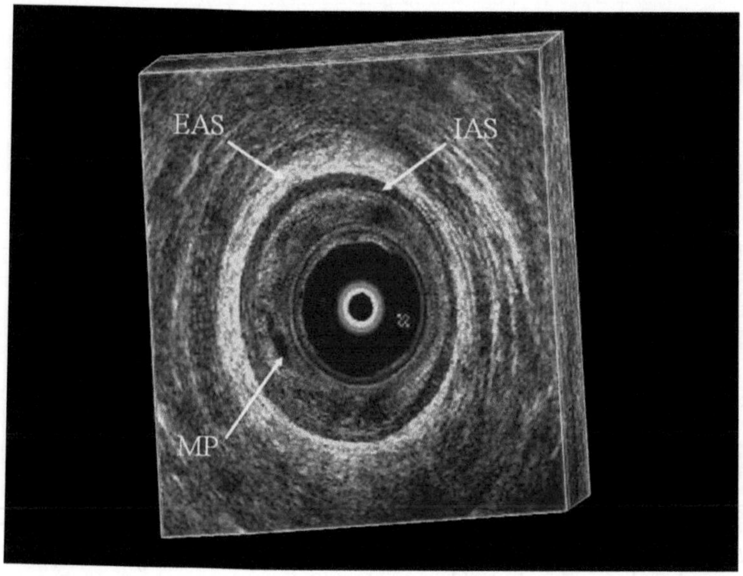

Fig. VI.11. Characteristic elliptical morphology of the internal anal sphincter (IAS) in a patient with cinrcumferential mucosal prolapse. *EAS* external anal sphincter, *MP* mucosal prolapse

vector manometry, was significantly increased at rest, confirming that rectal prolapse alters mainly IAS functions.

Rectocele

Rectocele is defined as ventral displacement of the anterior rectal wall into the posterior vagina over a distance of at least 1 cm during straining to defecate in comparison with the resting tone. The pathogenesis of this disorder remains controversial [21–26]. The concept of the rectocele as a defect in the integrity of the rectovaginal septum has been reported by Richardson [22, 23] and DeLancey [24]; however, there is still controversy concerning the anatomical importance (or even the existence) of the rectovaginal septum [25, 26]. Recently, Aigner et al. [25] performed macroscopic dissections on embalmed human pelvis and plastination histology of 40 fetal and newborn pelvic specimens. By means of conventional and immunohistochemical staining methods using monoclonal and polyclonal antibodies for tissue analysis and neuronal labeling, the authors were able to demonstrate that the rectovaginal septum is formed of dense collagenous and elastic fibers and longitudinal smooth muscle bundles originating from the external longitudinal muscle layer of the ventral rectal wall. The septum constitutes an incomplete partition between the rectum and the vagina, and it is completed by the perineal body caudally [25]. Leffler et al. [26] reported that laterally, the rectovaginal septum attaches to the pelvic sidewall. They reported that a significant percentage of the specific defect in the rectovaginal fascia have been found to occur laterally, representing a detachment of the septum from the pelvic sidewall.

In normal women, the septum can be visualized by EAUS as a V-shaped hyperechoic layer dividing the vagina and the rectum (Fig. VI.12). The septum appears decreased in thickness (Fig. VI.13) in patients with rectocele, or it may appear interrupted in the midline (Fig. VI.14). A ventral displacement or a bulging of the anterior rectal wall during straining may also be visualized by EAUS (Fig. VI.15). Barthet et al. [13] reported that DAE is a reliable procedure for diagnosing rectocele, with a sensitivity of 86% and accuracy of 87%. The rate of concordance between DAE and defecography was 57%. Recently, Beer-Gabel et al. [18] assessed the feasibility of DTP-US in the diagnosis of pelvic floor disorders. Rectoceles, peritoneoceles, enteroceles, and rectoanal intussusception were readily identified using DTP-US. This technique will be described in a different chapter of this section.

The concept of the rectocele as a consequence of a primary abnormality of the rectal wall with

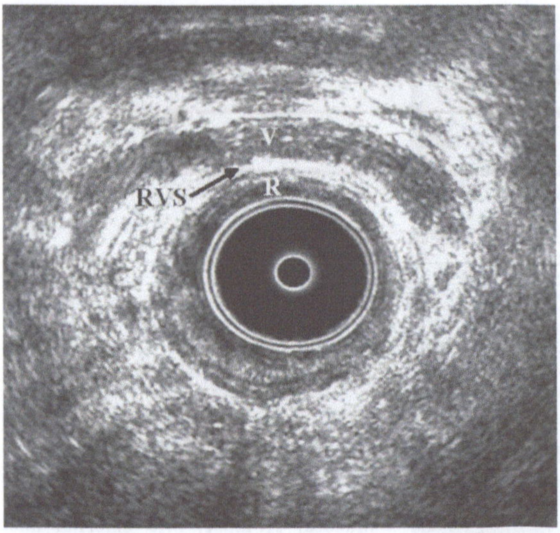

Fig. VI.12. In a normal woman, the septum (*RVS* rectovaginal septum) can be visualized as a V-shaped hyperechoic layer dividing the vagina (*V*) and the rectum (*R*)

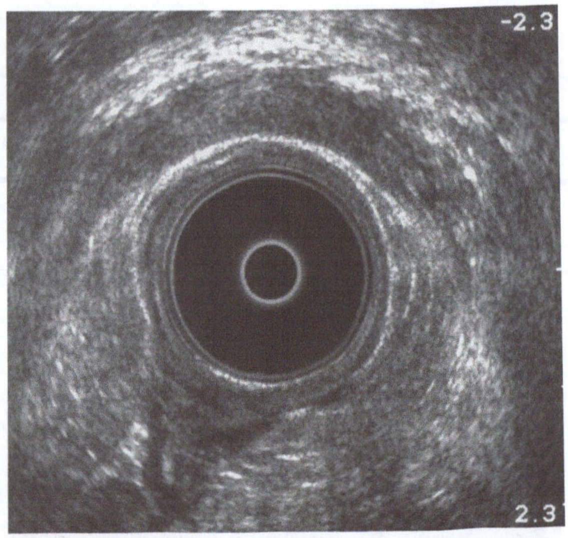

Fig. VI.13. The septum appears decreased in thickness in a patient with rectocele

a

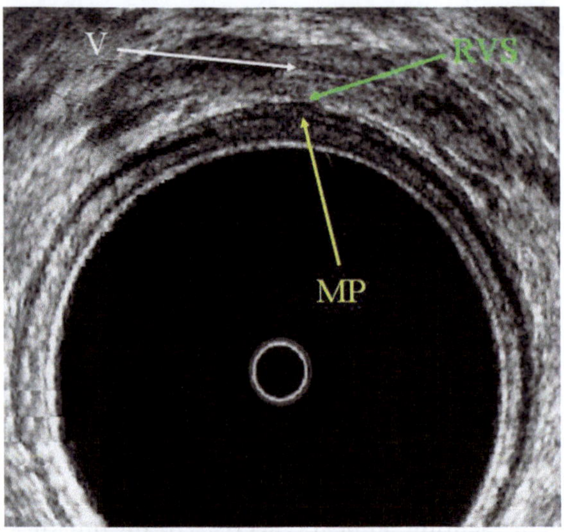

b

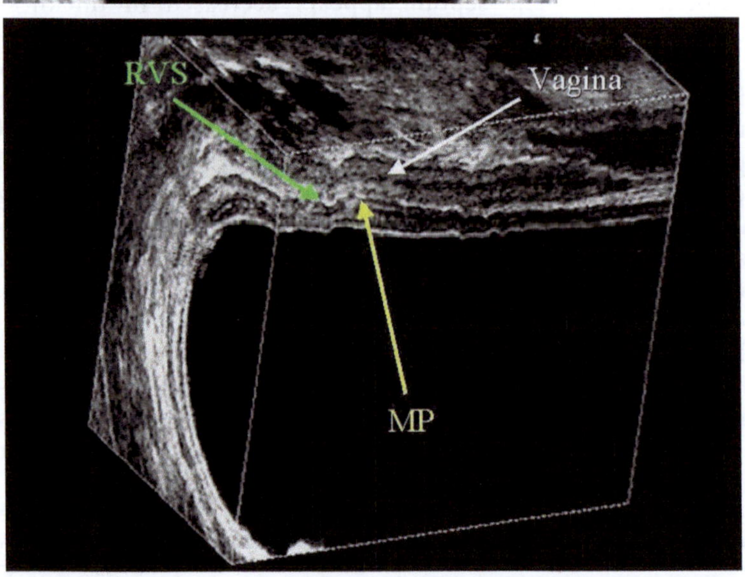

Fig. VI.14. The septum appears interrupted in the midline in a patient with rectocele (a). The characteristic five-layer structure of the rectal wall is disrupted: the mucosa exceeds the normal thickness, and the muscularis propria is irregular and interrupted. Three-dimensional reconstruction on the sagittal plane (b). *RVS* rectovaginal septum, *V* vagina, *MP* muscularis propria

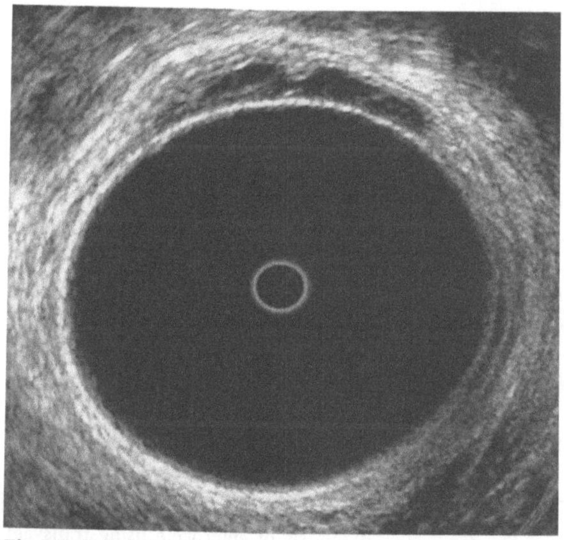

Fig. VI.15. Bulging of the anterior rectal wall during straining in a patient with rectocele

disruption of the muscularis propria layer has been recently reported [27]. Interestingly, in women with rectocele, ERUS has been able to demonstrate that, along with the discontinuity of the rectovaginal septum, the characteristic five-layer structure of the rectal wall is disrupted: the mucosa exceeds the normal thickness, and the muscularis propria is irregular and interrupted (Fig. VI.14).

Enterocele

An enterocele is a hernia of intestinal loops into the cul-de-sac of Douglas, which protrudes into the vagina or the rectum. They may accompany other pelvic and anorectal disorders or cause outlet obstruction. EAUS has the capability of diagnosing small, occult enteroceles. Three-dimensional reconstructions on axial and sagittal planes provide images of intestinal loops entering into the rectogenital space in patients with rectocele (Fig. VI.16). By using rectal ultrasonography, Vierhout et al. [19] correctly confirmed the existence of an enterocele in 27 of the 29 patients with this condition. Halligan et al. [15] examined 17 women with vaginal endosonography to diagnose enterocele, and the findings were compared with proctography. A diagnosis of enterocele was confirmed if bowel prolapsed into the rectogenital space during straining, obscuring the rectum (Fig. VI.17). The authors reported a sensitivity of 100% and specificity of 82%, with a positive predictive value of 75% and negative predictive value of 100%. Karuas et al. [12] investigated the use of DAE to detect this disorder. In patients with enterocele, the pouch of Douglas opened during straining, and intestinal loops moved toward the anus (Fig. VI.18). The diagnosis of enteroceles was confirmed in all patients by defecography, giving a specificity of 100%.

a

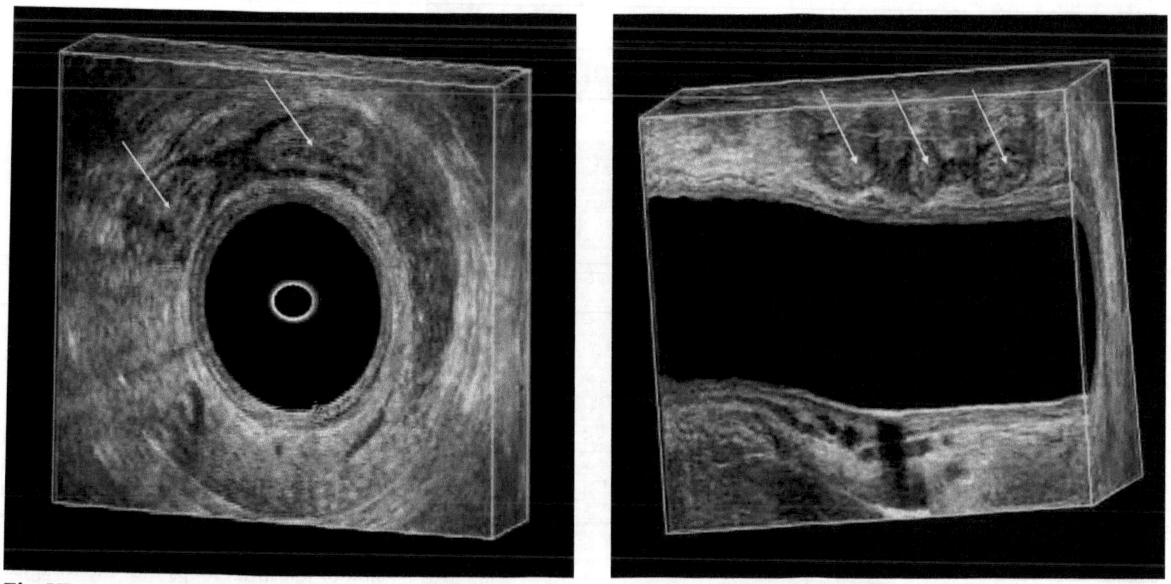

b

Fig. VI.16. Intestinal loops (*arrows*) visualized by endorectal ultrasonography in a patient with rectocele. Three-dimensional reconstruction on axial (**a**) and sagittal (**b**) planes

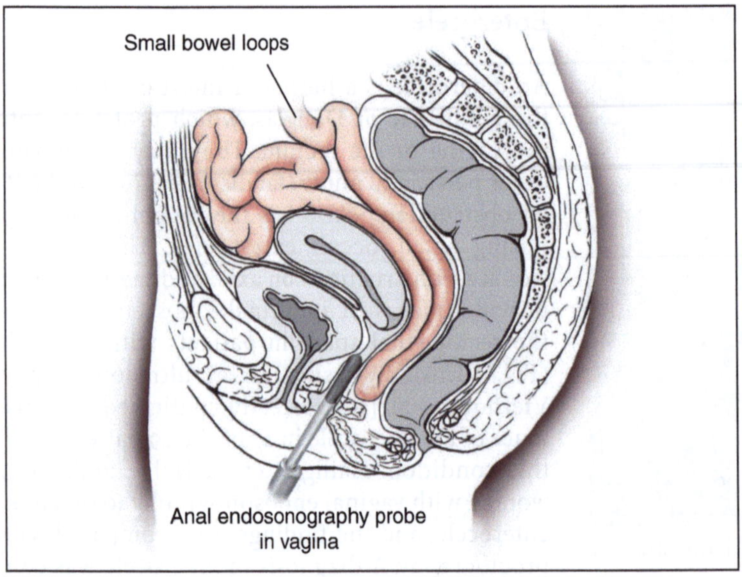

Fig. VI.17. Schematic representation of diagnosis of enterocele using transvaginal ultrasonography

a
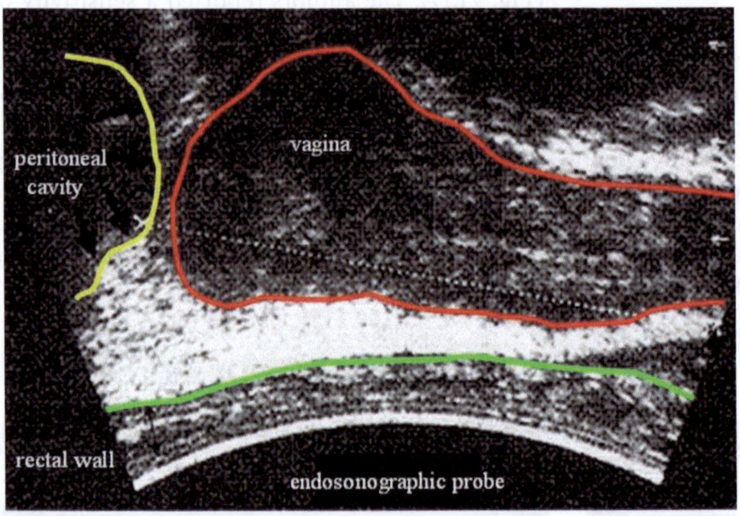

b
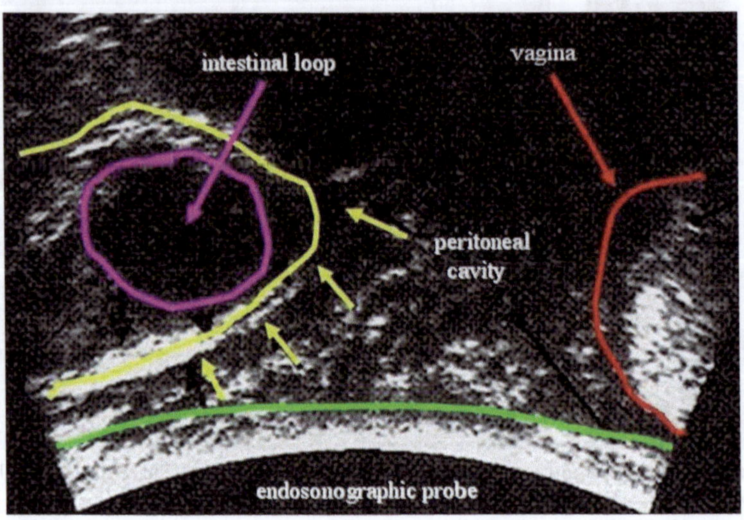

Fig. VI.18. Endosonographic sagittal scan of a normal women during maximal straining (a). Endosonographic scan of a patient with an enterocele during maximal straining showing the deep protrusion of intestinal loops into the Douglas, pushing the vagina in a horizontal position (b). (Modified from [12])

Pelvic Floor Dyssynergy

Pelvic floor dyssynergy is the most prevalent functional cause of dyschezia [2]. The patient does not sufficiently relax and sometimes even paradoxically contracts the anal sphincter muscles and puborectalis during straining to defecate. Dynamic ultrasound examination has been proved valuable in diagnosing this disorder [14]. Van Outryve et al. [14] evaluated 20 patients with a medical history of dyschezia. They found that the anal sphincter became paradoxically shorter and/or thicker during straining (versus the resting state) in 85% of patients but in only 35% of control subjects. Changes in sphincter length were statistically significantly different (p<0.01) in patients compared with control subjects. In the patients with dyschezia, a decrease in length (from 41 mm to 38 mm) and increase in thickness (from 8 mm to 10 mm) of the puborectalis was demonstrated during straining versus the resting state. Both the changes in length and thickness of the puborectalis were significantly different (p<0.01) in patients versus control subjects. These data indicate that in patient with pelvic floor dyssynergy, not only the anal sphincter but also the puborectalis muscle paradoxically contract instead of relaxing during a straining effort. The anorectal angle does not increase, preventing the descent of feces from the rectum into the anal canal.

References

1. Rasmussen OO, Sorensen M, Tetzeschner T, Christiansen J (1993) Dynamic anal manometry in the assessment of patients with obstructed defecation. Dis Colon Rectum 36:901–907
2. Fucini C, Ronchi O, Elbetti C (2001) Electromyography of the pelvic floor musculature in the assessment of obstructed defecation symptoms. Dis Colon Rectum 44:1168–1175
3. Felt-Bersma RJF, Luth WJ, Janssen JJWM, Meuwissen SGM (1990) Defecography in patients with anorectal disorders. Which findings are clinically relevant? Dis Colon Rectum 33:277–284
4. Rentsch M, Paetzel Ch, Lenhart M et al (2001) Dynamic magnetic resonance imaging defecography. A diagnostic alternative in the assessment of pelvic floor disorders in proctology. Dis Colon Rectum 44:999–1007
5. Burnett SJ, Spence-Jones C, Speakman CT et al (1991) Unsuspected sphincter damage following childbirth revealed by anal ultrasound. Br J Radiol 64:225–227
6. Woods R, Voyvodic F, Schloithe AC et al (2002) Anal sphincter tears in patients with rectal prolapse and incontinence. Colorectal Dis 5:544–548
7. Nielsen MB, Rasmussen OO, Pedersen JF, Christiansen J (1993) Anal endosonographic findings in patients with obstructed defecation. Acta Radiol 34:35–38
8. Halligan S, Sultan A, Rottenberg G, Bartram CI (1995) Endosonography of the anal sphincters in solitary rectal ulcer syndrome. Int J Colorectal Dis 10:79–82
9. Poen AC, de Brauw M, Felt-Bersma RJ et al (1996) Laparoscopic rectopexy for complete rectal prolapse. Clinical outcome and anorectal function tests. Surg Endosc 10:904–908
10. Dvorkin LS, Chan CLH, Knowles CH et al (2004) Anal sphincter morphology in patients with full-thickness rectal prolapse. Dis Colon Rectum 47:198–203
11. Damon H, Henry L, Roman S et al (2003) Influence of rectal prolapse on the asymmetry of the anal sphincter in patients with anal incontinence. BMC Gastroenterol 3:23–29
12. Karuas M, Neuhaus P, Wiedenmann B (2000) Diagnosis of enteroceles by dynamic anorectal endosonography. Dis Colon Rectum 43:1683–1688
13. Barthet M, Portier F, Heyries L (2000) Dynamic anal endosonography may challenge defecography for assessing dynamic anorectal disorders: results of a prospective pilot study. Endoscopy 32:300–305
14. Van Outryve SM, Van Outryve MJ, De Winter BY, Pelckmans PA (2002) Is anorectal endosonography valuable in dyschesia? Gut 51:695–700
15. Halligan S, Northover J, Bartram CI (1996) Vaginal endosonography to diagnose enterocele. Br J Radiol 69:996–999
16. Tunn R, Petri E (2003) Introital and transvaginal ultrasound as the main tool in the assessment of urogenital and pelvic floor dysfunction: an imaging panel and practical approach. Ultrasound Obstet Gynecol 22:205–213
17. Kleinubing H Jr, Jannini JF, Malafaia O et al (2000) Transperineal ultrasonography: new method to image the anorectal region. Dis Colon Rectum 43:1572–1574
18. Beer-Gabel M, Teshler M, Barzilai N et al (2002) Dynamic transperineal ultrasound in the diagnosis of

pelvic floor disorders. Pilot study. Dis Colon Rectum 45:239–248

19. Vierhout ME, van PD (2002) Diagnosis of posterior enterocele. Comparison of rectal ultrasonography with intraoperative diagnosis. J Ultrasound Med 21:383–387
20. Piloni V, Spazzafumo L (2005) Evacuation sonography. Tech Coloproctol 9:119–126
21. Zbar AP, Lienemann A, Fritsch H (2003) Rectocele: pathogenesis and surgical management. Int J Colorectal Dis 18:369–384
22. Richardson AC (1993) The rectovaginal septum revisited: its relationship to rectocele and its importance in rectocele repair. Clin Obstet Gynaecol 36:976–983
23. Richardson AC (1995) The anatomic defects in rectocele and enterocele. J Pelvic Surg 1:214–221
24. DeLancey JO (1999) Structural anatomy of the posterior pelvic compartment as it relates to rectocele. Am J Obstet Gynecol 180:815–823
25. Aigner F, Zbar AP, Ludwikowski B et al (2004) The rectogenital septum: morphology, function and clinical relevance. Dis Colon Rectum 46:131–140
26. Leffler KS, Thompson JR, Cundiff GW et al (2001) Attachment of the rectovaginal septum to the pelvic sidewall. Am J Obstet Gynecol 185:41–43
27. Boccasanta P, Venturi M, Stuto A et al (2004) Stapled transanal rectal resection for outlet obstruction: a prospective, multicenter trial. Dis Colon Rectum 47:1285–1297

VI.3. Clinical Dynamic Transperineal Ultrasonography in Proctologic Practice: the Case for its Use in Patients Presenting with Evacuatory Difficulty

A.P. Zbar, M. Beer-Gabel

Dynamic transperineal ultrasonography (DTP-US) is a relatively simple technique that has only recently been exploited to assess the component parts of the anterior, middle, and posterior pelvic compartments and their interaction during provocative maneuvers such as straining and simulated defecation in patients presenting to gynecologists or coloproctologists with evacuatory dysfunction [1, 2]. This approach provides comparative images to those achieved with axial endoanal ultrasound (EAUS) transducers for the assessment of morphologic integrity of both the internal (IAS) and external (EAS) anal sphincters; [3] however, our group and others have defined a clinical role for DTP-US in dynamic mode during forcible straining as a principal adjunct to the clinical evaluation of patients presenting to specialized clinics with evacuatory difficulty and obstructed defecation [4, 5].

There is generally a poor correlation between the symptoms attributed to pelvic floor dysfunction and radiologically demonstrable findings [6], where most studies have shown that virtually all patients presenting with evacuatory difficulty have a multiplicity of pathologic problems ranging across each pelvic compartment [7]. Traditionally, evacuation proctography (or one of its extended techniques, including opacification of the small bowel, bladder, vagina, and even the peritoneal cavity), has been used to define the presence of major morphological anomalies – most notably, rectocele, enterocele, rectoanal intussusception, rectal prolapse, and descending perineum syndrome – which are then attributed by the clinician as relatively dominant pathologies implicated in the evacuatory symptomatology and then accordingly treated [8]. What is clear is that a multidisciplinary approach, involving gastroenterologists, surgeons, gynaecologists, urologists, and biofeedback technologists, is required for these patients with multicompartmental disease [9] and that even within defined disorders such as rectocele, the preoperative assessment using different modalities may subcategorize patients into groups with different management solutions [10].

This chapter defines the indications, experience, and pitfalls of DTP-US, describing the basic technique, advantages, and limitations in specific pelvic floor disorders and accuracy in those patients presenting to a pelvic floor dysfunction unit with primary disorders of rectal evacuation.

Technical Features of DTP-US

The technique is simple when compared with endoluminal sonography although its interpretation is comparatively difficult, with a substantial leaning curve. No specific preparation is required, and it is wise if facilities exist to videotape the procedure for retrograde and orthograde scrolling akin to that routinely used in defecography. DTP-US is performed with a curvilinear 7.5 or 10 MHz probe after liberal application of acoustic gel to the perineum. It is wise to insert by Luer syringe a minimum of 50 ml intravaginally as well as into the rectum. Here, there have been claims that excessive distension of either organ may create a "crowded pelvis syndrome" [11] and obscure some diagnoses of clinical importance, most notably rectocele and enterocele, but this has not been our experience, where the amount of intravisceral gel has been varied without an effect on the principal diagnoses. For the diagnosis of both enterocele and peritoneocele, it is advisable that the patient ingest 100 ml of water-soluble Gastrografin (Schering, UK) diluted 1:1 with tap water 1 h prior to the examination. For sterility, the probe may be covered by an oversized condom instilled with acoustic gel, or with a latex glove. Patients are traditionally examined in the left lateral position (although it is recognized that this position, along with its use for provocative maneuvers such as gel evacuation or forcible straining, is not physiological), as it provides a standardized interpretation of images for all pelvic floor compartments. Comparison between this technique and dynamic magnetic resonance imaging (MRI) for patients presenting with evacuatory difficulty has not been performed, but here, conditions that appear at the end of defecation, (such as rectal prolapse and rectoanal intussusception) will be poorly diagnosed because of

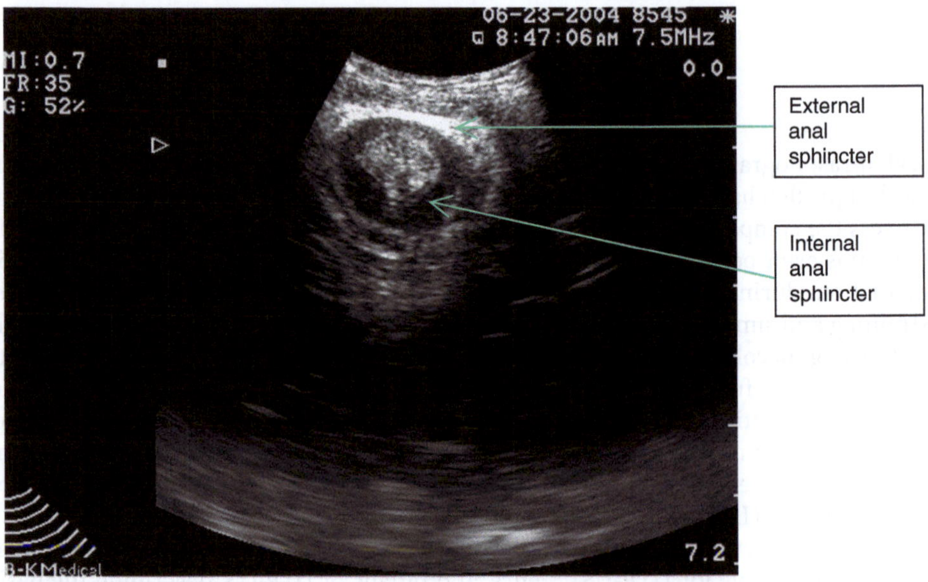

a

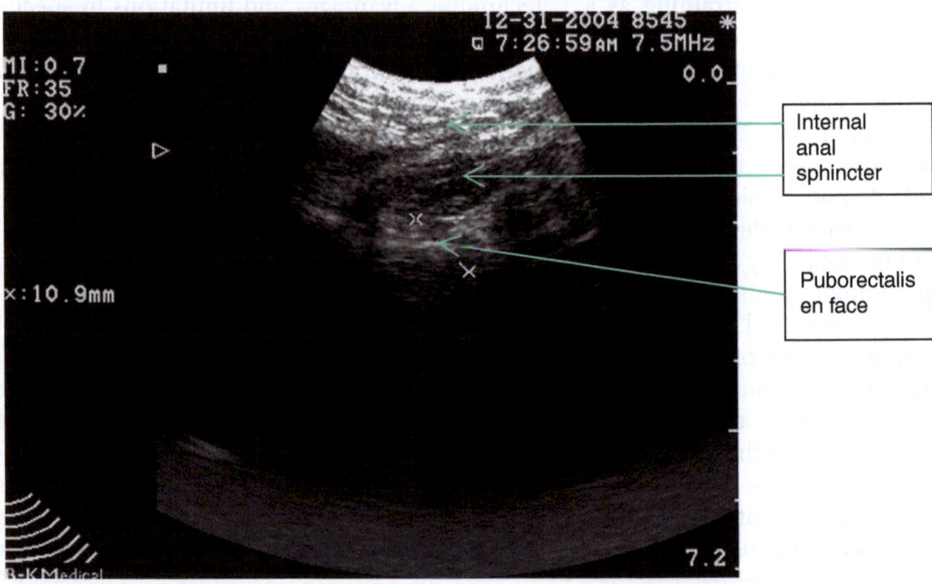

b

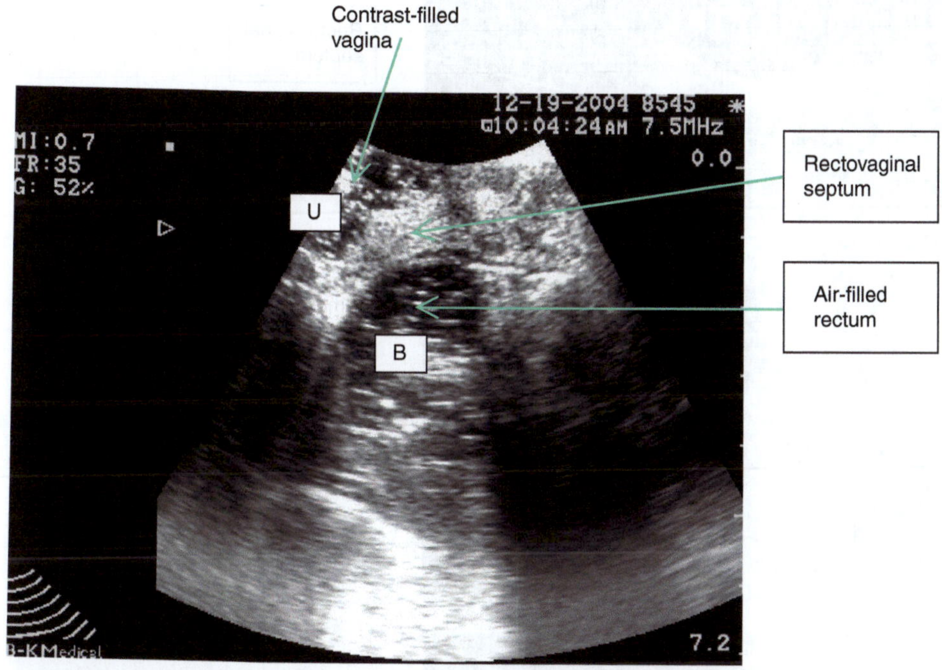

c

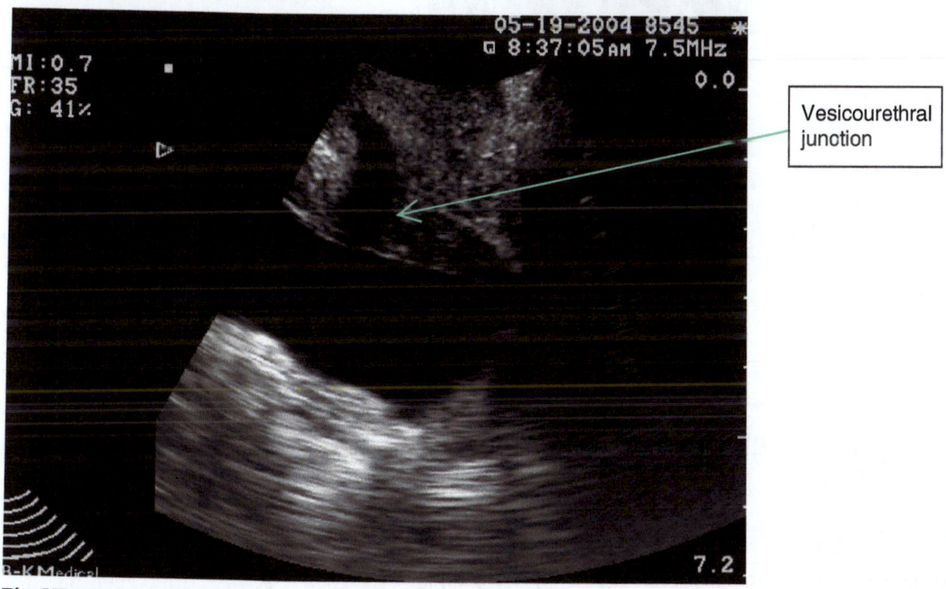

d

Fig. VI.19. Axial transperineal sonogram showing the complete hypoechoic ring of the internal anal sphincter (IAS) and the hyperechoic flattened external anal sphincter (**a**). Sagittal transperineal ultrasound (TP-US) showing the hypoechoic IAS in profile as a continuation of the air-filled rectum. The puborectalis muscle is seen as a bright elliptical structure *en face* (**b**). Transperineal ultrasound of the anterior perineal compartment showing the vesicourethral junction (**c**) (*B* bladder, *U* urethra). TP-US showing the normal rectovaginal septum as the territory between the vagina (containing acoustic gel) and the air-filled rectum (**d**)

the nonphysiological position. Comparative studies between conventional and upright DTP-US or with open-architecture MRI are awaited [12].

Examination of the anus is made with the transducer initially applied transversely to the perineal body, identifying the axial view of the anus using the landmark of the hypoechoic ring of the IAS in an image similar to that obtained in the midanal canal using endoanal ultrasonography (Fig. VI.19a). The transducer is then turned 180° to

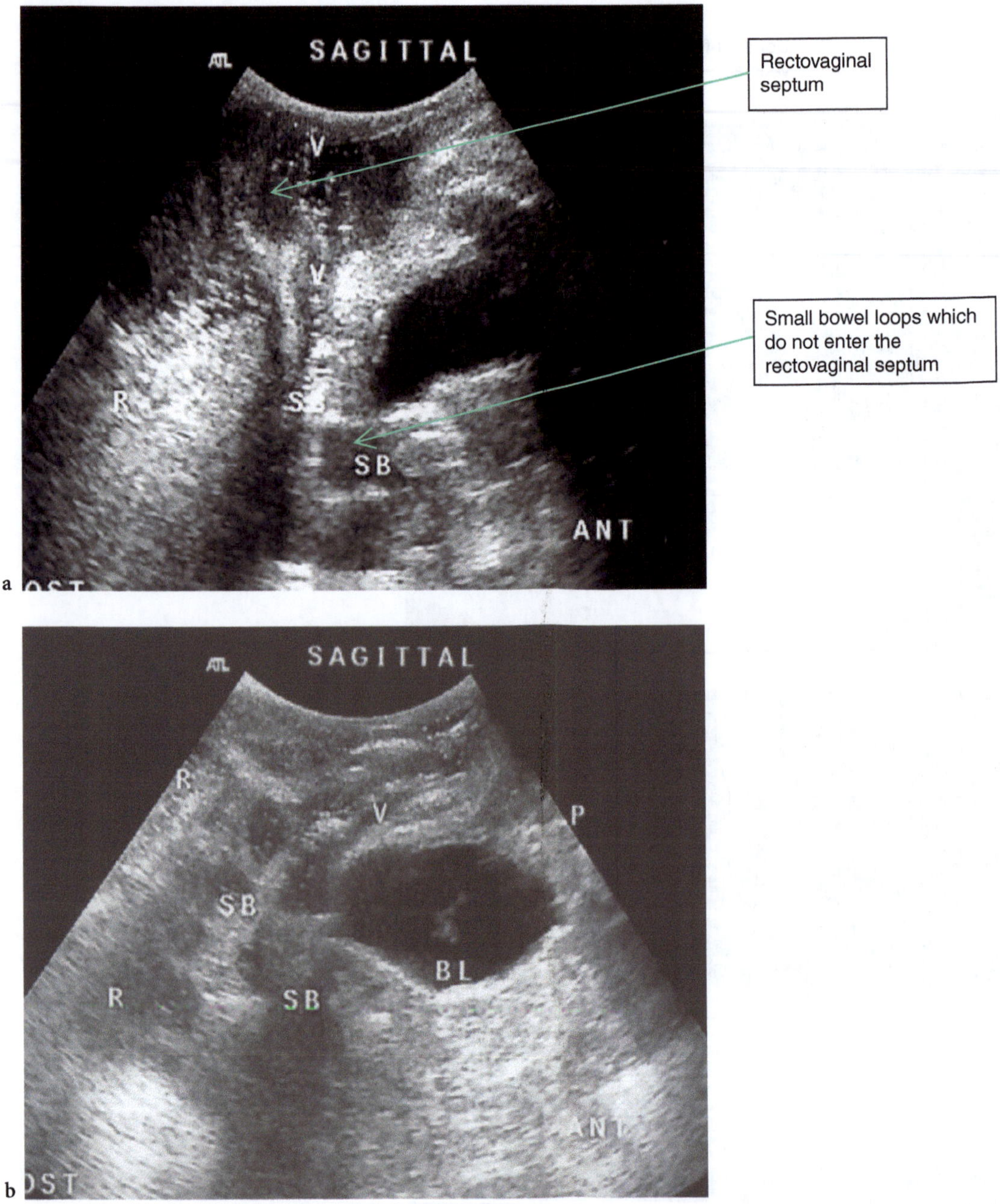

Fig. VI.20. In order to diagnose a peritoneocele, the rectovaginal septum is expanded beyond 2 cm in maximal diameter but is empty (**a**). An enterocele is defined by the presence of peristaltic, contrast-filled, enteric loops occupying the expanded rectogenital septum (**b**) (*R* rectum, *SB* small bowel, *V* vagina, *BL* bladder)

obtain a sagittal view of the contrast-filled rectum, with extension of the hypoechoic internal anal sphincter appearing above and below the anal canal in profile. The anorectal junction is well seen, with the bright hyperechoic elliptical bundle of the puborectalis sling demonstrable in relief (Fig. VI.19b). In the sagittal mode, the examination should proceed to identify the brilliantly hyperechoic pubis and is then worked back by downward movement of the transducer against the perineum to locate the hypoechoic bladder and the urethrovesical junction (Fig. VI.19c), the position and movement of which will be dependent upon the filling status of the bladder at the time of the investigation [13]. Transperineal sonography has been used definitively along with transintroital sonography for the objective diagnosis of urinary stress incontinence [14, 15]. The middle compartment is identified by focusing on the contrast-filled vaginal vault, with broad assessment of the depth and content of the rectogenital septum (Fig. VI.19d). Although standardized measurements of this septum are unavailable for DTP-US at this point [16], enlargement of this space beyond 2 cm. is regarded as abnormal, with an ultrasonographic diagnosis of peritoneocele if the space is enlarged but empty [17] and an enterocele if the space is filled either at rest or during forcible straining with contrast-filled enteric peristaltic loops on real-time sonography (Figs. VI.20a and b).

The anal canal has already been identified in the initial ultrasound sweep for landmarks but is now examined in more detail during forcible straining and simulated evacuation of the intrarectal acoustic gel. Here, definitive diagnoses may be made of rectocele, rectoanal intussusception (including its grade), perineal descent, and rectal prolapse. The technique has provided a number of specific landmarks for the determination of the anorectal angle (ARA) as well as for specific movement during straining of the anorectal junction (ARJ) using the pubococcygeal line akin to that seen in conventional defecography. Bony landmarks are more obvious with DTP-US since they can sometimes be obscured in proctography by film glare. Although it is recognized that these measurements have no clinical significance and are quite complex to perform with moderate interobserver variation [18], they do provide some validation of the DTP-US technique when compared with defecography in patients presenting with evacuatory difficulty. Our group has shown a high correlation between ARA and ARJ values both at rest and during maximal straining using the two modalities in blinded fashion [19]. In general, ARA during straining is greater, and ARJ is higher at rest with defecography, a finding probably related to the inherent positional differences using the two techniques [20]. Figures VI.21a and b show a Bland-Altman curve of agreement for ARA at rest and ARJ during straining between defecography and DTP-US in those patients presenting with evacuation difficulty, using defecography as the gold standard for positional assessment [21]; both show a high level of agreement. The mean ARA at rest obtained by proctography and by DTP-US were nearly identical, and the mean difference between techniques (proctography minus DTP-US) was not statistically different from zero (p=0.92). The mean ARA during straining measure by proctography was higher than that measured by DTP-US (123.3° ±4.vs. 116.4°±3.32°, respectively), with the average difference nearly reaching statistical significance (p=0.09). Bland-Altman plots were constructed for comparative ARA values at rest and during straining (Figs. VI.21a and b), with an SD at rest of 23.13° and during straining of 22.46°. The limits of agreement at rest ranged from −65° to +26 ° and during straining from −36° to +62°, with significant outliers yielding much higher proctographic values than ultrasonography.

Clinical Indications and Pitfalls of DTP-US in Evacuatory Dysfunction

The clinical indications for DTP-US are controversial, but it provides a validated alternative to dynamic MRI, which is frequently not available for functional anorectal studies. DTP-US has the advantage of rapid real-time demonstration of the interaction of the pelvic floor and soft-tissue compartments without complex algorithms or irradiation for use in young patients, including children. Specific advantage of DTP-US lies in the objective delineation of rectocele and in the decision making of its surgical repair when it is deemed to be the dominant clinical finding in patients who present with incomplete evacuation and the need for perineal or transvaginal manipulation [22, 23]. Here, measurement may be made of the rectocele depth by projection on transperineal ultrasonography (TP-US) images of the anterior rectal wall, showing high correlation with defecographic measurements [19] although it is recognized that emptying capacity does not specifically correlate with functional outcome after rectocele repair, however that is attempted [24, 25]. In this regard, larger nonemptying rectoceles do appear to be associated with more symptoms than do smaller ones, which tend to empty on defecography [23, 26]. Figure VI.22a shows the preoperative appearance of a rectocele in sagittal-mode DTP-US where a subjective interpretation may be made of the emptying capacity during forcible straining and evacuation. This dynamic sonography is useful in equating the contribution the rectocele makes to the overall pelvic floor dysfunction and may be quantified for postoperative comparison (Fig. VI.22b) with clinical outcome after operative repair. The presence of a coincident enterocele will dictate an alternative surgical approach to avoid

a

b

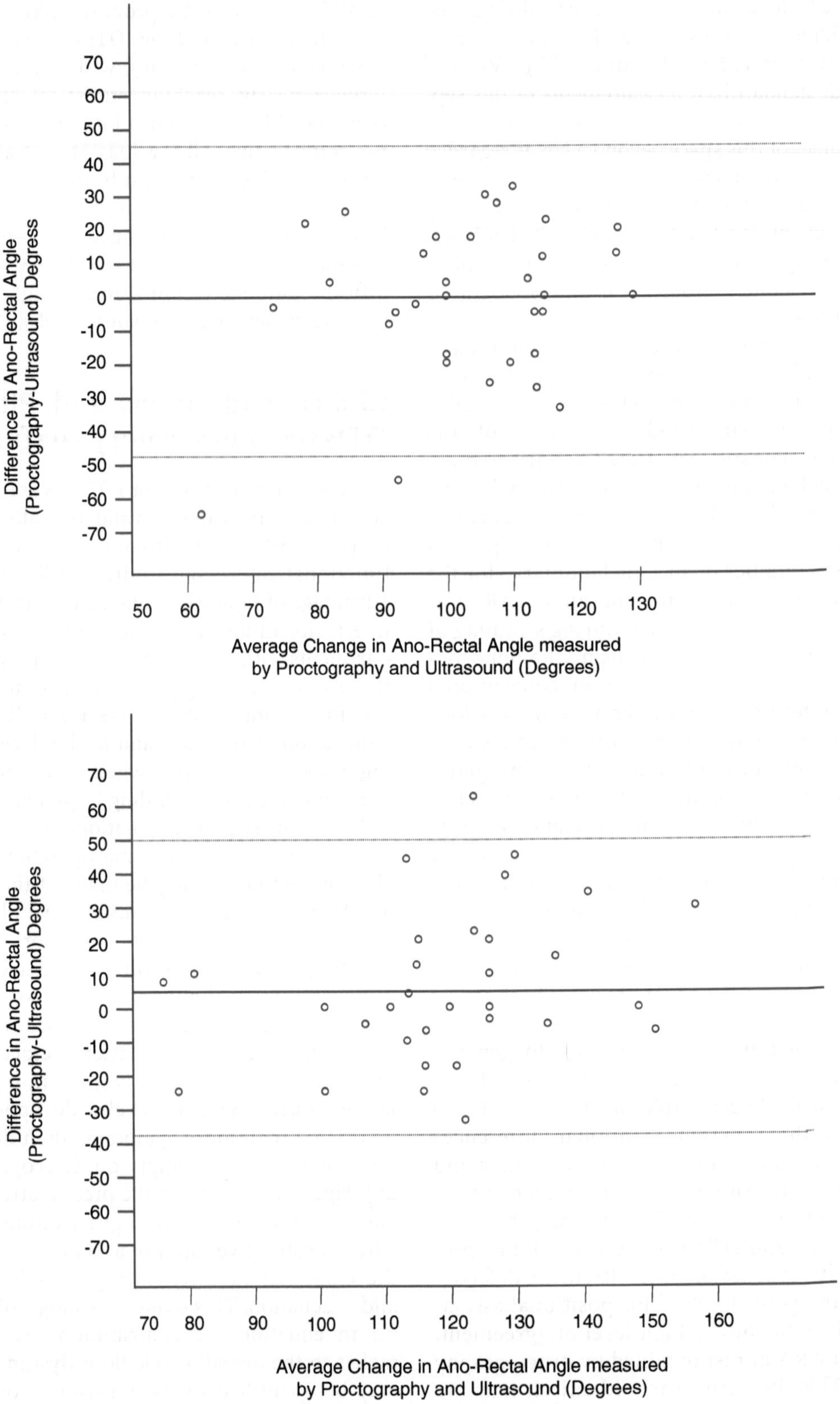

Fig. VI.21. Bland-Altman graph for anorectal angle at rest between defecography and dynamic transperineal ultrasonography using defecography as the gold standard, showing a high level of agreement between measurements (**a**). Similar agreement levels are achieved for anorectal junction movement between the two techniques during maximal straining (**b**). The solid line represents the mean of the measurement differences and the dashed lines represent two standard deviations from the mean

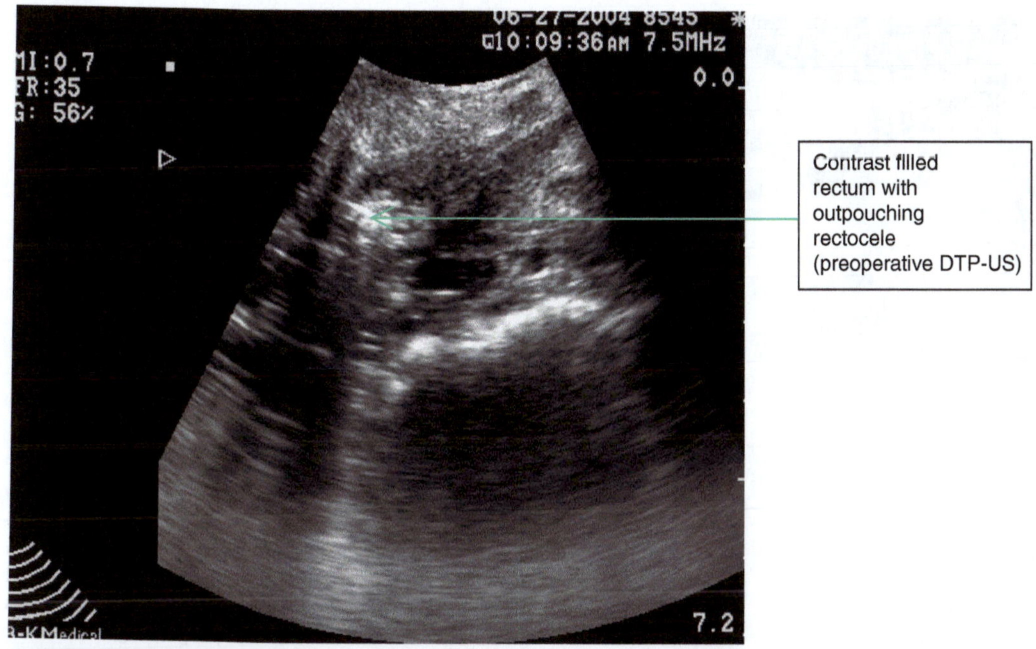

a

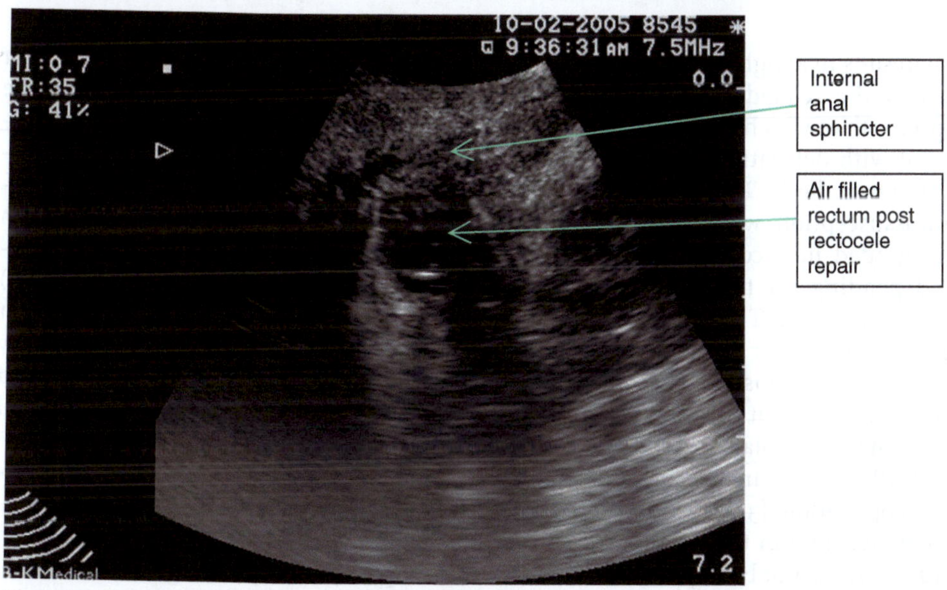

b

Fig. VI.22. Transperineal sonogram of a nonemptying rectocele. This is seen on sagittal scanning as an outpouching of the normal projected contour of the anal canal as seen in profile. The depth of these rectoceles as measured using dynamic transperineal ultrasonography (DTP-US) correlates closely with that measured on defecography (**a**). Postoperative DTP-US of the same patient after endorectal rectocele repair (**b**)

postoperative symptoms, where it is deemed that rectocele repair is indicated.

In a recent study of patients who had proven rectoceles, more enteroceles were diagnosed using DTP-US when compared with defecography [19, 27] and who presented with objectively scored evacuatory difficulty exceeding 6 months in duration (<1 bowel movement ever 4 days or longer or if ≥25% of bowel movements were accompanied by excessive straining), with a higher multiplicity of diagnosed pathologies of clinical importance using DTP-US, particularly in the posthysterectomy patient. In the latter circumstance, failure of routine culdosuspension (sacrocolpopexy) at the

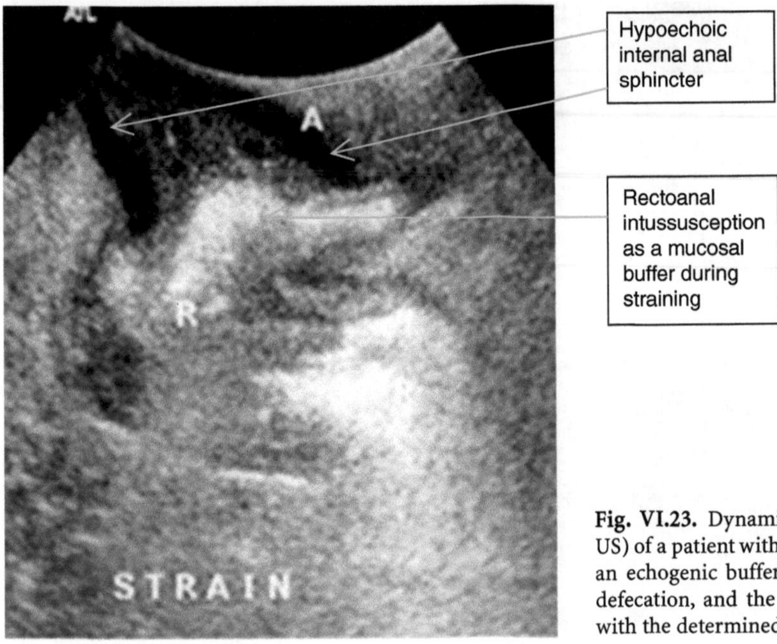

Fig. VI.23. Dynamic transperineal ultrasonography (DTP-US) of a patient with rectoanal intussusception. This is seen as an echogenic buffer appearing intraluminally on attempted defecation, and the grade as defined on DTP-US correlates with the determined clinical/endoscopic grading. *R* rectum

time of hysterectomy results in a higher incidence of both enterocele and the related problem of vaginal-vault prolapse, both of which may present to the coloproctologist with defecation difficulty [28–30]. Figure VI.23 shows the DTP-US appearance of rectoanal intussusception, which may be ultrasonographically graded in accordance with the clinical grade, depending on the extent of descent toward the anal canal. This typically appears as a bright echogenic buffer on straining, occupying the anal canal in the absence of contrast evacuation, an appearance that has similarity to rectal internal mucosal prolapse (RIMP). DTP-US grading of RIMP, too, appears to correlate with its clinical endoscopic grade [31, 32]. At present, DTP-US, although accurate in the diagnosis of both of these conditions, has not been prospectively validated as part of the treatment algorithm in terms of its impact on surgical management based on the preoperative ultrasonographic grade.

Clinical effects on anorectal function after hysterectomy are controversial and at present poorly studied [33, 34], and DTP-US requires validation in the objective assessment in comparison with the clinical grading of coincident uterovaginal prolapse [35, 36]. Finally, DTP-US may be of benefit in the delineation of some cases where there is a mechanical block to defecation, as shown in Fig. VI.24, where a postchemoradiation recurrence of an anal squamous cell carcinoma was shown in the rectovaginal septum but was not demonstrable using endoanal sonography. We had similar experience with the TP-US demonstration of retrorectal tumors [37] and in rare rectal duplications, which have both resulted in primary presentations to our pelvic floor unit with defecation block. Its role in the assessment of congenital anorectal anomalies (and their aftermath) has been poorly studied [38], but we have found it of some clinical use in the assessment of low anomalies with delineation of anovestibular and anocutaneous fistulas in infants suitable for anal cutback or transposition procedures (Fig. VI.25).

There are several pitfalls of the DTP-US technique in coloproctologic practice. It is time consuming and difficult to learn, requiring between 20–40 min to perform, depending on the level of one's expertise. Although no accreditation programs are established, it is likely that a minimum of 100 examinations are required to make the clinician relatively proficient. As stated, the position adopted for the performance of DTP-US is nonphysiological for most disorders that appear at the end of defecation, and there is no advanced data on what anatomic anomalies are detected in specific patient groups (posthysterectomy and uterovaginal prolapse), either in comparison with clinical or operative findings. The proximity of the operator's hand and the probe may create some patient reticence to strain adequately on request and limit the diagnostic capacity of the

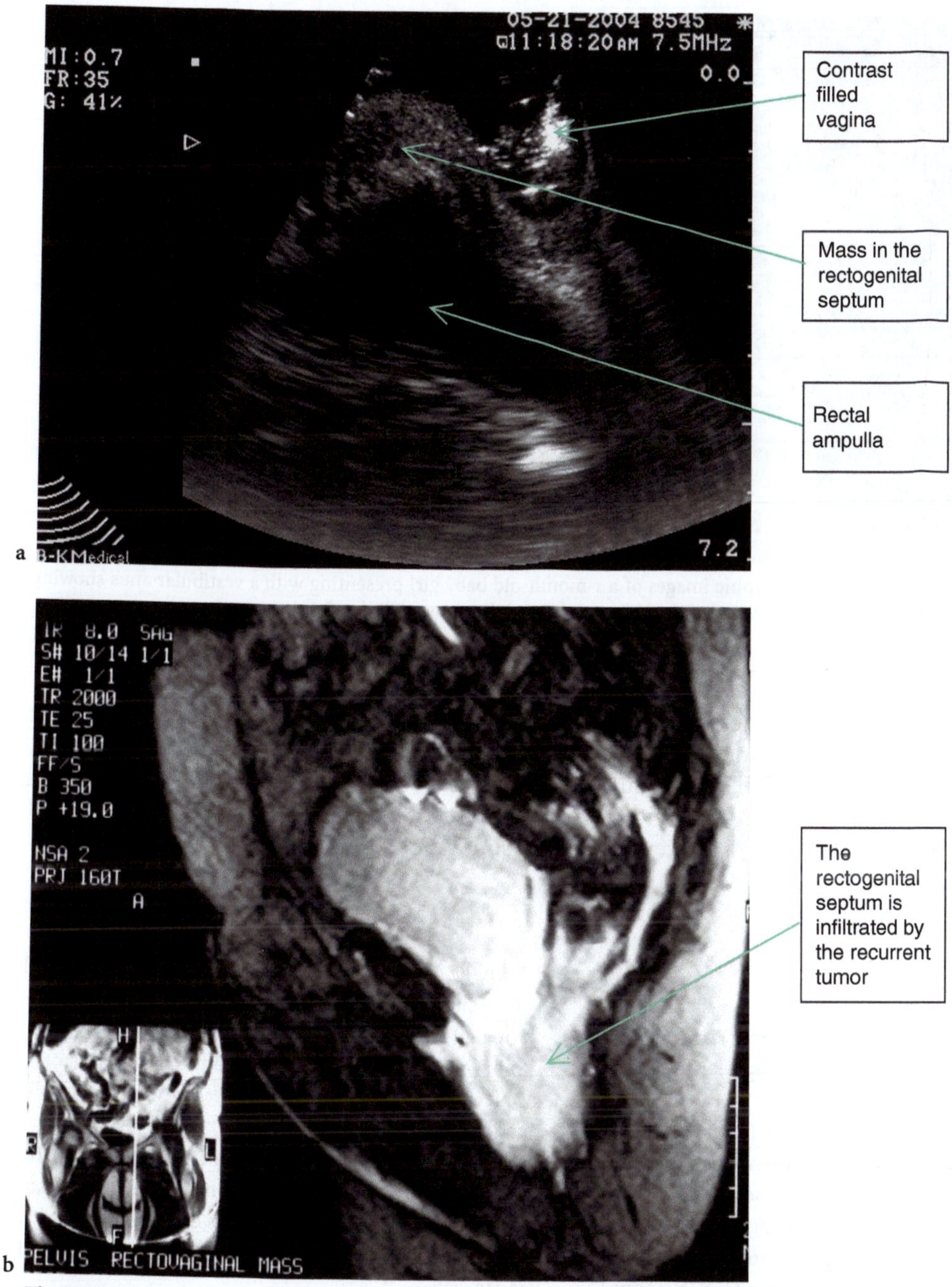

Fig. VI.24. Transperineal ultrasound of a patient presenting with defecation block showing a mass in the rectovaginal septum. This was a recurrence of an anal canal squamous cell carcinoma following initial chemoradiation (**a**). T1-weighted sagittal magnetic resonance image of the mass (**b**)

technique in the same way as may occur in some scrutinized patients during proctography. Also, its use in men or obese women is frequently impaired because of the sheer bulk of the buttocks and the inability to properly position the probe on the perineum [39].

In summary, the ready availability of ultrasound, lack of irradiation, portability, and repeatability make DTP-US an exciting novel technique for use in patients where the indications and contraindications of the procedure are still being determined in those presenting with evacuation difficulty. It provides dynamic, multiplanar imaging capacity for a multidisciplinary

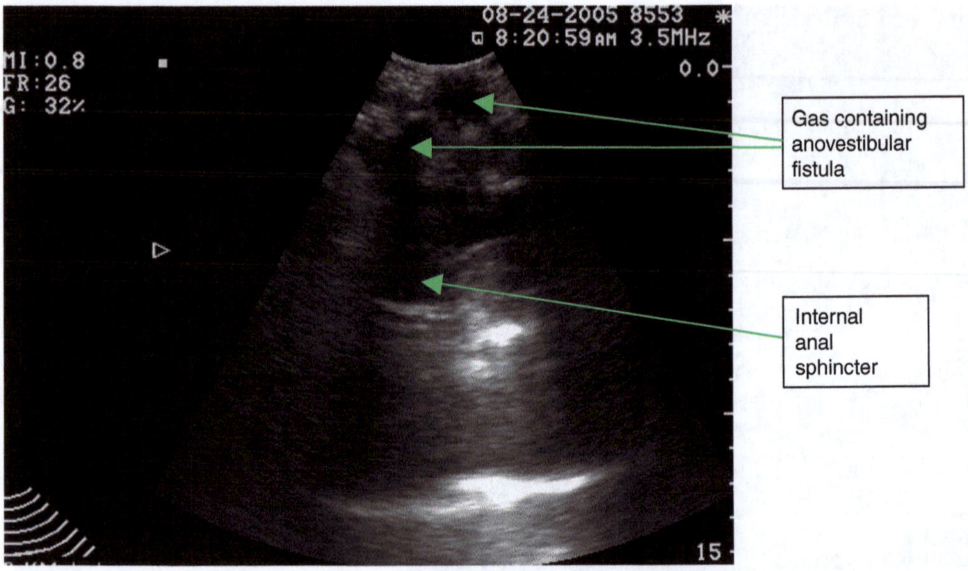

Fig. VI.25. Axial transperineal ultrasonographic images of a 1-month-old baby girl presenting with a vestibular anus showing an intact internal anal sphincter over the covered anus with a gas-containing anovestibular fistula

approach toward pelvic floor disorders and confirms the clinical impression of rectocele, enterocele, cystourethrocele, and genital descensus. Sagittal views may also afford definition (either intra- or postoperatively) of the rostral extent of sphincter damage in those patients who present with combined incontinence and constipation, without the requirement for complex and expensive software utilized in 3-dimensional endosonography [40–42].

References

1. Dietz HP, Broome J, Haylen BT (2001) Ultrasound quantification of uterovaginal prolapse. Ultrasound Obstet Gynecol 18:511–514
2. Beer-Gabel M, Frudinger A, Zbar A (2005) Dynamic transperineal ultrasound and transvaginal sonography. In Wexner SD, Zbar AP, Pescatori M (eds) Complex anorectal disorders: investigation and management. Springer, London, pp 246–262
3. Kleinübing H Jr, Jannini JF, Malafaia O et al (2000) Transperineal ultrasonography: new method to image the anorectal region. Dis Colon Rectum 43:1572 1574
4. Piloni V (2001) Dynamic imaging of the pelvic floor with transperineal sonography. Tech Coloproctol 5:103–105
5. Beer-Gabel M, Teshler M, Barzilai N et al (2002) Dynamic transperineal ultrasound in the diagnosis of pelvic floor disorders: pilot study. Dis Colon Rectum 45:239–248
6. Maglinte DD, Kelvin FM, Fitzgerald K, Hale DS, Benson T (1999) Association of compartment defects in pelvic floor dysfunction. AJR Am J Roentgenol 172:439–444
7. Rotholtz NA, Efron JE, Weiss EG et al (2002) Anal manometric predictors of significant rectocele in constipated patients. Tech Coloproctol 6:73–77
8. Shorvon PJ, McHugh S, Diamant NE et al (1989) Defecography in normal volunteers: results and implications. Gut 30:1737–1749
9. Davila GW, Ghoniem GM, Kapoor DS, Contreras-Ortiz O (2002). Pelvic floor dysfunction management practice patterns: a survey of members of the International Urogynecological Association. Int Urogynecol J 13:319–325
10. Dietz HP, Steensma AB (2005) Posterior compartment prolapse on two-dimensional and three-dimensional pelvic floor ultrasound: the distinction between true rectocele, perineal hypermobility and enterocele. Ultrasound Obstet Gynecol 26:73–77
11. Kelvin FM, Maglinte DD (1997) Dynamic cystoproctography of female pelvic floor defects and their interrelationships. AJR Am J Roentgenol 369:769–774
12. Schoenenberger AW, Debatin JF, Guldenschuh I et al (1998) Dynamic MR defecography with a superconducting MR system. Radiology 206:641–646
13. Dietz HP, Clarke B (2001) The influence of posture on

perineal ultrasound imaging parameters. Int Urogynecol J Pelvic Floor Dysfunct 12:104–106
14. Koebl H, Bernascheck G, Deutinger J (1990) Assessment of female urinary incontinence by introital sonography. J Clin Ultrasound 18:370–374
15. Schaer GN, Koechli GR, Schleussler B, Haller U (1995) Perineal ultrasound for evaluating the bladder neck in urinary stress incontinence. Obstet Gynecol 85:220–224
16. Aigner F, Zbar AP, Ludwikowski B et al (2004) The rectogenital septum: morphology, function and clinical relevance. Dis Colon Rectum 47:131–140
17. Lieneman A, Anthuber C, Baron A, Resier M (2000) Diagnosing enteroceles using dynamic magnetic resonance imaging. Dis Colon Rectum 43:205–213
18. Felt-Bersma RJ, Luth WJ, Janssen JJ, Meuwissen SG (1990) Defecography in patients with anorectal disorders: which findings are clinically relevant? Dis Colon Rectum 33:277–284
19. Beer-Gabel M, Teshler M, Schechtman E, Zbar AP (2004) Dynamic transperineal ultrasound versus defecography in patients with evacuatory difficulty: a pilot study. Int J Colorectal Dis 19:60–67
20. Jorge JM, Ger GC, Gonzales I, Wexner SD (1994) Patient position during cinedefecography: influence on perineal descent and other measurements. Dis Colon Rectum 37:927–931
21. Bland JM, Altman DG (1986) Statistical methods for assessing agreement between two methods of clinical measurement. Lancet 1:307–310
22. Ayabaca SM, Zbar AP, Pescatori M (2002) Anal continence after rectocele repair. Dis Colon Rectum 45:63–69
23. Zbar AP, Lienemann A, Fritsch H et al (2003) Rectocele: pathogenesis and surgical management. Int J Colorectal Dis 18:369–384
24. Ting KH, Mangel E, Eibl-Eibesfeldt B, Muller-Lissner SA (1992) Is the volume retained after defecation a valuable parameter at defecography? Dis Colon Rectum 35:762–768
25. Halligan S, Bartram CI (1995) Is barium trapping in rectoceles significant? Dis Colon Rectum 38:764–768
26. Heslop JH (1987) Piles and rectoceles. Aust NZ J Surg 57:935–938
27. Zbar AP, Aslam M, Gold DM et al (1998) Parameters of the rectoanal inhibitory reflex in patients with idiopathic fecal incontinence and chronic constipation. Dis Colon Rectum 41:200–208
28. Cruiskshank SH (1991) Sacrospinous fixation – should this be performed at the time of vaginal hysterectomy? Am J Obstet Gynecol 164:1072–1076
29. Backer MH (1992) Success with sacrospinous suspension of the prolapsed vaginal vault. Surg Gynecol Obstet 175:419–420
30. McCall ML (1997) Posterior culdoplasty: surgical correction of enterocele during vaginal hysterectomy. A preliminary report. Obstet Gynecol 10:596–602
31. Pescatori M, Quandamcarlo C (1999) A new grading of rectal internal mucosal prolapse and its correlation with diagnosis and treatment. Int J Colorectal Dis 14:245–249
32. Pescatori M, Boffi F, Russo A, Zbar AP (2005) Complications and recurrence after excision of rectal internal mucosal prolapse for obstructed defecation. Int J Colorectal Dis 7:107–108
33. Kelly JL, O'Riordain DS, Jones E et al (1998) The effect of hysterectomy on ano-rectal physiology. Int J Colorectal Dis 13:116–118
34. Saclarides TJ, Brubaker L (2005) Evacuatory dysfunction following gynecologic surgery. In: Wexner SD, Zbar AP, Pescatori M (eds) Complex anorectal disorders: investigation and management. Springer, London, pp 532–545
35. Bump RC, Mattiasson A, Bo K et al (1996) The standardization of terminology of female pelvic organ prolapse and pelvic floor dysfunction. Am J Obstet Gynecol 175:10–17
36. Digesu GA, Khullar V, Cardozo L et al (2005) P-QOL: a validated questionnaire to assess the symptoms and quality of life of women with urogenital prolapse. Int Urogynecol J 16:176–181
37. Wolpert A, Beer-Gabel M, Lifschitz O, Zbar AP (2002) The management of presacral masses in the adult. Tech Coloproctol 6:43–49
38. Kim I-O, Han TI, Kim WS, Yeon KM (2000) Transperineal ultrasonography in imperforate anus: identification of the internal fistula. J Ultrasound Med 19:211–216
39. Kapoor DS, Davila GW, Rosenthal RJ, Ghoneim GM (2004) Pelvic floor dysfunction in morbidly obese women: pilot study. Obes Res 12:1104–1107
40. Gold DM, Bartram CI, Halligan S et al (1999) Three dimensional endoanal sonography in assessing anal canal injury. Br J Surg 86:365–370
41. Williams AB, Cheetham MJ, Bartram CI et al (2000) Gender differences in the longitudinal pressure profile of the anal canal related to anatomical structure as demonstrated on three-dimensional anal endosonography. Br J Surg 87:1674–1679
42. Beer-Gabel M, Zbar AP (2002) Dynamic transperineal ultrasonography (DTP-US) in patients presenting with obstructed defecation. Tech Coloproctol 6:141

VI.4.
Defecographic Study of Rectal Evacuation in Constipated Patients

S.A. Taylor

Constipation is a very common problem, with up to 20% of the population regularly affected [1]. Although some patients will have a recognizable precipitating cause, many do not and are often classified as having idiopathic or functional constipation. The pathophysiology of this condition is complex and not yet fully understood, but a simple and clinically useful division is between those with prolonged colonic transit and those with difficulties in rectal evacuation (obstructed defecation). Clearly, with such a simple classification, there are many patients with overlapping symptomatology.

Patients diagnosed clinically with predominantly obstructed defecation often complain of ineffectual rectal emptying, a sensation of rectal fullness, and chronic straining. Up to 50% of patients with chronic constipation may have evidence of obstructive defecation [2]. This patient group can usefully be further subdivided into those with structural abnormalities such as excessive pelvic floor descent [3], rectoceles or intussusception [4], functional pelvic incoordination (anismus) [5], or both.

Evaluation of rectal evacuation in constipated patients involves a detailed clinical history and physical examination in combination with a variety of investigations, including anorectal manometry, balloon expulsion tests, and electrophysiology. Defecography, or evacuation proctography, is now well established and plays an important diagnostic role although, as will be discussed, the significance of findings are not always clearcut, and the examination must be interpreted carefully both by the reporting radiologist and referring clinician alike.

Technique

Defecography describes the utilization of fluoroscopic screening to record the evacuation of radio-opaque material from the rectum. Rather than actually reproducing the physiological process of normal defecation, defecography is a study of voluntary evacuation, hence the term "evacuation proctography" is often preferred [6] and will be used for the rest of this chapter.

The concept of radiological investigation of rectal evacuation in constipated patients is not new [7] although the proctographic technique widely practiced today is based on the initial description of Mahieu in the early 1980s [8].

Basic Technique

Proctography is a potentially embarrassing and stressful procedure for the patient, and the first part of any examination should include a careful and sensitive explanation of the test. Around 45 min prior to the actual procedure, patients are asked to drink a dilute barium solution (150 ml 100 w/v barium sulphate mixed with 150 ml of water) in order to outline the small bowel. In the author's experience, addition of 10–20 ml of meglumine diatrizoate aids intestinal transit, shortening the time patients must spend in the X-ray department.

Administration of two glycerin suppositories to empty the rectum is useful (although not obligatory) and helps standardize the technique, as well as increasing test acceptably both for patients and operators [9]. The patient is then escorted into the fluoroscopy suite, and after further explanation, lies on the left side on the X-ray table. The consistency of the contrast introduced into the rectum should mimic that of normal stool, and potato starch or methylcellulose mixed with barium sulphate are acceptable. However, in the author's experience, commercially available barium pastes are preferred, being both convenient and producing reliable results [10]. The paste is introduced either via a pressure injector or manually using bladder syringes. There is no real consensus as to the optimal volume of contrast introduced although it is advisable that a standard protocol is followed by any particular institution to assure consistency between examinations. Although some advocate up to 300 ml of paste [11], a volume between 120 and 200 ml is usually adequate [6]. Injection should continue as the syringe is withdrawn to outline the anal canal. Most authors consider proctography to be more physiological when performed with the patient in the seated position although in immobile or incontinent patients, the procedure may successfully be performed with the patient in the left lateral decubitus position [12]. Indeed, comparative studies suggest that although static findings differ, dynamic patterns are essentially similar [13].

When performing upright proctography, the patient is asked to step off the fluoroscopy table, which is then tilted to the upright position. A commode is then placed on the footrest and the patient seated such that the lateral rectum will be imaged. Specialized commodes have been developed [14] and are recommended. In particular, filtration with either wood or Perspex is necessary to reduce radiographic flare [15]. Once the patient is seated, many authors recommend spot images of the lateral rectum at rest, on straining, and on maximum squeezing [9] although there is little data on the clinical value of these images, and their diagnostic value has been questioned [6]. The patient is then asked to voluntarily empty the rectum to completion, thereby expelling the radio-opaque paste. Fluoroscopic recording can be achieved using video or 105 mm cut film although the former is preferred due to lower radiation dose and the ability to playback and review the process [16]. The radiation dose delivered during standard proctography is in the region of 3–7 mSv [17]. Continuous fluoroscopy is usually not necessary beyond the first 20–30 s, after which intermittent screening is adequate if the rectum is not yet empty [6]. Indeed, with digital equipment, evacuation can be recorded using filtered static images at one frame per second, lowering radiation dose and yet maintaining diagnostic accuracy [18]. Near the end of evacuation, it is sometimes useful to turn the patient on the commode and obtain straining images in the AP projection, notably to clarify the presence of intussusception (see below).

Modification of the Technique

Abnormalities of the anterior and middle pelvic compartments can only really be inferred using the basic protocol as outlined above. Contrast administration into the bladder and vagina provides a more comprehensive assessment of the pelvic organs [19] and has been labeled "dynamic cystoproctography" [20]. The bladder is first filled and static images obtained during rest and maximum stain. The bladder is then emptied and the vagina filled with 20 ml of barium solution prior to introduction of the rectal paste. A tampon may split the vagina and use is therefore not recommended [21]. The examination then proceeds largely as described above. Clearly more invasive than basic proctography, dynamic cystoproctography has the advantage of providing a more detailed assessment of pelvic floor dysfunction. However as discussed elsewhere, dynamic magnetic resonance imaging (MRI) has found an increasing role in imaging pelvic organ prolapse [22].

Interpretation

Normal Study

Rest

At rest, the anal canal is closed, and the rectum assumes its normal upright configuration. The position of the pelvic floor is often inferred by reference to the pubococcygeal line (inferior margin of pubic symphysis to the sacrococcygeal junction) although the side of the commode or inferior margins of the ischial tuberosities are useful approximations. Perineal decent is measured from this line to the anorectal junction and may be up to 1.8 cm at rest [11] (although usually less in younger patients [23] and often greater in the elderly [24]). Some pelvic floor descent during evacuation is considered normal, and a decent of up to 3 cm from the rest position to anal canal opening is acceptable [6, 11].

The anorectal angle (ARA) has received considerable attention although absolute measurements are of questionable clinical use. It is most commonly defined as the angle between the anal canal axis and the posterior rectal wall [8, 25] and on average is around 90° (Fig. VI.26). However, there is a wide range of normality (up to 140°), particularly in men [26], and measurement interobserver agreement is poor [27]. Overall, as discussed below, qualitative assessments of changes in the ARA in individual patients are more useful than absolute angle measurements.

The puborectalis muscle impression is often visible at rest (Fig. VI.26). The puborectalis length (PRL) can be estimated by measuring the distance between the ARA and symphysis pubis [11]. However, as for the ARA, qualitative assessment of the PRL in individuals is of greater use than reliance on absolute measurements.

Evacuation

The emptying phase of the proctogram gives important information about rectal structure and function. Mahieu et al. [8] originally described five elements to a normal proctogram: increase in the ARA, obliteration of the puborectalis impression, wide opening of the anal canal, evacuation of rectal contents, and lack of significant pelvic floor descent. Although later refined, this initial description remains a very useful baseline against which to judge normality. In the normal patient, the anal canal should open fully within a couple of seconds, and evacuation should then proceed promptly and to completion. It is important to remember that in essence, only contrast below the first rectal fold is expected to be evacuated during the examination; retained contrast above the first fold is a normal finding [6]. Typically, the ARA should increase by around 20–30°, and the PRL should increase by around 3–4 cm [11] although, as already stressed, absolute measurements are of limited value for individual patients. The rate and degree of contrast emptying is highly relevant in the diagnosis of functional disorders of defecation (see below).

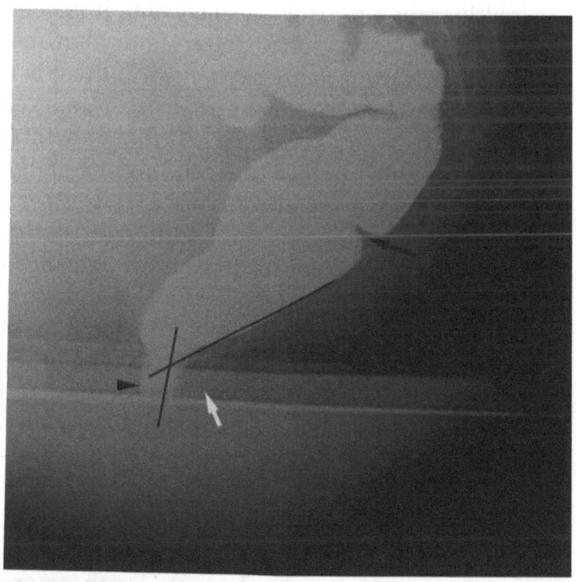

Fig. VI.26. Lateral view showing the normal resting rectal configuration. Note the position of the anal canal (*arrowhead*) in relation to the inferior ischial tuberosity (*white arrow*), a useful landmark for the normal position of the pelvic floor. A posterior puborectal impression (*black arrow*) is normal. The lines denote the anorectal angle (measured form the axis of the anal canal and posterior rectal wall)

Recovery

After evacuation is complete, the anal canal should close, the ARA recover, and the pelvic floor return to its normal baseline position. Posttoilet imaging may be required, particularly in those suspected of retained barium within rectoceles (see below).

Abnormal Study

Structural Abnormalities

1. *Pelvic floor descent*: Excessive pelvic floor decent, or perineal descent syndrome, has been attributed to pudendal neuropathy [28] although more recent data questions a causal relationship [29]. Although perineal descent can be assessed clinically, evacuation proctography is more reliable, not least because patients are seated and strain maximally to the point of anal canal opening. Pelvic floor descent (defined as the distance moved by the ARA at rest to the point of anal canal opening) is considered abnormal if it exceeds 3 cm. It is important to note the resting position of pelvic floor. In those with fixed pelvic floor descent at rest, the anorectal junction commonly lies 4 cm below the pubococcygeal line although moves little during evacuation [30] (Fig. VI.27).

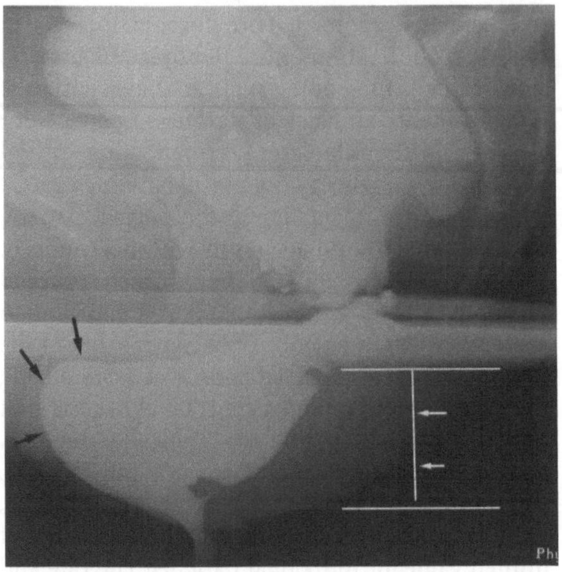

Fig. VI.27. Lateral view in the resting position demonstrates abnormal pelvic floor descent. *White lines* mark the position of the normal level of the pelvic floor and the actual position of the anorectal junction. The distance between these lines (*white arrows*) is 4 cm. Note the associated rectocele (*black arrows*)

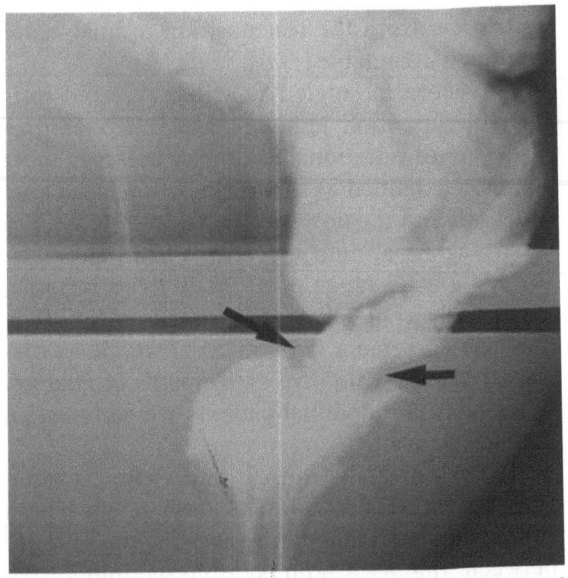

Fig. VI.28. Lateral view demonstrates infolding of the rectal wall (*black arrows*) in keeping with intrarectal intussusception. Note the width of the infolded rectal wall is greater than 3 mm, helping to distinguish it from normal folds

Excessive pelvic floor decent is suggestive of pelvis floor weakness although the exact etiology and significance remains controversial. There is a well-described association with anterior mucosal prolapse [31] (a proctological diagnosis characterized by persistent bulging of the anterior rectal wall often causing bleeding, pain, and tenesmus), and prolonged straining is suggested as the underlying common etiology for both conditions. However, excessive perineal descent is also found in up to 75% of patients with incontinence as well as those who chronically strain [11]. It is more common in women who have had multiple births [32] and in the elderly [23], and there are also reported associations with both rectal prolapse [33] and solitary rectal ulcer syndrome [34].

On balance, excessive pelvic floor descent is a common proctographic finding although its exact significance and cause is not yet fully elucidated. Although often secondary to global pelvic floor weakness, there is clear association with chronic straining and mucosal prolapse, and as such in some patients, its presence may indicated an underlying evacuatory disorder.

2. *Intussusception and prolapse*: Intussusception refers to infolding of the rectal wall into the rectal lumen. It may be described as intrarectal, intraanal, or external to form a complete rectal prolapse. There is often no identifiable cause in adults although it is more common in multiparous women [35], suggesting it may be a sign of more global pelvic floor damage. Based on early proctographic work, there is a common belief that most prolapse commences around 6–8 cm upstream of the anorectal junction [36] before descending caudally. Some degree of rectal intussusception is seen in normal volunteers [37] although symptomatic patients tend to have more advanced findings [38]. The categorization of intussusception into intrarectal and intra-anal is of doubtful utility, as it seems likely that all intussusception commences in the rectum and descends toward the anal canal. Furthermore, there is no clear definition of purely intrarectal intussusception [6].

The proctographic diagnosis is not clear cut, and there is often difficulty in distinguishing from normal mucosa descent. Furthermore, nonuniformity of rectal collapse may mean normal folds mimic intussusception in the lateral view [39], and repeat examination in the AP projection may be required. A relatively useful indicator of true intussusception is the

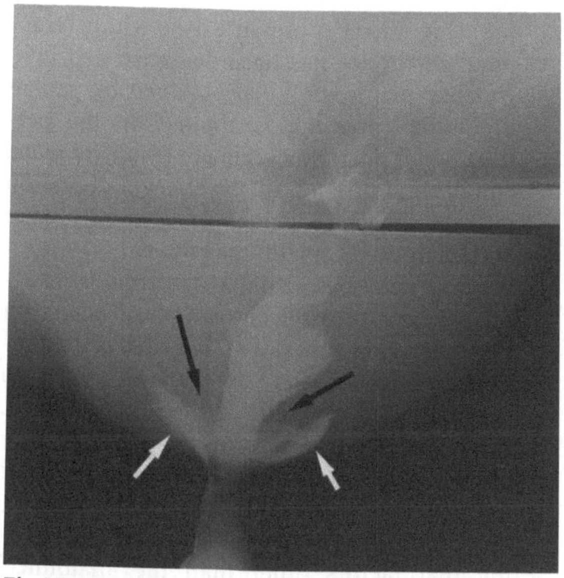

Fig. VI.29. Lateral view demonstrating high-grade intussusception. Note the intussusceptum (*black arrow*) and the widened intussuscipiens (*white arrows*)

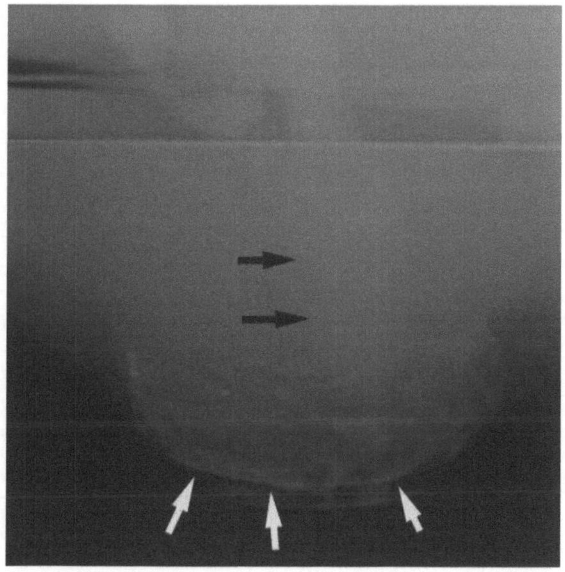

Fig. VI.30. Lateral view demonstrates the features of full rectal prolapse. The prolapsed rectum is seen as a rounded, barium-coated structure situated outside the pelvis (*white arrows*). Note the associated enterocele (*black arrows*)

presence of abnormally wide invaginating rectal folds measuring more than 3 mm (Fig. VI.28) although using this cutoff will diagnose prolapse in a significant minority of normal individuals [37]. Perhaps a more robust method has been recently described whereby the ratio of the intussuscipiens diameter and intussusceptum lumen diameter are calculated [40]. A ratio of more than 2.5 is highly suggestive of true intussusception. An advantage of this technique is the relative nonambiguity of the intussuscipiens and intussusceptum borders and the nondependence on technical factors (Fig. VI.29). Once the intussusception enters the anal canal, diagnosis is more clear cut. The canal is seen to splay both on the lateral and AP views, as it is filled by the descending intussusceptum. Full rectal prolapse is easily diagnosed, as the intussusceptum continues its descent and becomes exteriorized as a barium-coated "mass" beyond the anal canal (Fig. VI.30).

Although originally postulated as a cause of obstructed defecation [41], intussusception seems more likely a secondary phenomenon, occurring as it does at the end of evacuation rather than preceding it. There is, however, a very strong association with solitary rectal ulcer syndrome (SRUS), a condition related to chronic straining. Patients with SRUS present with rectal bleeding, mucus discharge, and symptoms of obstructed defecation. Proctoscopy reveals a rectal ulcer, and biopsy reveals characteristic histological changes. Evacuation proctography can demonstrate the associated intussusception in SRUS but importantly may also reveal an underlying functional defecatory disorder (see below). This has important therapeutic implications, as failure to respond to rectopexy is strongly related to delayed evacuation on preoperative proctography [42].

3. *Rectocele*: Rectocele diagnosis on evacuation proctography is straightforward and can be defined as any anterior rectal bulge [43]. The depth of a rectocele is measured from the anterior border of the anal canal to the anterior border of the rectocele. A distance of <2 cm is classified as small, 2–4 cm as moderate, and >4 cm as large. Using these definitions, it is clear that a small rectocele is essentially a normal finding in many women [37]. The condition is more common in multiparous women (particularly those who have undergone instrumental delivery), and a defect in the rectovaginal septum as been suggested as the causal mechanism [44]. There is also a clear association with symptoms of obstructed

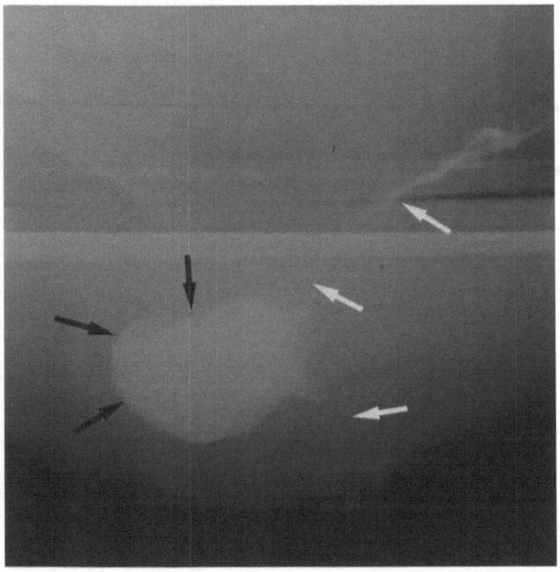

Fig. VI.31. Lateral view demonstrates significant barium trapping in a moderately sized rectocele. The rectum proper has emptied (*white arrows*), with significant retention of barium in the associated rectocele (*black arrows*)

defecation [45] although in itself, the mere presence of a rectocele has limited clinical meaning [46]. Of more relevance, however, is barium trapping at the end of evacuation (defined as retention of >10% of the area [47], and this itself is related the size of the rectocele [48] (Fig. VI.31). A pressure drop within "trapping" rectoceles has been demonstrated [47], which explains the relief obtained by patient digitation (pressure is applied on the perineum and posterior vagina to complete rectal emptying) [49]. Indeed, the effect of digitation may be imaged during proctography after careful discussion with the patient.

Proctography has an important role in triaging patients for surgical treatment. Those with an underlying functional disorder of defecation (see below) tend to respond poorly to surgery and benefit from biofeedback. Interestingly, however, even patients who obtain symptomatic relief from surgical repair may still have proctographic evidence of a rectocele on postoperative imaging [50], suggesting that factors other than the anatomical abnormality give rise to symptoms. Rarely, the rectum may be herniated in a posterolateral direction through a defect in the levator ani, commonly related to childbirth.

4. *Enterocele*: An enterocele is diagnosed when small bowel loops enter the peritoneal space between the rectum and vagina (rectogenital space). As discussed above, diagnosis of an enterocele on proctography is only really possible if oral contrast has been administered before the examination. The rectogenital space

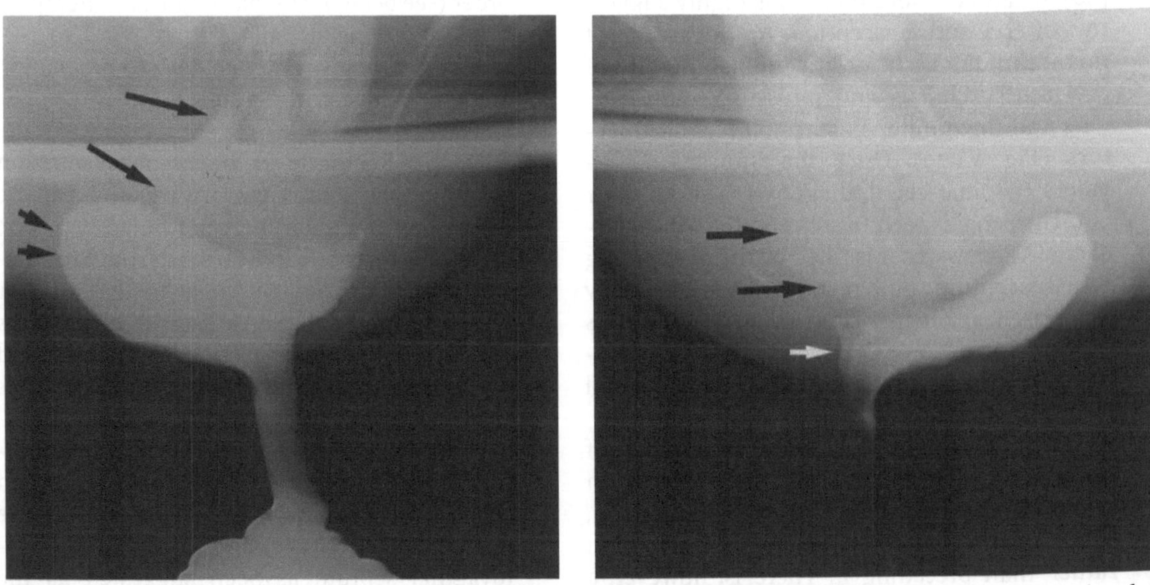

a b

Fig. VI.32. Lateral view acquired during evacuation shows the formation of a moderate anterior rectocele (*short arrows*) and an early enterocele (*long arrows*) (a). As evacuation proceeds, the rectocele empties (*white arrow*), allowing a dramatic increase in size of the enterocele (*black arrows*) (b)

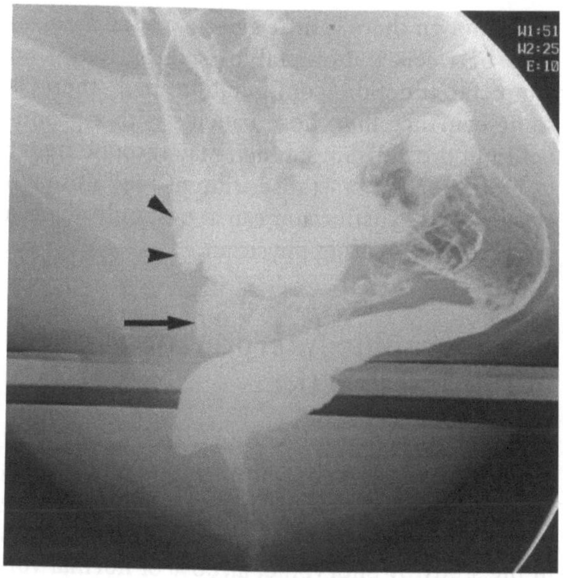

Fig. VI.33. Lateral rectal view demonstrates herniation of small bowel (enterocele) (*short arrows*) and sigmoid (sigmoidocele) (*long arrow*) into the rectogenital space anterior to the lower rectum

widens after evacuation when pressure from the adjacent full rectum is reduced, and as such, enteroceles are usually diagnosed at the end of the procedure. Formation can be prevented by filling of the rectogenital space with any other structure (such as a cystocele or large rectocele) (Fig. VI.32), and for this reason, the bladder should be emptied prior to rectal evacuation when performing extended proctography. Enteroceles may also only become apparent after repeated straining, and some authors recommend posttoilet strain images to increase diagnosis [20]. Indeed, Kelvin et al. found over 40% of enteroceles were diagnosed only on the posttoilet images [51].

Prior hysterectomy is a major precipitating cause of enteroceles, but there is an association with multiparity, age, and obesity. Patients typically complain of pelvic pressure or dragging, but it is increasing clear that, contrary to popular belief, enteroceles are not a cause of obstructed defecation [52].

Herniation of the sigmoid into the rectogenital space (sigmoidocele) is significantly less common than an enterocele although symptoms may be more severe. Diagnosis is based on the barium-filled sigmoid (or fecal contents within the sigmoid) anterior to the rectum (Fig. VI.33). Unlike enteroceles, there is some evidence that large sigmoidoceles can in themselves cause obstructed defecation. In a study of 24 patients, Jorge et al. demonstrated good correlation between the severity of the sigmoidocele and patient symptoms and the response to colonic resection [53].

The advent of newer MRI techniques hold considerable promise in the diagnoses of enteroceles and other forms of pelvic herniation and are discussed elsewhere.

Functional Abnormalities

There is undoubtedly a large group of constipated patients who complain bitterly of inability to evacuate but in whom no significant underlying structural abnormality is found [54]. Clinically, they are often recognized by their inability to evacuate a rectal balloon [55], and this patient group may outnumber those with slow-transit constipation by two to one [56]. The phenomenon has been variously labeled anismus, spastic pelvic floor syndrome, and paradoxical puborectalis syndrome [16], reflecting the as yet obscure etiology. Electromyographic data suggest these patients may inappropriately contract their pelvic floor muscles on evacuation [57] although this has also been documented both in normal and incontinent patients [58]. Indeed, more recent data questions whether this finding is real and not merely a test artifact [59]. Other workers have suggested that abnormality in pelvic floor innervation may be responsible or an inability to raise intra-abdominal pressure [46]. However, the frequent success of biofeedback therapy is good evidence that the condition is both real and, in part, behavioral in origin. It is thus an important diag-

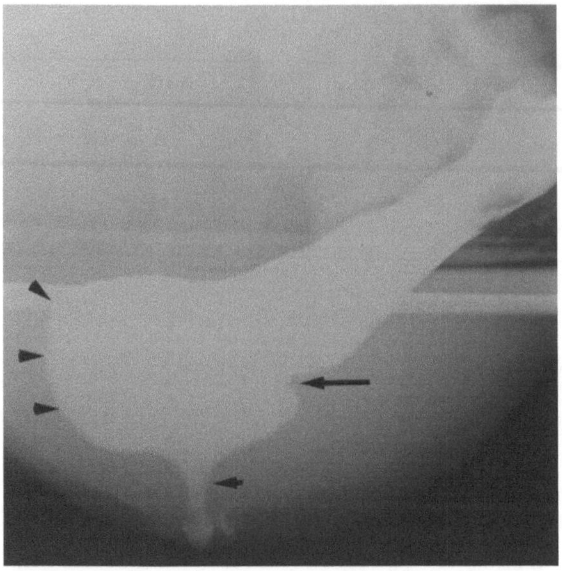

Fig. VI.34. Lateral rectal view demonstrating the proctographic features of the anismus. The patient is straining against a closed anal canal (*short arrow*) with a prominent puborectal impression (*long arrow*), with abnormally slow anal canal opening and evacuation. Note the formation of a rectocele (*arrowheads*) likely secondary to the underlying functional disorder

nosis to make in constipated patients with symptoms of rectal obstruction.

Although the diagnosis of animus may be suggested by tests of anorectal physiology, proctography has an important diagnostic role. Various proctographic abnormalities have been described, including prominent puborectal impression, a narrow anal canal, and acute anorectal angulation [60] (Fig. VI.34). However, these observations may be found in normal controls and are in themselves unreliable distinguishing features [61]. A more reliable assessment is based on the rate and completeness of evacuation. As already discussed, a normal patient evacuates rapidly and completely in within 30 seconds [62]. Those with anismus classically demonstrate delay in anal canal opening and prolonged, incomplete evacuation [61]. Evacuation may eventually proceed to completion in some patients, but only after repeated straining. Care must always be taken, however, when diagnosing anismus simply on the presence of prolonged evacuation. Inadequate straining and patient embarrassment may both simulate the condition and should be recognized by the radiologist. If there is any doubt, repeat fluoroscopic examination after the patient has been sent to evacuate in the privacy of the bathroom is often helpful.

Although there is little evidence of an association between puborectal muscle activity and anorectal junction configuration [63], there is some evidence that those patients with a prominent puborectalis impression may respond better to biofeedback than those without [64] although clearly such a distinction can at best only act as a guide for the treating physician.

Proctographic Interpretation in Clinical Practice

Although proctography is in itself a relatively straightforward procedure, interpretation is fraught with difficulty. There is a large overlap between normality and abnormality. For example, in the study by Shorvon et al, 80% of normal volunteers demonstrated rectal intussusception, of whom 80% also had a rectocele [37]. Furthermore, the descriptively useful division of proctographic abnormality into structural and functional is somewhat arbitrary, and the two frequently coexist. For example, rectoceles may be present in up to 45% of patients with anismus, and 71% of patients with rectoceles may also demonstrate anismus [65]. The clinical usefulness of proctography has therefore been questioned [66] [67] although recent data suggest that 90% of referring clinicians find the test useful [68].

In the author's opinion, the major function of proctography is not merely to document evacuatory abnormalities but also to classify those abnormalities into those potentially surgically relevant, those likely to benefit from behavioral biofeedback therapy alone, or, indeed, those that are incidental. Exact measurements of the ARA, PRL, etc. are useful in the context of research but offer little to the interpretation of individual examinations. A more global interpretation of the examination is more relevant.

The surgeon has a vast array of operative procedures at his or her disposal to correct underlying structural abnormalities such as rectoceles or intussusception although it is important to realize that such abnormalities are often secondary to an underlying functional disorder rather than the primary cause of the patient's symptoms. Surgery may therefore be inappropriate in many such patients [69]. For example, an apparently large symptomatic rectocele may be secondary to a prior obstetric tear in a functionally normal woman or due to chronic straining in a patient with underlying anismus. Clearly, while surgery may be indicated in the first scenario, it will be of little value in the second, where biofeedback therapy is more appropriate. Similarly, surgical repair of intussusception may not relieve the patient's underlying symptoms, suggesting it may be secondary to an underlying functional problem [70].

Summary

Evacuation proctography or defecography is a long-established and relatively straightforward diagnostic procedure for the investigation of those with symptoms of rectal outlet obstruction. Controversy exists as to the interpretation and clinical utility of the technique largely due to absent or imperfect reference standards for comparison. However, when interpreted sensibly, proctography still has a very important role in patient management, particularly in therapeutic triage. A simplistic (but effective) interpretative approach is to firstly assess the speed and completeness of evacuation (abnormality of which largely suggests an underlying functional problem) and then to describe any structural problems, documenting whether they are likely primary or secondary.

References

1. Drossman DA, Sandler RS, McKee DC et al (1982) Bowel patterns among subjects not seeking health care. Use of a questionnaire to identify a population with bowel dysfunction. Gastroenterology 83:529–534
2. Wald A, Caruana BJ, Freimanis MG et al (1990) Contributions of evacuation proctography and anorectal manometry to evaluation of adults with constipation and defecatory difficulty. Dig Dis Sci 35:481–487
3. Hudson CN (1988) Female genital prolapse and pelvic floor deficiency. Int J Colorectal Dis 3:181–185
4. Bartolo DC, Roe AM, Virjee J et al (1988) An analysis of rectal morphology in obstructed defaecation. Int J Colorectal Dis 3:17–22
5. Preston DM, Lennard-Jones JE (1985) Anismus in chronic constipation. Dig Dis Sci 30:413–418
6. Bartram C (2003) Dynamic evaluation of the anorectum. Radiol Clin North Am 41:425–441
7. Ekengren K, Snellman B (1953) Roentgen appearances in mechanical rectal constipation. Acta Radiol 40:447–456
8. Mahieu P, Pringot J, Bodart P (1984) Defecography: I. Description of a new procedure and results in normal patients. Gastrointest Radiol 9:247–251
9. Mezwa DG, Feczko PJ, Bosanko C (1993) Radiologic evaluation of constipation and anorectal disorders. Radiol Clin North Am 31:1375–1393
10. Ikenberry S, Lappas JC, Hana MP et al (1996) Defecography in healthy subjects: comparison of three contrast media. Radiology 201:233–238
11. Jorge JM, Habr-Gama A, Wexner SD (2001) Clinical applications and techniques of cinedefecography. Am J Surg 182:93–101
12. Poon FW, Lauder JC, Finlay IG (1991) Technical report: evacuating proctography – a simplified technique. Clin Radiol 44:113–116
13. Jorge JM, Ger GC, Gonzalez L et al (1994) Patient position during cinedefecography. Influence on perineal descent and other measurements. Dis Colon Rectum 37:927–931
14. Bernier P, Stevenson GW, Shorvon P (1988) Defecography commode. Radiology 166:891–892
15. Ginai AZ (1990) Evacuation proctography (defecography). A new seat and method of examination. Clin Radiol 42:214–216
16. Halligan S, Bartram CI (1995) The radiological investigation of constipation. Clin Radiol 50:429–435
17. Goei R, Kemerink G (1990) Radiation dose in defecography. Radiology 176:137–139
18. Hare C, Halligan S, Bartram CI et al (2001) Dose reduction in evacuation proctography. Eur Radiol 11:432–434
19. Maglinte DD, Kelvin FM, Hale DS et al (1997) Dynamic cystoproctography: a unifying diagnostic approach to pelvic floor and anorectal dysfunction. AJR Am J Roentgenol 169:759–767
20. Kelvin FM, Maglinte DD (2003) Dynamic evaluation of female pelvic organ prolapse by extended proctography. Radiol Clin North Am 41:395–407
21. Archer BD, Somers S, Stevenson GW (1992) Contrast medium gel for marking vaginal position during defecography. Radiology 182:278–279
22. Roos JE, Weishaupt D, Wildermuth S et al (2002) Experience of 4 years with open MR defecography: pictorial review of anorectal anatomy and disease. Radiographics 22:817–832
23. Pinho M, Yoshioka K, Ortiz J et al (1990) The effect of age on pelvic floor dynamics. Int J Colorectal Dis 5:207–208
24. Oettle GJ, Roe AM, Bartolo DC et al (1985) What is the best way of measuring perineal descent? A comparison

of radiographic and clinical methods. Br J Surg 72:999–1001
25. Jorge JM, Wexner SD, Marchetti F et al (1992) How reliable are currently available methods of measuring the anorectal angle? Dis Colon Rectum 35:332–338
26. Skomorowska E, Hegedus V (1987) Sex differences in anorectal angle and perineal descent. Gastrointest Radiol 12:353–355
27. Ferrante SL, Perry RE, Schreiman JS et al (1991) The reproducibility of measuring the anorectal angle in defecography. Dis Colon Rectum 34:51–55
28. Parks AG, Porter NH, Hardcastle J (1966) The syndrome of the descending perineum. Proc R Soc Med 59:477–482
29. Jorge JM, Wexner SD, Ehrenpreis ED et al (1993) Does perineal descent correlate with pudendal neuropathy? Dis Colon Rectum 36:475–483
30. Shorvon PJ, Stevenson GW (1989) Defaecography: setting up a service. Br J Hosp Med 41:460–466
31. Tsiaoussis J, Chrysos E, Glynos M et al (1998) Pathophysiology and treatment of anterior rectal mucosal prolapse syndrome. Br J Surg 85:1699–1702
32. Karasick S, Spettell CM (1997) The role of parity and hysterectomy on the development of pelvic floor abnormalities revealed by defecography. AJR Am J Roentgenol 169:1555–1558
33. Allen-Mersh TG, Henry MM, Nicholls RJ (1987) Natural history of anterior mucosal prolapse. Br J Surg 74:679–682
34. Snooks SJ, Nicholls RJ, Henry MM et al (1985) Electrophysiological and manometric assessment of the pelvic floor in the solitary rectal ulcer syndrome. Br J Surg 72:131–133
35. Karasick S, Spettell CM (1999) Defecography: does parity play a role in the development of rectal prolapse? Eur Radiol 9:450–453
36. Broden B, Snellman B (1968) Procidentia of the rectum studied with cineradiography. A contribution to the discussion of causative mechanism. Dis Colon Rectum 11:330–347
37. Shorvon PJ, McHugh S, Diamant NE et al (1989) Defecography in normal volunteers: results and implications. Gut 30:1737–1749
38. Dvorkin LS, Gladman MA, Epstein J et al (2005) Rectal intussusception in symptomatic patients is different from that in asymptomatic volunteers. Br J Surg 92:866–872
39. McGee SG, Bartram CI (1993) Intra-anal intussusception: diagnosis by posteroanterior stress proctography. Abdom Imaging 18:136–140
40. Pomerri F, Zuliani M, Mazza C et al (2001) Defecographic measurements of rectal intussusception and prolapse in patients and in asymptomatic subjects. AJR Am J Roentgenol 176:641–645
41. Wallden L (1953) Roentgen examination of the deep rectogenital pouch. Acta Radiol 1953; 39:105–116
42. Halligan S, Nicholls RJ, Bartram CI (1995) Proctographic changes after rectopexy for solitary rectal ulcer syndrome and preoperative predictive factors for a successful outcome. Br J Surg 82:314–317
43. Stoker J, Halligan S, Bartram CI (2001) Pelvic floor imaging. Radiology 218:621–641
44. Gill EJ, Hurt WG (1998) Pathophysiology of pelvic organ prolapse. Obstet Gynecol Clin North Am 25:757–769
45. Van Dam JH, Ginai AZ, Gosselink MJ et al (1997) Role of defecography in predicting clinical outcome of rectocele repair. Dis Colon Rectum 40:201–207
46. Halligan S, Thomas J, Bartram C (1995) Intrarectal pressures and balloon expulsion related to evacuation proctography. Gut 37:100–104
47. Halligan S, Bartram CI (1995) Is barium trapping in rectoceles significant? Dis Colon Rectum 38:764–768
48. Kelvin FM, Maglinte DD, Hornback JA et al (1992) Pelvic prolapse: assessment with evacuation proctography (defecography). Radiology 184:547–551
49. Siproudhis L, Dautreme S, Ropert A et al (1993) Dyschezia and rectocele – a marriage of convenience? Physiologic evaluation of the rectocele in a group of 52 women complaining of difficulty in evacuation. Dis Colon Rectum 36:1030–1036
50. Van Laarhoven CJ, Kamm MA, Bartram CI et al (1999) Relationship between anatomic and symptomatic long-term results after rectocele repair for impaired defecation. Dis Colon Rectum 42:204–210
51. Kelvin FM, Hale DS, Maglinte DD et al (1999) Female pelvic organ prolapse: diagnostic contribution of dynamic cystoproctography and comparison with physical examination. AJR Am J Roentgenol 173:31–37
52. Halligan S, Bartram C, Hall C et al (1996) Enterocele revealed by simultaneous evacuation proctography and peritoneography: does "defecation block" exist? AJR Am J Roentgenol 167:461–466
53. Jorge JM, Yang YK, Wexner SD (1994) Incidence and clinical significance of sigmoidoceles as determined by a new classification system. Dis Colon Rectum 37:1112–1117
54. Turnbull GK, Bartram CI, Lennard-Jones JE (1988) Radiologic studies of rectal evacuation in adults with idiopathic constipation. Dis Colon Rectum 31:190–197
55. Barnes PR, Lennard-Jones JE (1985) Balloon expulsion from the rectum in constipation of different types. Gut 26:1049–1052
56. Wexner SD, Jorge JM (1994) Colorectal physiological tests: use or abuse of technology? Eur J Surg 160:167–174
57. Womack NR, Williams NS, Holmfield JH et al (1985)

New method for the dynamic assessment of anorectal function in constipation. Br J Surg 72:994–998
58. Jones PN, Lubowski DZ, Swash M et al (1987) Is paradoxical contraction of puborectalis muscle of functional importance? Dis Colon Rectum 30:667–670
59. Voderholzer WA, Neuhaus DA, Klauser AG et al (1997) Paradoxical sphincter contraction is rarely indicative of anismus. Gut 41:258–262
60. Kuijpers HC, Bleijenberg G (1985) The spastic pelvic floor syndrome. A cause of constipation. Dis Colon Rectum 28:669–672
61. Halligan S, Bartram CI, Park HJ et al (1995) Proctographic features of anismus. Radiology 197:679–682
62. Bartolo DC, Bartram CI, Ekberg O et al (1988) Symposium. Proctography. Int J Colorectal Dis 3:67–89
63. Thorpe AC, Williams NS, Badenoch DF et al (1993) Simultaneous dynamic electromyographic proctography and cystometrography. Br J Surg 80:115–120
64. Park UC, Choi SK, Piccirillo MF et al (1996) Patterns of anismus and the relation to biofeedback therapy. Dis Colon Rectum 39:768–773
65. Johansson C, Nilsson BY, Holmstrom B et al (1992) Association between rectocele and paradoxical sphincter response. Dis Colon Rectum 35:503–509
66. Hiltunen KM, Kolehmainen H, Matikainen M (1994) Does defecography help in diagnosis and clinical decision-making in defecation disorders? Abdom Imaging 19:355–358
67. Ott DJ, Donati DL, Kerr RM et al (1994) Defecography: results in 55 patients and impact on clinical management. Abdom Imaging 19:349–354
68. Harvey CJ, Halligan S, Bartram CI et al (1999) Evacuation proctography: a prospective study of diagnostic and therapeutic effects. Radiology 211:223–227
69. Orrom WJ, Bartolo DC, Miller R et al (1991) Rectopexy is an ineffective treatment for obstructed defecation. Dis Colon Rectum 34:41–46
70. Christiansen J, Zhu BW, Rasmussen OO et al (1992) Internal rectal intussusception: results of surgical repair. Dis Colon Rectum 35:1026–1028

VI.5. Dynamic MR Imaging in the Evaluation of Outlet Obstruction

N. Bolog, D. Weishaupt, B. Marincek

Constipation is a heterogeneous condition, being one of the most common digestive complaints [1]. The prevalence of constipation within the population varies between 2% and 28% [1–5]. Currently, three types of constipation are differentiated: slow-transit colonic constipation, outlet obstruction, and a combination of both [6]. The term "outlet obstruction" encompasses all pelvic floor dysfunctions or abnormalities that are responsible for an incomplete evacuation of fecal contents from the rectum. It has been estimated that outlet obstruction may be observed in half of constipated patients [7]. Different pathophysiological mechanisms, including morphological and functional causes, may lead to outlet obstruction (Table VI.2).

Detailed history and thorough physical examination still represent the cornerstone of clinical evaluation of patients with outlet obstruction. Depending on the local situation and availability, different anorectal physiology testing and imaging examinations are recommended for diagnostic and treatment planning. Traditionally, conventional defecography or evacuation proctography has played an important role in the radiological assessment of these patients. Conventional defecography allows for reliable assessment for a variety of morphological and functional causes associated with outlet obstruction, including rectocele, enterocele, internal rectal prolapse, and anismus. Although conventional defecography has its value in diagnostic assessment, the technique has some significant limitations. There is a considerable irradiation associated with conventional evacuation proctography, with a mean effective radiation dose of up to 4.9 mSv [8, 9]. Moreover, the technique is limited from a practical point of view by its projectional nature and its inability to detect soft tissue structures.

Over recent years, dynamic magnetic resonance imaging (MRI), also called MR defecography, has gained increasing interest for assessment

Table VI.2. Causes of outlet obstruction

Functional Causes of Outlet Obstruction (muscular hypertonicity)	Morphological Causes of Outlet Obstruction
Anismus	Rectocele
Hirschprungs' disease	Enterocele
Chagas' disease	Rectal prolapse
Hereditary internal sphincter myopathy	Descending perineum syndrome
Central nervous system lesions	Rectal tumors
	Posttherapeutical stenosis of the anorectum

of pelvic floor abnormalities. Dynamic pelvic MRI may be performed in closed- and open-configuration MR systems and allows for evaluation of the pelvic floor in different positions. The free selection of imaging planes, the good temporal resolution, and the excellent soft tissue contrast transformed this method into the preferred imaging modality in the evaluation of patients with pelvic floor dysfunction. In this chapter, we describe the technique of dynamic MRI for evaluation of outlet obstruction. Special attention is directed to the MR appearance of abnormalities associated with outlet obstruction as well as the current role of dynamic pelvic MRI in its clinical assessment and management.

Technical Considerations

Dynamic pelvic imaging may be performed in closed-configuration conventional MR systems in the supine position or in open-configuration MR systems in the sitting position. Although open-configuration MR systems allow for a more physiological approach of the examination when considering patient positioning, the use of such systems is limited by the lack of their world-wide availability. Since Bertschinger et al. [10] have shown that no clinically significant findings were missed when comparing dynamic pelvic MR in the supine position with dynamic pelvic MR in the sitting position, MR in the supine position may be considered a reliable pelvic floor imaging modality. In our experience, performing the exam using state-of-the-art technique – which means MR imaging at rest, at maximal contraction of the anal sphincter (squeezing), and at straining as well as imaging during evacuation – is probably more important than the patient position. In particular, MRI during defecation is of paramount importance since relevant findings may be missed when dynamic pelvic MR encompasses imaging at rest, at squeeze, and at straining only [11].

Although there is general agreement that no premedication and or oral or intrarectal preparation for bowel cleansing is necessary when dynamic pelvic MRI is performed, there is considerable variation in the literature with regard to the optimal examination protocol. For evaluation of the posterior compartment (i.e., the anorectum), all authorities agree that the rectum should be filled with a contrast agent. Regular water is not suitable for that purpose since the viscosity of the enema should be somehow similar to that of normal rectum content. The rational of using an enema with a stool-like viscosity seems to be important considering the fact that the manifestations of outlet obstruction vary with every change of fecal consistency [12]. When performing dynamic pelvic MR, most authors use ultrasound gel for rectal enema [11, 13–15]. Other authors proposed the use of the mashed potatoes spiked with a small amount of gadolinium chelate for filling the rectum [10, 16–18]. With the increasing use of dynamic MRI, it has been realized that patients with abnormalities of the posterior pelvic compartment often show concomitant disorders involving the anterior as well as the middle compartment [19]. Therefore, some authors propose also to tag the middle compartment (i.e., vagina) and the anterior pelvic compartment (i.e., bladder) in order to visualize the vagina as well as the bladder and urethra [13, 14, 18, 20, 21]. In our institution, we do not routinely administer contrast agent either in the vagina or in the bladder. However, we always administer a rectal enema.

Dynamic Pelvic MRI in the Sitting Position

Dynamic MRI of the pelvic floor in the sitting position requires a vertically open-configuration MR system such as the 0.5 T superconducting open-configuration MR system Signa SP (GE Medical Systems, Milwaukee, WI, USA). A wooden chair, which fits into the open space between the two magnet rings, allows imaging in the sitting position (Fig. VI.35). Before the patient is placed on the seat, the rectum is filled with 300 ml of a contrast agent solution consisting of a suspending agent (mashed potatoes) spiked with 1.5 ml of an extracellular gadolinium chelate contrast agent (377mg/ml). A flexible transmit/receive radiofrequency coil is wrapped around the pelvis. On the basis of axial localizing images, a 15-mm thick multiphase T1-weighted spoiled gradient-echo (GRE) sequence that transverses the rectal canal in the midsagittal plane is planned. An image update is provided every 2 s. Images are obtained at rest, at maximal sphincter contraction, during straining, and during defecation in the midsagittal plane. The images are analyzed on a workstation in cine loop presentation. Additional GRE images are used in axial and coronal planes when a lateral rectocele or an internal rectal prolapse is suspected.

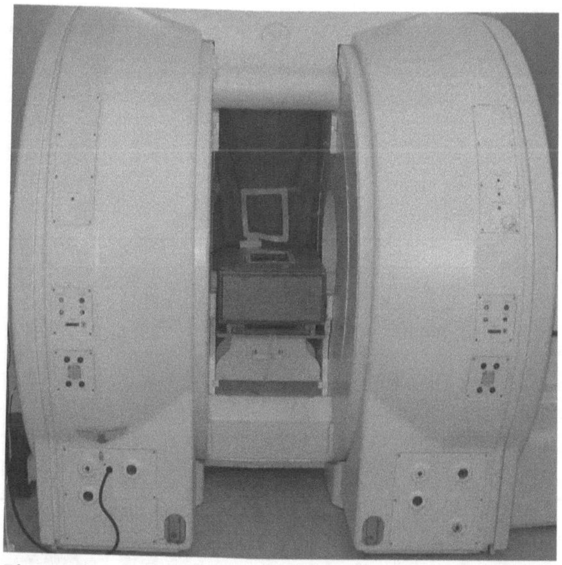

Fig. VI.35. The 0.5 T superconducting, open-configuration magnetic resonance system used for dynamic pelvic examinations. A wooden chair that functions as a toilet allows imaging in the sitting position

Dynamic Pelvic MRI in the Supine Position

Dynamic pelvic MRI may also be performed in the supine position using nearly all commercially available closed- or open-configuration MR systems with horizontal access. When dynamic pelvic MRI is performed in these MR systems, the patient is placed in the supine position, and a pelvic phased array coil is used for signal transmission and/or reception. After filling the rectum, the examination starts with a localizer sequence similar to that described above. For dynamic MRI in the different positions, various MR sequences can be used with similar results. The basic requirement for the sequence is the necessity for a fast imaging update. Some authors have used T2-weighted single-shot fast-spin-echo sequences (SSFSE) in the midsagittal plane obtained at rest, at squeezing, at straining, and during defecation [11, 22–24]. Alternatively, steady state free precession (SSFP) sequences may be used for this purpose. Our current protocol includes SSFP sequences obtained at rest, at squeezing, straining, and after evacuation. For assessment of defecation, we prefer the use of a T1-weighted multiphase GRE sequence since it offers an imaging window long enough for continuous imaging the evacuation even in patients with a prolonged evacuation time. The choice of the enema depends on the MR sequence used for dynamic imaging of the pelvic floor. For SSFSE and SSFP sequences, ultrasound gel is most suitable [10, 13, 22, 23]. If the dynamic sequences are performed with some sort of T1 weighting, the rectum is filled with an enema consisting of ultrasound gel or mashed potatoes mixed with a small amount of gadolinium chelate, as described above.

MR Findings in Patients with Outlet Obstruction

Rectocele

An anterior rectocele is the most frequent anatomical abnormality in patients with pelvic floor disorders and is defined as a rectal wall protrusion or bulging during defecation. The anterior wall is most commonly involved, but a rectocele may also be located in the posterior rectal wall (Fig. VI.36). Posterior rectoceles are also referred to as a posterior perineal hernia by some authors based on the fact that the bulging is through a puborectalis muscle defect [25, 26].

Rectoceles are more frequently found in women. The pathogenetic mechanisms include chronic straining during evacuation and weakness of the rectovaginal septum (congenital or after an obstetric trauma). Although the clinical importance of a rectocele is still debatable since the finding was demonstrated in 20% of asymptomatic women [27], it is recognized that large rectoceles (i.e., >2 cm in sagittal diameter) may result in outlet obstruction, and the retention of stool leads to the need of digital maneuvers in order to empty the rectum [27, 28]. A clinically significant rectocele should be considered based on the following criteria [29]:

- Patient history
- Size exceeding 2 cm in sagittal diameter
- Retention of contrast medium
- Reproducibility of the patient's symptoms of outlet obstruction
- The need for evacuation assistance.

The physical examination detects most of the rectoceles, but valuable information such as size and emptying are not provided based on physical examination. Therefore, dynamic pelvic imaging is helpful in providing this information. Dynamic MRI enables an accurate assessment of size, loca-

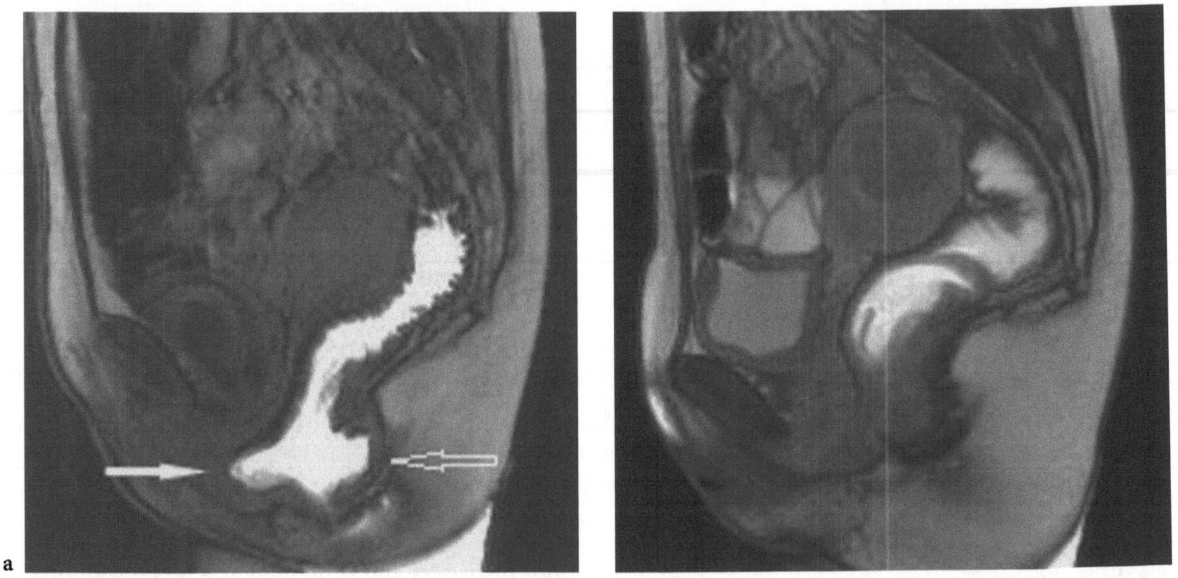

Fig. VI.36. A 42-year-old woman with clinical symptoms of outlet obstruction. The examination was performed with the patient in supine position using a closed-configuration conventional magnetic resonance (MR) system. T1-weighted spoiled gradient-echo MR image during defecation enables the identification of an anterior (*arrow*) and posterior (*empty arrow*) rectocele (**a**). Steady state free precession image obtained after evacuation shows a complete evacuation of both rectoceles (**b**)

tion, and degree of emptying of a rectocele, which are important factors for treatment strategy. Using dynamic pelvic MRI, an anterior rectocele may be classified with regard to its size, expressed as the depth of wall protrusion beyond the expected margin of the normal anterior rectal wall, into small (<2 cm), moderate [2–4 cm (Fig. VI.37)], and large (>4 cm) [17]. In addition, rectoceles are classified into those with complete evacuation (Fig. VI.36) and those with incomplete evacuation (Fig. VI.37) depending on the contrast material retention at the end of defecation.

Treatment decision in patients with rectocele highly depends on associated imaging findings. It is known that anterior rectocele as a solitary finding is rare [19]. Anismus, internal rectal prolapse, and enterocele are often associated with the presence of a rectocele [30–32], and therefore, the treatment should be tailored according to the imaging findings in order to achieve an optimal outcome [33, 34].

Enterocele

Enterocele is defined as an internal herniation of the peritoneal sac below the pubococcygeal line (PCL) into the rectovaginal space. The PCL is defined as the line that joins the inferior border of the symphysis pubis to the last coccygeal joint on midsagittal images (Fig. VI.38) [27, 35].The PCL is used as the reference line for pelvic floor weakness evaluation [14, 36]. Along this line, which is independent of the pelvic position, the pelvic floor muscle and pubovesical ligament attach [37]. The prevalence of enteroceles in patients with pelvic floor disorders is between 17-37% [38–40], with women being more frequently affected. In addition, there is a high correlation between pelvic surgery (e.g., hysterectomy) and enteroceles formation [41, 42]. Enteroceles most frequently occur at the end of evacuation and can be filled with omental fat (peritoneocele), small bowel (enterocele), or sigmoid colon (sigmoidocele). The extent of an enterocele is measured at 90° to the PCL from the lowest margin of herniation content (e.g., small-bowel loop) during evacuation effort on defecography [36]. They are classified as small if they extend less than 3 cm below the PCL, moderate if they extend from 3 to 6 cm below this line (Fig. VI.39), and large if they extend 6 cm or more below this line [14]. Large enteroceles slipping over the anal canal lead to outlet obstruction and a feeling of incomplete evacuation due to rectal compression [43, 44]. Clinical symptoms are poor and nonspecific, and

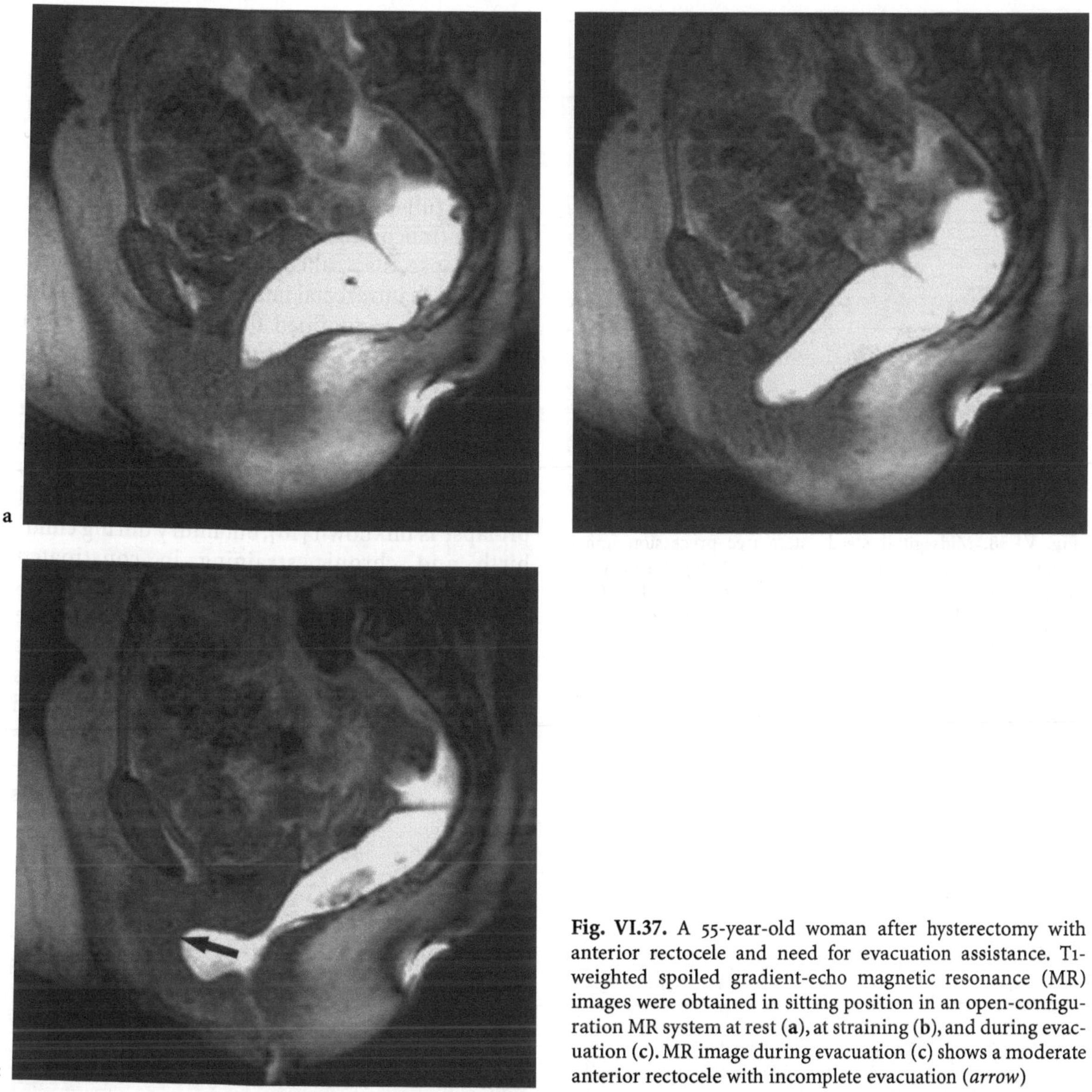

a b c

Fig. VI.37. A 55-year-old woman after hysterectomy with anterior rectocele and need for evacuation assistance. T1-weighted spoiled gradient-echo magnetic resonance (MR) images were obtained in sitting position in an open-configuration MR system at rest (**a**), at straining (**b**), and during evacuation (**c**). MR image during evacuation (**c**) shows a moderate anterior rectocele with incomplete evacuation (*arrow*)

physical examination is insufficient for an accurate assessment. Hence, enteroceles are often missed at clinical examination [45].

Dynamic pelvic MRI is the method of choice in the evaluation of enteroceles, being superior to conventional proctography even when additional opacification of vagina and bowel is performed during fluoroscopic examination. At conventional defecography, separation of the vagina and the rectum during defecation suggests an enterocele, but the diagnosis of a small enterocele is difficult since a distance of 2–3 cm between rectum and vagina does not allow the differentiation from a thickened rectal wall [40]. MRI is useful especially in these cases and can influence the surgical procedure since an operative closure is necessary if surgery is performed [14]. An undetected small enterocele may result in progressive symptoms and the need for another intervention [39].

MRI, with its excellent soft tissue contrast, also enables an accurate differentiation between peritoneocele, enterocele, and sigmoidocele without filling the small or large bowel with contrast agents. Although sigmoid colon herniation is less common compared with small-bowel herniation, sigmoidoceles are more frequently associated with constipation, and sigmoidectomy may be performed (Fig. VI.40) [46, 47].

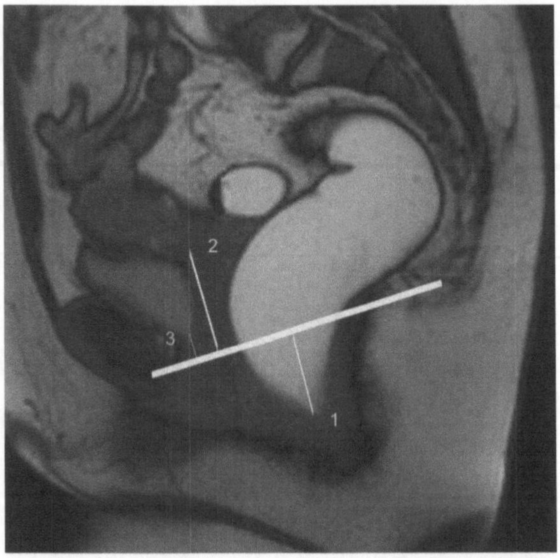

Fig. VI.38. Midsagittal steady state free precession image obtained in a patient in supine position. The pubococcygeal line defined as the line that joins the inferior border of the symphysis pubis to the last coccygeal joint. Pubococcygeal line is used to measure the extent of the enterocele as well as to express the position of the anorectal junction (*1*, posterior compartment), the position of the vaginal vault (*2*, middle pelvic compartment), and the position of the bladder base (*3*, anterior pelvic compartment)

Rectal Prolapse

Rectal prolapse is an invagination of the rectal wall and may be classified as internal or external [21]. The location may be anterior, posterior, or circumferential and may involve all rectal wall layers (full-thickness prolapse) or only the mucosa (mucosal prolapse) [17]. The internal rectal prolapse, also called intussusception, may be classified as intrarectal internal prolapse when the invagination is confined to the rectum or as an intra-anal internal prolapse when its apex penetrates the anal canal and remains in it during straining (Fig. VI.41). The external rectal prolapse is an invagination of the rectal wall beyond the anal canal (Fig. VI.42). External rectal prolapse is a clinical diagnosis. The etiology of internal rectal prolapse is unknown [16], but injury during childbirth and chronic straining in constipated patients seem to be possible concomitant factors [48, 49]. Although small internal prolapses are common findings in asymptomatic patients it has been demonstrated that internal rectal prolapse is present twice as often in patients with impaired defecation in comparison with asymptomatic volunteers [50]. The mean frequency of internal rectal prolapse is between 12% and 27% in patients

a 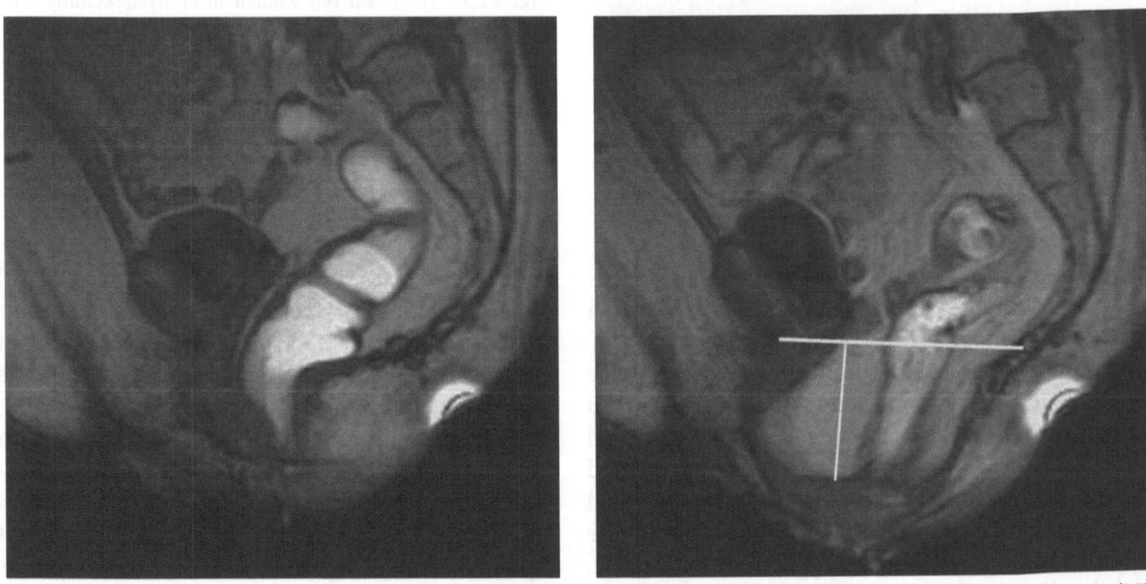 b

Fig. VI.39. A 74-year-old woman with a history of hysterectomy. T1-weighted spoiled gradient-echo magnetic resonance (MR) images obtained at rest (**a**) and during evacuation (**b**) with the patient sitting in an open-configuration MR system. During evacuation (**b**), herniation of the peritoneal sac below the pubococcygeal line (PCL) is seen. The sac contains peritoneal fat (peritoneocele) and extends more than 3 cm below the PCL, being classified as a moderate enterocele. In addition, the patient has a moderate rectal descent

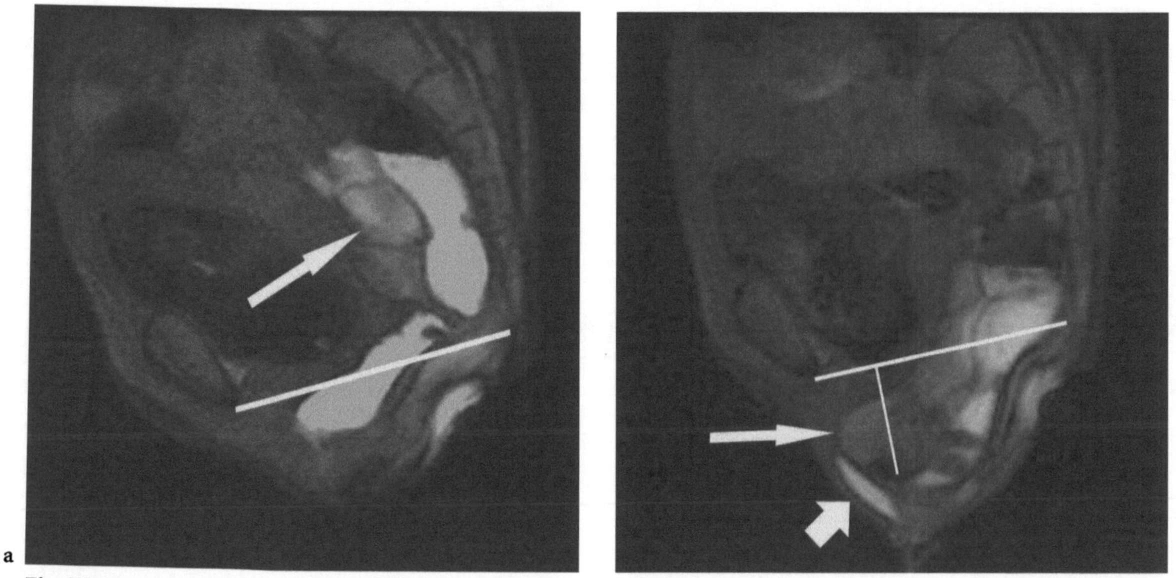

Fig. VI.40. A 28-year-old woman with chronic constipation. T1-weighted spoiled gradient-echo magnetic resonance image obtained in sitting position and at rest (**a**). The sigmoid colon is well delineated in normal position (*arrow*). During evacuation (**b**), a moderate enterocele protrudes into the rectovaginal space below the pubococcygeal line. The herniation consists exclusively of sigmoid colon (*arrow*). In addition, an anterior rectocele with incomplete evacuation is evident (*small arrow*)

with evacuation disorders [51], and the most frequent clinical manifestation is the feeling of incomplete evacuation [45]. Dynamic MRI is useful for the diagnosis of internal rectal prolapse. One major advantage of MRI over conventional proctography is represented by an accurate appreciation of the wall layers. Dynamic MRI enables differentiation between a mucosal internal prolapse (Fig. VI.43) and a full-thickness internal prolapse (Fig. VI.41) [16], which is of clinical importance since the treatment is different [52]. Internal rectal prolapse is often associated with other anatomical abnormalities, including enterocele and rectocele.

Pelvic Floor Descent

Pelvic floor descent, or descending perineal syndrome, is an excessive caudad movement of the pelvic floor during evacuation [36]. This abnormality is most likely the result of a pudendal nerve injury from a combination of obstetric trauma and chronic straining [53–55]. Pelvic floor descent is the most common finding in patients with outlet obstruction and is associated with pelvic pain and a feeling of incomplete evacuation. Incomplete evacuation is followed by more straining, which leads to increasing denervation of anal and puborectalis muscles and over time to fecal incontinence [56]. Although clinical examination and electrophysiological tests play a significant role in diagnosis, dynamic MRI provides the most accurate assessment.

Outlet obstruction may be associated with a descent of any of the three pelvic compartments (i.e., posterior, middle, or anterior). The landmark for the posterior compartment is the anorectal junction. There are different quantification or grading systems in the literature, but in our clinical practice, we prefer to measure the descent of the anorectal junction with respect to the PCL [10]. A small rectal descent is considered when the anorectal junction is less than 3 cm below the PCL, a moderate descent when the distance between anorectal junction and PCL is between 3 and 6 cm (Fig. VI.44), and a large rectal descent when the distance between the anorectal junction and PCL is more than 6 cm [10]. Even in the case of patients with clinical manifestations attributable to the posterior compartment, an isolated rectal descent is rarely present. Pelvic floor weakness is generalized and frequently involves multiple sites especially in constipated patients (Fig. VI.45) [26, 35]. Cystoceles are expression of the descent of the anterior compartment, and descent of the vaginal vault (or any part of the remaining cervix in case of hysterec-

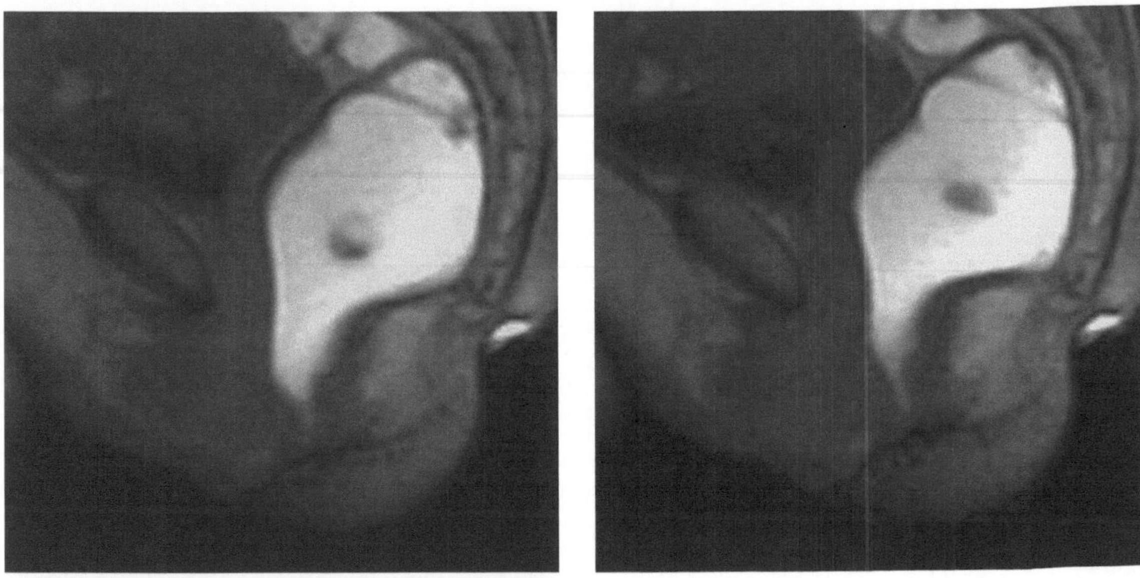

a b

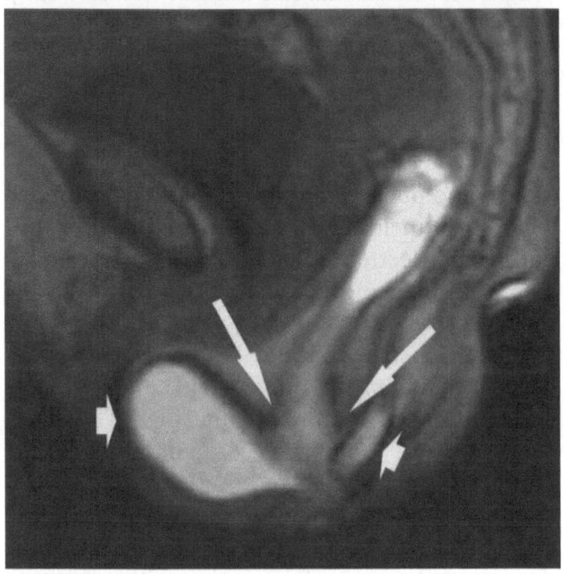

c

Fig. VI.41. A 47-year-old woman with constipation and diffuse pelvic pain. T1-weighted spoiled gradient-echo magnetic resonance (MR) images obtained at rest (**a**), at straining (**b**), and during evacuation (**c**) with the patient sitting in an open-configuration MR system. During evacuation (**c**), all layers of the rectal wall protrude through the anal canal (*arrow*) with formation of a full-thickness internal intra-anal prolapse. The rectum is incompletely evacuated. Associated anterior and posterior rectoceles are evident (*small arrows*)

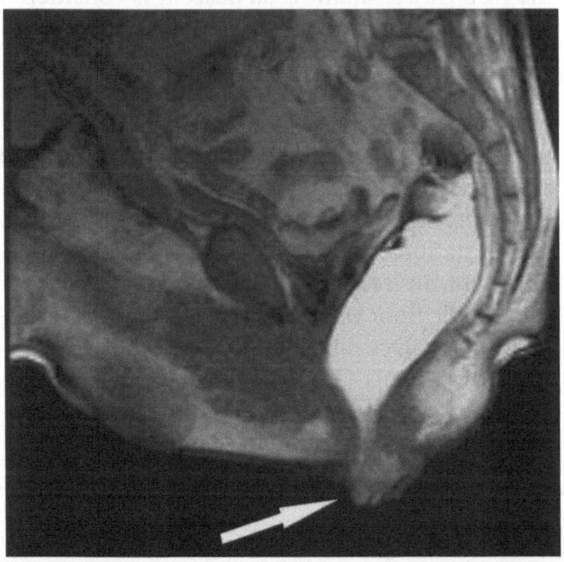

Fig. VI.42. A 58-year-old man with chronic constipation and incomplete evacuation. Sagittal T1-weighted spoiled gradient-echo magnetic resonance image with the patient in sitting position and obtained during defecation shows a full-thickness external rectal prolapse (*arrow*)

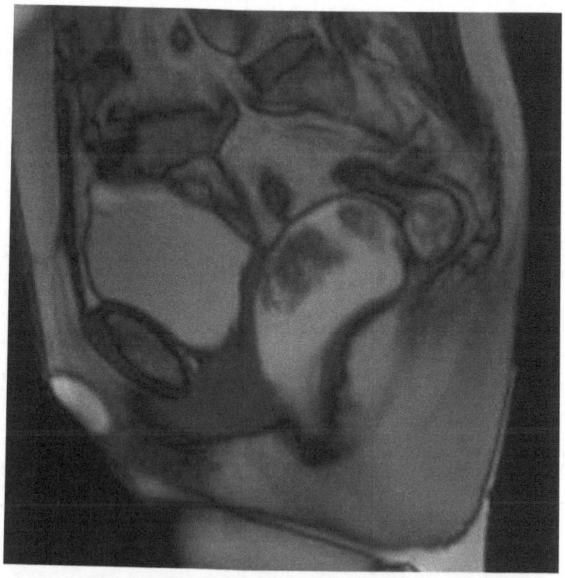

a

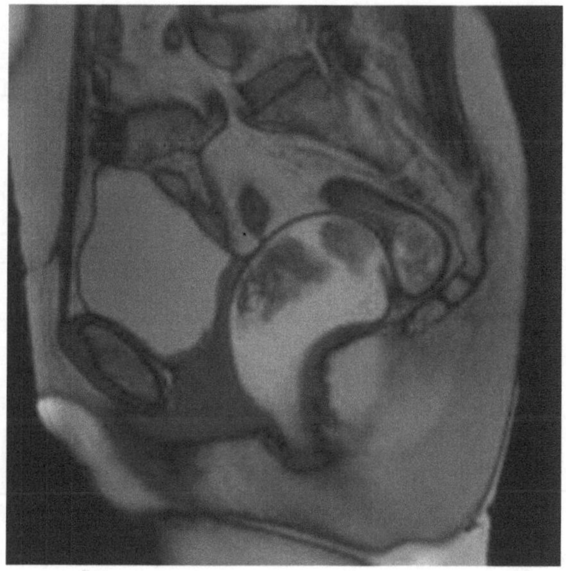

b

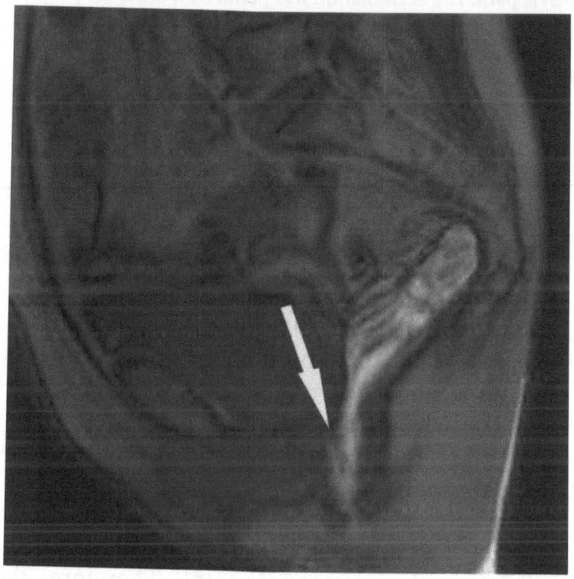

c

Fig. VI.43. A 71-year-old woman with feeling of incomplete evacuation. Steady state free precession (SSFP) sequence was used at rest (**a**) and at squeezing (**b**). During defecation (**c**), dynamic T1-weighted spoiled gradient-echo image shows a thin hypointense anterior infolding through the anal canal (*arrow*) consistent with the typical appearance of an intra-anal internal mucosal prolapse

tomy) represents descent of the middle compartment. The descent of the anterior and middle compartments are quantified relative to the PCL in a similar fashion as described for the posterior compartment [14].

Anismus

Anismus is an outlet obstruction characterized by difficulties in rectal evacuation due to an abnormal activity of pelvic floor musculature. In the literature, anismus is also known as spastic pelvic floor syndrome [17, 45], dyskinetic puborectalis muscle [41], and pelvic floor dyssynergia [57]. During normal defecation, the pelvic floor descends, the internal and external sphincters relax, and the anorectal junction opens due to the puborectalis muscle reflex inhibition. A paradoxical contraction or an insufficient relaxation of the puborectalis or external sphincter muscles are the causes of obstruction and, in most cases, these dysfunctions are not confined to a single muscle [58]. The etiology of obstruction is unknown, but a morphological lesion of the nerves or muscles is unlikely since at least two thirds of patients are able to relax the pelvic floor muscles during biofeedback training [59]. However, there seems to be an association between anismus and pelvic surgery, previous sexual abuse, anxiety, and/or psychological stress [57, 60]. Although it was reported that anismus may be the main cause of

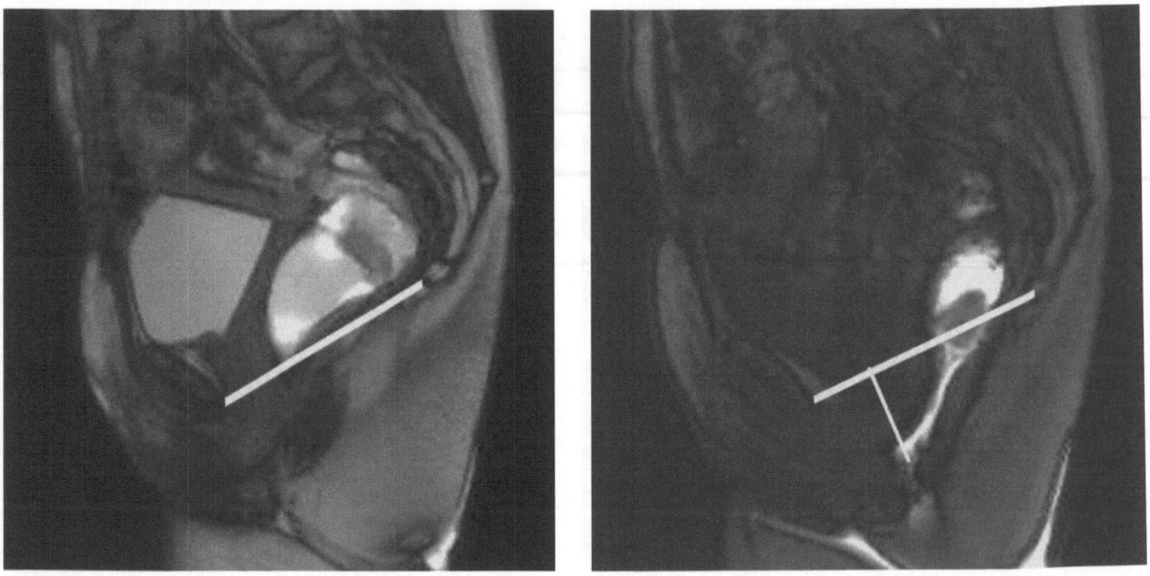

Fig. VI.44. A 55-year-old woman with chronic constipation and pelvic pain. The examination was performed in supine position and using a closed-configuration conventional magnetic resonance (MR) system. Steady state free precession sequence obtained at rest shows no abnormality (**a**). T1-weighted spoiled gradient-echo MR image during defecation demonstrates a moderate rectal descent (**b**). The anterior and middle pelvic compartments are normal

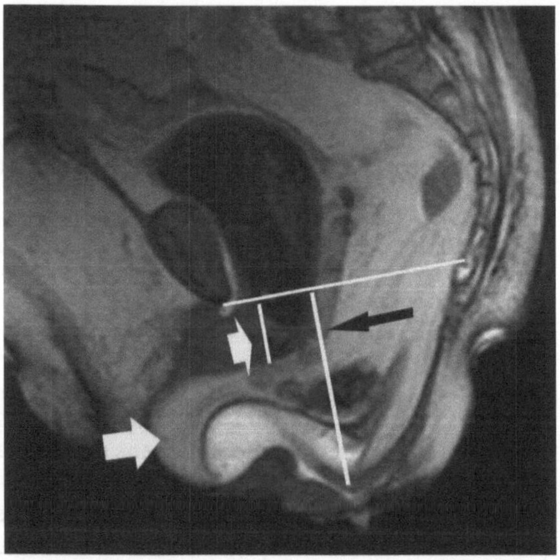

Fig. VI.45. A 67-year-old constipated woman after hysterectomy. T1-weighted spoiled gradient-echo magnetic resonance image during evacuation with patient in sitting position reveals a generalized pelvic floor weakness involving all pelvic compartments: a large posterior compartment descent with the distance between anorectal junction and pubococcygeal line more than 6 cm (*black arrow*) and a small cystocele, which is the expression of the anterior compartment weakness (*small arrow*). In addition, the rectovaginal space is enlarged and is occupied by a large enterocele (*large arrow*) that contains fat, small bowel, and sigmoid

outlet obstruction in almost half of constipated patients [61], the real prevalence is difficult to assess, being known that false positive and false negative results are common with different tests including anorectal manometry, balloon expulsion, and electromyography [7, 62]. Similar, electromyographic findings were described in either normal or constipated patients [63], and anorectal manometry showed that nearly 80% of patients suspected of anismus had appropriate sphincter relaxation during straining [7]. Therefore, the diagnostic requires a combination of tests, both physiological and radiological.

Dynamic pelvic MRI provides valuable information in patients with anismus regarding functional as well as morphological abnormalities of the pelvic floor during defecation. Using dynamic pelvic MRI, various signs may be seen in patients with anismus. In our experience, the best single finding of functional outlet obstruction is represented by a prolonged attempted defecation and incomplete evacuation (Fig. VI.46). It has been demonstrated that an evacuation time longer than 30s is highly suggestive for anismus, having a positive predictive value of 90% [64]. In that study, Halligan et al. compared patients with proven anismus with controls, and a prolonged evacua-

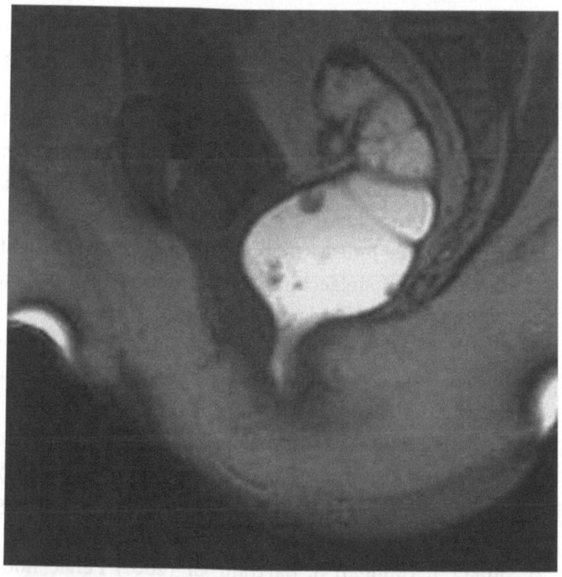
a

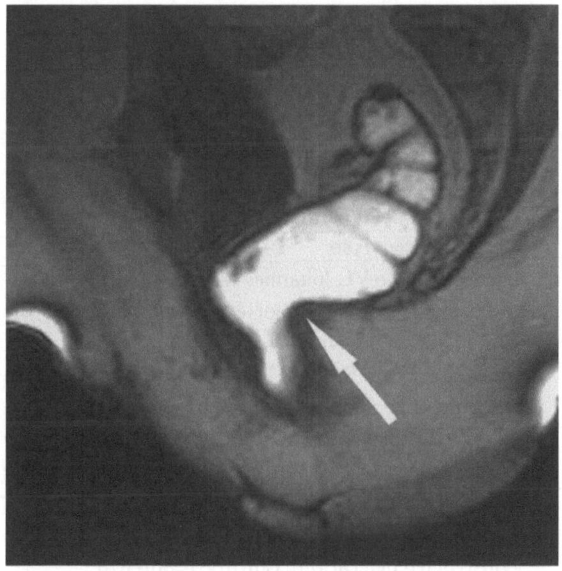
b

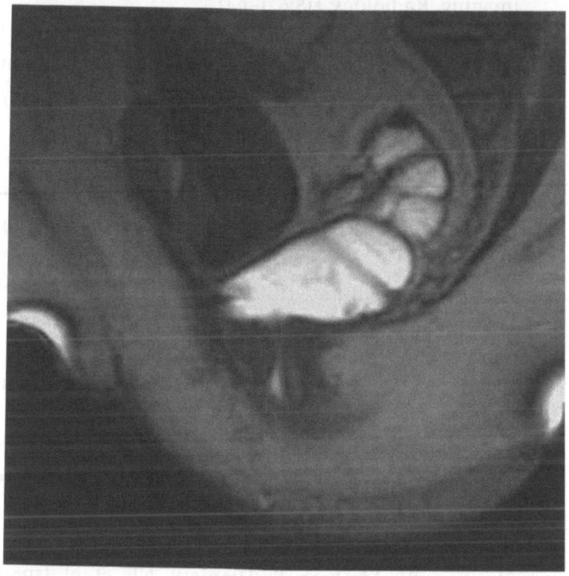
c

Fig. VI.46. A 40-year-old woman with clinical suspicion of anismus. T1-weighted spoiled gradient-echo magnetic resonance (MR) images obtained in sitting position obtained at rest (**a**), at squeezing (**b**), and during evacuation (**c**). The puborectalis impression is visible on MR image at squeezing as a result of puborectalis muscle contraction (*arrow*) (**b**). MR image obtained 40 s after several attempts at defecation shows no rectal evacuation (**c**). The final diagnostic of anismus was established based on clinical, radiological, and physiological findings

tion time was present in 83% of patients compared with none of the control group.

Another MR sign used for diagnosis of anismus is the behavior of the anorectal angle. Normal value of the anorectal angle at rest is between 90° and 110° [36], decreases during the squeeze, and increases during defecation as a result of puborectalis relaxation. In patient with anismus, during evacuation, the anorectal angle becomes more acute instead of obtuse, and it was considered an indicator of the lack of puborectalis muscle relaxation [45, 65]. However, there is data in the literature that showed that the configuration of rectum and anorectal junction is irrelevant to the diagnosis, and this finding cannot differentiate patients with functional outlet obstruction from asymptomatic subjects [66].

Conclusion

Dynamic pelvic MRI using either closed-configuration or open-configuration MR systems is a rapidly evolving technique that is considered an alternative to conventional evacuation proctography. In patients with outlet obstruction, the technique may reveal various findings associated with outlet obstruction.

References

1. Sonnenberg A, Koch TR (1989) Epidemiology of constipation in the United States. Dis Colon Rectum 32:1–8
2. Drossman DA, Li Z, Andruzzi E et al (1993) U.S. householder survey of functional gastrointestinal disorders. Prevalence, sociodemography, and health impact. Dig Dis Sci 38:1569–1580
3. Everhart JE, Go VL, Johannes RS et al (1989)A longitudinal survey of self-reported bowel habits in the United States. Dig Dis Sci 34:1153–1162
4. Jones R, Lydeard S (1992) Irritable bowel syndrome in the general population. BMJ 304:87–90
5. Talley NJ, Zinsmeister AR, Van Dyke C et al (1991) Epidemiology of colonic symptoms and the irritable bowel syndrome. Gastroenterology 101:927–934
6. Bruch HP, Fischer F, Schiedeck TH et al (2004) [Obstructed defecation]. Chirurg 75:861–870
7. D'Hoore A, Penninckx F (2003) Obstructed defecation. Colorectal Dis 5:280–287
8. Zonca G, De Thomatis A, Marchesini R et al (1997) The absorbed dose to the gonads in adult patients undergoing defecographic study by digital or traditional radiographic imaging. Radiol Med 94:520–523
9. Goei R, Kemerink G (1990) Radiation dose in defecography. Radiology 176:137–139
10. Bertschinger KM, Hetzer FH, Roos JE et al (2002) Dynamic MR imaging of the pelvic floor performed with patient sitting in an open-magnet unit versus with patient supine in a closed-magnet unit. Radiology 223:501–508
11. Vanbeckevoort D, Van Hoe L, Oyen R et al (1999) Pelvic floor descent in females: comparative study of colpocystodefecography and dynamic fast MR imaging. J Magn Reson Imaging 9:373–377
12. Mibu R, Hotokezaka M, Kai T et al (2001) A simplified defaecographic procedure for the assessment of faecal incontinence or obstructed defaecation. Colorectal Dis 3:328–333
13. Lienemann A, Anthuber C, Baron A et al (1997) Dynamic MR colpocystorectography assessing pelvic-floor descent. Eur Radiol 7:1309–1317
14. Kelvin FM, Maglinte DD, Hale DS, Benson JT (2000) Female pelvic organ prolapse: a comparison of triphasic dynamic MR imaging and triphasic fluoroscopic cystocolpoproctography. AJR Am J Roentgenol 174:81–88
15. Fletcher JG, Busse RF, Riederer SJ et al (2003) Magnetic resonance imaging of anatomic and dynamic defects of the pelvic floor in defecatory disorders. Am J Gastroenterol 98:399–411
16. Dvorkin LS, Hetzer F, Scott SM et al (2004) Open-magnet MR defaecography compared with evacuation proctography in the diagnosis and management of patients with rectal intussusception. Colorectal Dis 6:45–53
17. Roos JE, Weishaupt D, Wildermuth S et al (2002) Experience of 4 years with open MR defecography: pictorial review of anorectal anatomy and disease. Radiographics 22:817–832
18. Lamb GM, de Jode MG, Gould SW et al (2000) Upright dynamic MR defaecating proctography in an open configuration MR system. Br J Radiol 73:152–155
19. Maglinte DD, Kelvin FM, Fitzgerald K et al (1999) Association of compartment defects in pelvic floor dysfunction. AJR Am J Roentgenol 172:439–444
20. Healy JC, Halligan S, Reznek RH et al (1997) Dynamic MR imaging compared with evacuation proctography when evaluating anorectal configuration and pelvic floor movement. AJR Am J Roentgenol 169:775–779
21. Stoker J, Halligan S, Bartram CI (2001) Pelvic floor imaging. Radiology 218:621–641
22. Comiter CV, Vasavada SP, Barbaric ZL et al (1999) Grading pelvic prolapse and pelvic floor relaxation using dynamic magnetic resonance imaging. Urology 54:454–457
23. Gufler H, Laubenberger J, DeGregorio G et al (1999) Pelvic floor descent: dynamic MR imaging using a half-Fourier RARE sequence. J Magn Reson Imaging 9:378–383
24. Pannu HK, Kaufman HS, Cundiff GW et al (2000) Dynamic MR imaging of pelvic organ prolapse: spectrum of abnormalities. Radiographics 20:1567–1582
25. Kelvin FM, Maglinte DD (2001) Extended proctography. Imaging 13:448–457
26. Maglinte DD, Kelvin FM, Hale DS et al (1997) Dynamic cystoproctography: a unifying diagnostic approach to pelvic floor and anorectal dysfunction. AJR Am J Roentgenol 169:759–767
27. Shorvon PJ, McHugh S, Diamant NE et al (1989) Defecography in normal volunteers: results and implications. Gut 30:1737–1749
28. Siproudhis L, Dautreme S, Ropert A et al (1993) Dyschezia and rectocele – a marriage of convenience? Physiologic evaluation of the rectocele in a group of 52 women complaining of difficulty in evacuation. Dis Colon Rectum 36:1030–1036
29. Pfeifer J, Oliveira L, Park UC et al (1997) Are interpretations of video defecographies reliable and reproducible? Int J Colorectal Dis 12:67–72
30. Mahieu P, Pringot J, Bodart P (1984) Defecography: II Contribution to the diagnosis of defecation disorders Gastrointest Radiol 9:253–261
31. Sarles JC, Arnaud A, Selezneff I, Olivier S (1989) Endorectal repair of rectocele. Int J Colorectal Dis 4:167–171
32. Johansson C, Nilsson BY, Mellgren A et al (1992)

Paradoxical sphincter reaction and associated colorectal disorders. Int J Colorectal Dis 7:89–94
33. Mellgren A, Anzen B, Nilsson BY et al (1995) Results of rectocele repair. A prospective study. Dis Colon Rectum 38:7–13
34. Marti MC, Roche B, Deleaval J (1999) Rectoceles: value of videodefaecography in selection of treatment policy. Colorectal Dis 1:324–329
35. Healy JC, Halligan S, Reznek RH et al (1997) Patterns of prolapse in women with symptoms of pelvic floor weakness: assessment with MR imaging. Radiology 203:77–81
36. Lowry AC, Simmang CL, Boulos P et al (2001) Consensus statement of definitions for anorectal physiology and rectal cancer. Colorectal Dis 3:272–275
37. Yang A, Mostwin JL, Rosenshein NB, Zerhouni EA (1991) Pelvic floor descent in women: dynamic evaluation with fast MR imaging and cinematic display. Radiology 179:25–33
38. Hock D, Lombard R, Jehaes C et al (1993) Colpocystodefecography. Dis Colon Rectum 36:1015–1021
39. Kelvin FM, Maglinte DD, Hornback JA, Benson JT (1992) Pelvic prolapse: assessment with evacuation proctography (defecography). Radiology 184:547–551
40. Hauck R (1993) Enterocele. In: Buchmann P, Brühlmann W (eds) Investigation of anorectal functional disorders. Springer, Berlin Heidelberg New York, pp 170–189
41. Karasick S, Karasick D, Karasick SR (1993) Functional disorders of the anus and rectum: findings on defecography. AJR Am J Roentgenol 160:777–782
42. Kelvin FM, Hale DS, Maglinte DD et al (1999) Female pelvic organ prolapse: diagnostic contribution of dynamic cystoproctography and comparison with physical examination. AJR Am J Roentgenol 173:31–37
43. Hilfiker PR, Debatin JF, Schwizer W et al (1998) MR defecography: depiction of anorectal anatomy and pathology. J Comput Assist Tomogr 22:749–755
44. Stoker J, Bartram CI, Halligan S (2002) Imaging of the posterior pelvic floor. Eur Radiol 12:779–788
45. Kelvin FM, Maglinte DD, Benson JT (1994) Evacuation proctography (defecography): an aid to the investigation of pelvic floor disorders. Obstet Gynecol 83:307–314
46. Fenner DE (1996) Diagnosis and assessment of sigmoidoceles. Am J Obstet Gynecol 175:1438–1442
47. Jorge JM, Yang YK, Wexner SD (1994) Incidence and clinical significance of sigmoidoceles as determined by a new classification system. Dis Colon Rectum 37:1112–1117
48. Keigley M, et al (1992) Rectal prolapse. In: Henry MM, Swash M (eds) Coloproctology and the pelvic floor, 2nd edn. Butterworth-Heinemann, Oxford, pp. 316–350
49. Kodner IJ, Fry RD, Fleshman JW (1992) Rectal prolapse and other pelvic floor abnormalities. Surg Annu 24:157–190
50. Goei R (1990) Anorectal function in patients with defecation disorders and asymptomatic subjects: evaluation with defecography. Radiology 174:121–123
51. Pomerri F, Zuliani M, Mazza C et al (2001) Defecographic measurements of rectal intussusception and prolapse in patients and in asymptomatic subjects. AJR Am J Roentgenol 176:641–645
52. Tsiaoussis J, Chrysos E, Glynos M et al (1998) Pathophysiology and treatment of anterior rectal mucosal prolapse syndrome. Br J Surg 85: 1699–1702
53. Parks AG, Porter NH, Hardcastle J (1966) The syndrome of the descending perineum. Proc R Soc Med 59:477–482
54. Henry MM, Parks AG, Swash M (1982) The pelvic floor musculature in the descending perineum syndrome. Br J Surg 69:470–472
55. Snooks SJ, Swash M, Henry MM, Setchell M (1986) Risk factors in childbirth causing damage to the pelvic floor innervation. Int J Colorectal Dis 1:20–24
56. Locke GR 3rd, Pemberton JH, Phillips SF (2000) AGA technical review on constipation. American Gastroenterological Association. Gastroenterology 119:1766–1778
57. Whitehead WE, Wald A, Diamant NE et al (1999) Functional disorders of the anus and rectum. Gut 45 (Suppl 2):55–59
58. Marshall M, Halligan S (2001) Evacuation proctography. Imaging 13:440–447
59. Rao SS, Welcher KD, Pelsang RE (1997) Effects of biofeedback therapy on anorectal function in obstructive defecation. Dig Dis Sci 42:2197–2205
60. Leroi AM, Berkelmans I, Denis P et al (1995) Anismus as a marker of sexual abuse. Consequences of abuse on anorectal motility Dig Dis Sci 40:1411–1416
61. Wald A, Caruana BJ, Freimanis MG et al (1990) Contributions of evacuation proctography and anorectal manometry to evaluation of adults with constipation and defecatory difficulty. Dig Dis Sci 35:481–487
62. Jorge JM, Wexner SD, Ger GC et al (1993) Cinedefecography and electromyography in the diagnosis of nonrelaxing puborectalis syndrome. Dis Colon Rectum 36:668–676
63. Jones PN, Lubowski DZ, Swash M, Henry MM (1987) Is paradoxical contraction of puborectalis muscle of functional importance? Dis Colon Rectum 30:667–670
64. Halligan S, Malouf A, Bartram CI et al (2001) Predictive value of impaired evacuation at proctography in diagnosing anismus. AJR Am J Roentgenol 177:633–636
65. Kuijpers HC, Bleijenberg G (1985) The spastic pelvic floor syndrome. A cause of constipation. Dis Colon Rectum 28:669–672
66. Halligan S, Bartram CI, Park HJ, Kamm MA (1995) Proctographic features of anismus. Radiology 197: 679–682

Invited Commentary

J. B. Kruskal

The preceding chapters highlight the current state of the art for imaging pelvic outlet obstruction using the trio of currently available dynamic studies: ultrasound, defecography, and magnetic resonance imaging (MRI). Each of these techniques provides different and possibly complementary information to the ordering physician, and few studies have compared the relative information provided by each of these imaging techniques. For instance, endoanal ultrasound is routinely used for evaluating the integrity of the internal and external anal sphincters, but many operators continue to be challenged when trying to accurately define the precise location and integrity of the external anal sphincter. The reason for this limitation is that the decussating fibers that compromise the external sphincter do not form a uniform hypoechoic ring such as is routinely seen with the internal sphincter and are less difficult to confidently image with endosonography. Similarly and of relevance to patient management, abnormalities of the internal sphincter are not likely to result in any specific surgical management whereas only those of the external sphincter might ultimately require surgical repair. For this reason, attention should focus primarily on the more challenging external sphincter when performing anal evaluation with endosonography.

Transperineal dynamic ultrasound is not widely used around the world but does provide an alternative approach to imaging of the sphincters. Little data exist describing clinical impact and accuracy of transperineal anal sphincter imaging or comparative studies of this and endoluminal imaging. Such studies would be important areas of focus on. Given that transperineal imaging is not widely employed, the transperineal technique should only be used when the operating surgeons are likely to use this information from trusted, experienced endosonographers performing the studies.

In terms of video defecography or voiding proctography, this technique is routinely performed for evaluating the complex inter-related mechanisms of rectal evacuation in constipated patients. The technique is also useful when evaluating patients with fecal incontinence. Defecography provides entirely different information to endoanal ultrasonography since the mechanisms of defecation, including puborectalis function and the presence of internal hernias, are not likely to be confidently seen with endosonography. Also, the two techniques image entirely different anatomic regions. In our experience, defecography is likely to provide additional and complementary information to endoanal ultrasonography, and this information might be useful to the operating surgeon when planning the procedure. For instance, tears of the external sphincter might be associated with additional abnormalities, such as enteroceles or sigmoidoceles. Such information is important if surgical repair is contemplated, in which case the additional abnormalities documented during defecography might be repaired at the same time. Again, from our experience of imaging patients with constipation or fecal incontinence, defecography provides useful additional and complementary information to the results of endoanal sonography, and this information is helpful to the physician evaluating and managing the patient. What is important, however, is that defecography be performed correctly by radiologists trained to perform and interpret the study. It is important to recognize that soaked tampons should not be used to outline the vaginal anatomy since these alter the mechanics of defecation and can produce misleading results. Many institutions still rely on this method, and it is hoped that the excellent techniques described in the preceding chapters will be used by physicians learning to perform these diagnostic studies.

An important component of the defecography study is to continue imaging the patient for at least 2 min once the rectal vault has emptied. The study should not be terminated when the vault is empty; the presence and occurrence of clinically relevant sigmoidoceles and enteroceles might depend in part on the anatomic space occupied by the distended rectal vault being emptied first, permitting descent of these internal hernias into the pelvis. Another important technical requirement is to record the dynamic events; interpretation of a defecogram cannot be made on captured static images since these do not display transient dynamic events that are essential for correct interpretation of the study.

Dynamic MRI of pelvic organ prolapse is being increasingly used throughout the world. The ability to image pelvic muscles and structures in axial, sagittal, and coronal planes during dynamic motion provides not only anatomic detail but also dynamic information relating to defecation and outlet obstruction. From my own experience, it is important that radiologists interpreting the MRI studies are familiar with the mechanisms of defecation, and we find the most helpful interpretations are rendered by those who are well versed in performing defecography studies. Opportunities for further study include comparisons of MRI with fluoroscopic defecography as well as examining the impact of MRI with the patient in the supine versus erect positions. It is still not certain to what extent dynamic MRI in the supine position might lead to underestimation of pelvic floor abnormalities, but it would be an important question to answer.

In conclusion, the preceding chapters have summarized the current state of dynamic pelvic floor imaging. Further advances are likely to come in evaluating complementary abnormalities of complexes of associated findings, but ultimately, the clinical impact both on choice and success of subsequent patient management will need to be studied.

SECTION VII

Anorectal Physiology Testing

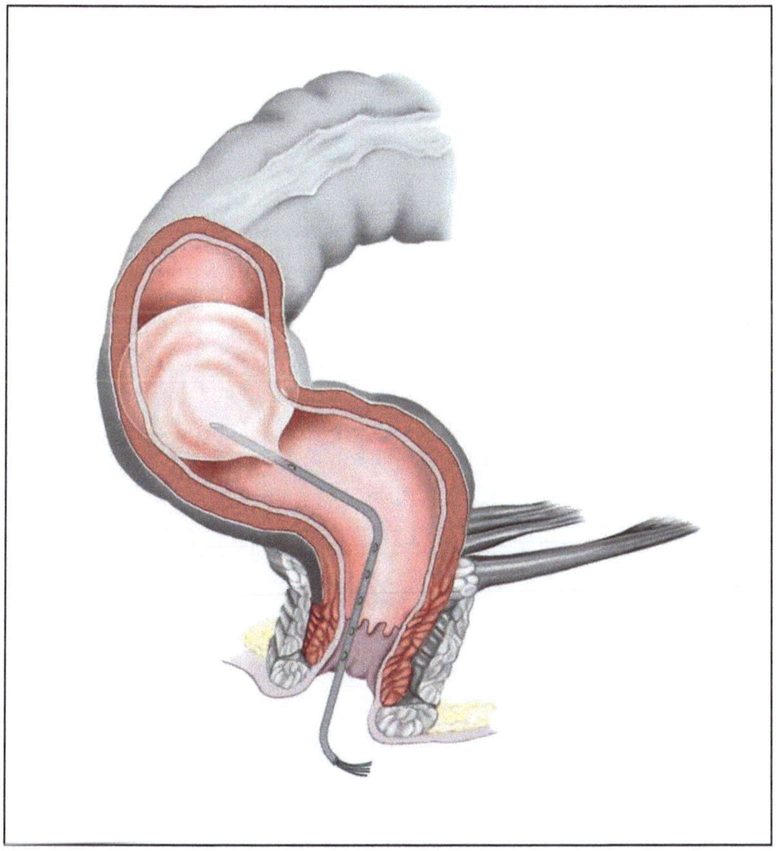

VII.1. Introduction

G.A. Santoro, B. Salvioli

Anorectal benign disorders affect 10–20% of the population [1], and an extensive investigation is necessary to characterize defecation disturbances. Currently, several diagnostic and sophisticated physiological tests are available for assessing anorectal function, and interpretation is based on the integration of all data obtained [2]. Anorectal manometry, electromyography, and pudendal nerve terminal motor latency are widely accepted as diagnostic tools, but their clinical utility and application are limited by lack of standardized protocols and wide range of normal values. Nevertheless, they add important information about pathophysiology of anorectal dysfunction, providing indications in the management of these disorders and are mainly suggested in a diagnostic flowchart of fecal incontinence and constipation. Their indications, however, have diminished over time, being replaced by more sophisticated, accurate, and noninvasive techniques, such as endoanal, transvaginal, and transperineal ultrasonography.

In this section, the technical issues of these different physiological anorectal testing will be described in detail along with normal and abnormal findings and correlated to clinical conditions. It will follow a critical review on which tests we really need in the treatment of benign anorectal disease.

Continence Mechanisms

Maintenance of fecal continence depends on anatomical factors and complex sensory and motor interaction between the rectum, the anus, and the sphincteric mechanism [3–5]; central and peripheral innervation; mental awareness; and physical ability to get to a toilet [6]. Continence is maintained by tonic contraction of the external and internal anal sphincters and acute angulation of the anorectum due to the tonic contraction of the puborectalis muscle [7]. When one of these structures is damaged, fecal continence is threatened [8].

Anal Sphincters and the Rectoanal Inhibitory Reflex

The anorectum consist of the rectum, the anorectal angle formed by the puborectalis muscle, and the internal and external sphincters surrounding the anal canal (Fig. VII.1). The rectum is the lower part of the intestine, about 12- to 15-cm long, between the sigmoid colon and the anal canal. The function of the rectum is to act as a reservoir for stools for a short period of time. The ampulla recti is normally completely empty of fecal material. The sensation of the urge to defecate is initiated when fecal material reaches the ampulla recti.

The anal canal is the terminal portion of the large intestine. The anal sphincters include the internal (IAS) and the external (EAS) anal sphincter muscles. The sphincters and the pelvic floor work as holding forces to maintain fecal continence. The IAS is the involuntary, thickened layer of the circular smooth muscle of the rectum. It is in a state of continuous contraction, maintained by myogenic tone and the intrinsic and extrinsic innervations (enteric , parasympathetic, and sympathetic nervous systems) [9]. Doubtless, this complex set of controls reflects the importance of the IAS in normal continence. The muscle has two excitatory innervations, one cholinergic and one

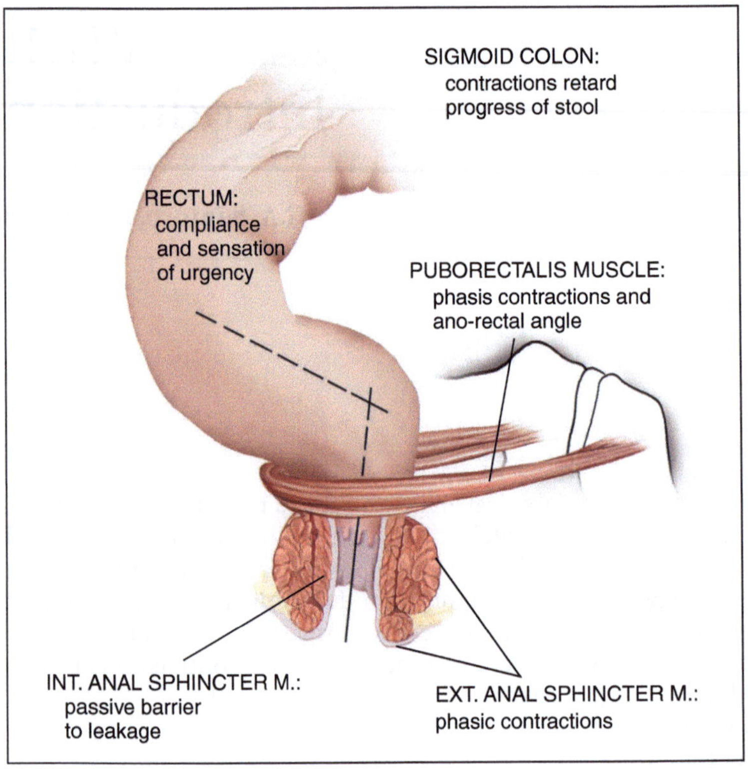

Fig. VII.1. Pelvic floor components involved in the mechanisms for preserving continence

adrenergic, and two inhibitory innervations, one adrenergic and the other nonadrenergic–noncholinergic [10]. The IAS relaxes during defecation and straining and in response to rectal distention [11], the so-called "rectoanal inhibitory reflex" (RAIR), which is mediated by intramural neural pathways independent of extrinsic control [12]. The role of the RAIR is to allow rectal contents to reach the sensitive mucosa of the anal canal and for this reason it is also termed "sampling reflex." The IAS contributes up to 70–80% of resting tone but less during a voluntary squeeze or during sudden increases in intra-abdominal pressure [13]. Episodes of spontaneous IAS relaxation occur in healthy individuals [14], but simultaneous contraction of the external anal sphincter provides an efficient protective barrier to the passage of stool. The sampling reflex occurs in all normal subjects at a rate of four per hour at rest in the alert state. The frequency of this reflex increases following daytime rectal motor activity, following meals, and prior to defecation. About 65% of these episodes are associated with a desire to pass flatus or feces.

The external anal sphincter is a striated muscle that surrounds the IAS and contributes to 20–30% of the resting tone [13] but is able to double the resting pressure during a squeeze [15]. Its importance in continence is to contract in reflex response to sudden rectal distention or increases in intra-abdominal pressure [16]. The EAS has a somatic innervation from the second, third, and fourth sacral roots via the pudendal nerve [17]. The EAS is capable of reflex contraction believed to be mediated by nerves related to Onuf's nucleus (at S2 in the ventral horn of the spinal cord) [18]. The EAS and puborectalis muscle act largely as a single unit. The contractile responses of these striated muscles, e.g., to raised intra-abdominal pressure (Valsalva maneuver, coughing) and rectal distension lasts only for about 1 min, after which the muscles fatigue [19].

Anorectal Angle

The levator ani muscle in the pelvic floor includes the puborectalis sling. The puborectalis muscle is responsible for the angle between the rectum and upper anal canal, which has an average value at rest of about 90° [19]. The angle is sharpened by a voluntary contraction of the pelvic floor muscles and made more obtuse by straining at defecation [20].

Rectal Compliance

The rectum has the ability to accommodate fecal volumes until defecation becomes convenient: this reservoir function maintains a low intraluminal pressure despite an increase in volume. The rectum is not only distensible but, following meals, can increase its tone [21]. Rectal accommodation is important for continence such that reduced capacity of the viscus will result in higher intraluminal pressures.

Rectal Sensation

Mechanoreceptors in the rectum are excited by movements of the mucosa [22] or by distension [23]. In the rectal mucosa, there are abundant nonmyelinated nerve fibers, but only one recognizable intraepithelial receptor ending has been identified [24]. Receptors are also believed to lie outside the rectum [18], and patients can still perceive rectal filling even after rectal excision and coloanal anastomosis [25]. Sensation travels in both the parasympathetic (through S2, S3, S4) and sympathetic (through the superior and inferior hypogastric plexuses, L1, L2) systems. The parasympathetic afferent nerves are thought to mediate rectal filling sensations. Rectal sensation is crucial for continence and is correlated to the contractile activity of the sphincters [26]. The EAS responds only when distention is perceived and the duration of sphincter contraction correlates to the duration of sensation [27].

Anal Sensation

The epithelium of the anal canal contains abundant free nerve endings [24] and specialized sensory organs (e.g., Krause, Golgi-Mazzoni, Pacini corpuscles) capable of perceiving different stimuli. Touch, pinprick, and temperature are readily felt by the perianal skin and within the anal canal to a level of 2.5–1.5 cm above the anal valves [24]. The sensitivity of this region, which is comparable to that on the tip of the index finger, has been postulated as a mechanism facilitating continence by discriminating between gas, liquid, and feces [28]. The concept of the sampling reflex helps explain the role of anal sensation in normal continence.

Stool Volume and Consistency

Stool consistency is an important determinant of continence/incontinence [29]. By history, most patients who fear loss of control of liquid stools have no similar concerns when feces are solid. Moreover, persons with intact mechanisms of continence may experience fecal incontinence if a large volume of liquid stools (e.g., diarrhea) arrives in the rectum.

Anorectal Physiology History

Despite the availability of a wide battery of tests [30], a careful physical examination is still deemed indispensable, as it identifies structural disorders (e.g., perineum descending syndrome, prolapse), gives estimation of anal canal pressures at rest and during squeeze, and assesses perineal sensation and reflex contraction of the EAS to perineal stimulation and cough [31].

An extremely accurate anorectal physiological history should be obtained. In fecal incontinence, the investigator should ask the patient the time defecation can be deferred (minutes), the presence of urgency, urge incontinence, difficulty wiping, postdefecation soiling, passive soiling, and events causing these symptoms. Control of flatus (good, variable, poor), ability to distinguish stool/flatus, nocturnal fecal incontinence, consistency of incontinence (solid, liquid, mucus only), how much is lost with fecal incontinence (no leakage, minor stain only, small amount, moderate amount, or large amount), need to wear a pad, and use of constipating medicines should always be questioned. Past medical history (including bowel, anal trauma, surgical, medical, psychological) and obstetric history (parity, use of forceps, other difficult deliveries, heaviest baby) should be evaluated. Information on bladder problems, such as stress incontinence, urge incontinence, voiding difficulty, and nocturnal enuresis should also be obtained.

In evacuation difficulties, important data are: urge to defecate felt, straining, unsuccessful visits to the toilet, sensation of incomplete evacuation, bloating, digitations (vaginally/anally to empty, anally to initiate defecation, external perineal support), pain, and sensation of rectal prolapse.

References

1. Drossman DA, Zhiming L, Andruzzi E et al (1993) US householder survey of functional gastrointestinal disorders: prevalence, sociodemography, and health impact. Dig Dis Sci 38:1569–1580
2. Bharucha AE (2004) Outcome measures for fecal incontinence: anorectal structures and function. Gastroenterology 126:S90–S98
3. Shafik A (1987) A concept of the anatomy of the anal sphincter mechanism and the physiology of defecation. Dis Colon Rectum 30:970–982
4. Ferguson GH, Redford J, Barrett JA et al (1989) The appreciation of rectal distention in fecal incontinence. Dis Colon Rectum 32:964–967
5. Bielefeldt K, Enck P, Erckenbrecht JF (1990) Sensory and motor function in the maintenance of anal continence. Dis Colon Rectum 33:674–678
6. Read NW, Celik AF, Katsinelos P (1995) Constipation and incontinence in the elderly. J Clin Gastroenterol 20:61–70
7. Duthie HL (1971) Anal continence. Gut 122:844–852
8. Shafik A (1980) A new concept of the anatomy of the anal sphincter mechanism and the physiology of defecation. IX. Single loop continence: a new theory of the mechanism of anal continence. Dis Colon Rectum 23:37–43
9. Jorge JMN, Wexner SD (1993) Etiology and management of fecal incontinence. Dis Colon Rectum 36:77–97
10. Christensen J (1994) The motility of the colon. In: Johnson LR (ed) Physiology of the gastrointestinal tract, 3rd edn. Raven, New York, pp 91–124
11. Swash M (1991) Pathophysiology of incontinence. In: Phillips SF, Pemberton JH, Shorter RG (eds) The large intestine: physiology and disease. Raven, New York, pp 697–708
12. Nagasaki A, Akeda K, Suita S et al (1984) Induction of rectoanal inhibitory reflex by electric stimulation. a diagnostic aid for Hirschsprung's disease. Dis Colon Rectum 27:598–601
13. Freckner B, Von Euler C (1975) Influence of pudendal block on the function of the anal sphincters. Gut 16:482–489
14. Read NW, Sun WM (1989) Anorectal manometry, anal myography and rectal sensory testing. In: Read NW (ed). Gastrointestinal motility: which test? Wrightson Medical, Petersfield, pp 227–241
15. Coller JA (1987) Clinical application of anorectal manometry. Gastroenterol Clin North Am 16:17–33
16. Goligher JC, Hughes ESR (1951) Sensibility of the rectum and colon. Its role in the mechanism of anal continence. Lancet 543–547
17. Devroede G (1991) Functions of the anorectum: defecation and continence. In: Phillips SF, Pemberton JH, Shorter RG (eds) The large intestine: physiology and disease. Raven, New York, pp 115–140
18. Wood BA (1985) Anatomy of the anal sphincters and pelvic floor. In: Henry MM, Swash M (eds) Coloproctology and the pelvic floor: pathophysiology and management. Butterworth-Heinemann, London, pp 3–21
19. Phillips SF, Edwards AW (1965) Some aspects of anal continence and defecation. Gut 6:396–406
20. Ekberg O, Nylander G, Fork FT (1985) Defecography. Radiology 155:45–48
21. Bell AM, Pemberton JH, Hanson R et al (1991) Variations in muscle tone of the human rectum: recordings with an electromechanical barostat. Am J Physiol 260:G17–25
22. Garry RC (1933) The responses to stimulation of the caudal end of the large bowel in the cat. J Physiol (London) 78:208–224
23. Schuster MM, Hundrix TR, Mendeloff AI (1963) The internal anal sphincter response: manometric studies on its normal physiology, neural pathways, and alteration in bowel disorders. J Clin Invest 42:196–207
24. Duthie HL, Gairns FW (1960) Sensory nerve-endings and sensation in the anal region of man. Br J Surg 47:584–594
25. Lane RHS, Parks AG (1977) Function of the anal sphincters following colo-anal anastomosis. Br J Surg 63:596–599
26. Sun WM, Read NW (1989) Anorectal function in normal human subjects. Effect on gender. Int J Colorectal Dis 4:188–196
27. Sun WM, Read NW, Miner PB (1990) Relation between rectal sensation and anal function in normal subjects and patients with fecal incontinence. Gut 31:1056–1061
28. Duthie HL, Bennett RC (1963) The relation of sensation in the anal canal to the functional anal sphincter: a possible factor in anal continence. Gut 4:179–182
29. Ambroze WL, Pemberton JH, Bell AM et al (1991) The effect of stool consistency on rectal and neorectal emptying. Dis Colon Rectum 34:1–7
30. Hallan RI, Marzouk DEMM, Waldron DJ et al (1989) Comparison of digital and manometric assessment of anal sphincter function. Br J Surg 76:973–975
31. Felt-Bersma RJF, Klinkenberg-Knol EC, Meuwissen SGM (1998) Investigation of anorectal function. Br J Surg 75:53–55

VII.2. Manometric and Myographic Evaluation of the Anal Sphincters Morphology and Function

C. Ratto, G.A. Santoro

Anorectal disorders determining alterations of morphology and function of all pelvic floor structures, including sphincters, need to be studied accurately. Only an adequate diagnostic approach can attempt to overcome lack of knowledge still existing today on defecation and continence physiology and then significantly help clinicians in the diagnosis of anorectal disturbances [1–3]. Manometry is a traditional method of investigation of anal sphincters (measuring pressures derived from their muscle activity in the anal canal) and rectal wall (recording rectal compliance and sensations) [4]. Under the terms of *myographic* or *electromyographic*, examinations are comprised of a few tests evaluating not only sphincter muscle activity but also nerve function in the pelvis using electrical recording and stimulation so that *anorectal electrophysiology* should better define this type of diagnostic approach [5].

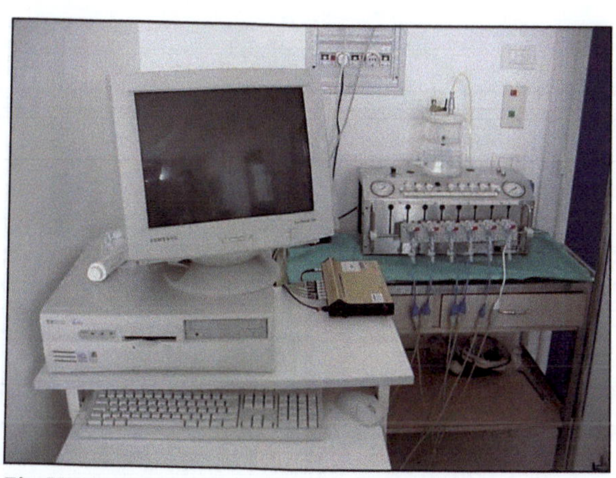

Fig. VII.2. Water-perfused manometry system

Anorectal Manometry

Since the 1960s, anorectal manometry has played a major role in the physiological investigation of anorectal functional disorders. It is a simple and noninvasive procedure well tolerated by the patient. Even if there are differences in the procedure at different centers, it allows the physician to obtain peculiar information about the physiology of continence and defecation [4].

Technique of Anorectal Manometry

A significant evolution of instruments, accessories, and techniques of examination has occurred in the last few decades [1–4]. The ultimate models of anorectal manometer include a multichannel catheter connected to pressure transducers that direct signals to a computerized recording system (polygraph). A dedicated software allows conversion of these signals in digitized traces visible on a screen, and analysis of manometrically recorded data (Fig. VII.2). Polygraphs commercially available today are usually computerized and equipped with software dedicated to anorectal manometry, with the possibility of adding urodynamic or gastroesophageal diagnostics (Fig. VII.3).

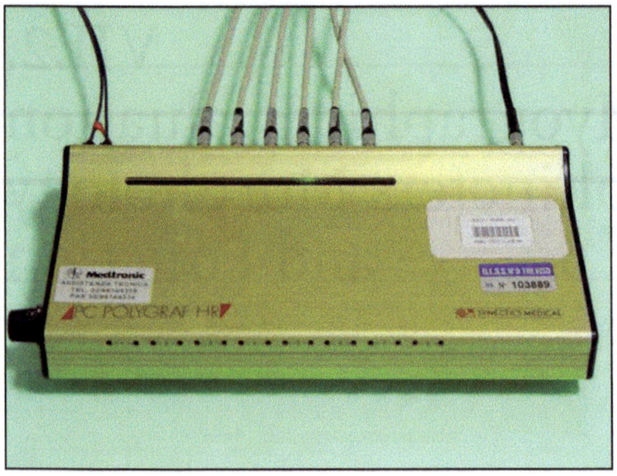

Fig. VII.3. Polygraph (Medtronic)

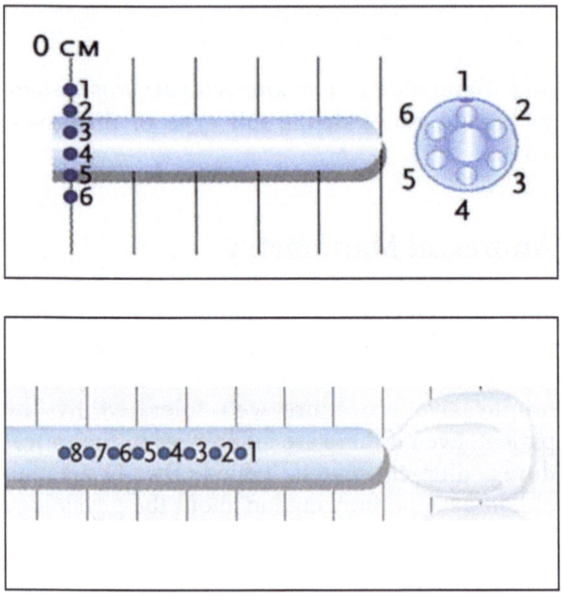

a

b

Fig. VII.4. Anorectal manometry catheters: with radial side holes (**a**) or with longitudinal side holes (**b**)

Several models of catheters are available, and no agreement exists as to which type is to be preferred. However, the majority of investigators prefer perfused, multichannel catheters with side openings: they are well tolerated by patients because they are thin and flexible. The number of openings varies, ranging from four to eight (less frequently, only one opening is preferred). According to the preference of each investigator, openings can be located in different configurations, i.e., radial or helicoidal. During the examination, the radial configuration allows pressure measurement at the same anal canal level in different sites of the anal canal circumference. The helicoidal configuration measures, at the same time, pressures at different anal canal levels (each 0.5–1 cm) in different sites of the anal canal circumference (Fig. VII.4).

Perfusion must be constant during the entire examination. The catheter can be perfused with deionized water by a standard pneumohydraulic perfusion pump (Fig. VII.5) or a simpler (and less expensive) pressure-inflated cuff. Actually, water perfused in the rectum and anal canal might cause distortion of pressures measured due to the elicitation of abnormal rectoanal reflexes. Usually, an adjunctive channel within the catheter allows the inflation or deflation (with air or water) of a small balloon placed on the tip of the catheter (at least 1 cm distally to the most distal catheter opening) in order to elicit the rectoanal inhibitory reflex and rectal sensations or to perform the balloon expulsion test (Fig. VII.6).

Sleeve catheters represent an alternative to perfused catheters: they provide a nonradial measurement along the anal canal but do not differentiate pressure influences of internal (IAS) and external anal sphincters (EAS), being more useful for prolonged recordings than standard investigation.

A balloon catheter, more frequently used in the past, is constituted by an inflated microballoon placed on the tip of the catheter and connected to the transducer. It allows a pressure measurement as the sum of all pressures exerted on the probe from the entire anal canal area. The absence of perfused water reduces possible artefacts; however, the presence of the microballoon is perceived by the anal mucosa, and anal sphincter tone could be modified.

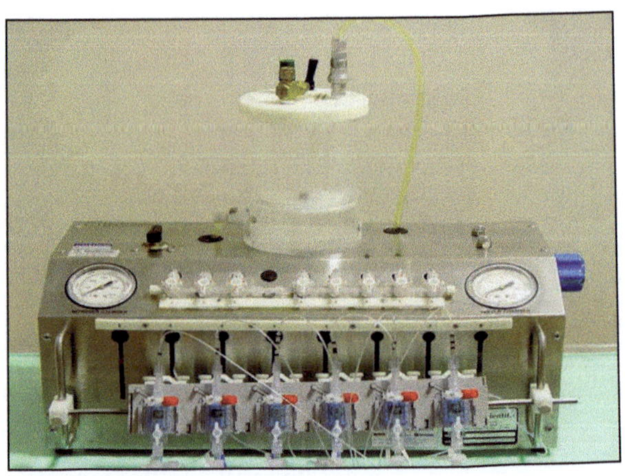

Fig. VII.5. Water perfusion pump (MUII)

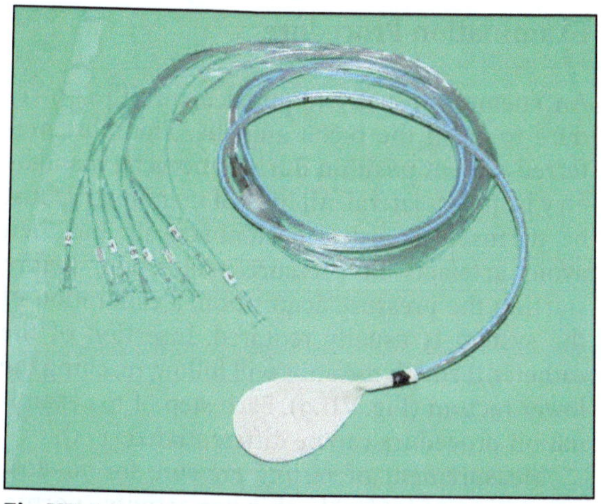

Fig. VII.6. Anorectal catheter with balloon tied at the proximal end

A new kind of catheter, different from solid-state and water-perfused systems, is the Latitude (Clinical Innovations) single-use, air-charged catheter. Body diameter is 2.5 mm, and all four sensors are circumferential (Fig. VII.7).

Finally, more sophisticated probes equipped with microtransducers should avoid artefacts due to the water infusion used in perfused catheters. They are thinner but fragile, more expensive, and need a special disinfection procedure. They can record the finest pressure variations for better assessment of sphincteric function and can be connected to a portable data recorder, allowing prolonged anorectal pressure recordings of >24 h (Fig. VII.8). During the recordings, all subjects are fully ambulant at home and instructed to press a button on the data recorder to mark the time of events such as eating, walking, and sleeping. Data are then transferred from the portable data recorder to a personal computer for further analysis.

Even if anorectal manometry is the oldest procedure in the functional diagnosis of anorectal disorders, a number of controversies still exist about the correct modality of examination [1–4]. There is no agreement between pressure units (millimeters of mercury, mmHg or centimeters of water, cmH_2O) and due to the variability between different instruments, normality values have to be

a

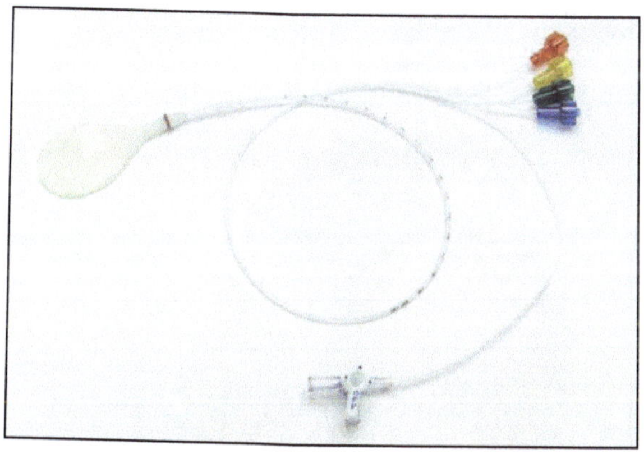

c

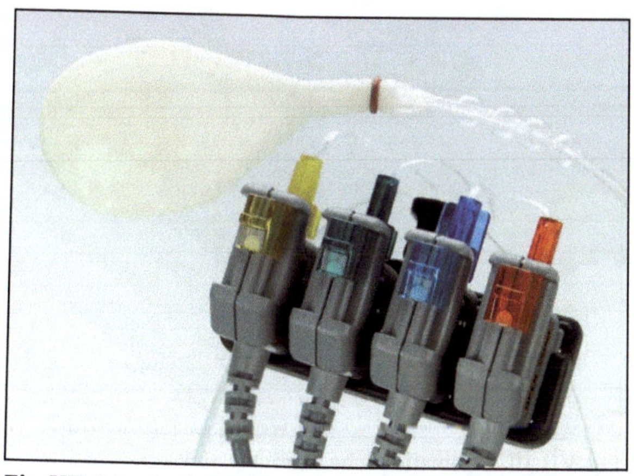

b

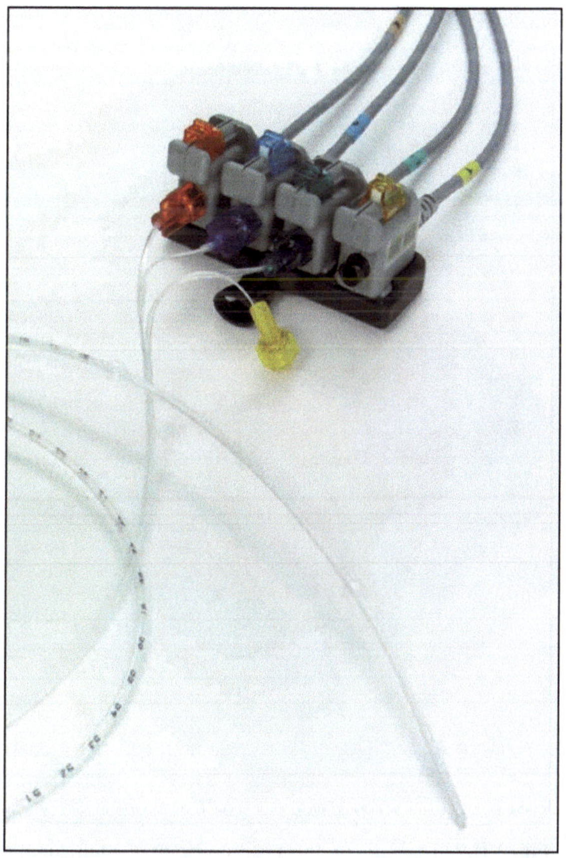

Fig. VII.7. Latitude single-use, air-charged catheter (Clinical Innovations) (a–c)

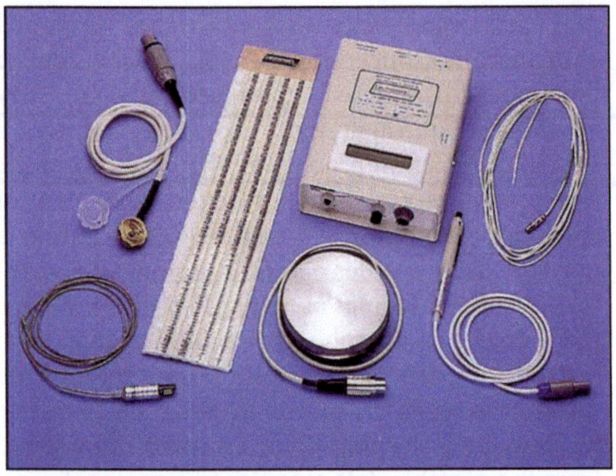

Fig. VII.8. Ambulatory manometry device with monitoring box for prolonged (24-h) recordings

derived from a number of normal subjects examined in each center so that a wide spread in reference values exists between investigators, with consequent problems in comparing and interpreting similar clinical condition.

Examination Procedure

An enema is usually required before the procedure to clean the rectal ampulla. The most preferred patient position during anorectal manometry is the left lateral. All lines of manometry must be perfused in order to eliminate air and then avoid artefacts in pressure acquisition. Before starting the pressure acquisition, a calibration of the system is usually required. Insertion of the catheter through the anus will follow, reaching the lower rectum (Fig. VII.9). Each step of the examination procedure can be differentiated [1–4].

Measurement of *resting pressure* for 70–80% expression of internal sphincter activity (normal range: 40–80 mmHg) can be performed by rapid or slow pull-through of the catheter; an automatic puller can be provided, maintaining a constant speed of catheter extraction (Fig. VII.10). A pressure profile of the anal canal pressure is obtained, and the *high pressure zone* (HPZ) can be identified (Fig. VII.11). The HPZ, defined as the length of the internal sphincter in which pressures are greater

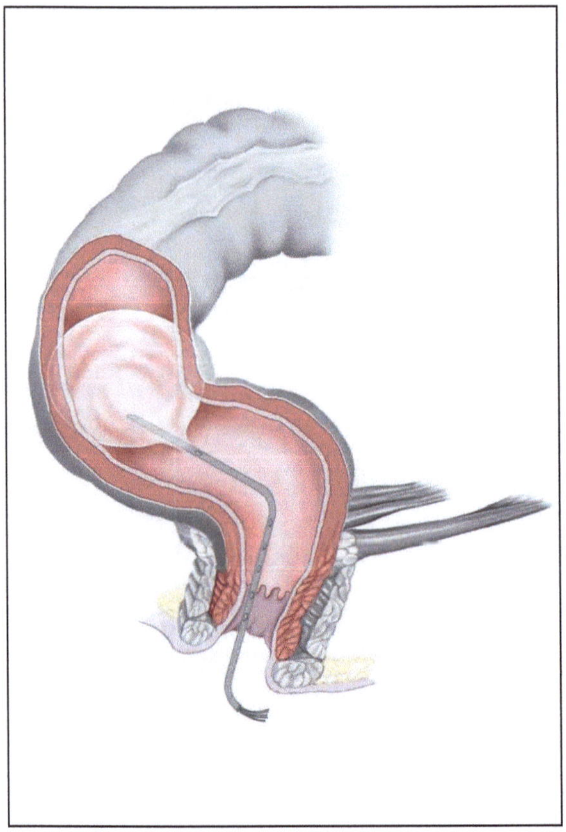

Fig. VII.9. Diagram of the positioning of a multichannel anorectal catheter with longitudinal side holes

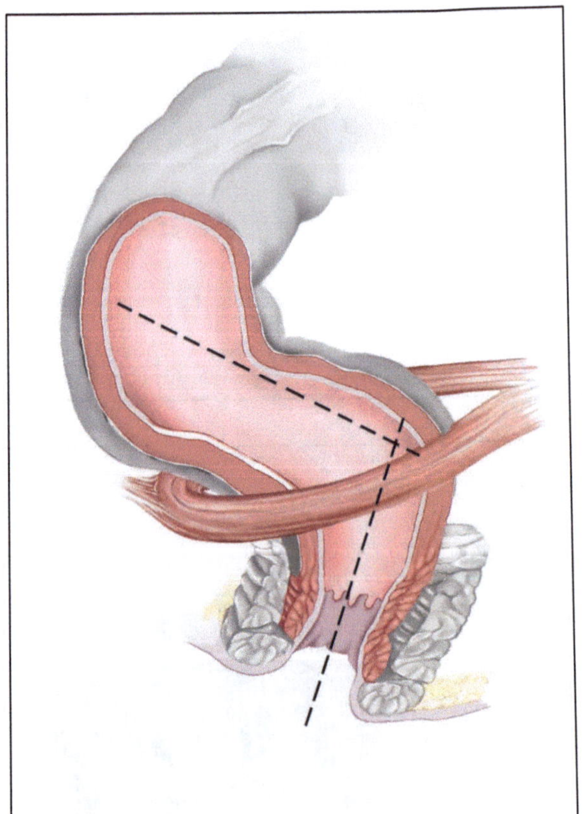

Fig. VII.10. Automatic probe extractor

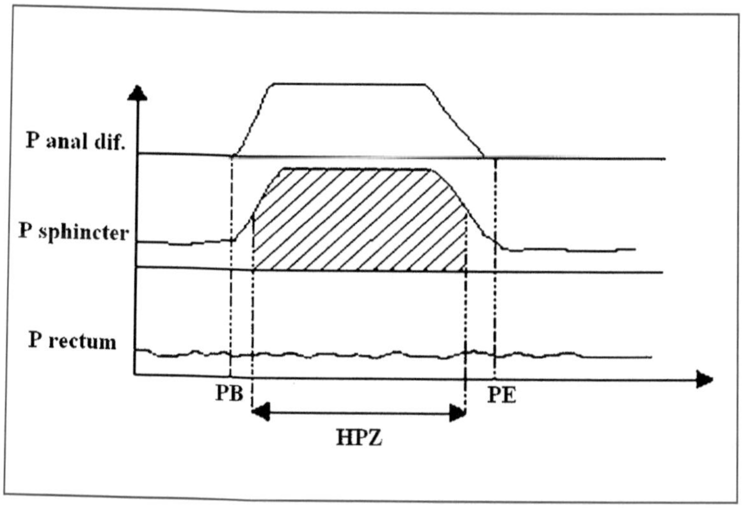

Fig. VII.11. Measurement of resting pressure and high-pressure zone (*HPZ*). *PB* pressure begin, *PE* pressure end

than half of the maximum pressure at rest, is generally about 2–3 cm in length in women and about 2.5–3.5 cm in men. The maximum and mean resting pressure is calculated, as well as the *functional anal canal length.* Several other parameters are allowed by the computerized system of pressure analysis concerning different segments of the anal canal. A vector manometry profile of all pressures acquired along the anal canal can be obtained showing, in a three-dimensional view, the areas and levels of the anal canal with increased or decreased pressures (Fig. VII.12).

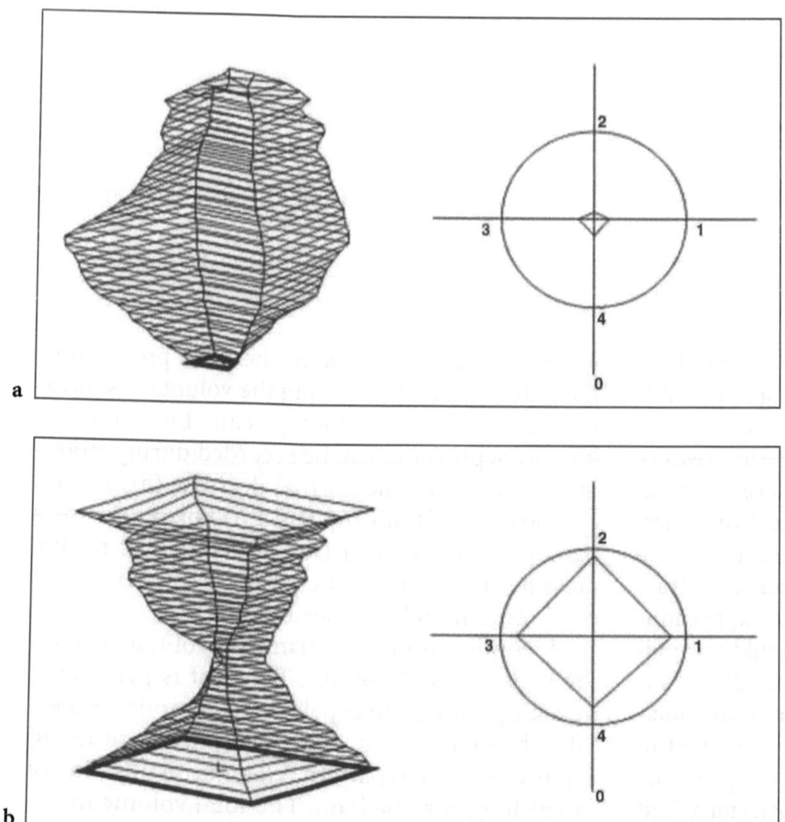

Fig. VII.12. Vector manometry profile obtained during anorectal manometry. It refelects all the pressures acquired along the anal canal showing, in a three-dimensional view, the areas and levels of anal canal with increased or decreased pressures. In (**a**) the vector profile is the expression of all pressures registered. in (**b**) it represents the "resistence" offered by the anal canal to the water pressure during manometric measurements

a

b

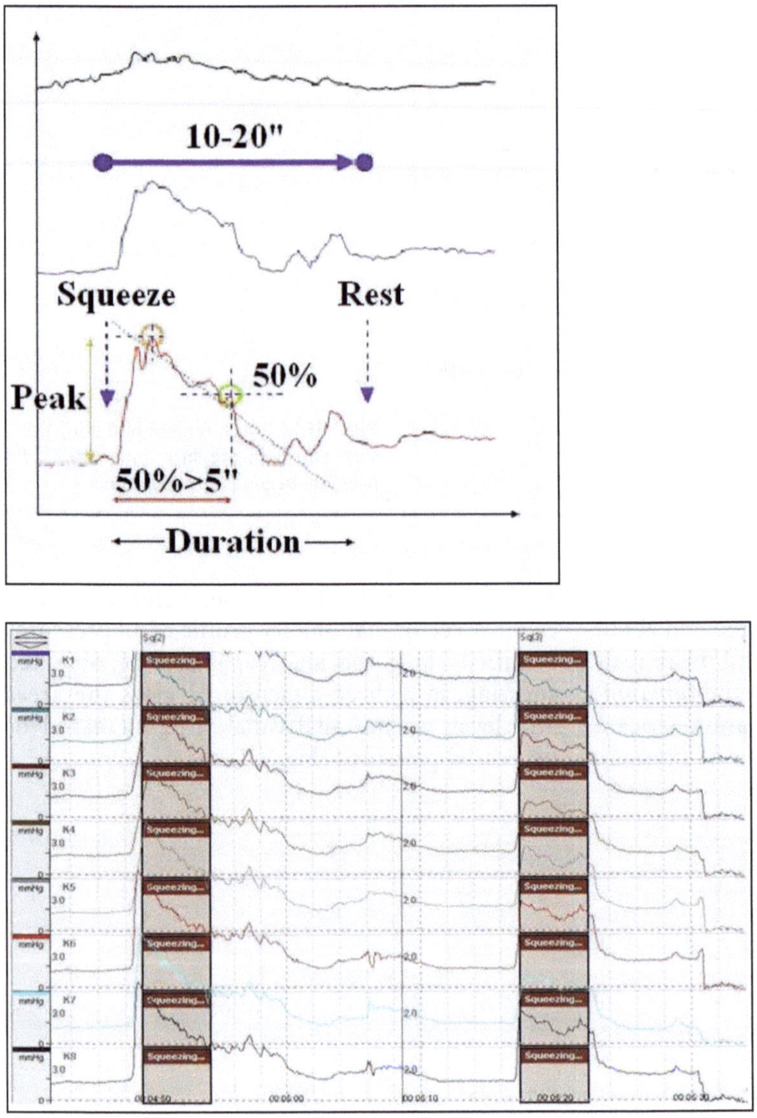

Fig. VII.13. Measurement of squeezing pressure (**a, b**)

With the catheter placed in the HPZ, the patient is asked to squeeze as much and as long as possible in order to calculate *maximum squeeze pressure*. The estimated characteristics of squeeze pressure are essentially the absolute pressure level (normal range: 90–180 mmHg), the difference from basal pressure (normal range: two to three times the baseline resting value), and the duration of contraction (Fig. VII.13). These parameters are expressions of striated muscle activity. The EAS should normally stay contracted for at least 3–5 s. Less than 3 s is considered abnormal. Squeeze pressure is unequally distributed. The pressures are radially equal in the middle of the anal canal while in the proximal anal canal, the pressure is highest posteriorly and lowest anteriorly because of the force provided by the puborectalis. Also during the voluntary squeezing, a vector manometry can be obtained. Moreover, pressures can be recorded during straining to investigate the normal decrease (expression of relaxation of both IAS and EAS) or, otherwise, a paradoxical increase or lack of decrease of resting pressure in pathological conditions (anismus and pelvic floor muscles incoordination).

A confirmation of anismus is obtained with the *balloon expulsion test*. This test is performed by asking patients to expel on a commode a water-filled balloon placed in the rectum in order to explore defecation pattern. Water is instilled into a 10-cm-long latex balloon. The total volume intro-

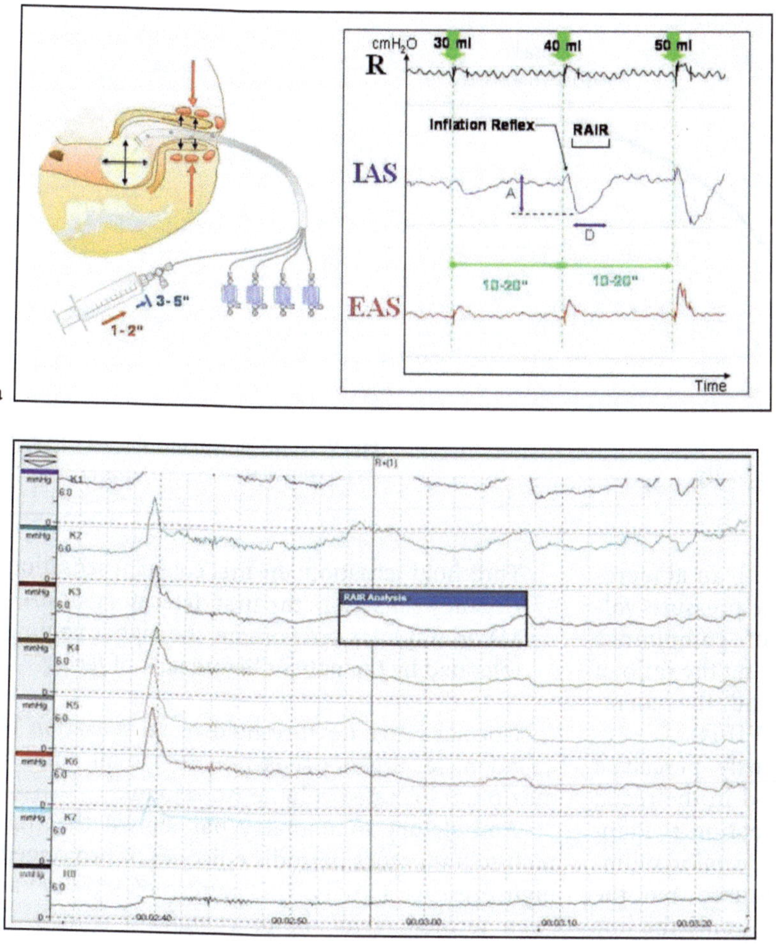

a

b

Fig. VII.14. Rectoanal inhibitory reflex (RAIR): rectal balloon inflation elicits inhibition of the internal anal sphincter (*IAS*) with decreasing of resting tone and contractile response of the external anal sphincter (*EAS*). *R* rectum, *A* amplitude, *D* duration (**a**). The graph shows a normal RAIR (**b**)

duced is the minimum required to induce sustained desire to defecate. The test is considered normal if the balloon can be expelled in <60 s. It is important to individualize the volume of water used to fill the balloon because a sustained feeling of defecation is necessary to start the defecatory maneuver. The use of a volume insufficient to achieve a constant desire to defecate would overdiagnose anismus.

The study of *rectoanal inhibitory reflex* (RAIR) is usually performed with the catheter within the HPZ (measuring anal canal pressures during reflex) and the balloon located in the rectum. The operator rapidly inflates the balloon with air (or water), eliciting the following events (Fig. VII.14):

- Rectal contraction consequent to the perception of the balloon, which mimics stools; this contraction induces the balloon to proceed to the anal canal reaching the sensitive mucosa
- Relaxation of the IAS, with a prompt decrease of resting pressure proportional in amplitude and duration to the intensity of the stimulus. Usually, this relaxation does not proceed to a complete weakness of the anus in order to avoid lack of feces, the physiologic meaning being only to ascertain the presence of stools to be evacuated (sampling reflex)
- Contraction of the EAS, sending back the balloon into the rectum and recovering the previous anal resting pressure; physiologically, this phase allows the patient to delay defecation in an appropriate time and condition.

The minimal volume required to elicit the IAS relaxation (decrease in pressure 10–15 mmHg) is defined (n.v.: present with volumes of 10–20 ml). Increasing the inflation of air or water, the RAIR threshold and the best relaxation/contraction profile can be determined.

Rectal compliance is studied with the balloon placed in the rectum and the catheter within the

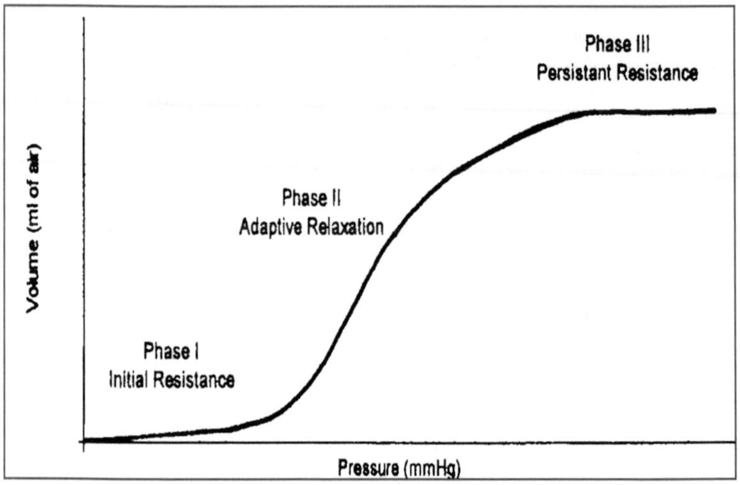

Fig. VII.15. The sigmoid-shaped curve of rectal compliance

anal HPZ. The balloon is inflated with air at increments of 30–60 ml. The slope of the pressure-volume curve allows calculation of compliance ($\Delta V/\Delta P$), maximum compliance being the ratio of the maximal tolerable volume and the corresponding measured pressure (Fig. VII.15).

Rectal sensations are consciously perceived during inflation of a balloon placed in the rectal ampulla. This phase of the examination is inappropriately named as a part of anorectal manometry because no pressure is measured, but the same catheter can be used. Actually, only the line connected to the balloon is needed: the balloon is slowly and progressively inflated with air (or water), and the patient is asked to indicate the following three levels of rectal sensation:

- Threshold sensation: the first constant sensation
- Urgency sensation: the first defecatory desire
- Maximum tolerated volume: the higher volume tolerated by the patient before lack of feces.

Normal range for threshold rectal sensation is 40–70 ml, for urgency sensation 60–130 ml, and for maximum tolerated volume 150–230 ml.

Ambulatory manometry has shown that the rectum undergoes periodic episodes of prolonged high-pressure activity. This pattern of activity has been termed *rectal motor complexes* (RMC). A typical RMC consists of a burst of regular pressure fluctuations from 20 to 60 mmHg with a frequency of three or six cycles per minute and duration from 3-to 30 min (Fig. VII.16). The nature and the function of this activity is poorly under-

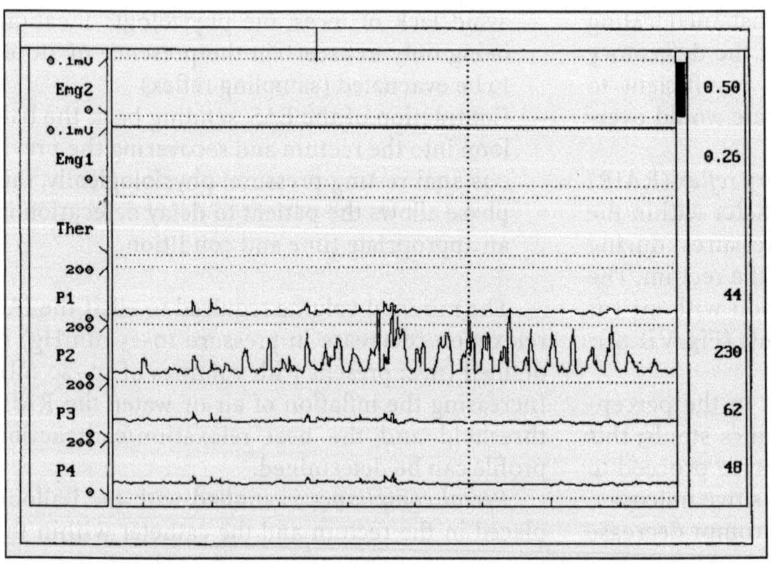

Fig. VII.16. Typical rectal motor complex

stood. Sleep results in a reduction of rectal motor activity whereas a meal provides a stimulus for increased rectal motor activity.

Indications for Anorectal Manometry and Findings

Patient history and physical examination (particularly digital) can indicate the need of performing anorectal manometry. Several symptoms could be suggestive of anorectal functional disorders: constipation (particularly obstructed defecation and rectal prolapse), incomplete evacuation, straining during defecation, necessity of digitation to evacuate, anal pain, tenesmus, minor or major incontinence, pruritus ani, previous anorectal trauma, surgery, malformation, central or peripheral nervous diseases, or metabolic diseases with suspected secondary anorectal disorders.

At the digital examination (at rest and during squeezing and straining), a few characteristics could indicate anorectal manometry: a tight or patulous anus with apparent hypertonic or hypotonic sphincters, respectively; lack of normal perianal plication; scars (including those located in the perivulvar/vaginal area); anal fissure; descent perineum; paradoxical sphincter contraction during straining; decreased squeezing; rectal prolapse.

Other procedures can be indicated in conjunction with anorectal manometry: anoscopy, endoscopy, myography, endoanal ultrasound (EAUS) and radiologic tests [defecography, computed tomography (CT) scan, magnetic resonance imaging (MRI)]. In most patients, only a multidisciplinary diagnostic evaluation allows the highest accuracy in clinical assessment, this being the appropriate way of planning effective treatment [1–4].

The only functional disease in which anorectal manometry has a primary role in diagnosis is Hirschsprung's disease. In this clinical condition, frequent in children presenting with constipation due to aganglionosis of the bowel, manometry demonstrates the absence of RAIR irrespective of volumes of air inflated. Similar manometric (and functional) features can be observed in patients with a significantly reduced number of bowel ganglia.

Increased resting pressure is the most frequently associated manometric finding in patients with an anal fissure; it can be observed also in patients with constipation, either idiopathic or associated with other pelvic floor disorders (obstructed defecation, rectocele, enterocele, internal intussusception, anismus, internal sphincter hypertrophia). The resting pressure profile should be accurately evaluated (distinguishing total or distal hypertonic anal canal) to explain pathophysiology of the disorder and choose the appropriate therapy. On the other hand, a decreased resting pressure can be found in patients with minor (soiling or seepage, incontinence to flatus) or major incontinence (to liquid or solid stools), idiopathic, secondary to anal traumatic or surgical (not only for anal diseases but, unfortunately, also due to obstetric causes) events, or neurogenic and metabolic diseases; moreover, IAS atrophy shows reduced resting pressure.

Detailed analysis of pressures recorded from each channel as well as data from vector manometry can be of help in identifying the site of a possible sphincter lesion. However, even if study of the pressure profile is of primary importance in the diagnostic assessment, manometric data should be related to other diagnostic findings, particularly from EAUS or MRI, which seems more accurate in locating site(s) and extent of sphincter defect(s).

A decreased squeeze pressure is a manometric sign of reduced activity of striated muscle (including EAS, puborectalis muscle, and, at large, levator ani muscle). It could be due to an EAS lesion (secondary to trauma or obstetric or anal surgery) or to idiopathic or neurogenic muscle insufficiency. Also, in case of reduced squeeze pressure, analysis of pressure profile characteristics and vector manometry is useful, as well as the myographic evaluation, but EAUS or MRI are more accurate in determining the precise morphology of sphincter lesions.

As mentioned above, the balloon expulsion test is a simple and meaningful phase of manometric study, identifying patients with impairment of normal defecation during straining. Inability to push out the balloon may reflect lack of sphincter relaxation (functional outlet constipation) or mechanical obstruction. This test has not been proved to be of clinical value, but it helps to identify patients with pelvic dyssynergia, defined as paradoxical contraction or failure to relax the pelvic floor muscles during attempts to defecate.

Abnormalities of functional anal canal length can be frequently observed: higher values in hypertonic anal canal; lower values in patients with sequelae of anal surgery or fecal incontinence. These features need to be correlated to other manometric and nonmanometric findings.

Except for Hirschsprung's disease, just what diagnostic role should be attributed to the modifications of RAIR characteristics (threshold, rate and duration of relaxation, and contraction) is not well defined. Especially, loss of proportionality between intensity of the stimulus and amplitude and duration of RAIR, eventually associated with abnormalities of rectal sensation, or the absence or significant reduction of anal contraction during voluntary squeeze may indicate central neurologic disease. Rectal compliance presents increased values in patients with rectal hypotonia while it can be decreased when a prevalence of fibrosis of the rectal wall is present (inflammatory bowel disease or chronic sequelae of high-dose pelvic radiation therapy).

Abnormalities of rectal sensations play a major role in several functional disorders of defecation. Increased levels of rectal sensation parameters can be frequently found in patients with chronic constipation; in these cases, a larger amount of feces is necessary to elicit awareness of defecation need, and, consequently, the patient delays evacuation too long. Similar manometric alterations are also frequently found in patients with megarectum or obstructed defecation in presence of rectocele, internal intussusception, or rectal prolapse. Pathophysiology of these abnormalities involves the afferent/efferent nerve supply to the rectal wall and perirectal space, particularly nerve endings (thought as desensitized) and nerve fibers (toward the pudendal nerves, which could be altered by muscle and nerve stretching that occur frequently during straining). Moreover, chronically constipated patients (in particular, older and institutionalized subjects) could present increased rectal sensation with pseudoincontinence due to the passive passage of liquid stools (not perceived because of too high a threshold of rectal sensation) between rectal wall and large and hard, solid stools in the rectal lumen. Also, decreased rectal sensations are frequently observed, in particular in subjects with hypersensitized nerve receptors. This condition is typical of patients with inflammatory bowel disease or treated with high-dose pelvic radiation therapy and who complain of frequent tenesmus as well as soiling or transient episodes of major incontinence.

No univocal alterations of rectal sensation (increased or decreased levels) can be recorded in patients presenting with similar clinical condition, either constipation or incontinence. This is possibly due to a secondary deregulation of the physiologic balance between the different nervous systems (sympathetic, parasympathetic, somatic, motor, sensory, etc.) involved in the complex defecation (and voiding) functions. Damage of one system could impact the others with prevalence of their functions. Pelvic nerve damage secondary to pelvic surgery (frequently for gynecologic reasons or rectal tumors) is more frequently associated with higher levels of rectal sensations and subsequent constipation (and urinary retention). Also, patients with partial or complete spinal cord injury could present increased rectal sensation parameters associated with constipation (and urinary retention). A number of patients with neurogenic fecal incontinence not due to sphincteric lesions present different patterns of rectal sensations, including increased, decreased, or even normal levels. These clinical and manometric conditions are under investigation in order to elucidate more detailed aspects of the influence of sensory functions on normal and altered defecation and the impact of specific therapies (i.e., sacral neuromodulation) on their improvement.

Anorectal Electrophysiology

This diagnostic approach includes a few tests directed to patients already investigated with history and physical assessment and other procedures (mainly manometry and ultrasound) in whom pelvic muscular and/or nervous functions seem to be altered. Electrophysiological tests used to study the anorectum are derived from myographic and nerve conduction examinations performed in other parts of the body, and over the last 20 years an evolution of instruments, techniques of examination, and indications has been registered [5]. These tests add important additional information on the physiology of defecation and continence [1–3, 5].

Technique of Anorectal Electrophysiology

Electrophysiological studies are usually carried out using a neuromyography system equipped with software dedicated to anorectal physiological evaluation (Fig. VII.17). The examination includes tests evaluating electrical muscle activity and nerve functionality [5]. In performing such tests,

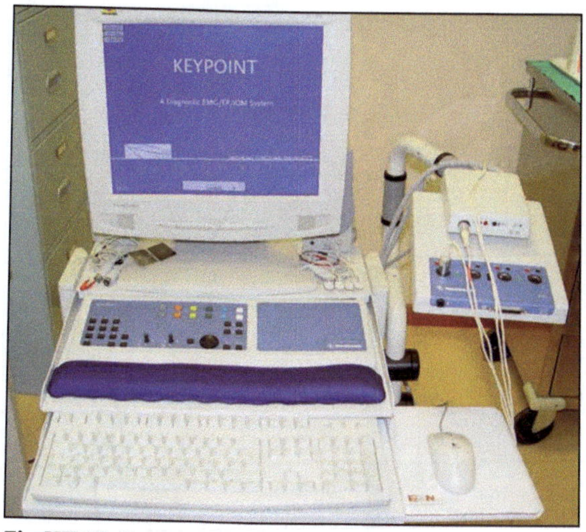

Fig. VII.17. Keypoint electromyographic system (Medtronic)

either a recording function or an electrostimulating function or both can be requested. The neuromyographic instrument needs to be connected to dedicated cables and electrodes. As with anorectal manometry, before anorectal electrophysiology, an enema is usually required to clean the rectal ampulla; thus, when available, both examinations could be performed in the same session (electrophysiology must follow manometry in order to avoid sphincters manipulation before measurements of resting pressures). The most preferred patient position during this procedure is the left lateral, and a ground electrode soaked in normal saline is placed around the thigh.

The purpose of *electromyography* (EMG) is to investigate electrical activity of the EAS and the other striated pelvic floor muscles at rest and during squeezing and straining. Over time, four different types of electrodes have been developed: concentric needle, monopolar wire, single-fiber electrode, and surface electrode (Fig. VII.18). The concentric needle electrode consists of a thin needle (0.1 mm in diameter) covered by an insulating resin, which is able to uptake electrical activity of the small area into which it has been inserted; this needle is unable to record single muscle fiber action potentials. Under the guidance of digital anal exploration, the needle must be inserted into the EAS or puborectalis muscle; recordings from the four anal canal quadrants should be obtained (Fig. VII.19). This procedure is quite uncomfortable for the patient; the electrode could slide in a different position during trace acquisition and, even if multiple recording samples are taken, the mapping obtained is far from being considered sufficient to delineate accurately the area of normal and abnormal muscle. The monopolar wire should reduce the patient's discomfort and avoid the electrode sliding because it is kept in site by a small hook placed at the electrode tip. The single-fiber electrode is thinner than the monopolar wire and is able to record individual motor unit potentials. An appropriate amplification of the signals recorded is necessary. Also, fiber density can be calculated based on 20 different recordings from each anal hemisphere. Evaluation with the single-fiber electrode is more accurate than the two electrodes previously described but remains uncomfortable. Surface electrodes, mounted on an endoanal plug or a small external adhesive plaque, are able to record gross muscle activity but unable

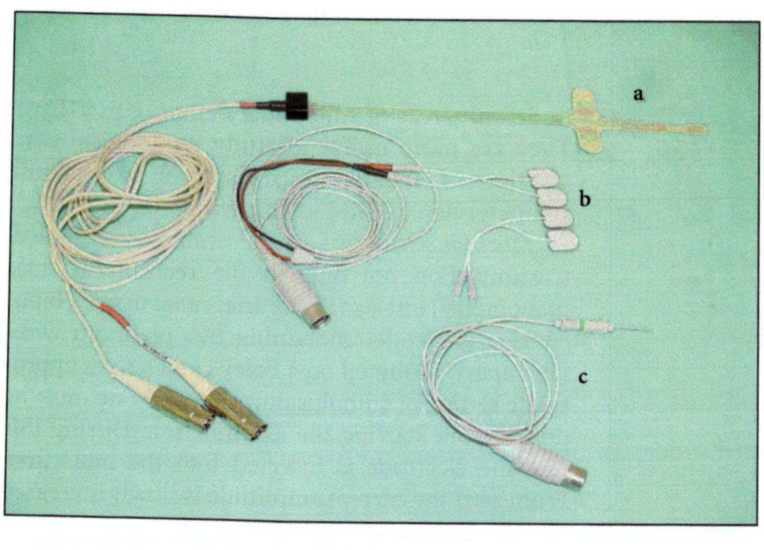

Fig. VII.18. St. Mark's pudendal electrode (**a**), surface electrodes (**b**), and needle electrode (**c**)

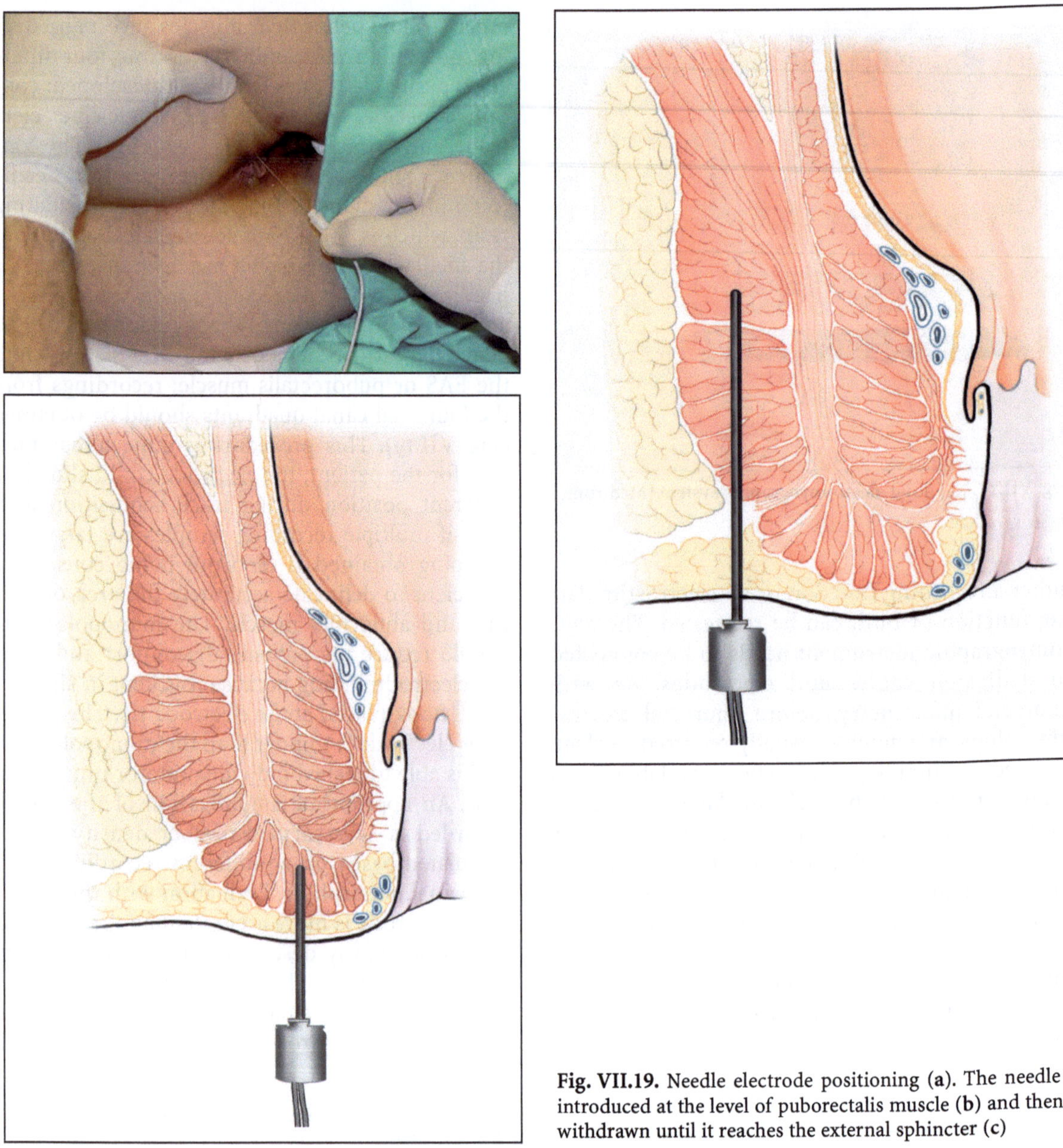

a

b

c

Fig. VII.19. Needle electrode positioning (**a**). The needle is introduced at the level of puborectalis muscle (**b**) and then is withdrawn until it reaches the external sphincter (**c**)

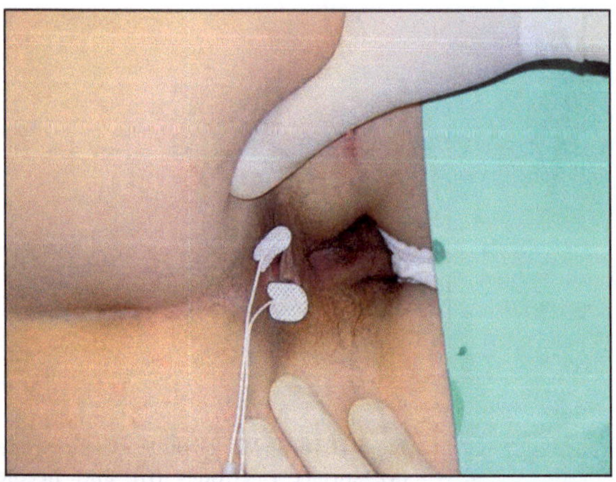

Fig. VII.20. Surface electrodes positioning

to delimit areas of functional deficit (Fig. VII.20). They are more useful to study paradoxical contraction of striated muscles than to evaluate sphincter damage in incontinent patients.

Mucosal sensitivity can be evaluated with electrostimulation not only in the rectum (as does manometry) but also in the anal canal using a bipolar ring electrode (containing two platinum wires 1 cm apart) mounted on a Foley catheter. An appropriate setting of stimulus duration and rate must be done before starting the examination. During this test, the electrode is inserted into the anus first. From zero, the current amplitude is slowly increased

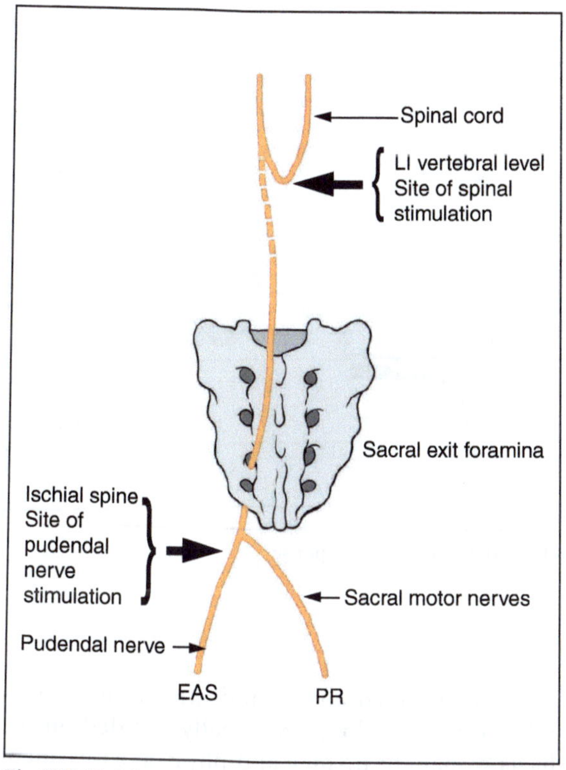

Fig. VII.21. Schematic representation of anal sphincter innervation. *EAS* external anal sphincter, *PR* puborectalis muscle

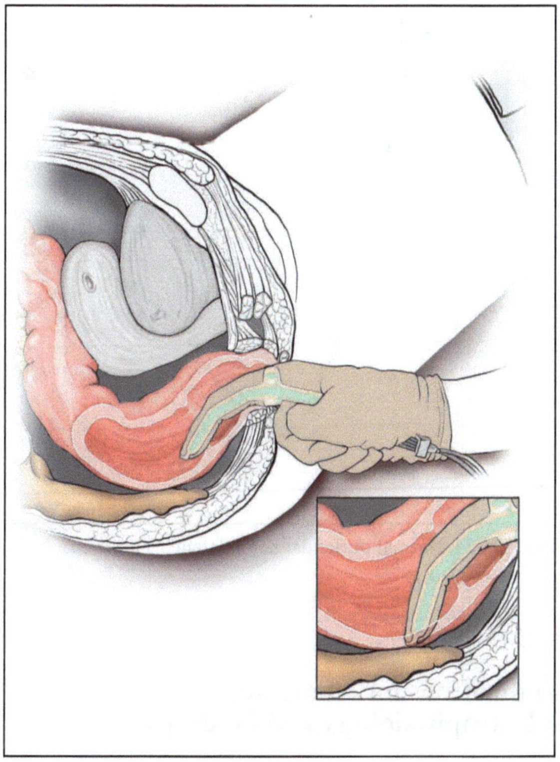

Fig. VII.23. Schematic representation of pudendal nerve stimulation

until the patient feels a buzzing or tingling sensation in the anus. At least three measurements need to be taken, choosing the lower threshold value for the report. A similar procedure is used for mucosal sensitivity analysis in the rectum. Rectal ampulla must be reached by the electrode; under slowly increasing current (parameters setting is different than that used for the anal sensitivity test), three values should be obtained, taking the lowest as the rectal threshold sensation to be reported.

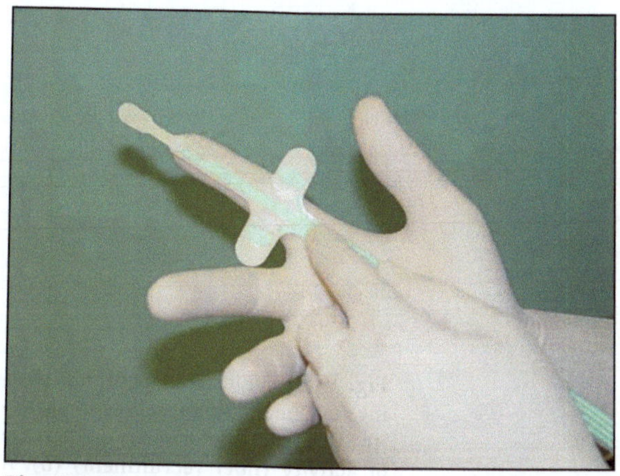

Fig. VII.22. St. Mark's pudendal electrode (13L40, Dantec Electronics, Bristol, UK) used for recording pudendal motor nerve latencies

Finally, *pudendal nerve terminal motor latency* (PNTML) is measured, allowing the evaluation of pelvic floor neuromuscular integrity (Fig. VII.21). A disposable St. Mark's pudendal electrode is used, mounted onto the volar side of the examiner's gloved index finger (Fig. VII.22). The index finger is inserted into the rectum, the finger tip reaching the course of each pudendal nerve and the proximal phalanx sited within the anal canal (Fig. VII.23). During this test, both electrostimulation and recording function need to be activated. Four cables run within the electrode, conveying stimuli (0.1 or 0.2 ms duration, 1 s. interval, not exceeding 15 mA) from the machine to the finger tip (to the anode and cathode) in order to stimulate the pudendal nerve fibers and from the finger tip to the machine to record the striated muscle response visualized on the screen. The latency (expressed in milliseconds) from the onset of the stimulus to the first deflection of the response is calculated for each pudendal nerve (n.v.: 2.0±0.2 ms) (Fig. VII.24).

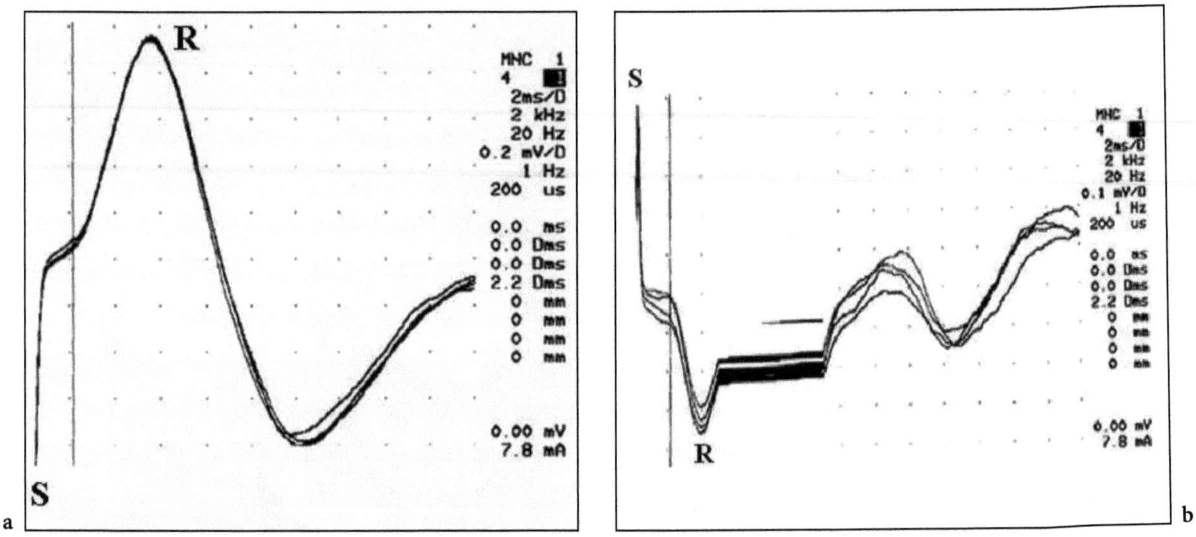

Fig. VII.24. Normal pudendal nerve latencies on the right (**a**) and left (**b**). *S* stimulus, *R* response

Indications for Anorectal Electrophysiology and Findings

In healthy subjects, the introduction of a needle electrode is followed by a reactive discharge of motor unit potentials. The pelvic floor muscles, which include the levator ani, the puborectalis muscle, and the EAS, have continuous tonic EMG activity at rest. Squeeze determines an increase of activity (fiber recruitment) while a decrease or electrical silence is observed during attempted defecation (push) (Fig. VII.25).

As mentioned above, indications for anorectal electrophysiology are usually decided on the basis of patient history and physical assessment if pelvic muscular and/or nervous disorders are hypothesized; moreover, data from other diagnostic procedures (mainly manometry and ultrasound) should confirm the need to submit the patient to the anorectal electrophysiology [1–3, 5].

In constipated patients, EMG is used to demonstrate a paradoxical puborectalis contraction or lack of relaxation. In this condition, stri-

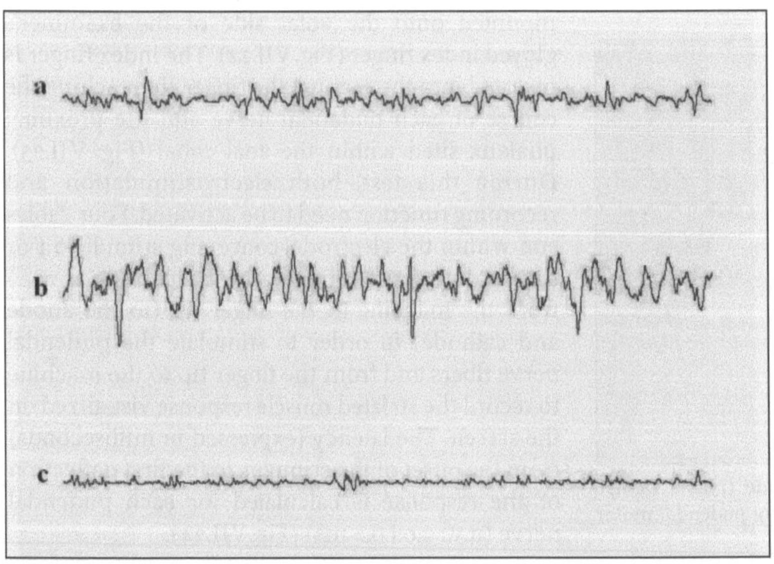

Fig. VII.25. Electromyographic findings in a healthy subject. Resting activity (**a**). Squeeze determines an increase of activity (fiber recruitment) (**b**). A decrease or electrical silence is observed during attempted defecation (**c**)

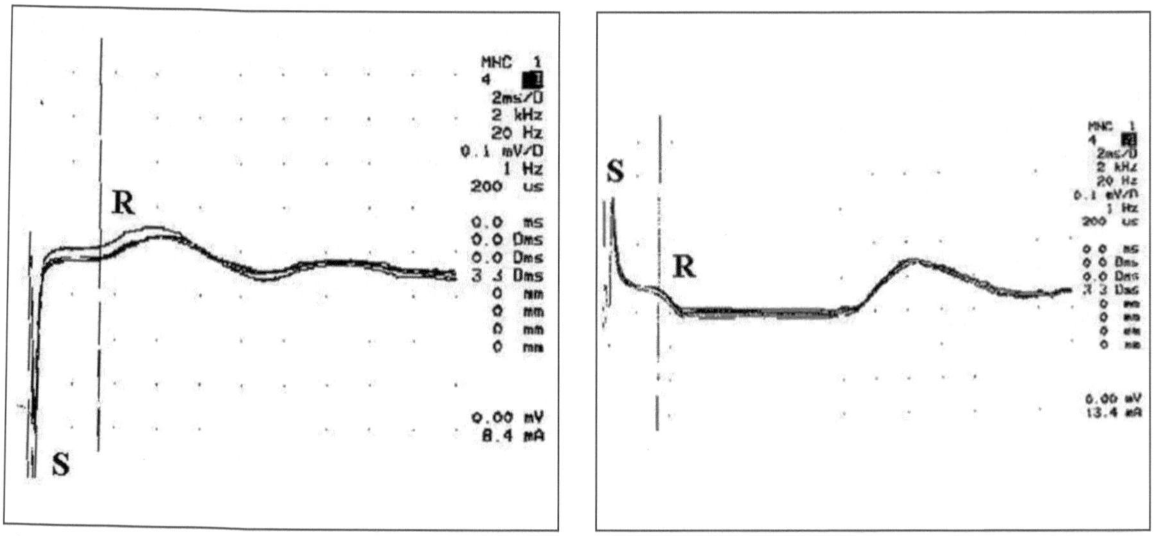

a b

Fig. VII.26. Abnormal prolonged pudendal nerve latencies on the right (**a**) and left (**b**). *S* stimulus, *R* response

ated muscle activity recorded during straining is either increased or not changed when compared with at-rest activity. These findings could be related to a paradoxical increase or unchanging anal pressure during straining observed with manometry. EMG features of pelvic floor incoordination is frequently observed even if a large number of false positive results need to be considered; indeed, a significant number of patients with this EMG result do not complain of relevant constipation, so that it needs to be critically evaluated. In cases of constipation and EMG demonstration of anismus, cinedefecography could also be useful.

In patients with sphincter lesions, no electrical activity can be found in case of wide, complete replacement of normal muscular tissue with scar or, more frequently, polyphasic potentials as signs of a reinnervation process may be registered. Polyphasic potentials present multiple spikes of muscle activity, prolonged in duration, and an increased fiber density. In evaluating sphincter injury, EAUS has higher sensitivity and specificity compared with EMG in mapping the lesion; however, only EMG can assess neuromuscular integrity. In this respect, these two procedures are complementary.

Evaluation of anal mucosal electrosensitivity could have clinical relevance in some clinical conditions. Apart from the alterations registered in patients with prolapsing hemorrhoids (higher threshold levels), in neurogenic incontinence, a wide spectrum of findings can be observed, probably related to the degree of pudendal neuropathy. Also, rectal sensation measurements by electrophysiology study are meaningful. In patients suffering constipation, threshold levels are frequently higher than normal even if this is not the rule. In incontinent patients with only sphincter lesion, mucosal electrosensitivity can be normal, whereas in those with neurogenic incontinence, a wide variability of findings can be found. Concerning manometric rectal sensation measurement, its meaning must be carefully interpreted and correlated with results from other tests.

The utility of PNTML measurements remains questionable; sensitivity and specificity are uncertain, and reproducibility between different examiners or on different days is unknown. Alterations of PNTML are identified in relation to patient age, being more frequent in older subjects. This is probably due to several reasons, including chronic straining in constipated patients, causing a perineal descent for continuous stretching of pudendal nerves. However, this feature is inconstant, and the direct relationship between pudendal neuropathy and constipation is not demonstrated. In a large number of patients with fecal incontinence (with or without urinary incontinence) and rectal prolapse, the PNTML is abnormally prolonged (Fig. VII.26). PNTML levels are thought to have a predicting value in patients undergoing treatment, but this assumption remains controversial.

References

1. Kamm MA (1994) Pelvic floor tests. In: Kamm MA, Lennard-Jones JE (eds) Constipation. Wrightson Biomedical, Hampshire, pp 145–153
2. Lubowski DZ, Kennedy ML (1997) Physiologic investigations. In: Nicholls RJ, Dozois RR (eds) Surgery of the colon and rectum. Churchill Livingstone, New York, pp 167–194
3. Moreira H, Wexner SD (1998) Anorectal physiology testing. In: Beck D, Wexner SD (eds) Fundamentals of anorectal surgery. WB Saunders, London, pp 37–53
4. Read NW, Sun WM (1990) Anorectal manometry. In: Henry MM, Swash M (eds) Coloproctology and the pelvic floor, 2nd edn. Butterworth Heinemann, pp 119–145
5. Swash M (1990) Electromyography in pelvic floor disorders. In: Henry MM, Swash M (eds) Coloproctology and the pelvic floor, 2nd edn. Butterworth Heinemann, pp 187–198

VII.3. What Studies do we Really Need in the Treatment of Benign Anorectal Diseases?

B. Cola, D. Cuicchi, R. Lombardi, P.F. Almerigi

Correct clinical management of benign anorectal disorders depends on a detailed understanding of the underlying physiopathological mechanisms. Technological innovations provide the specialist with functional investigation techniques and increasingly sophisticated imaging methods thanks to which the clinical examination, with its subjective nature, is backed up by the acquisition of information that makes it possible to quantify the physiological parameters and to observe the anatomical structures with a high degree of definition. The contribution of modern methods has been further expanded by their integration although there is as yet no agreement on the best combination of diagnostic tools to be used for the various individual conditions.

The aim of this chapter is to identify, based on the features of the various benign anoperineal disorders, a diagnostic standard justified by evidence that demonstrates their true clinical significance and the direct consequences on therapeutic management of patients.

Anal fissures and hemorrhoids are not dealt with due to the substantial simplicity of the diagnostic approach unanimously considered to be necessary. For both these disorders, diagnostic integration has very little influence on the indication for surgery, which is mostly determined by clinical assessment. It is, on the other hand, important in excluding associated diseases, such as tumors and inflammatory bowel disease, in documenting preoperative functional or organic alterations, and also for forensic purposes. Attention will therefore focus on three disorders of particular interest as regards diagnostic integration and its effects on therapy: perianal sepsis, fecal incontinence (FI), and obstructed defecation (OD).

Perianal Sepsis and Fistula-in-ano

The two most important failures of surgical treatment of anorectal sepsis are recurrences, due to an incomplete drainage of collections, and postoperative FI that may be caused by extensive surgical intervention [1]. The art of fistula surgery is therefore based on the right balance between treatment of the sepsis (eradication of tracks and drainage of any associated abscesses) and preservation of anal continence [2]. The key to achieving this aim is careful preoperative assessment directed at defining the topography of the fistula (the internal opening, the external opening, the course of the primary track, the presence of any secondary extensions) and its relationship with the anal sphincter complex.

Clinical history and physical examination are often sufficient for diagnosis. Anal exploration can be also carefully carried out under general anesthesia [examination under anesthesia (EUA)] immediately before the surgical approach (Fig. VII.27). In this way, fistula probing is less painful and clinical evaluation is more accurate than that performed in awake patients [3]. However, digital palpation may fail to depict complex fistulas or may lead to incorrect classification and determination of the height of the track [4]. It may also be difficult, in the case of recurrence, to distinguish the woody tissue caused by chronic sepsis from scar tissue [4].

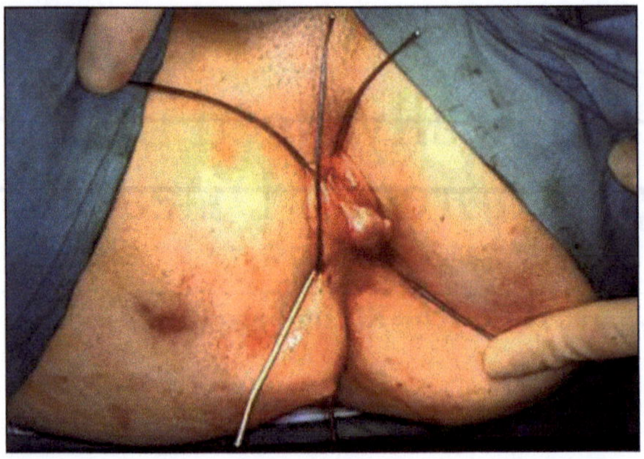

Fig. VII.27. Multiple fistula probing in perianal Crohn's disease

The main aim of preoperative imaging is to identify unsuspected areas of sepsis so that they can be targeted for subsequent treatment and to define their relationship with the anal sphincter complex more accurately.

Fistulography

Fistulography is the most traditional radiological technique for defining fistula anatomy. It is not expensive and is readily available, but its results are difficult to interpret for two main reasons: (1) the relationship between the fistula and the sphincter muscle and, above all, the level of internal opening can be only guessed because the sphincter complex is not visualized (Fig. VII.28), and (2) secondary extensions can be missed if they are plugged with purulent secretions. Fistulography can be helpful when an extrasphincteric fistula is suspected in the presence of an external opening distant from the anus and without abnormality of the anal canal.

In a retrospective study comparing fistulographic and operative findings in 25 patients, Kuijpers and Schulpen [5] reported that fistulography allowed a correct interpretation in only 16% of cases, with an accuracy of 24% in recognizing an internal opening into the anal canal. Fistulography has been shown to be an inaccurate and unreliable method of investigation in defining fistula anatomy and today has only a historical value.

Computed Tomography Scanning

Computed tomography (CT) scanning has not acquired an important role in the assessment of perianal sepsis. The main reason is the poor intrinsic tissue contrast: the pelvic muscles are not well identified, and their relationship with tracks can only be inferred [6] (Fig. VII.29). CT is also an expensive technique, and it is hampered by risks related to the use of ionizing radiations and contrast media.

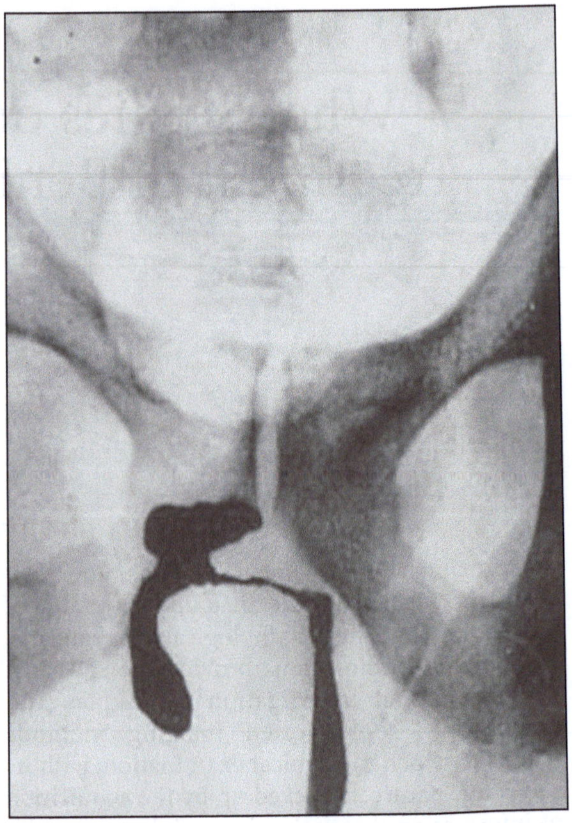

Fig. VII.28. Horseshoe fistula with secondary extension toward upper level

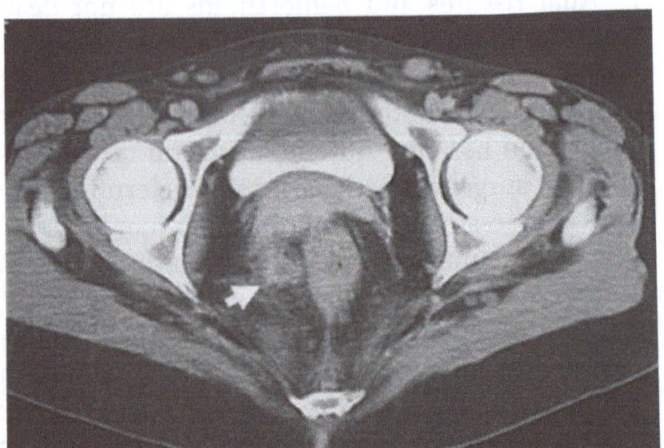

Fig. VII.29. Right lateral pelvirectal abscess (*arrow*)

Endoanal Ultrasonography

Endoanal ultrasonography (EAUS) is based on ultrasound reflection at the interface between tissues with different densities of acoustic impedance [7]. The use of EAUS in the study of anoperineal suppurative disorders was revised after the initial enthusiasm. In the early 1990s, Choen et al. [8] reported a degree of accuracy that was no higher than the clinical evaluation carried out by expert operators although at that time the criteria for interpreting ultrasonography findings had still not been clearly defined. The contribution of several studies published subsequently made it possible to increase the accuracy of the method through identification of validated criteria [9, 10].

The method does, however, have some significant limitations, such as the difficulty in differentiating scar areas from active lesions and the limited visual field that makes it difficult to identify secondary extensions far away from the probe. The use of hydrogen peroxide (H_2O_2) as a contrast media inside the fistula tracks and abscesses, described for the first time in 1993 by Cheong et al., [11] has reduced these limitations and made identification of the internal opening easier, making EAUS one of the main techniques used to distinguish perianal sepsis (Fig. VII.30).

Poen et al. [12] compared intraoperative findings in 21 patients with results of the clinical examination, the standard scan, and the hydrogen peroxide enhanced ultrasound (HPUS). With the use of the contrast medium, the fistula track was identified in 95% of patients compared with 62% at the standard EAUS scan and 38% at the clinical examination while localization of the internal opening was possible in only 48% of cases.

In a more recent study, Navarro-Luna et al. [13] compared surgical findings with results of HPUS in 80 patients with complex or recurrent fistulas. The percentage of agreement as regards identification of fistula level and internal opening and detection of chronic fistula tracks was 91%, 85%, and 75%, respectively. The authors concluded HPUS performed by colorectal surgeons with appropriate experience makes it possible to achieve excellent results in the preoperative assessment of anal fistulas.

Buchanan et al. [14] reviewed the diagnostic value of H_2O_2 in distinguishing recurrent and complex fistulas and found no statistically significant differences between three-dimensional (3-D) EAUS with and without H_2O_2 as regards identification of the internal opening (p=1), level of the fistula track (p=0.072), and secondary extensions (p=1).

In a study on 102 patients with cryptogenic anal fistulas undergoing EAUS-guided surgery, Ratto et al. [15] reported a recurrence rate of 2% and no case of postoperative incontinence. Basing their surgical decisions on US findings, they report that it is possible to perform curative surgery in a significantly high number of patients without impairing sphincteral continence.

Endoanal ultrasound is a simple method, quick to perform, inexpensive, safe, and widely available. For all these reasons, it must be considered the first study to be carried out in distinguishing perianal sepsis, and in expert hands, it also plays an important part in the assessment of complex and recurrent fistulas.

Magnetic Resonance Imaging

Magnetic resonance imaging (MRI) has acquired growing importance in distinguishing perianal sepsis thanks to the excellent intrinsic tissue contrast and the multiple scanning planes (Fig. VII.31). This method accurately defines the topography of the septic process and, by identifying the septic areas missed with EUA, it is also able to modify the surgical approach in a significant number of patients [4].

In an attempt to quantify the added clinical value of MRI with respect to anal EUA alone, Beets-Tan et al. [16] reported changes to the surgical approach in 21% of cases. This percentage rose to 24% in the group of patients with recurrent fistulas and to 40% in the group with perianal Crohn's disease while only 8% of subjects with simple fistulas benefited from the additional information provided by MRI.

In a study performed in 71 patients with recurrent fistulas in which the results of MRI were revealed at the end of the surgical operation, Buchanan et al. [17] reported agreement between MRI and EUA findings in 25 patients (35%). In the remaining cases, the decision to perform an MR-guided surgical revision was left to the discretion of the surgeon: in 15 patients (21%), an in-depth clinical examination was decided on, leading to further agreement between the two assessments, showing a true therapeutic impact of the method in these cases, while in the remaining 31 patients (44%), the sur-

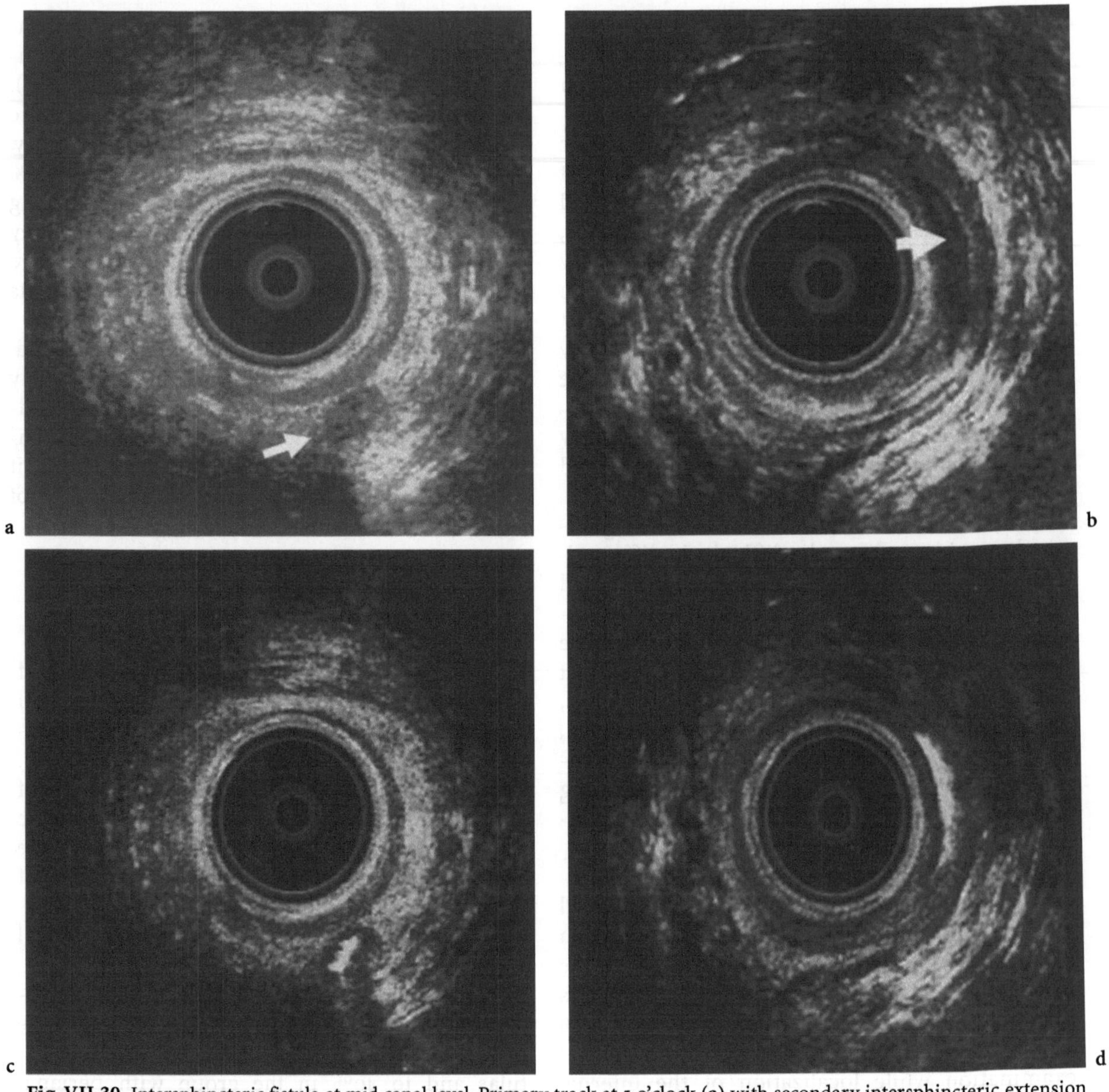

Fig. VII.30. Intersphincteric fistula at mid canal level. Primary track at 5 o'clock (a) with secondary intersphincteric extension (b) (*arrows*). After hydrogen peroxide enhancement both primary and secondary tracks are more clearly visible (c, d)

gical approach was not changed and the disagreement between MRI and EUA remained. At a mean follow-up of 1 year, only 13% of patients (5/40) in whom the two assessments agreed developed a recurrence compared with 52% (16/31) of cases in which the disagreement remained (p=0.0005). In addition, in this last group, all recurrences developed at sites indicated by preoperative MRI. This study demonstrated that, with regard to recurrent fistulas, MR-guided surgery can reduce the rate of recurrence by approximately 75%.

In a more recent prospective study, the same authors [18] applied the same study design to a sample of 30 patients with simple fistulas. MRI guided the surgical revision in only three patients (10%), showing the presence of two internal openings missed during the initial surgery, while surgical revision was not performed in 12 cases (40%) despite the disagreement between MRI and EUA. At a mean follow-up of 12 months, no recurrences were observed, suggesting a lesser clinical impact of MRI in the assessment of simple fistulas.

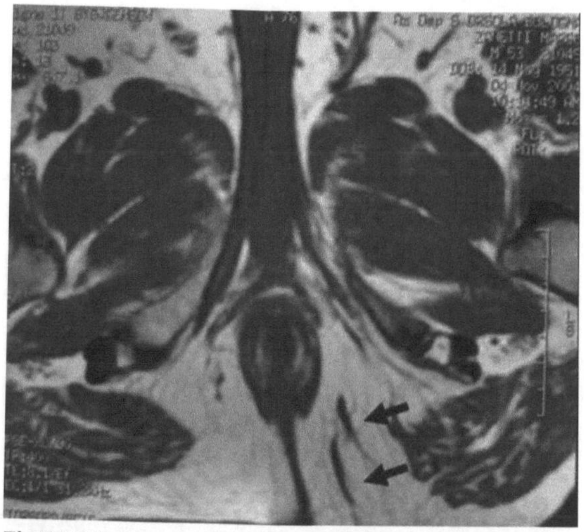

Fig. VII.31. Scar tissue in left ischioanal fossa (*arrows*)

Evidence [16, 17] shows that MRI is a powerful and validated diagnostic tool that, especially in complex and recurrent fistulas, is able to increase the percentage of success of surgical treatment.

Magnetic Resonance Imaging with an Endoanal Coil

The use of an endoluminal coil makes it possible to obtain images in which fistula tracks inside the sphincter complex and the site of the internal opening are displayed with greater resolution than with an external coil. However, since image definition decreases as the distance from the coil increases, this method is less accurate in distinguishing tracks that are far away from the anal sphincter [4]. This method has two other significant limitations: it is not widely available, and it is quite expensive [2].

Diagnostic Integration

In the preoperative assessment of perianal sepsis, EAUS and MRI should be considered as complementary rather than antagonistic techniques (Fig. VII.32) [4]. A number of studies have compared the results of MRI and EAUS in distinguishing perianal septic lesions; however, only two studies used a more accurate gold standard than the mere surgical specimen, thus being more precise. In 19 patients with complex Crohn's disease fistulas, Schwartz et al. [19] compared the accuracy of biplanar ultrasound, MRI, and EUA, considering as the gold standard the unanimous agreement reached by operators in cases of initial disagreement between the three assessments. The study showed almost identical accuracy: ultrasound and surgical assessment correctly identified 91% of lesions and MRI 87%. Since a combination of any two studies achieved almost 100% accuracy, and considering that 53% of patients required surgery, the authors suggest that EUA should be combined with one of the two imaging techniques.

Buchanan et al. [1] recently evaluated the accuracy of the clinical examination, EAUS, and MRI, considering the outcome of MR-guided surgery as the reference gold standard in the event of agreement between radiological method and EUA and the clinical follow-up in the event of disagreement, following the principle whereby healing of a fistula represents the only guarantee of complete eradication of the septic sites. In a series of 108 patients (27% simple fistulas and 73% complex fistulas, 9% of which were Crohn's fistulas) it emerged that clinical examination, EAUS, and MRI correctly classified the primary tracks in 61%, 81%, and 90% of cases and the internal openings in 78%, 91%, and 97% of cases, respectively. The accuracy of the three methods decreased in identifying abscesses and horse-shoe secondary extensions (36%, 70%, and 88% respectively). The authors concluded that EAUS is closer in accuracy to MRI than are clinical examination and that EAUS is particularly useful in defining primary tracks and internal openings. On the contrary, it is less precise in identifying secondary lesions.

In conclusion, evidence suggests that EAUS should be considered a first-level investigation method in distinguishing perianal sepsis. Although clinical examination is often sufficient for low and simple fistulas, the low cost, simplicity and ability to identify preexisting sphincter defects justify the use of EAUS even in these patients. The high degree of accuracy of MRI in identifying secondary tracks and in differentiating fibrosis from sepsis makes this method particularly useful in distinguishing complex lesions and recurrent fistulas (Fig. VII.33 and 34).

Fecal Incontinence

Fecal incontinence (FI) is a symptom common to various disorders that can alter one or more of the mechanisms involved in maintaining continence

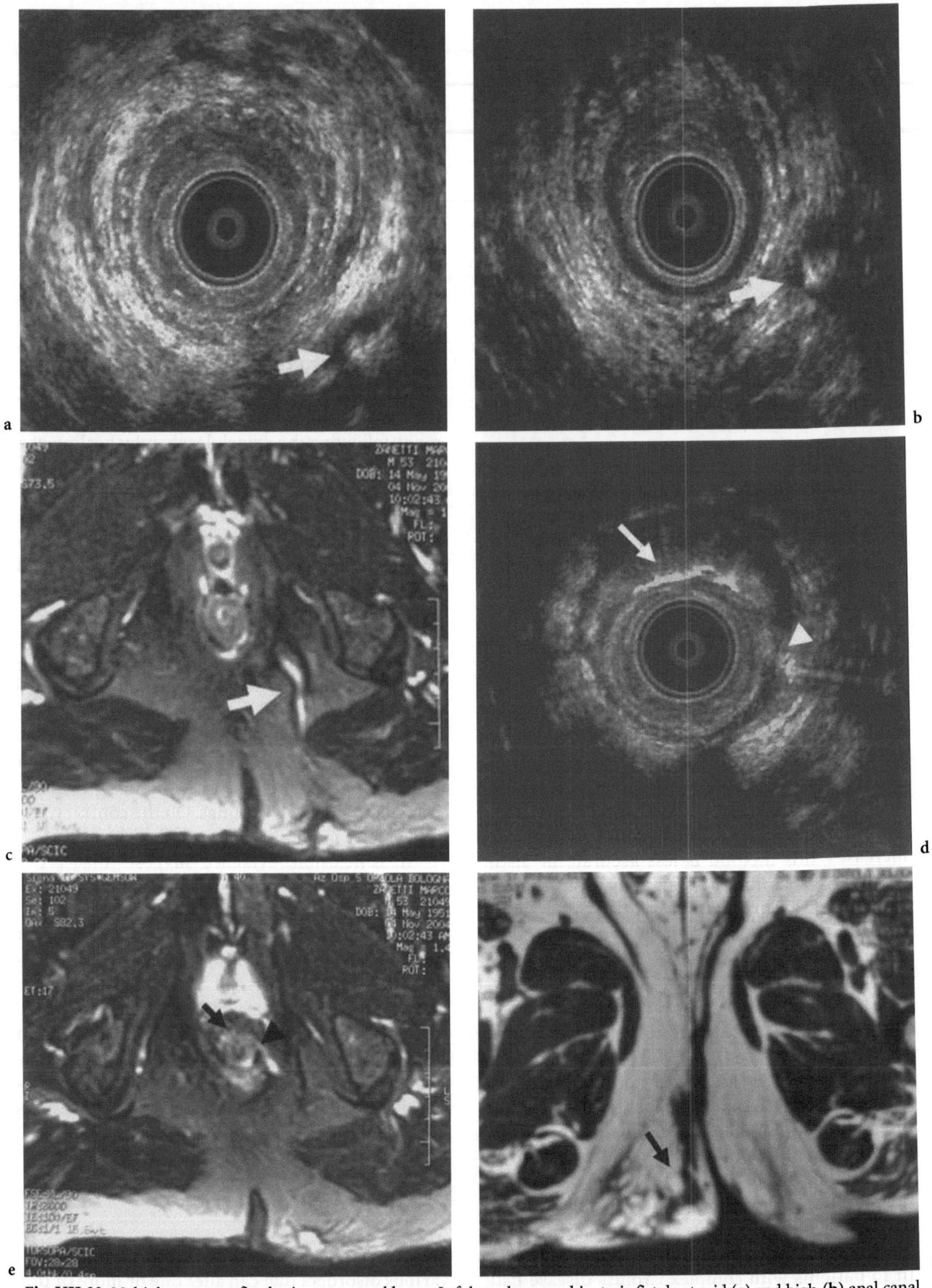

Fig. VII.32. Multiple recurrent fistulas in a 54-year-old man. Left lateral suprasphincteric fistula at mid (**a**) and high (**b**) anal canal level after administration of hydrogen peroxide on endoanal ultrasound (*arrows*). The same primary fistula on magnetic resonance imaging (MRI) (*arrow*) (**c**). Supralevator anterior horseshoe extension (*arrow*) with internal opening in the left anterior quadrant (*arrowhead*) on endoanal ultrasound (**d**) and MRI (**e**). Area of fibrosis located far from the sphincter on MRI (*arrow*) (**f**)

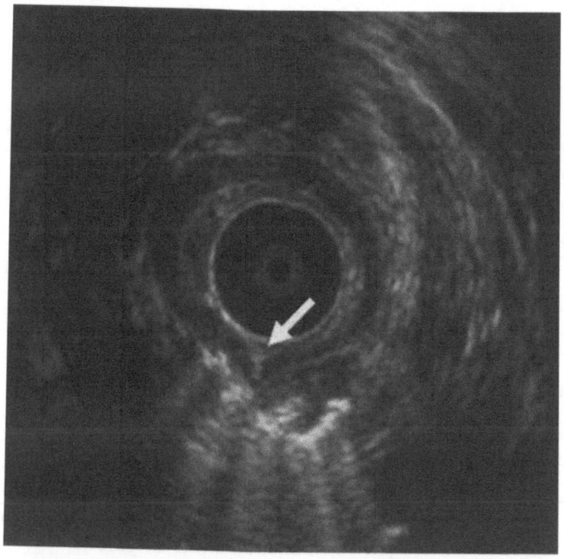
a

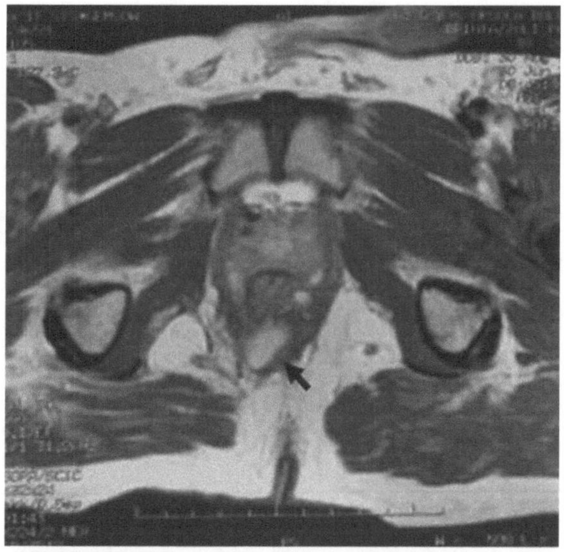
b

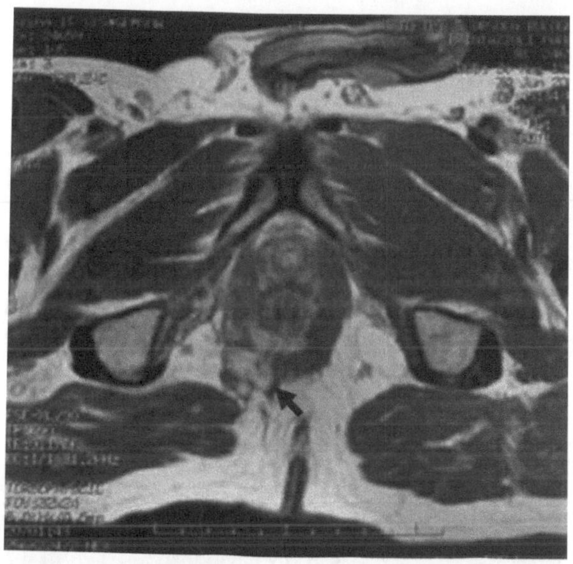
c

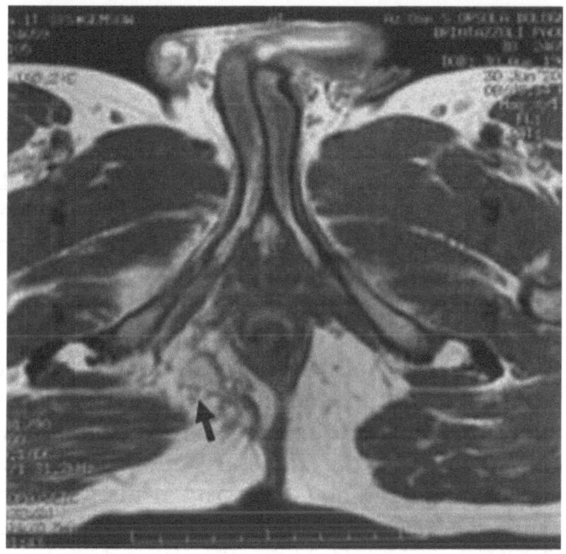
d

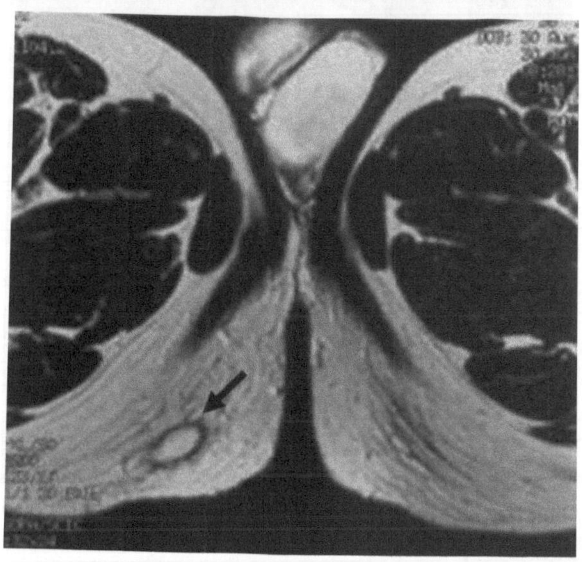
e

Fig. VII.33. Posterior suprasphincteric fistula drained with loose seton in a 39-year-old man who complained of pain underneath the right ischial tuberosity. Primary fistula with internal opening at 6 o'clock at the high anal canal level after hydrogen peroxide enhancement without evidence of secondary extensions on endoanal ultrasound (*arrow*) (**a**). Primary fistula (**b**) and secondary track that reaches the right ischial tuberosity (**c, d**) and ends in the subcutaneous fat (**e**) on magnetic resonance imaging (*arrows*)

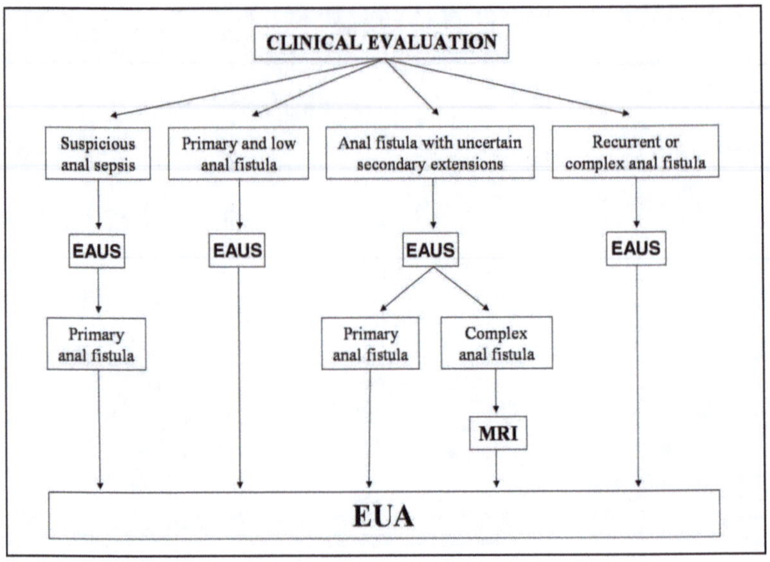

Fig. VII.34. Diagnostic flow chart for perianal sepsis and fistula in ano. *EAUS* endonal ultrasonography; *MRI* magnetic resonance imaging; *EUA* examination under anesthesia

to the extent of invalidating the compensation provided by the remaining unimpaired structures [20]. The cause of incontinence is often multifactorial [21]: in fact, in a prospective study, Rao et al. [22] demonstrated that in 80% of patients, alterations of more than one factor were present.

A careful clinical assessment of the patient combined with anorectal instrumental diagnostics provides useful information in defining the contribution of the individual etiopathogenetic factors, determining the severity of the problem, and establishing the impact of FI on quality of life [23]. It is only by combining these complementary data that the problem can be classified in its entirety and the most appropriate therapeutic option be selected, be it medical or surgical.

History taking alone is, in fact, not sufficient to determine the causes of incontinence while digital exploration only permits a qualitative assessment of resting and contraction endoanal pressure. Detailed diagnostic investigation is based on a series of examinations that can be divided into two main categories:

1. Morphological examinations, such as EAUS, defecography, and pelvic MRI (static, dynamic, and with an endoanal coil)
2. Functional examinations, such as anorectal manometry, sensory tests, study of pudendal nerve terminal latency, and electromyography.

The use of endoscopy is limited to cases of incontinence associated with recent bowel movement alterations, above all diarrhea, in order to exclude organic lesions or intestinal inflammatory conditions in which specific treatment could probably resolve the problem of continence (Fig. VII.35) [24].

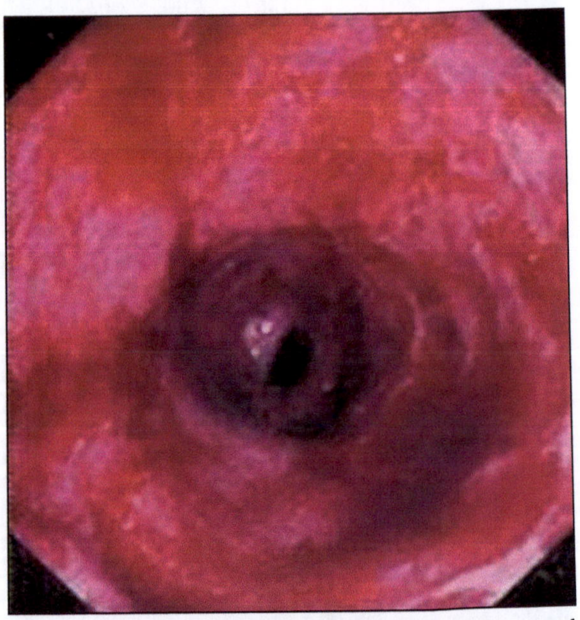

Fig. VII.35. Radiation proctitis characterized by rectal mucosal friability

Endoanal Ultrasound

Endoanal ultrasound (EAUS) allows evaluation of the thickness and anatomical integrity of the internal (IAS) and external (EAS) anal sphincter and detection of the presence of scar tissue with a high degree of accuracy [25]. This method has been validated both by in vivo and in vitro studies [26] and has demonstrated an almost 100% sensitivity and specificity in determining the topography of sphincter defects, thus completely replacing electromyography (EMG) [27]. EAUS makes it possible to foresee the complexity of the mechanisms involved in FI, showing sphincter defects in patients considered to be affected by neuropathic incontinence, not revealing significant anatomical alterations in women strongly suspected of suffering from obstetric sphincter damage, or showing muscular lesions in completely asymptomatic subjects.

The importance of this method in the diagnosis of FI is due to the fact that sphincter defects are responsible in most cases of incontinence, particularly in women, in whom obstetric sphincter damage is the most frequent cause (Fig. VII.36). Although the anatomical variations of the EAS in the upper third of the anal canal in women can lead to an overestimation of the incidence of this etio-

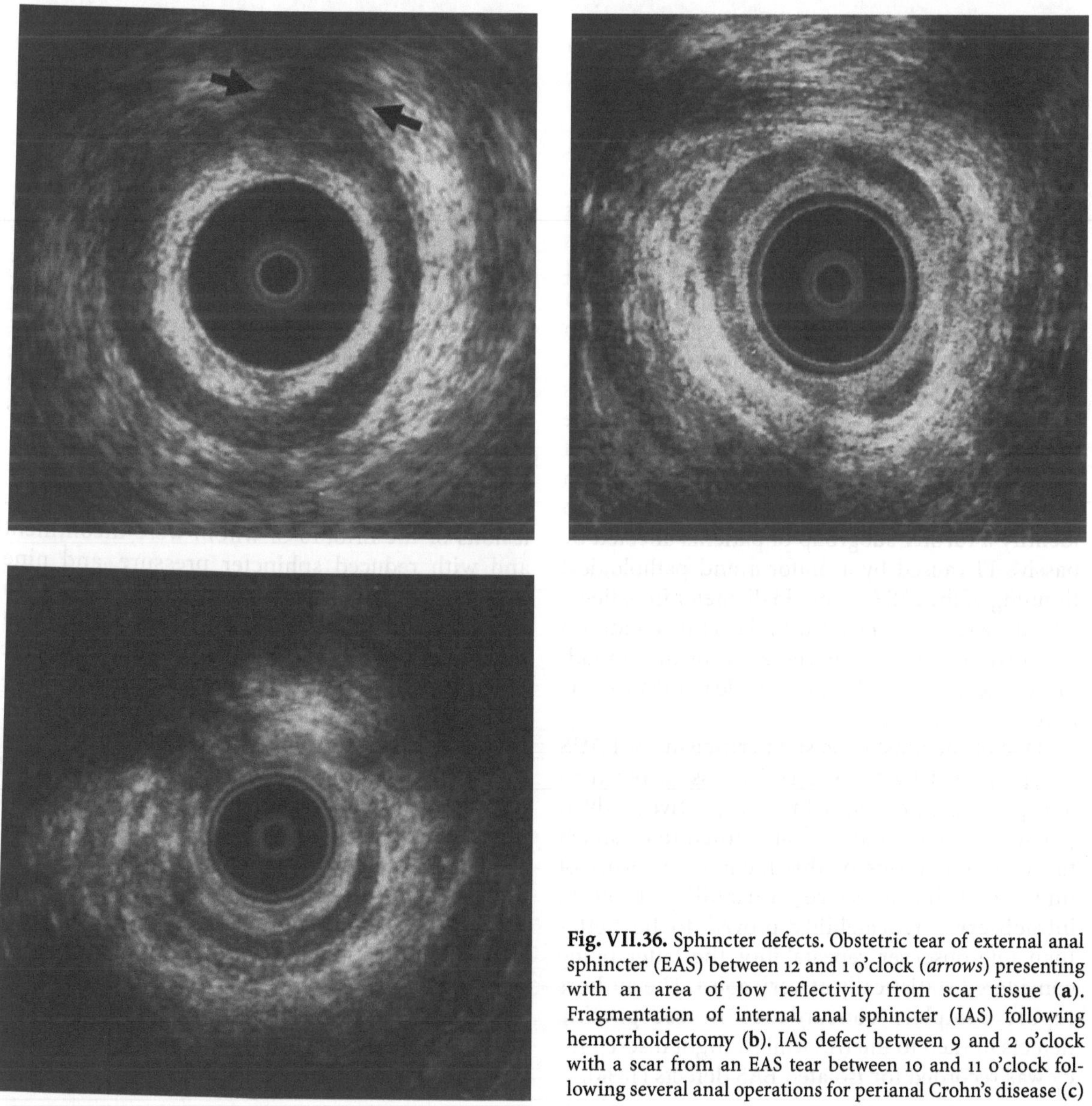

a

b

c

Fig. VII.36. Sphincter defects. Obstetric tear of external anal sphincter (EAS) between 12 and 1 o'clock (*arrows*) presenting with an area of low reflectivity from scar tissue (**a**). Fragmentation of internal anal sphincter (IAS) following hemorrhoidectomy (**b**). IAS defect between 9 and 2 o'clock with a scar from an EAS tear between 10 and 11 o'clock following several anal operations for perianal Crohn's disease (**c**)

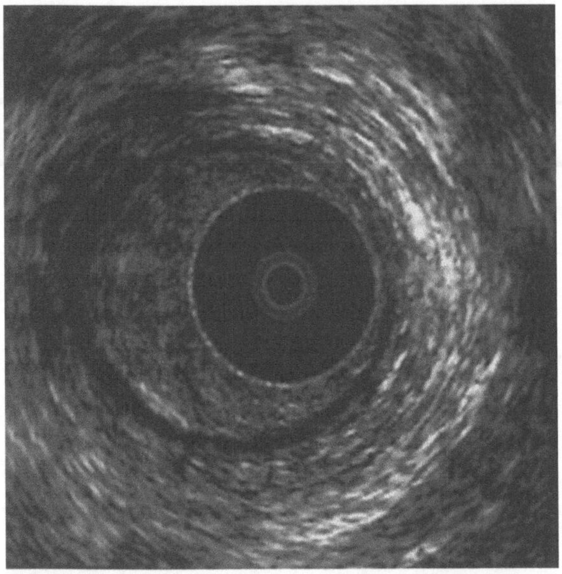

Fig. VII.37. Internal sphincter degeneration. Thinning of internal sphincter abnormal for the age of the patient (69 years) measuring 1.3 mm

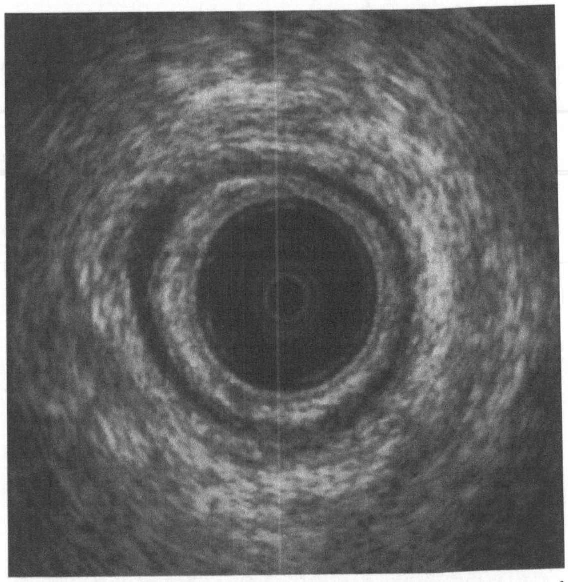

Fig. VII.38. External sphincter atrophy. Thinning of internal sphincter and poor definition of outer border of external sphincter

logical factor, their importance is nevertheless unquestionable, as shown by a recent meta-analysis on a sample of 717 women [28]. The authors report a 26.9% incidence of occult sphincter defects in primipara women and new muscular damage in 8.5% of pluripara women who delivered vaginally. In addition, although only 29.7% of the patients with sphincter defects were symptomatic in the immediate postpartum period, the probability of FI onset in the long-term is high (76.8–82.8%). In the absence of sphincter defects, EAUS is able to identify a further subgroup of patients affected by passive FI caused by a uniform and pathological thinning of the IAS (<2 mm in diameter in patients over the age of 50) (Fig. VII.37). This rare condition is known as primary degeneration of the smooth muscle cells of the IAS and was described for the first time in 1997 [29].

One of the most consistent criticisms of EAUS is represented by the subjectiveness involved in interpreting the findings. In a prospective study of 51 patients, Gold et al. [30] attempted to establish the true limitations of this method in terms of inter- and intraobserver variability. Overall, intraobserver repeatability proved to be better than interobserver repeatability, the latter being considered statistically as very good. The authors report complete concordance in recognizing defects limited to the IAS while a slight discrepancy was recorded for isolated EAS defects (18%).

Another considerable limitation of this method is the difficulty in identifying the neurogenic atrophy of EAS (Fig. VII.38). Since neurological damage causes the loss of functional tissue and its consequent replacement with adipose tissue, it is in fact difficult to identify the interface that separates the EAS from the fat of the ischioanal space and consequently the precise measurement of the thickness of the striated muscle [25] Williams et al. [31] carried out a prospective study on 25 patients without EAUS-detectable lesions of the EAS, 16 of whom were incontinent and with reduced sphincter pressure, and nine healthy controls, performing MRI with an endoanal coil and EMG. The authors showed that the loss of definition of the EAUS interface at the outer margin of the striated muscle and the thinning of the IAS identified EAS atrophy with a positive predictive value of 74%.

The high degree of definition of the anal canal and the accuracy in characterizing any sphincter defects make EAUS an indispensable examination in the assessment of patients with incontinence and also in confirming the integrity of the sphincters in cases of suspected neuropathic incontinence. The relationship between structural damage and clinical symptoms must nevertheless be clarified by carrying out additional tests in view of the numerous factors that can be involved in causing FI.

Magnetic Resonance Imaging

Compared with EAUS, MRI offers a series of advantages in the study of patients with FI, in particular, a wider visual field and above all the possibility of performing a dynamic study of the pelvic floor [32]. The use of endoanal coils has made it possible to achieve a high definition of the sphincter complex, thus opening the road to an entire series of studies comparing MRI with EAUS.

In a retrospective study in 22 women suffering from FI and undergoing surgery, Rociu et al. [33] compared operative findings with the results of EAUS with a 7-MHz rotating probe and endoanal MRI. The authors reported MRI as being more accurate: the defects localized at the EAS were identified at EAUS and MRI in 16 (73%) and 20 cases (91%), respectively and alterations of the IAS in 15 (68%) and 17 (77%). MRI also determined the correct surgical indication in 95% of patients compared with 77% with EAUS.

A second prospective randomized study on 52 symptomatic patients [34] suggests that EAUS and MRI are comparable in defining defects involving the EAS but that EAUS is better in evaluating IAS defects. Overall, ultrasound proved wrong in the localization of IAS defects in only one case versus the 12 incorrectly evaluated at MRI (p=0.002); the errors concerning the EAS were, on the other hand, almost identical (p=1.0). According to the authors, the above-mentioned study by Rociu et al. presents a statistical flaw connected with the selection of the sample since the reference gold standard was surgery, for which only the subjects with external sphincter lesions were candidates. Moreover, in the study by Rociu et al., a 7-MHz probe was used, which generates images in which the IAS is less well defined than with 10-MHz probes.

The superiority of MRI in assessing EAS atrophy is not, on the contrary, questioned. The loss of muscular tone and its replacement with adipose tissue are accurately defined, thanks to the different intensity of the signal emitted by the two tissues. Considering the histological examination as the reference gold standard, endoanal MRI has a sensitivity and specificity of 89% and 94%, respectively, in determining the presence or absence of atrophy of the external sphincter [35].

Williams et al. [31] performed a prospective study on 25 patients without EAUS-detected lesions of the EAS. The sample included two groups: 16 incontinent patients with reduced anal pressure under contraction and nine healthy control subjects. All subjects underwent MRI with an endoanal coil and EMG. The authors showed that women with normal anal pressure under contraction presented a greater area of the EAS measured at MRI on coronal sections (p=0.01) and a lower mean content of fat (p<0.001) compared with subjects with low contraction pressure. A significant correlation was also found between contraction pressure, area of the EAS (p=0.02), and fat content (p<0.001). Since the last two parameters are associated with EAS atrophy, the authors drew up a radiological classification of the degree of atrophy.

Assessment of the degree of any EAS atrophy is important if sphincteroplasty is considered. Briel e al. [36] demonstrated a positive correlation (p=0.001) between sphincter area measured on MR coronal sections and postoperative functional outcome. Patients with a surface area measuring less than 360 mm^2 had a worse outcome. As regards interobserver variability in identifying sphincter defects, a "moderate" level of agreement was recorded for endoanal MRI, which was, however, less than with EAUS. This mainly reflects the different level of experience of examiners of this new method rather than differences in the images [37].

Although the role of endoanal MRI in assessing sphincter defects is still being studied, its superiority with respect to EAUS in identifying EAS atrophy has, on the other hand, now been confirmed. This method should therefore be considered as a complementary examination to ultrasound in patients with EAS lesions who may be candidates for surgery.

Defecography

The use of defecography in assessing patients with FI is justified by the fact that the possible causes of this disorder are rectal prolapse (Fig. VII.39) and rectocele, conditions which, moreover, present with continence alterations in around 50–70% and 33% of cases, respectively [38, 39]. The American Gastroenterological Association (AGA) does not recommend its routine use, suggesting that this method should be limited to cases in which there is evidence of a rectocele or strong clinical suspicion of rectal intussusception [24].

Anorectal Manometry

Anorectal manometry is the basic examination for studying anorectal function, as it allows objective evaluation of the barrier pressure generated by sphincter activity, rectoanal inhibitory reflex, and rectal sensitivity and compliance [32]. The sensitivity and specificity of this method in distinguishing incontinent and continent patients have been investigated in a number of studies. Felt-Bersma et al. [40] used anorectal manometry and continence tests with perfusion of saline solution in the rectum to assess 350 patients affected by defecation disorders, 170 of whom had a history of incontinence. Among the manometric parameters considered, only maximum contraction pressure showed significant accuracy in distinguishing between incontinent patients and healthy controls. Using a cutoff value of 60 mmHg in women and 120 mmHg in men, sensitivity and specificity were 90% and 78% and 67% and 67%, respectively. The authors were, however, of the opinion that anorectal manometry is not able to accurately predict the degree of continence. In a similar study, Sun et al. [21] compared 302 incontinent patients with 65 healthy controls, confirming the high degree of sensitivity and specificity of maximum contraction pressure (92% and 97%) in distinguishing between the two groups. Most patients also presented more than one alteration at the tests used (anorectal manometry, rectal sensory testing, and EMG) and, stressing the concept of the multifactorial etiology of incontinence, the authors thus suggested that the various diagnostic techniques should be combined in order to identify all pathogenetic mechanisms involved and plan the most effective therapeutic strategy.

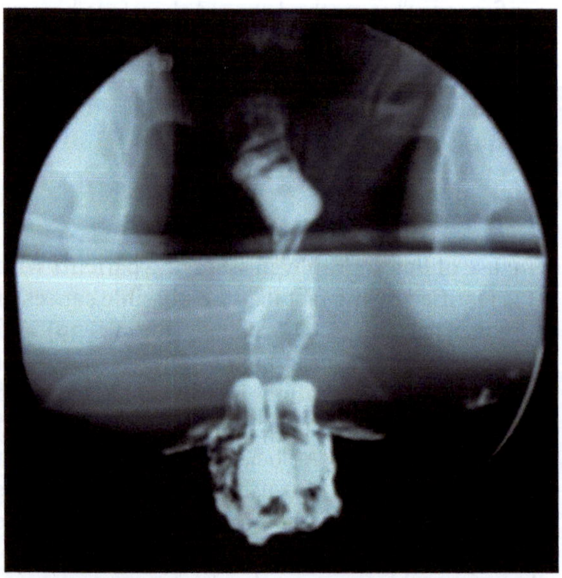

Fig. VII.39. Complete rectal prolapse in a 65-year-old man

The AGA recommends the use of manometry to quantify the functional deficit of the sphincters and predict the response to treatment [24]. Anal pressure vectography is a development of traditional manometry and is used to assess any functional asymmetry associated with sphincter defects [24]. Yang and Wexner [41] performed a prospective study on 50 patients with FI, assessing the concordance of the method with EAUS and EMG. Of the 27 patients with sphincter defects identified at EAUS, vectography localized the lesion in the same quadrant shown by EAUS in only three cases. Similar results were obtained by comparing vectography with EMG (5/38). In a study on 69 female patients with functional evacuation disorders, Perry et al. [42] quantified the pressure symmetry of the anal canal by means of the "vector symmetry index." In asymptomatic women, this parameter was on average 0.76 while in incontinent patients with known sphincter defects, it was around 0.33 (p=0.0001) and in any case always less than 0.60. In the group of incontinent women without known sphincter defects but with a positive history of episiotomy, the vector symmetry index was less than 0.60 in 57% of cases, thus suggesting a sphincter lesion in half the patients. Although these data seem to credit vectography with some value as a possible guide to surgery, EAUS is still the preferred examination in studying patients with sphincter defects, particularly for those who are candidates for surgical treatment [24].

The fact remains, however, that anorectal manometry has two important limitations: the lack of a standardization of the technique and the disagreement between experts regarding the significance of manometric parameters [20]. Nevertheless, although sphincter pressure is not strictly correlated with continence, manometry should be performed in incontinent patients since it allows an objective assessment of anorectal function and monitoring of the outcome after pharmacological, rehabilitative (biofeedback), or surgical therapy.

Sensory Testing

Rectal sensitivity and compliance are measured by progressive distention of the rectal wall through inflation of a balloon positioned in the lumen. In incontinent patients, it is possible to observe both rectal hypo- and hypersensitivity [43]. A lowering of the threshold of rectal distention perception (hypersensitivity) can be observed in inflammatory disorders of the intestine, in radiation proctitis, and in irritable bowel syndrome, conditions that can present with an urgency to defecate [32]. Conversely, an increase in the threshold of rectal perception (hyposensitivity) can contribute to FI in patients with organic and/or functional alterations of the rectal reservoir, such as megarectum, descending perineum syndrome, autonomic neuropathies (diabetes mellitus), and congenital anorectal malformations [43].

The AGA upholds the validity of rectal sensory testing not only in identifying conditions of hypersensitivity and reduced rectal compliance, which can influence the therapeutic strategy, but also in monitoring patients undergoing rehabilitation (biofeedback), the success of which is correlated with the reduction/normalization of the threshold of rectal distention perception [24].

Anal sensitivity tests provide information on the integrity of the sensitive nerve endings of the anal canal by electrical or thermal stimulation. The AGA does not number these tests among those with true clinical value although it recommends their use in cases in which it is necessary to distinguish between idiopathic and neurological disorders (e.g., diabetes mellitus and amyloidosis) [24].

Neurophysiological Tests

Neurophysiological assessment of incontinent patients includes measurement of pudendal nerve terminal motor latency (PNTML) and EMG. PNTML measures neuromuscular integrity between the terminal portion of the pudendal nerve and the anal sphincter. A prolonged nerve latency time, albeit physiological as age increases, suggests the presence of a pudendal neuropathy, and its measurement can be important in distinguishing between weakness of the sphincter due to pudendal neuropathy or to an anatomical defect of the muscle [24]. A normal PNTML does not, on the contrary, allow exclusion of the presence of a pudendal neuropathy since just a few intact nerve fibers are sufficient to give a normal result [32].

Kiff and Swash [44] were the first to report a prolonged latency time in patients with idiopathic incontinence compared with healthy controls although subsequent studies have questioned the true value of this finding. Wexner et al. [45] showed that approximately 50% of patients with normal contraction pressure presented a prolonged PNTML. In a similar retrospective study on 2,067 patients [46], 31% presented a maximum contraction pressure within the normal range despite having signs of bilateral neuropathy, and on the contrary, 49% of patients with a normal PNTML and intact sphincter showed lower than normal pressure values.

As regards the ability of PNTML to predict the surgical result, a recent review of eight case-control studies [47] reported that the group of patients with high PNTML values presented a worse outcome than the cases without signs of neuropathy. This finding was, however, disproved by other evidence, which found no relationship between the condition of the pudendum and surgical outcome [48].

The AGA does not recommend the use of PNTML since its results correlate poorly with symptoms and histology findings, do not distinguish the true cause of muscular weakness, and has poor sensitivity and specificity; the method is also operator dependent and does not predict surgical outcome [24].

The use of needle EMG in studying incontinent patients is not currently recommended by the AGA [24]. EAUS has, in fact, proved to be more sensitive and accurate in localizing sphincter defects and is also less invasive [49]. On the contrary, surface EMG may be indicated in functional assessment of the striated sphincter in cases in which the muscular weakness cannot be explained by the ecographic morphological finding. This method is also valid in biofeedback as a control during rehabilitation [24].

Diagnostic Integration

The numerous anorectal tests available have undoubtedly contributed to understanding the etiopathogenetic mechanisms of FI; it is, however, necessary to question their true clinical impact, i.e., we must ask ourselves if and to what extent these tests can affect therapeutical decisions.

A number of studies have, in fact, shown that the integration of instrumental tests with respect to clinical evaluation alone provides additional information in identifying the cause of FI in a percentage of cases ranging from 19% to 55% [50–53] and is able to modify the treatment in 10–20% of cases [51, 52, 54]. In a recent prospective study, Liberman et al. [54] carried out an in-depth clinical evaluation of 90 patients suffering from FI following which the subjects were divided into two groups according to the therapeutic indication: medical or surgical. The patients were then studied by means of anorectal manometry, EAUS, and PNTML. Finally, a panel of four colorectal surgeons reclassified the patients into two treatment groups on the basis of the information obtained from the instrumental assessment. The therapeutic indication was modified in nine patients (10%): five patients were transferred from the medical group to the surgical group, three from the surgical group to the medical group, and the type of surgery was altered in one patient. Without the information provided by the diagnostic integration, 11% (5/45) of patients in the medical group would not have been able to benefit from necessary surgical treatment, and in the same way, 7% (3/45) of patients in the surgical group would have undergone avoidable surgery and 2% (1/45) an inappropriate surgical procedure. By revealing sphincter defects in all five patients moved to the surgical group and excluding anatomical damage in two of the three patients initially in the surgical group, EAUS proved the only method able to modify the treatment plan. Neither manometry nor PNTML did, in fact, have any effect on the initial therapeutic decision. The authors conclude by claiming that clinical assessment by expert colorectal surgeons is sufficiently reliable and is confirmed by physiological tests in most cases. Among the tests available, moreover, EAUS is the only one that has a true impact on therapeutic choice and should therefore be routinely performed in the assessment of patients with FI.

In conclusion, although there are no standardized protocols for the morphofunctional characterization of patients with FI, EAUS and the physiological tests should be considered first-level methods for investigating the problem. An in-depth diagnostic assessment with additional instrumental tests, such as defecography, MRI, endoscopy, and neurophysiological tests, must be guided by the clinical assessment (suspicion of a particular etiology, diarrhea, age, severity of symptoms, impact on quality of life, response to medical treatment).

Obstructed Defecation

Obstructed defecation (OD) characterizes a category of patients affected by persistent constipation in which ineffective emptying of the rectum represents the main pathogenetic element as opposed to the so-called "colon constipation" or *inertia coli*, which is, instead, caused by a slowing down in intestinal transit [55]. The two forms of constipation do not exclude each other and can both be present in the same subject, probably connected by a cause-effect relationship [56, 7]. It is, however, necessary to point out that the majority of patients classified as constipated on the basis of Rome II criteria [57] are affected by another form of constipation characterized by normal intestinal transit and by the absence of objective defecation disorders, which typically respond to dietary–behavioral therapy or osmotic laxatives [58]. It should also be taken into account that constipation may be secondary to other conditions, such as tumors of the colon, some endocrinal disorders (e.g., hypothyroidism), neurological diseases (e.g., multiple sclerosis), the use of some drugs (analgesics, antidepressants, etc.), and psychiatric disorders (e.g., depression, anorexia). Thus, after seeing a failure of dietary–behavioral therapy and excluding the causes of possible secondary constipation, there is still a subgroup of patients affected by severe constipation that is probably caused either by *inertia coli* or by OD, or even by a combination of both forms. The aim of this section is identification of the methods that are of use and necessary in distinguishing between constipation due to OD and slow intestinal transit .

Accuracy of clinical assessment in identifying disorders that may be responsible for OD was investigated in a prospective study in 50 patients [59], which showed the negative predictive value of clinical assessment in identifying rectocele, anismus, and intussusception was 96%, 96%, and 80%, respectively. In other words, these results tell us that clinical assessment is of value above all in identifying patients in whom it is possible to reasonably avoid performing further diagnostic tests. On the contrary, a positive clinical assessment requires instrumental confirmation. Similar conclusions were also reached by Karlbom et al. [60] in a more recent study on the accuracy of clinical evaluation in the diagnosis of rectal intussusception.

No examination alone can be considered sufficient in characterizing patients with OD, and it is therefore necessary to combine the information obtained from a number of tests [61]. The diagnostic tools available consist of:

1. Imaging methods, such as defecography, colpocystoproctography, MRI, EAUS, and intestinal transit time
2. Functional tests, such as anorectal manometry, the balloon expulsion test, and EMG.

Intestinal Transit Time

The study of intestinal transit time with radioopaque markers provides an objective assessment of the peristaltic activity of the colon and thus represents the most useful method of identifying intestinal sluggishness in patients with persistent constipation (Fig. VII.40) [24]. This examination also allows an objective check of the symptoms reported by the patient, who may lie or not assess intestinal activity correctly [61]. On the contrary, in the presence of symptoms suggesting dysmotility, if the transit time is normal, it is advisable to repeat the examination [62].

Although marker retention at the level of the sigmoid colon/rectum can be associated with evacuation difficulties, the study of intestinal transit time can only show the presence or absence of colic dysmotility and does not discriminate between the two forms of constipation. Even in the event of a positive test result, additional studies are therefore necessary to identify or exclude OD [24]. In the event of a documented combination of slow transit and OD, the patient, who may also be a candidate for surgical correction of the expulsion problem, should be informed that if this correction is successful, it will improve evacuation but cannot shorten the transit time of the fecal bolus in the large intestine.

Finally, it should be remembered that there is another procedure, colon scintigraphy, that is able to provide even more accurate information on regional transit. This method is, however, more complex and has not demonstrated any clear advantage compared with the use of radioopaque markers [63].

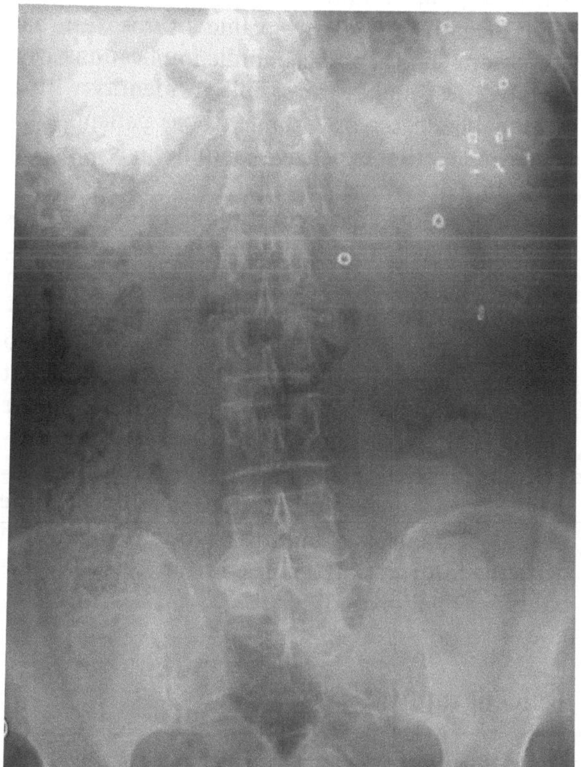

Fig. VII.40. Slow colonic transit in a middle-aged woman with obstructed defecation (markers retained in left colon on day 8)

Anorectal Manometry

Anorectal manometry can provide important information in the assessment of patients with chronic constipation. The nonreduction of endoanal pressure or its paradoxical increase during the attempt to simulate defecation is highly suggestive of pelvic floor anismus. To be able to diagnose anismus, however, it is necessary to show that the described pressure alterations are the result of an irregular contraction activity of the striated muscles (EAS and puboanal), and manometry alone does not provide this type of information. For this purpose, diagnostic integration by means of a combination of tests, such as surface EMG, defecography, or balloon expulsion test, can prove useful in increasing diagnostic accuracy [24].

The failure of the IAS to relax during dilation of the rectum is highly indicative of Hirschsprung's disease, which can, however, only be definitively diagnosed histologically. On the contrary, the presence of a normal inhibitory anorectal reflex makes it possible to exclude this disease. Finally, it should be remembered that there are "pseudoabsence" forms of this reflex, as occurs, for example, in megarectum in which a high degree of rectal distention is necessary to induce the relaxation of the IAS [24].

There are few studies on the ability of anorectal manometry to affect the management of patients with defecation disorders. In a recent review of the literature, the percentage of patients in whom manometry provided additional information to the extent of modifying the treatment was 65–67%.[64]. According to the AGA, anorectal manometry has a true clinical value in identifying patients with Hirschsprung's disease and is useful in assessing patients with anismus, especially if this diagnosis is supported by other evidence (EMG, defecography, balloon expulsion test). The method is also a valid contribution in monitoring the outcome of rehabilitation therapy [24].

The results of anorectal manometry cannot, however, be predicted on the basis of the clinical examination or the results of imaging methods. This was confirmed by a recent study we performed with the collaboration of G. Bazzocchi, from the Department of Gastroenterology of University of Bologna, not yet published, in which 47 women affected by OD underwent anorectal manometry and defecography. In the 33 patients with a radiological diagnosis of rectocele, the mean value of the maximum radial tone varied and was totally unpredictable. Conversely, 16 of the 18 women who had a higher-than-normal mean value of the maximum radial tone presented rectocele at defecography ($p<0.001$). Likewise, in the 22 women with radiological diagnosis of rectocele and intussusception, the value of the vectogram volume varied and was totally unpredictable while nine of the 13 patients with a higher-than-normal value of the vectogram volume presented rectocele and intussusception ($p<0.001$).

Electromyography

EMG is used for the functional assessment of patients with constipation in order to evaluate the presence of an appropriate relaxation of the pelvic muscles during defecation [24]. In a study designed to evaluate the role of paradoxical contraction of the puborectalis muscle in constipated patients, the electromyographic pattern of anismus correlated with the inability to expel a balloon containing 50 ml of water from the rectum in 82% of cases [65]. On the contrary, a subsequent study of 24 patients affected by constipation and 11 control subjects in whom EMG, defecography, and anorectal manometry were performed showed no correlation of the electromyographic results with the ability to evacuate or the symptoms reported by the patient. The authors thus concluded that EMG cannot be used as the only method in diagnosing OD [66].

Surface EMG is of practical use in rehabilitation therapy with biofeedback, indicated in patients with pelvic floor anismus [24].

Balloon Expulsion Test

The balloon expulsion test is a very simple procedure used to demonstrate an alteration of evacuation in patients affected by chronic constipation. In a recent prospective study, Minguez et al. [67] divided 130 patients with functional constipation into two groups, with and without pelvic floor dyssynergia, on the basis of Rome II criteria and manometric and defecographic findings. The balloon expulsion test showed sensitivity, specificity, a positive predictive value, and a negative predictive value of 87.5%, 89%, 64%, and 97%, respectively, in identifying patients with dyssynergia. On the basis of these results, the authors consider the test to have a low degree of accuracy in diagnosing dyssynergia while stressing its important role in excluding this condition. They also claim that the high negative predictive value of the test has important clinical and economic implications, as a negative test makes it possible to identify with a reasonable degree of certainty those patients who can avoid further expensive examinations aimed at excluding dyssynergia.

Other studies have contradicted these results, showing that a number of patients with pelvic floor dyssynergia are able to expel the balloon normally. According to the authors of these studies, the method is not sufficient on its own to make a diagnosis of dyssynergia [68]. A recent review of the literature showed that although the inability to expel the balloon suggests the possibility of dyssynergia, a positive result of the procedure does not exclude this possibility, and the results of the tests should therefore be integrated with the information obtained from other anorectal functional procedures [64].

Defecography

Defecography, or evacuation proctography (EP), is a relatively simple and rapid radiological method that can provide anatomofunctional information on the structures involved in the evacuation process. Radiological findings do, in fact, include anatomical alterations of the rectum and pelvic floor (rectorectal intussusception, rectal prolapse, rectocele, pelvic floor descent) and functional evacuation abnormalities, i.e., the inability to empty the rectum quickly and completely [7].

Defecography represents the gold standard for the diagnosis of rectocele (Fig. VII.41) [7] although the clinical significance of this anatomical abnormality is still far from being clear. Shorvon et al. [69] showed the presence of rectocele in 96% of asymptomatic women studied by means of defecography. The authors also suggest considering 2 cm as the limit below which the protrusion of the anterior wall of the rectum should be considered as an anatomical alteration of little clinical significance. The size of the rectocele should not, however, be considered the only parameter able to identify the clinical value and to predict the surgical outcome [70]. In this sense, a case history of digitations associated with defecographic phenomenon of "barium trapping" is of greater value [71]. The results of surgical treatment are, moreover, strictly dependent on the identification and treatment of a possible functional disorder often associated with rectoceles [72].

In rectal prolapse, EP is usually indicated when the diagnosis is suspected but not proved by clinical examination. The method is also of use in identifying the degree of intussusception (Fig. VII.42) and the presence of associated alterations. In this case, too, however, the anatomical abnormality does not always have a clinical equivalent, as reported by Shorvon et al. [69] who found intussusception of the rectum in 22 out of 44 (50%) healthy volunteers who underwent EP.

If associated with opacification of the intestinal loops, EP is useful in identifying the presence of enterocele, another possible cause, or concomitant cause, of OD [25]. Defecography is the most accurate method for determining the position of the pelvic floor at rest and its excursion during defecation. The method is therefore of value in diagnosis of the descending perineum syndrome [73].

Finally, although the impression of the puborectal muscle and the nonopening of the anorectal angle are considered typical signs of pelvic floor dyssynergia, some authors have revised their discriminating value [74]. Halligan et al. [75] reported that the inability to evacuate more than two thirds of 120 ml of rectal contrast medium in less than 30 s is the main indicator of anismus, with a positive predictive value of 90%. The excessive interest in searching for anatomical abnormalities in patients with OD can distract attention from assessment of an underlying anismus, of which these alterations could constitute epiphenomena [7].

The true clinical value of defecography in assessing patients with OD has been questioned by the AGA [24]. The authors ascribe a high interobserver variability to the method, especially as

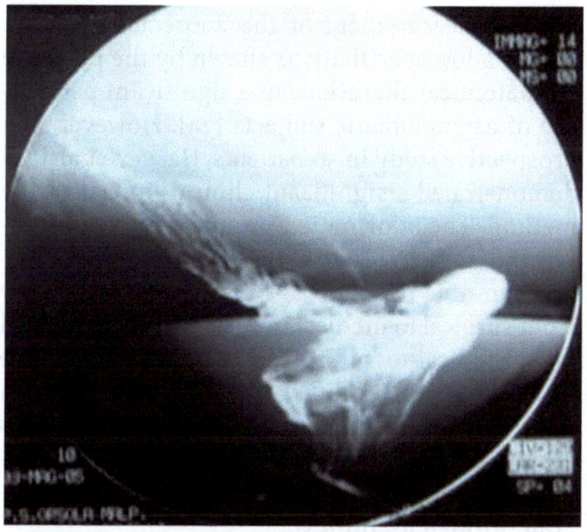

Fig. VII.41. Anterior rectocele in a 54-year-old man with obstructed defecation and digital assistance

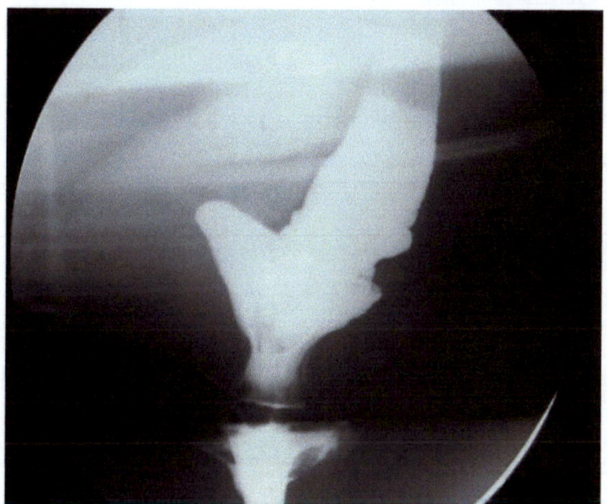

Fig. VII.42. High-grade intussusception with circumferential rectal infolding during evacuation low in the rectum

regards measurement of the anorectal angle, as well as a low specificity, as shown by the presence of anatomical alterations in a significant percentage of asymptomatic subjects [24]. However, in a prospective study in 50 patients, Harvey et al. [76] demonstrated a significant clinical impact of the method. The information provided by defecography did, in fact, lead to a modification of the diagnosis in nine patients (18%), a change in therapy from surgical to medical in seven cases (14%), and from medical to surgical in two cases (4%). The procedure also modified the type of surgery in 10% of cases. Finally, 94% of the clinicians who reassessed the cases in the light of the defecographic findings judged the method to be of moderate-to-high usefulness.

Colpocystoproctography

Colpocystoproctography allows dynamic assessment of the pelvic organs by identifying the morphological alterations during evacuation (Fig. VII.43) [77]. The usefulness of a complete study of the pelvis lies in evidence that associates weakness of the pelvic floor with multiple alterations of the organs contained within the pelvic cavity [78]. In this connection Maglinte et al. [79] compared the results of colpocystoproctography with the symptoms reported by 100 women with pelvic floor disorders, showing that 95% of the patients presented alterations in all three pelvic compartments although the reported symptoms were attributable to only one of them.

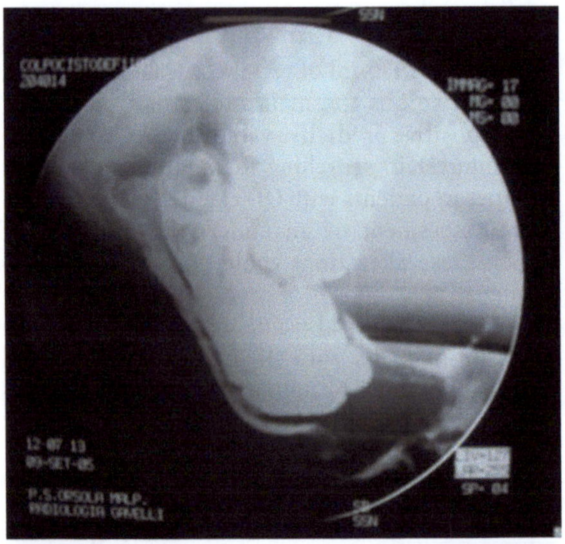
a

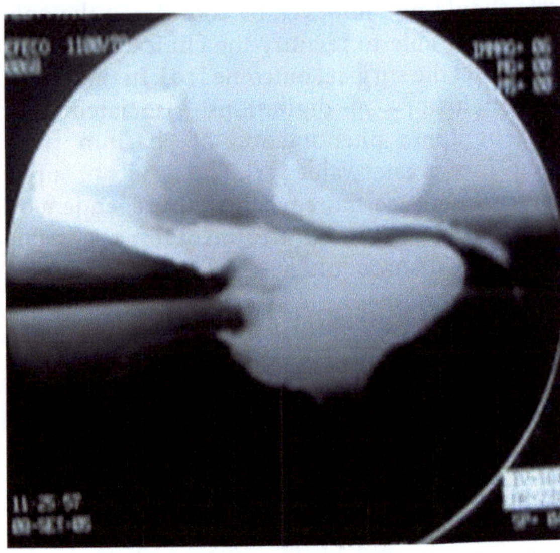
b

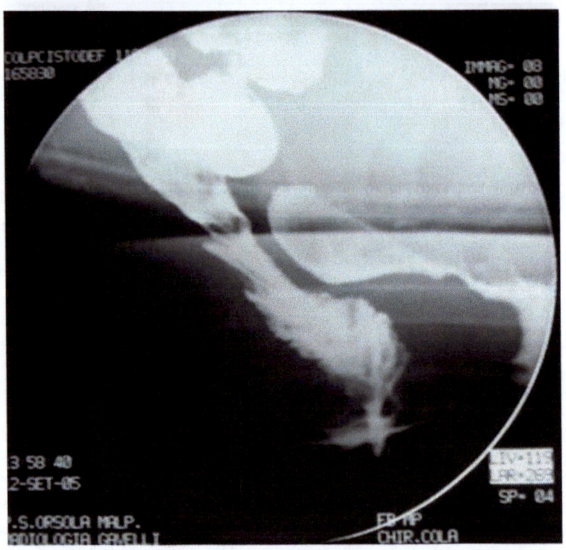
c

Fig. VII.43. Colpocystodefecography with opacification of small bowel. Postevacuation image shows a large enterocele in rectovaginal space (**a**), barium trapping in a large rectocele (**b**), and rectal intussusception (**c**) in three women with obstructed defecation

The possibility of preoperatively identifying all pelvic floor alterations allows a more precise planning of the surgical procedure, choosing the best approach and repairing all the defects in a single operation [80]. According to some authors, in fact, the relatively high rate of redo pelvic floor surgery could be partly due to the nonrecognition of all the alterations present [78]. One study [81] showed that the clinical diagnosis of enterocele, rectocele, and cystocele was modified in 75% of patients on the basis of additional information provided by colpocystoproctography.

Dynamic Magnetic Resonance Imaging of the Pelvis

Dynamic MRI has recently been proposed as a useful procedure for studying the pelvic floor. The method has considerable advantages: it provides real-time visualization of the movement of the pelvic organs and of the descent of muscular planes; it does not foresee the use of ionizing radiations and identifies reference bone structures more precisely than with fluoroscopy. Multiplanar images and high tissue contrast also allow a better visualization of the pelvic musculature and support structures, making oral administration of barium and opacification of the bladder superfluous [78]. On the other hand, traditional MRI allows assessment of any morphological alterations of the pelvic organs during straining in a situation in which the patient is certainly not in a physiological position and expels nothing from the rectum. The *closed* configuration of the most common MR machines does, in fact, oblige the patient to be in a recumbent position, which does not allow abdominal pressure on the pelvic structures. To overcome these problems, the use of paramagnetic contrast medium to be inserted in the rectum has been proposed (Fig. VII.44), and above all, *open*-style magnets have been developed, thanks to which the patient can take up a more physiological position during the examination.

MRI has been compared with what is currently considered the gold standard procedure for the diagnosis of morphofunctional abnormalities of the pelvic organs, i.e., colpocystoproctography, only in small series and with contradicting results. MRI proved to be equivalent to or better than the fluoroscopic method in studies in which the patient was in a sitting position or in any case evacuated a contrast medium [82, 83].

In conclusion, assessment of the true accuracy of MRI requires studies with larger sample populations and a greater standardization of the method. Although its use promises a better understanding of the pathogenetic mechanisms involved, the low cost-efficacy ratio does not currently justify its routine use [78].

a

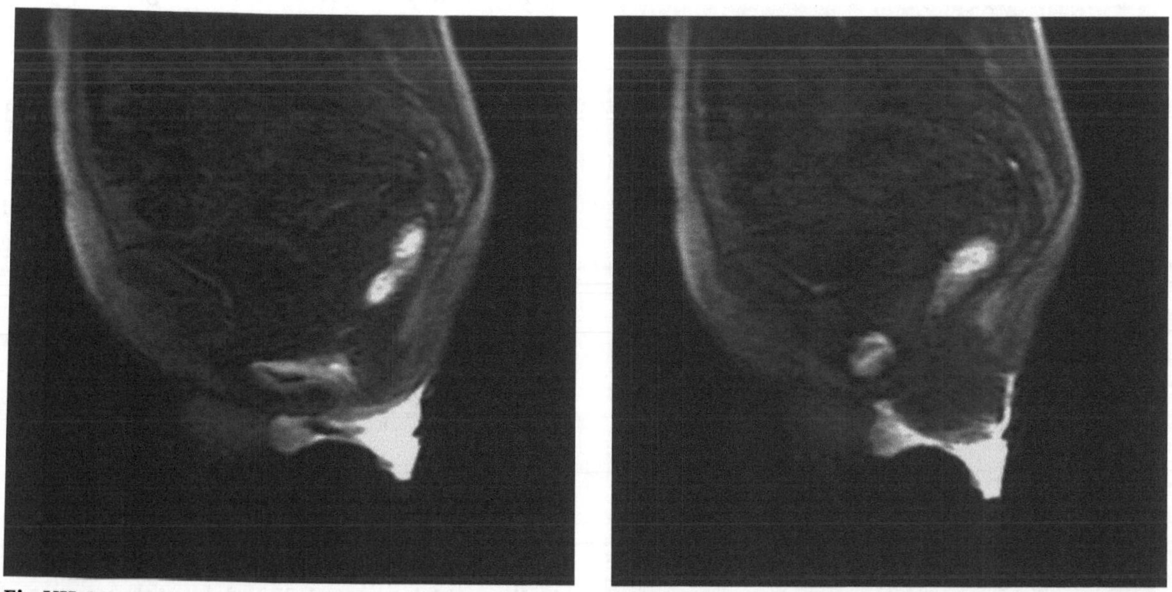

b

Fig. VII.44. Complete rectal prolapse in a 35-year-old woman. Dynamic magnetic resonance imaging at rest (**a**) and during evacuation (**b**)

Endoanal Ultrasound

The only disorder associated with OD in which EAUS plays a leading diagnostic role is hereditary IAS myopathy, a rare condition clinically characterized by constipation and proctalgia fugax and at ultrasound by a pathological thickening of the IAS of up to 1 cm (Fig. VII.45) [84]. Other conditions in which EAUS can be used, but with less diagnostic value, are solitary rectal ulcer syndrome, intussusception, and rectal prolapse. All three disorders are associated with a thickening of the IAS, albeit to a lesser extent with respect to hereditary myopathy [85, 7]. In solitary rectal ulcer, ultrasound can detect other features, such as hyperechoic fibrotic areas and multiple cysts in the submucosa, in the absence of an interruption in the layers of the rectal wall and of regional lymph nodes involvment (Fig. VII.46) [86]. Although in histologically doubtful cases these findings can suggest the benign nature of the lesion, the biopsy must be repeated for a definitive exclusion of a mucinous carcinoma. Finally, in patients with rectal prolapse, EAUS can reveal damage of the IAS secondary to the prolapse or to other causes [7].

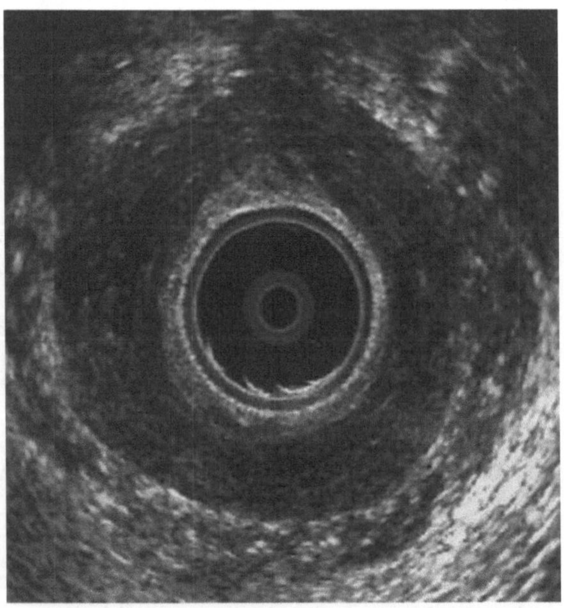

Fig. VII.45. Thickening of the internal sphincter in hereditary internal sphincter myopathy (8 mm)

Diagnostic Integration

Diagnostic study of a patient with OD is extremely complex due to multifactorial etiopathogenesis, aspecificity of symptoms, and frequent lack of a correlation between anatomical alterations and clinical symptoms. According to the AGA, anorectal manometry, intestinal transit times, and surface EMG should be considered worthwhile procedures in the diagnosis and management of patients with constipation while defecography, balloon expulsion tests, and sensory tests are procedures with a possible clinical value.

Some studies, however, attribute defecography with a greater clinical value. Halverson et al. [62] studied 98 patients affected by severe constipation, performing a detailed clinical assessment and a series of instrumental tests (anorectal manometry, transit times, defecography, PNTML, EMG and the balloon expulsion test) in order to identify the method with the greatest clinical impact from among those currently available. The authors reported little correlation between patients' symptoms and the causes of their constipation. Overall, the tests were necessary to obtain a correct diagnosis in 53% of cases. Transit times and, above all, defecography were the most useful methods in formulating a definitive diagnosis, and in the authors' opinion, these two methods should therefore be performed in all patients with severe constipation. The authors concluded by stating that since it is difficult to identify cases in which in-depth instrumental diagnostic tests should be performed due to poor predictability of clinical findings, all patients with severe constipation refractory to medical treatment should be systematically investigated with physiological and morphological tests.

We believe that the integration of defecography, anorectal manometry, and the study of intestinal transit times is mandatory in assessing patients with OD in order to identify the underlying functional etiology and the symptomatological value of anatomical alterations, guiding the clinician toward the choice of the most appropriate treatment.

Conclusions

Technological progress has provided specialists dealing with anorectal disorders with a series of morphological and functional tests which, used

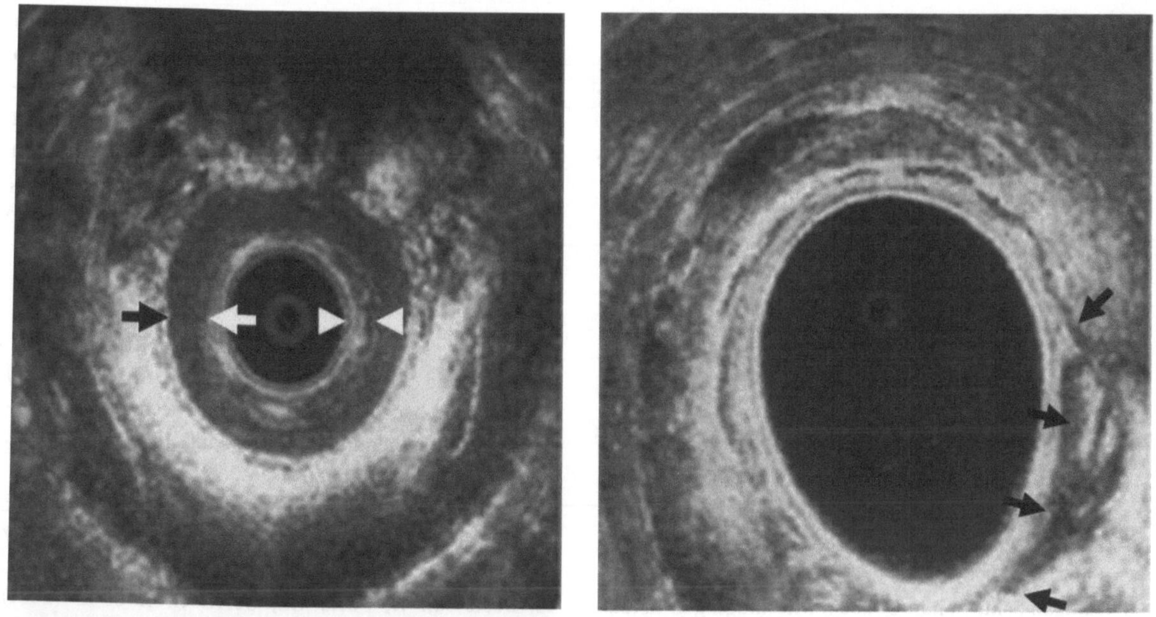

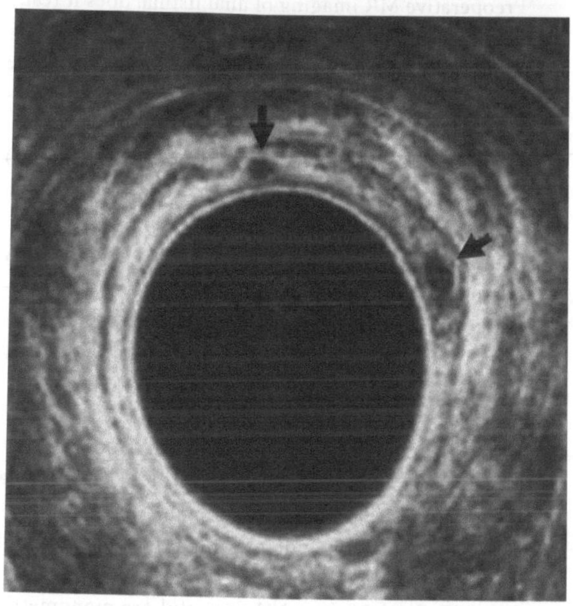

Fig. VII.46. Solitary polypoid rectal ulcer. Endoanal sonography showed thickening of the submucosal layer (*arrowheads*) and internal sphincter (*arrows*) (**a**). Endorectal sonography revealed hypoechoic lesions within the rectal muscle (*arrows*) (**b**). Multiple small cysts (*arrows*) were observed close to the main lesion (**c**)

together, have, on one hand, made it possible to understand the majority of etiopathogenetic mechanisms involved in the various disorders and, on the other hand, to consciously guide therapeutical choices.

This does not mean that clinical experience must now be considered less important than data provided by these modern methods of investigation: quite the reverse. It does, in fact, retain all its value, not only because it can provide data to be combined with those that emerge from morphofunctional tests but also because it is an essential element in the choice between the various procedures available and in interpreting the results they provide.

Development of new diagnostic techniques in the field of benign anorectal disorders has in the last few years been so overwhelming, and is still so, that it is not easy to draw up guidelines or diagnostic protocols that can stand up to criticism triggered by continuous new evidence. It is nevertheless indispensable to acknowledge the fact that it is no longer possible to take the risk of treating a patient with a benign anorectal disorder based solely on a clinical examination, as was the case for decades when diagnostic technological support was practically nonexistent.

Over and above a comparison of opinions as to one procedure being more useful with respect to another in assessing a certain benign anorectal disorder, the fact remains that there is a minimum diagnostic standard that must be maintained when preparing to treat a patient with anorectal sepsis, focal incontinence, or obstructed defecation.

References

1. Buchanan GN, Halligan S, Bartram CI et al (2004) Clinical examination, endosonography, and MR imaging in preoperative assessment of fistula in ano: comparison with outcome-based reference standard. Radiology 233:674–681
2. Halligan S, Buchanan G (2003) MR imaging of fistula-in-ano. Eur J Radiol 47:98–107
3. Seow Choen F, Burnett S, Bartram CI, Nicholls RJ (1991) A comparison between anal endosonography and digital examination in the evaluation of anal fistulae. Br J Surg 78:445–447
4. Bartram CI, Buchanan G (2003) Imaging anal fistula. Radiol Clin N Am 41:443–457
5. Kuijpers HC, Schulpen T (1985) Fistulography for fistula-in-ano: is it useful? Dis Colon Rectum 28:103–104
6. Guillamin E, Jeffrey RB, Shea WJ et al (1986) Perirectal inflammatory disease: CT findings. Radiology 161:153–157
7. Bartram CI, DeLancey JOL (2003) Imaging pelvic floor disorders. Springer, Berlin Heidelberg New York
8. Choen S, Burnett S, Bartram CI, Nicholls RJ (1991) Comparison between endosonography and digital examination in the evaluation of perianal fistulae. Br J Surg 78:445–447
9. Cho DY(1999) Endosonographic criteria for an internal opening of fistula-in-ano. Dis Colon Rectum 42:515–518
10. Bartram CI, Frudinger A (1997) A handbook of anal endosonography. Wrightson Biomedical Publishing, Petersfield
11. Cheong DM, Nogueras JJ, Wexner SD et al (1993) Anal endosonography for recurrent anal fistulas: image enhancement with hydrogen peroxide. Dis Colon Rectum 36:1158–1160
12. Poen AC, Felt-Bersma RJ, Eijsbouts QA et al (1998) Hydrogen peroxide-enhanced transanal ultrasound in the assessment of fistula-in-ano. Dis Colon Rectum 41:1147–1152
13. Navarro-Luna A, Garcia-Domingo MI, Rius-Macias J et al (2004) Ultrasound study of anal fistulas with hydrogen peroxide enhancement. Dis Colon Rectum 47:108–114
14. Buchanan GN, Bartram CI, Williams AB et al (2005) Value of hydrogen peroxide enhancement of three-dimensional endoanal ultrasound in fistula-in-ano. Dis Colon Rectum 48:141–147
15. Ratto C, Grillo E, Parello A et al (2005) Endoanal ultrasound-guided surgery for anal fistula. Endoscopy 37:722–728
16. Beets-Tan R, Beets GL, Gerritsen A et al (2001) Preoperative MR imaging of anal fistula: does it really help the surgeon? Radiology 218:75–84
17. Buchanan G, Halligan S, Williams A et al (2002) The effect of MRI on clinical outcome in recurrent fistula-in-ano. Lancet 360:1661–1662
18. Buchanan GN, Halligan S, Williams AB et al (2003) Magnetic resonance imaging for primary fistula in ano. Br J Surg 90:877–881
19. Schwartz DA, Wiersema MJ, Dudiak KM et al (2001) A comparison of endoscopic ultrasound, magnetic resonance imaging and exam under anesthesia for evaluation of Crohn's perianal fistulas. Gastroenterology 121:1064–1072
20. Rao SSC (2004) Diagnosis and management of fecal incontinence. Am J Gastroenterol 2:1585–1604
21. Sun WM, Donnely TC, Read NW (1992) Utility of a combined test of anorectal manometry, electromyography and sensation in determining the mechanism of idiopathic fecal incontinence. Gut 33:807–813
22. Rao SSC, Patel RS (1997) How useful are manometric tests of anorectal function in the management of fecal disorders? Am J Gastroenterol 92:469–473
23. Bharucha AE (2003) Fecal incontinence. Gastroenterology 124:1672–1685
24. Diamant NE, Kamm MA, Wald A et al (1999) AGA technical review on anorectal testing techniques. Gastroenterology 116:732–760
25. Bartram CI (2005) Functional anorectal imaging. Abdom Imaging 30:195–203
26. Sultan AH, Nicholls RJ, Kamm MA et al (1993) Anal endosonography and correlation with in vivo and in vitro anatomy. Br J Surg 80:508–511
27. Law PJ, Kamm MA, Bartram CI (1990) A comparison between electromyography and anal endosonography

in mapping external anal sphincter defects. Dis Colon Rectum 33:370–373
28. Oberwalder M, Connor J, Wexner SD (2003) Meta-analysis to determine the incidence of obstetric anal sphincter damage. Br J Surg 90:1333–1337
29. Vaizey CJ, Kamm MA, Bartram CI (1997) Primary degeneration of the IAS as a cause of passive faecal incontinence. Lancet 349:612–615
30. Gold SMD, Halligan S, Kmiot WA et al (1999) Intraobserver and interobserver agreement in anal endosonography. Br J Surg 86:371–375
31. Williams AB, Bartram CI, Modhawadia D et al (2001) Endocoil magnetic resonance imaging quantification of external anal sphincter atrophy. Br J Surg 88:853–859
32. Madoff RD, Parker SC, Varma MG et al (2004) Faecal incontinence in adults. Lancet 364:621–632
33. Rociu E, Stoker J, Eijkemans MJ et al (1999) Fecal incontinence: endoanal US versus endoanal MR imaging. Radiology 212:453–458
34. Malouf AJ, Halligan S, Williams AB et al (2000) Prospective assessment of accuracy of endoanal MR imaging and endosonography in patients with fecal incontinence. AJR Am J Roentegenol 175:741–745
35. Briel JW, Zimmerman DD, Stoker J et al (2000) Relationship between sphincter morphology on endoanal MRI and histopathological aspects of the external anal sphincter. Int J Colorectal Dis 15:87–90
36. Briel JW, Stoker J, Rociu E et al (1999) External anal sphincter atrophy on endoanal magnetic resonance imaging adversely affects continence after sphincteroplasty. Br J Surg 86:1322–1327
37. Malouf AJ, Halligan S, Williams AB et al (2001) Prospective assessment of interobserver agreement for endoanal MRI in fecal incontinence. Abdom Imaging 26:76–78
38. Ayabaca SM, Zbar AP, Pescatori M (2002) Anal continence after rectocele repair. Dis Colon Rectum 45:63–69
39. Andrews NJ, Jones DJ (1992) Rectal prolapse and associated conditions. Br Med J 305:243–245
40. Felt-Bersma RJ, Klinkeberg-Knol EC, Meuwissen SGM (1990) Anorectal functional investigation in continent and incontinent patients: differences and discriminatory value. Dis Colon Rectum 33:479–485
41. Yang Y, Wexner SD (1994) Anal pressure vectography is of no apparent benefit for sphincter evaluation. Int J Colorectal Dis 9:92–95
42. Perry RE, Blatchford GJ, Christensen MA et al (1990) Manometric diagnosis of anal sphincter injuries. Am J Surg 159:112–117
43. Tuteja AK, Rao SSC (2004) Review article: recent trends in diagnosis and treatment of faecal incontinence. Aliment Pharmacol Ther 19:829–840
44. Kiff ES, Swash M (1984) Slowed conduction in the pudendal nerves in idiopathic (neurogenic) faecal incontinence. Br J Surg 71:614–616
45. Wexner SD, Marchetti F, Salanga VD et al (1991) Neurophysiologic assessment of the anal sphincters. Dis Colon Rectum 34:606–612
46. Hill J, Hosker G, Kiff ES (2002) Pudendal nerve terminal motor latency measurements: what they do and do not tell us. Br J Surg 89:1268–1269
47. Olsen AL, Rao SSC (2001) Clinical neurophysiology and electrodiagnostic testing of the pelvic floor. Gastroenterol Clin N Am 30:33–54
48. Buie WD, Lowry AC, Rothenberger DA et al (2001) Clinical rather than laboratory assessment predicts continence after anterior sphincteroplasty. Dis Col Rectum 44:1255–1260
49. Tjandra JJ, Milsem JW, Schroeder I et al (1993) Endoluminal ultrasound is preferable to electromyography in mapping anal sphincter. Dis Colon Rectum 36:689–692
50. Wexner SD, Jorge JM (1994) Colorectal physiological test: use or abuse of technology? Eur J Surg 160:167–174
51. Keating JP, Stewart PJ, Eyers AA et al (1997) Are special investigations of value in the management of patients with fecal incontinence. Dis Colon Rectum 40:896–901
52. Speakman CT, Henry MM (1992) The work of an anorectal physiology laboratory. Baillieres Clin Gastroenterol 6:59–73
53. Ternent CA, Shashidharan M, Blatchford GJ et al (1996) Do anorectal physiology tests result in altered therapy for fecal incontinence [abstract]. Gastroenterology 110:A43
54. Liberman H, Faria J, Ternet CA et al (2001) A prospective evaluation of the value of anorectal physiology in the management of fecal incontinence. Dis Colon Rectum 44:1567–1574
55. Cheung O, Wald A (2004) Review article: the management of pelvic floor disorders. Aliment Pharmacol Ther 19:481–485
56. Karlbom U, Pahlman L, Nilsson S et al (1995) Relationship between defecographic findings, rectal emptying, and colonic transit time in constipated patients. Gut 36:907–912
57. Whitehead WE, Wald A, Diamant N et al (1999) Functional disorders of the anorectum. Gut 45:55–59
58. Lembo A and Camilleri M (2003) Chronic constipation. N Eng J Med 349:1360–1368
59. Siproudhis L, Ropert A, Vilotte J et al (1993) Clinical examination in diagnosing and quantifying pelvirectal disorders? a prospective study in a group of 50 patients complaining of defecatory difficulties. Dis Colon Rectum 36:430–438

60. Karlbom U, Graf W, Nilsson S et al (2004) The accuracy of clinical examination in the diagnosis of rectal intussusception. Dis Colon Rectum 47:1533–1538
61. D'Hoore A, Penninckx F (2003) Obstructed defecation. Colorectal Dis 5:280–287
62. Halverson AL and Orkin BA (1998) Which physiologic tests are useful in patients with constipation? Dis Colon Rectum 41:735–739
63. Van der Sijp JR, Kamm MA, Nighingale JM et al (1993) Radioisotope determination of regional colonic transit in severe constipation: comparison with radio opaque markers. Gut 44:77–80
64. Rao SSC, Ozturk R, Laine L (2005) Clinical utility of diagnostic tests for constipation in adults: a systematic review. Am J Gastroenterol 100:1605–1615
65. Jones PN, Lubowski DZ, Swash M et al (1987) Is paradoxical contraction of puborectalis muscle of functional importance? Dis Colon Rectum 30:667–670
66. Miller R, Duthie GS, Bartolo DC et al (1991) Anismus in patients with normal and slow transit constipation. Br J Surg 78:690–692
67. Minguez M, Herreros B, Sanchiz V et al (2004) Predictive value of the Balloon expulsion test for excluding the diagnosis of pelvic floor dyssynergia in constipation. Gastroenterology 126:57–62
68. Rao SSC, Mudipalli RS, Stessman M et al (2004) Investigation of the utility of colorectal function tests and Rome II criteria in dyssynergic defecation (anismus). Neurogastroenterol Motil 16:1–8
69. Shorvon PJ, McHugh S, Diamant NE et al (1989) Defecography in normal volunteers: results and implication. Gut 30:1737–1749
70. van Dam JH, Hop WC, Schouten WR (2000) Analysis of patients with poor outcome of rectocele repair. Dis Colon Rectum 43:1556–1560
71. Watson SJ, Loder PB, Halligan S et al (1996) Transperineal repair of symptomatic rectocele with Marlex mesh: a clinical physiological and radiologic assessment of treatment. J Am Coll Surg 183:257–261
72. Tjandra JJ, Ooi BS, Tang CL et al (1999) Transanal repair of rectocele corrects obstructed defecation if it is not associated with anismus. Dis Colon Rectum 42:1544–1550
73. Bartram C (2003) Dynamic evaluation of the anorectum. Radiol Clin N Am 41:425–441
74. Halligan S, Bartram CI, Park HJ et al (1995) The proctographic features of anismus. Radiology 197:679–682
75. Halligan S, Maoluf A, Bartram CI et al (2001) Predictive value of impaired evacuation at proctography in diagnosing anismus. AJR Am J Roentegenol 177:633–636
76. Harvey C, Halligan S, and Bartram CI (1999) Evacuation proctography: a prospective study of diagnostic and therapeutic impact. Radiology 221:223–227
77. Maglinte DDT, Kelvin FM, Hale DS et al (1997) Dynamic cystoproctography: a unifying diagnostic approach to pelvic floor and anorectal dysfunction. AJR Am J Roentegenol 169:759–767
78. Kelvin FM, Maglinte DDT (2003) Dynamic evaluation of female pelvic organ prolapse by extended proctography. Radiol Clin N Am 41:395–407
79. Maglinte DDT, Kelvin FM, Fitzgeralg K et al (1999) Association of compartment defects in pelvic floor dysfunction. AJR Am J Roentegenol 172:439–444
80. Benson JT (1992) Female pelvic floor disorders. Investigation and management. Norton, New York
81. Altringer WE, Saclarides TJ, Dominguez JM et al (1995) Four-contrast defecography: pelvic "floor-oscopy". Dis Colon Rectum 38:695–699
82. Kelvin FM, Maglinte DDT, Hale DS et al (2000) Female pelvic organ prolapse: a comparison of triphasic dynamic MR imaging and triphasic fluoroscopic cystocolpoproctography. AJR Am J Roentegenol 174:81–88
83. Lienemann A, Anthuber C, Baron A et al (1997) Dynamic MR colpocystorectography assessing pelvic-floor descent. Eur Radiol 7:1309–1317
84. Kamm MA, Hoyle CH, Burleigh DE et al (1991) Hereditary internal anal sphincter myopathy causing proctalgia fugax and constipation. A newly identified condition. Gastroenterology 100:805–810
85. Marshall M, Halligan S, Fortheringham T et al (2002) Predictive value of internal anal sphincter thickness for diagnosis of rectal intussusception in patients with solitary rectal ulcer syndrome. Br J Surg 89:1281–1285
86. Cola B, Cuicchi D, Dalla Via B et al (2005) Endosonographic pattern of solitary polypoid rectal ulcer. Tech Coloproctol 9:71–72

Invited Commentary

A. Shafik

The rectal neck (anal canal) is the terminal part of the gut. Its importance arises from the fact that it is the gateway to the whole gut; it is thus surrounded by sphincters and muscles that regulate the passage of the rectal content to the exterior. These muscles are responsible for fecal continence and defecation.

External Anal Sphincter

The external anal sphincter (EAS) is a triple-loop system consisting of top, intermediate, and base loops [1] (Fig. VII.47). Each loop is separated from the other by a fascial septum (Fig. VII.48) and has its individual attachment, direction of muscle bundles, and innervation. The top loop comprises the deep part of the external sphincter and puborectalis, which are intimately fused together. Its muscle bundles loop around the upper part of the rectal neck and are attached to the symphysis pubis. It sends a downward prolongation, which descends along the rectal neck and shares in the formation of the longitudinal muscle (Fig. VII.48). It is supplied by the inferior hemorrhoidal nerve [2, 3]. The intermediate loop embraces the midportion of the rectal neck and is innervated by the perineal branch of the fourth sacral nerve. The base loop encloses the lower rectal neck and is supplied by the inferior hemorrhoidal nerve. It consists of only loop fibers in its upper part and of inner-circular and outer-loop fibers in its lower part.

Mechanism of Action

The external sphincter induces voluntary continence by a double-fold action [4]: (a) prevention of internal sphincter relaxation on detrusor contraction, which I termed "voluntary inhibition reflex," and (b) direct compression of the rectal neck, or the "mechanical action."

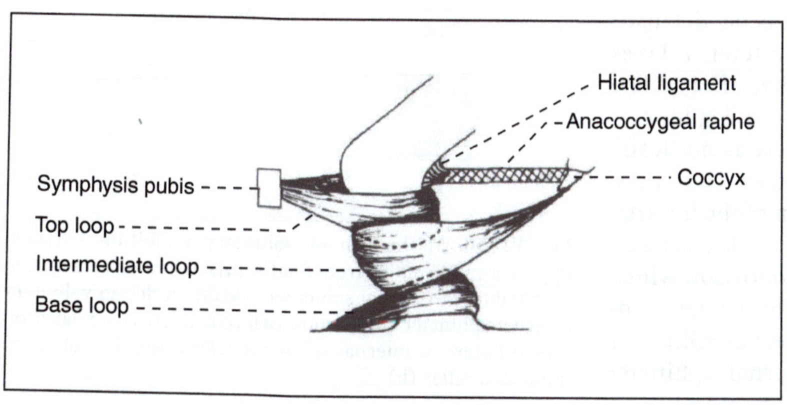

Fig. VII.47. Triple-loop system of the external anal sphincter (from Shafik [1])

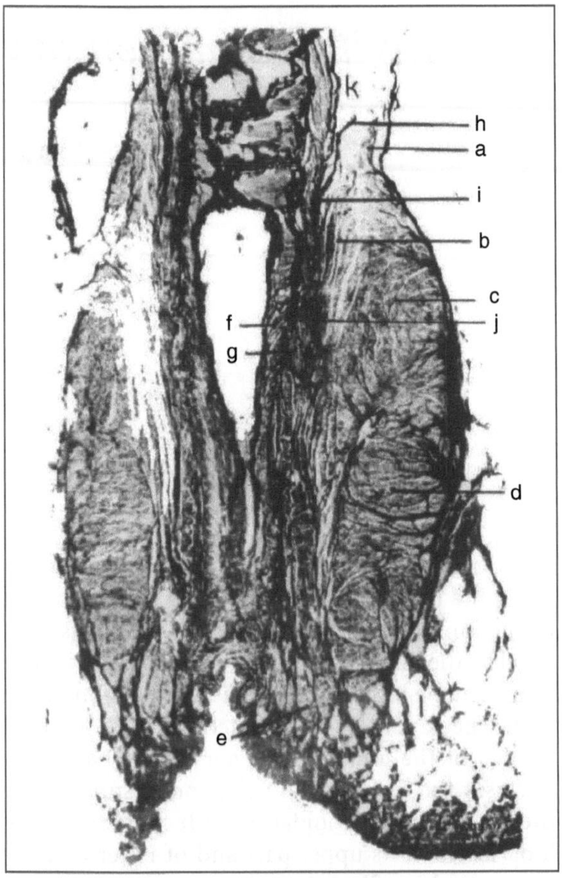

Fig. VII.48. Coronal section at the level of the midanal orifice shows the three loops of the external anal sphincter. It shows also the external anal fascia investing the whole sphincter and sending inward extensions between its loops. Verhoeff-van Gieson X7. (from Shafik [1]): levator plate (a), suspensory sling (b), top loop (fused puborectalis and deep external anal sphincter) (c), intermediate loop of external anal sphincter (d), base loop of external anal sphincter (e), internal anal sphincter (f), longitudinal anal muscle (g), fascia on pelvic surface of levator plate (h), hiatal ligament (i), tunnel septum (j), pelvirectal space (k), ischiorectal space (l)

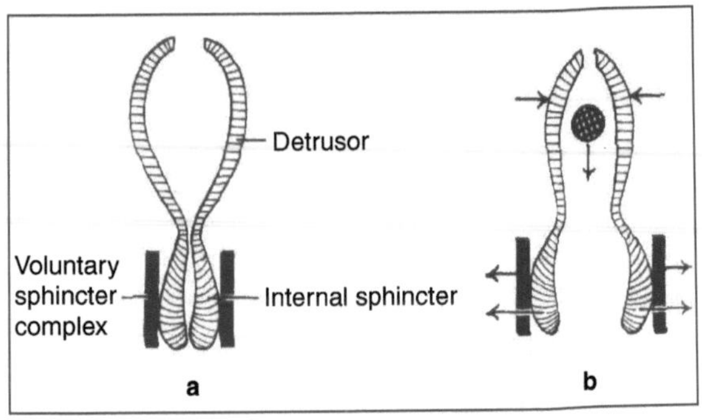

Fig. VII.49. External and internal sphincters at rest and during defecation: at rest – detrusor relaxed and internal sphincter involuntarily contracted (**a**); during defecation – detrusor contracted and external and internal sphincters relaxed (**b**) (from Shafik [4])

Voluntary inhibition reflex

As stools enter the rectum, the rectal detrusor contracts, and the internal sphincter relaxes reflexly to open the rectal neck (Fig. VII.49). The latter does not open unless the external sphincter relaxes voluntarily. However, if there is no desire to defecate, the external sphincter contracts, mechanically preventing relaxation of the internal sphincter. Failure of the latter to relax reflexly inhibits contraction of the rectal detrusor, which relaxes and dilates to accommodate the new contents (Fig. VII.50). Voluntary external sphincter contraction to inhibit reflex internal sphincter relaxation is the "voluntary inhibition reflex" [4]. This is the main action responsible for voluntary continence. Internal sphincter integrity is thus necessary not only for involuntary continence but also for voluntary continence, the voluntary inhibition reflex being mediated through it. For this reason, internal sphincter reconstruction should be considered as an essential step in rectal incontinence repair [5].

Voluntary mechanical action

Besides the voluntary inhibition reflex, external sphincter contraction firmly seals the rectal neck by mechanical compression (Fig. VII.51). Being striped, the external sphincter cannot contract for a long period to maintain continence mechanical-

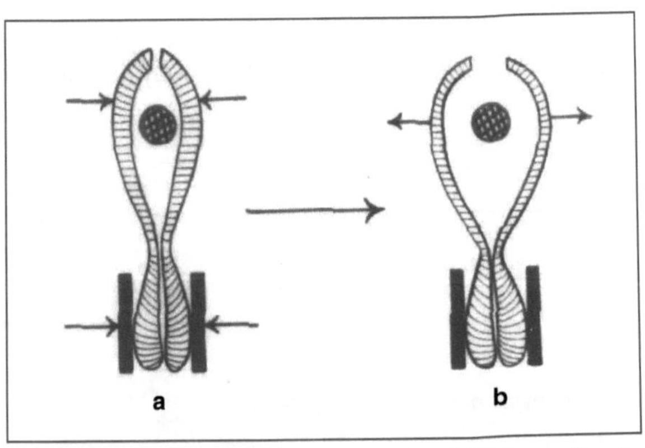

Fig. VII.50. Mechanism of voluntary inhibition reflex to oppose a call to stool (from Shafik [4]): detrusor contraction with failure of internal sphincter relaxation due to voluntary external sphincter contraction (**a**); reflex detrusor relaxation due to failure of internal sphincter relaxation, the voluntary inhibition reflex (**b**)

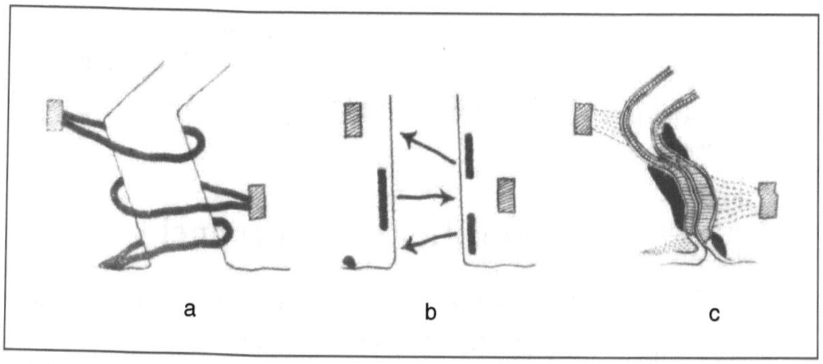

Fig. VII.51. Mechanism of anal occlusion by the mechanical compression of the triple-loop system of the external anal sphincter (from Shafik [1]): external sphincter relaxed (**a**), direction of contraction of external sphincter loops (**b**), external sphincter contracted causing air-tight anal occlusion (**c**)

ly. The mechanical compression action is thus momentary (40–60 s) and serves to occlude the rectal neck by the time the detrusor relaxes as a result of the voluntary inhibition reflex.

Stress Defecation

In internal sphincter damage, voluntary continence is induced only by the mechanical action of the external sphincter [4]. Voluntary inhibition reflex is lost. Being striped, the external sphincter cannot contract long enough to withstand the noninhibited, prolonged contraction of the loaded detrusor. Detrusor contraction continues despite external sphincter contraction until the latter fatigues and relaxes and the detrusor evacuates itself (Fig. VII.52). Hence, in cases of internal sphincter damage, once the desire to defecate is initiated, evacuation should occur. This condition, which I gave the name "stress defecation" [4], is observed in patients after internal sphincterotomy for anal fissure. It could also explain the impaired control of feces and flatus after internal sphincterotomy.

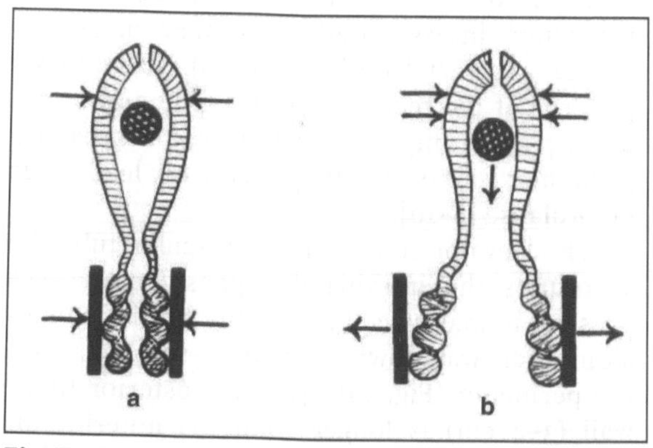

Fig. VII.52. Mechanism of stress defecation: detrusor contraction with external sphincter contraction – internal sphincter is damaged (**a**); detrusor continues contraction, uninhibited by the damaged internal sphincter – external sphincter fatigues, relaxes, and defecation occurs (**b**) (from Shafik [4])

Single-loop Continence

As a result of the separate arrangement of the three external sphincter loops, and since each loop has its own separate and bilateral innervation, any single loop can function as a sphincter [4]. External sphincter continent action can be achieved by a single-loop contraction and not necessarily by the three loops. This constitutes the basis of "single-loop continence" [4]. On contraction, a single loop induces continence by both the voluntary inhibition reflex and mechanical occlusion. The latter action is significantly tight in loop contraction, being effected not only by direct compression but also by rectal-neck kinking [1].

Anogenital Muscle

A recent study has demonstrated that the base loop of the EAS extends uninterrupted across the perineum to the bulb of the penis where it becomes continuous with the bulbocavernosus muscle [6]. While lying over the bulb, the muscle bundles were arranged into three groups: one median and two lateral (Fig. VII.53). Median fibers form the "retractor penis muscle," which is inserted into the corpora cavernosa, while lateral fibers, or the "compressor bulbae muscle," are inserted into the perineal membrane. Upon glans stimulation, both the EAS and the bulbocavernosus muscle contract synchronously with similar latency and action potentials [6]. The bulbocavernosus muscle is an integral part of the EAS, and the muscle in its entirety is appropriately named "anogenital muscle." The muscle plays a dual and syn-

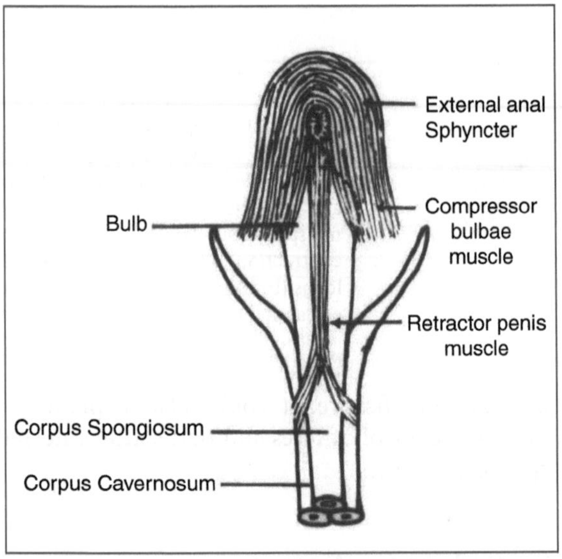

Fig. VII.53. Diagram showing the lateral fibers of the base loop of the external anal sphincter overlying the penile bulb and forming the compressor bulbae muscle while the median fibers proceed forward, forming the retractor penis muscle, which bifurcates on either side of the corpora cavernosa (from Shafik [6])

chronous role in fecal control and sexual response. It is suggested that external sphincter disorders lead to sexual dysfunction and vice versa.

Longitudinal Muscle

The longitudinal muscle consists of three layers: medial, intermediate, and lateral [7]. (Fig. VII.48). The medial longitudinal muscle is a continuation of the longitudinal rectal muscle coat. The intermediate muscle is the suspensory sling of the levator ani whereas the lateral muscle is the longitudinal extension of the top loop of the EAS [1]. The fleshy longitudinal muscle ends at the level of the lower border of the internal sphincter by giving rise to a fascial condensation called "central tendon" [7]. The latter splits into multiple fibrous septa. The medial septum attaches to the rectal-neck lining whereas the lateral passes into the ischiorectal fossa. The intermediate septa penetrate the external sphincter base loop, decussate to form the corrugator cutis, and insert in the perineal skin (Fig. VII.48). The longitudinal muscle plays an important role in the mechanism of defecation [7]. On contraction at stool, it shortens and widens the rectal neck. Furthermore, it helps to fix the rectal neck during straining at defecation, thus preventing rectal prolapse [7]. Subluxation of the longitudinal muscle shares in rectal prolapse genesis [8].

Levator Hiatus and Tunnel

The levator ani consists essentially of the pubococcygeus, the iliococcygeus being rudimentary in humans. The puborectalis is not a part of the levator; both differ in morphology, innervation, and function [9, 10]. The pubococcygeus is funnel shaped, with a transverse portion called "levator plate" and a vertical portion called suspensory sling [9, 10] (Fig. VII.48). The levator plate is an oval cone, which stretches across the pelvis; the levator hiatus occupies its anterior portion, and the rectococcygeal raphe exists posteriorly (Fig. VII.54). Two patterns of the rectococcygeal raphe could be identified: single and triple decussation (Fig. VII.55). The latter seems to give firmness to the levator plate and might be a factor in resisting rectal prolapse [9]. The "hiatal ligament" connects the medial border of the levator plate to the anorectal junction [9, 10]. The levator plate consists of two "crura" that bound the levator hiatus and of two "lateral masses" [10] (Fig. VII.54). Three crural patterns were identified: classic, crural overlap, and crural scissor (Fig. VII.56).

The levator ani is the principal muscle of defecation. On contraction at defecation, it opens the rectal neck for the stool to descend. Any interference with levator function results in disturbance of the defecation act and leads to levator dysfunction syndrome [11], which presents as descending perineum, intussusception, solitary ulcer syndrome, and rectal prolapse [8–10]. The different patterns of the rectococcygeal raphe and levator crura play an important role in rectal-neck support; their subluxation may eventually lead to rectal prolapse [8–10].

The "levator tunnel" is a muscular tube that surrounds the intrahiatal organs (rectal neck, prostate in males; vagina and urethra in females) along their way down from the levator hiatus to the perineum (Fig. VII.54). The posterior tunnel wall (3–4 cm) is longer than the anterior one (2.5–3 cm). The tunnel is double sheathed with an inner coat of the suspensory sling and an outer of the puborectalis. Both coats are of striped muscle bundles. The inner coat is a tunnel "dilator," which opens the rectal neck at defecation, whereas the

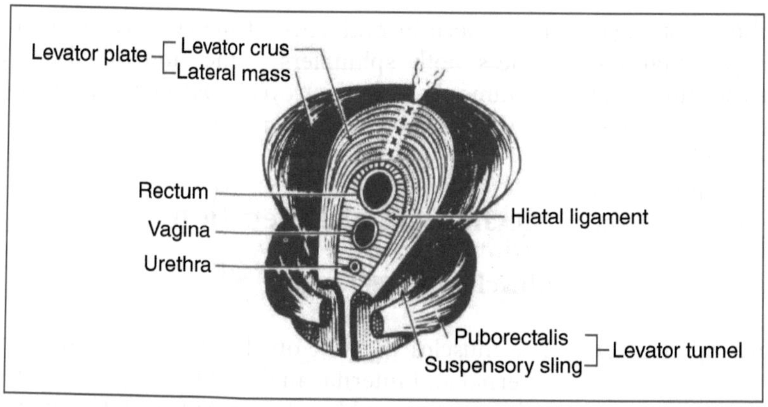

Fig. VII.54. Diagram illustrating the levator plate and tunnel (from Shafik [10])

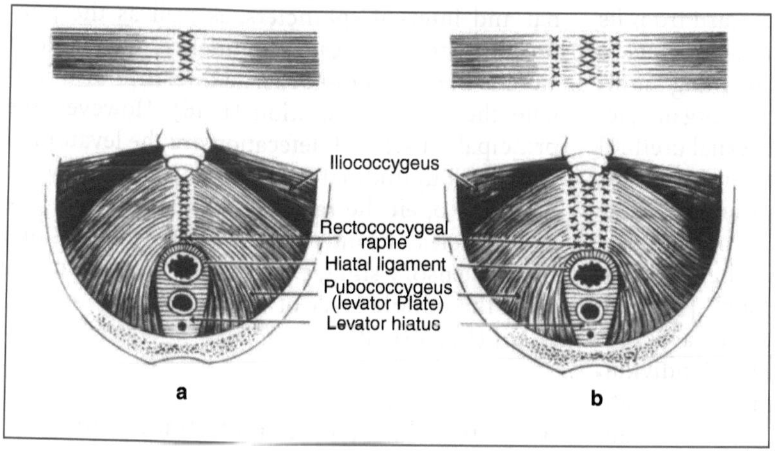

Fig. VII.55. Diagram illustrating decussation patterns of the rectococcygeal raphe (from Shafik [10]): single pattern (**a**), triple pattern (**b**)

outer coat is a tunnel "constrictor" [10]. The "tunnel septum," a grayish white membrane, lines the inner aspect of the levator tunnel and separates it from the fascia propria of the intrahiatal organs [10] (Fig. VII.48). It separates voluntary from involuntary components of the levator tunnel. It serves as an important landmark during mobilization of the intrahiatal organs from within the levator tunnel as in the operation of anorectal mobilization for rectal cancer [12, 13].

Hiatal Ligament

The levator plate is connected to the intrahiatal organs by a fascial condensation called the "hiatal ligament" [9, 10] (Fig. VII.48). It arises from the inner edge of the levator plate and splits fanwise into multiple septa to insert into the upper rectal neck, vesical neck, as well as into the upper vaginal end. Anteriorly, the ligament fills the gap between the two levator crura at their origin,

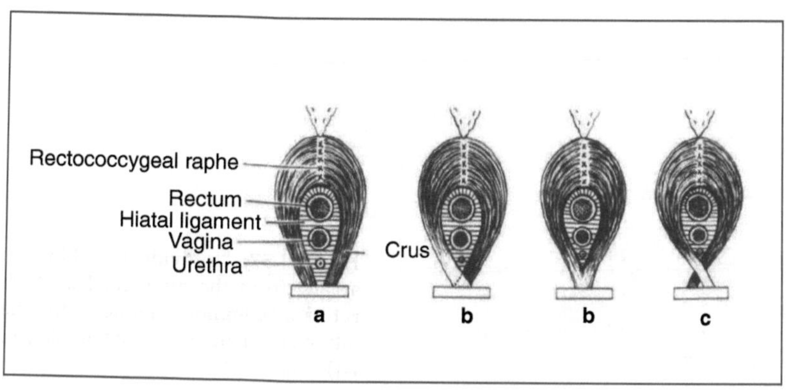

Fig. VII.56. Different crural patterns of the levator ani muscle (from Shafik [10]): classic pattern (**a**), crural overlap (**b**), crural scissor (**c**)

forming the puboprostatic or pubovesical ligament [9, 10]. The hiatal ligament plays a vital role in harmonizing the action between levator plate and intrahiatal organs during evacuation of their contents (defecation and urination). Hiatal ligament subluxation interferes not only with the act of evacuation but leads also to prolapse of the intrahiatal organs [8, 9, 14].

Puborectalis and the Double-Sphincter Control

The puborectalis, as it proceeds backward from its origin in the symphysis pubis, gives off muscle bundles to each intrahiatal organ, forming "individual" voluntary sphincters for these organs [10, 15] (Fig. VII.57). It gives rise to the external urethral sphincter and deep EAS in both genders, as well as to the vaginal sphincter in the female and prostatic sphincter in the male. However, the puborectalis and deep EAS were found fused together, the conjoint muscle being named "top loop" [1]. Each intrahiatal organ is thus provided with a double voluntary sphincteric apparatus: (a) an "individual" organ sphincter, derived from the puborectalis and specific for the organ, and (b) a "common" tunnel sphincter, the puborectalis itself, which acts on the intrahiatal organs collectively. This separate sphincteric activity for the individual organs under the control of a common continent muscle secures not only an immune sphincteric function to the organ but a harmonized action among the structures enclosed within the levator tunnel [16, 17]. Further, the double sphincteric mechanism provided to each organ could be a guarantee of functional maintenance in case either of the two sphincters is damaged. Injury of either sphincter alone does not induce incontinence of the concerned organ. Unless both sphincters – the "individual" and "common" – are destroyed, continence could be maintained by either [10, 15, 17].

Mechanism of Defecation

Muscles of Defecation

The muscles that act on the rectal neck are the external and internal anal sphincters, puborectalis, levator ani, and longitudinal muscle. The external and internal sphincters, as well as the puborectalis, are muscles of continence. Their role at stool is to contract in order to interrupt or terminate the act of defecation [1, 16]. However, the principal muscles of defecation are the levator ani and the longitudinal muscles [7, 9, 10]. They act jointly to open the rectal neck at defecation. The two muscles are interrelated due to the fact that the suspensory sling, a part of the levator, constitutes the middle layer of the longitudinal muscle [7, 10] (Fig. VII.48).

Anatomical Mechanism of Defecation

With knowledge of the physioanatomical aspects of the pelvic floor muscles and assisted by manometric EMG and barium enema studies, the precise mechanism of defecation could be explored [18, 19]. As stools enter the rectum, reflex detrusor contraction and internal sphincter relaxation occur. Continuation of defecation depends on two factors: (a) external sphincter relaxation, and (b) straining. If defecation is acceded to, the external sphincter is voluntarily relaxed. Straining is nec-

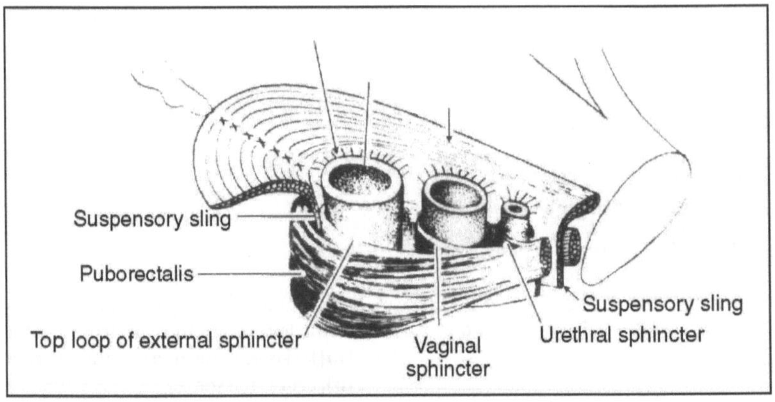

Fig. VII.57. "Individual" sphincters arising from the puborectalis, which act as a "common" sphincter for the intrahiatal structures (from Shafik [10, 15])

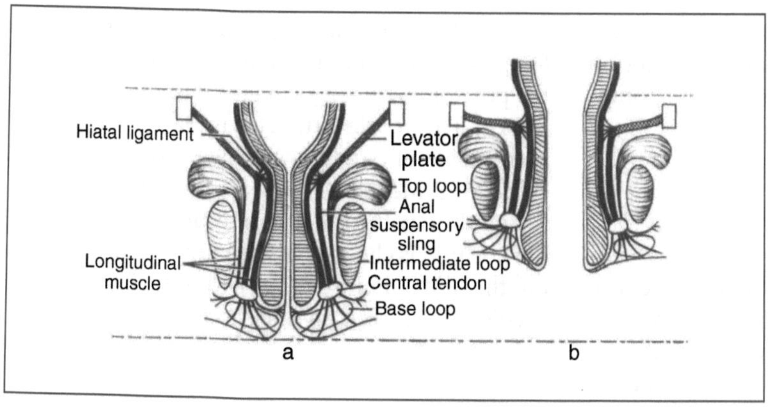

Fig. VII.58. Mechanism of defecation: at rest (**a**); at defecation – flattening of levator cone as well as suspensory sling contraction result in opening of anal canal (**b**) (from Shafik [4, 18])

essary to maintain defecation, as it raises the intra-abdominal pressure. This serves a double purpose: it compresses the detrusor, which helps evacuation, and it stimulates levator contraction through the straining-levator reflex [20]. Although the intra-abdominal pressure compresses the detrusor, the rectal neck is spared owing to its protected location below the levator plate. When the levator plate contracts, it moves from the cone to the flat position and is elevated and laterally retracted [9] (Fig. VII.58). This results in pulling on the hiatal ligament, which in turn pulls open the anorectal junction and partially opens the rectal angle. Simultaneously, the suspensory sling contracts and not only pulls up the base loop to unseal the anal orifice, but it also partially opens the rectal neck (Fig. VII.58).

The longitudinal muscle joins the detrusor in contraction, which results in shortening and opening of the rectal neck as well as in complete straightening of the rectal angle [7]. This brings the rectal neck into alignment with the detrusor so that efficient fecal pumping occurs. The final result of the joint contraction of the detrusor, longitudinal muscle, and levator is the opening of the rectal neck for the rectum to evacuate its contents.

Physiologic Mechanism of Defecation

The concerted functions of the anorectal musculature at defecation are initiated and harmonized by voluntary impulses and reflex actions, as demonstrated in recent communications [21–24]. When the rectal detrusor is distended with fecal mass and the stretch receptors are stimulated, the rectoanal inhibitory reflex [21] is initiated by which the rectal detrusor contracts and the internal sphincter relaxes. Detrusor contraction triggers two reflexes: the rectopuborectalis reflex [22] and the rectolevator reflex [23]. These two reflexes act simultaneously yet have opposite functions; on detrusor contraction, the rectolevator reflex effects a reflex levator contraction, which opens the rectal neck. At the same time, the reflex puborectalis contraction, actuated by the rectopuborectalis reflex, functions to close or keep closed the rectal neck as impulses reach the conscious level to probe the circumstances for defecation. If inopportune, the puborectalis continues voluntary contraction.

Voluntary puborectalis contraction evokes two reflex actions: (a) reflex levator relaxation through the levator-puborectalis reflex [24], and (b) reflex detrusor relaxation by means of the voluntary inhibition reflex [4]. Meanwhile, it aborts the rectoanal inhibitory reflex, which relaxes the internal sphincter. Hence, voluntary puborectalis contraction, through the voluntary inhibition reflex, prevents internal sphincter relaxation, which results in reflex detrusor relaxation and waning of the urge to defecate [4]. However, as soon as circumstances would allow defecation and the sensation of desire is felt, the puborectalis muscle relaxes voluntarily, and the detrusor evacuates its contents. This demonstrates that the act of defecation is under voluntary control despite the presence of reflex actions sharing in the mechanism of defecation. Thus, although the rectoanal inhibitory and rectolevator reflexes function to open the rectal neck, the rectopuborectalis and the levator-puborectalis reflexes keep the rectal neck closed until the decision for defecation has been made.

Straining at the start of defecation is a normal physiological process and as such is part of the mechanism of defecation. By elevating the intra-abdominal pressure, it triggers the straining-levator reflex [20], which effects levator contraction and the opening of the rectal neck for spontaneous evacuation of stools.

Anorectal Physiology Testing

As regards the studies needed in the treatment of benign anorectal disease, valuable information can be obtained from a physical workup, including neurologic and proctologic examination. Investigations comprise barium enema, colonoscopy and biopsy studies, defecography [25, 26], intestinal transit, anorectal manometry, balloon expulsion test [27], and defecometry [28], as well as electromyogram (EMG) of anal sphincters and levator ani muscle. This is in addition to endoanal ultrasonography (EAU) and magnetic resonance imaging (MRI). However, conventional examinations of the anorectum commonly reveal little correlation between subjective symptoms and investigative results. Although they offer valuable information regarding anorectal function, they are not representative of the act of defecation, and the range of normality is quite broad. Herein, we present new methods that can add to the diagnostic tools investigating the anorectum.

EMG: levator ani muscle

With the patient in the left lateral position, a concentric needle electromyographic electrode (type 13 L 49, DISA, Copenhagen, Denmark) of 65 mm in length and 0.65 mm in diameter is inserted through the perianal skin 2–2.5 cm lateral to the anal orifice [23, 29]. The needle is directed upward to an approximate depth of 2–2.5 cm. A standard EMG apparatus (type MES, Medelec, Woking, UK) is used to amplify and display the potentials recorded. Correct needle position is checked by the burst of activity heard on the EMG loudspeaker and visualized on the oscilloscope screen on muscle contraction.

Fecoflowmetry

Since the introduction of the fecoflowmeter, which we developed to obtain an authentic and detailed recording of the act of defecation [30–32], fecal flow rate can be studied from curves that represent the changes occurring in rate versus time. Fecal flow rate is the product of rectal detrusor action against outlet resistance. A 1-l enema is given, and the subject sits on the commode of the fecoflowmeter when he/she feels the desire to defecate. Fecoflowmetry provides quantitative and qualitative data regarding the act of defecation (Figs. VII.59 and 60). It is simple, easy, noninvasive, and nonradiological.

Determination of Residual Stools

Twenty healthy volunteers, mean age 35.7 years, and 25 patients with chronic idiopathic constipation (CIC), mean age 31.2 years, were evaluated for

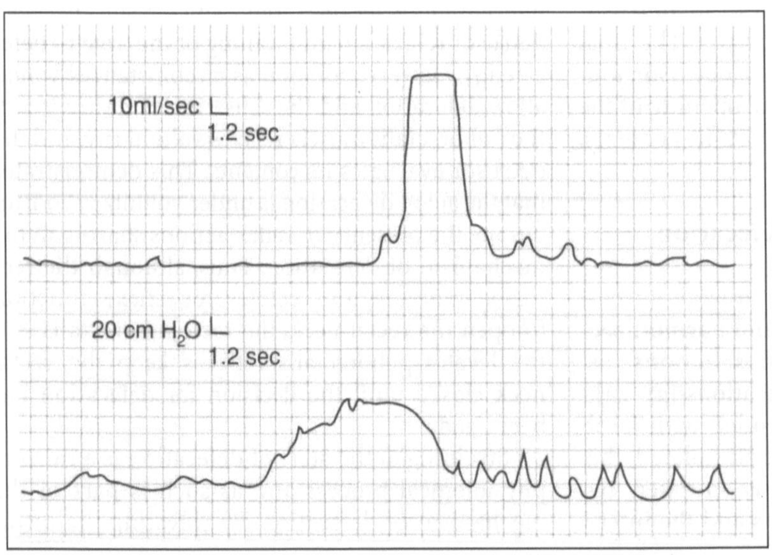

Fig. VII.59. Normal fecoflowmetry (*upper tracing*) and intra-abdominal pressure (*lower tracing*). Intra-abdominal pressure increased before the start of flow curve. When flow started, pressure dropped (from Shafik [31])

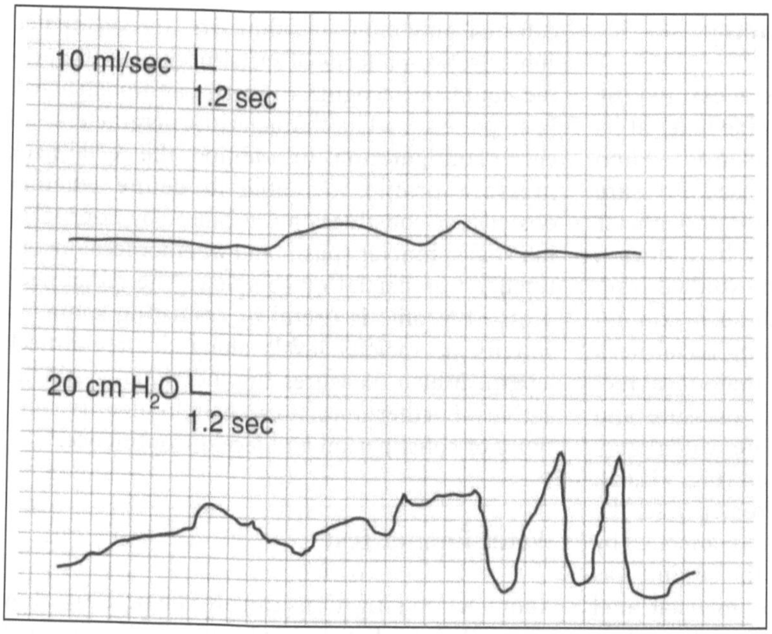

Fig. VII.60. Fecoflowmetry (*upper tracing*) and intra-abdominal pressure (*lower tracing*) in chronic constipation. Mean and maximum flow rate was small, and flow curve showed a plateau compared with normal flow curve. Flow was maintained as long as high pressure was maintained (from Shafik [31])

residual stools in the rectum after defecation [33]. The act of defecation was studied by fecoflowmetry. A 1-l water enema was administered, and fecoflowmetric studies were done while the subject was evacuating the enema. After evacuation, a rectal tube was introduced to evacuate the residual fluid for quantitative assessment. Six of the 20 healthy volunteers had a mean volume of residual fluid of 32.3 ml; the remaining subjects had no residual fluid. All constipated patients had a mean residual fluid of 370.6 ml.

Rectometry

Rectal volume, pressure, and compliance at first rectal and urge sensation are assessed in one test by a simple and noninvasive new parameter: rectometry [34]. The shape of the rectometrogram is also informative. Rectometry was performed on 36 subjects: 20 healthy volunteers and 16 patients with constipation. Carbon dioxide was infused into a balloon introduced into the rectum and connected to a pressure transducer. The rectal neck and intra-abdominal pressures were measured simultaneously. A rectometrogram was obtained (Fig. VII.61). It reads the volume of carbon dioxide infused and the intrarectal and detrusor pressure at both the first rectal and urge sensation. In addition to quantitative values, the curve configuration could differentiate between not only normal and constipated subjects but also obstructive and inertia-type constipation. Apart from its diagnostic value, rectometry can be used to monitor the effectiveness of pharmacotherapy on detrusor function.

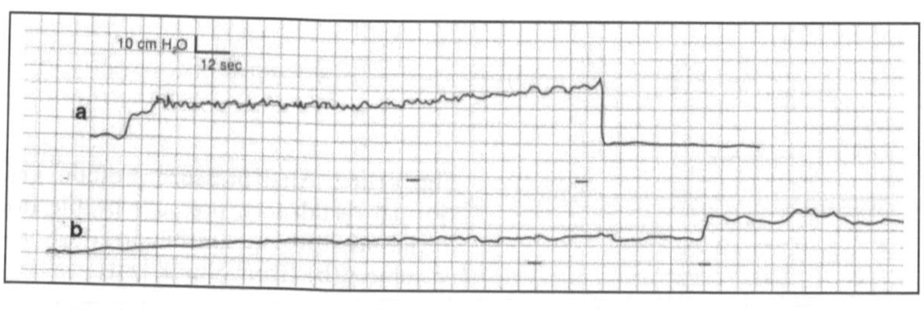

Fig. VII.61. Rectometrogram. Normal rectometrogram (**a**): *first dash* below curve denotes first rectal sensation, *second dash* denotes sensation of urge. Rectometrogram of constipation (**b**): Patient failed to expel the balloon (from Shafik [34])

Rectal-neck Pressure Profilometry

Rectal-neck pressure profile was measured by means of a catheter with a ring of side holes at its distal end [35]. After the catheter was inserted into the rectum, carbon dioxide was infused. Pressure in the rectal neck was recorded while the catheter was being withdrawn automatically by a device. Important parameters that could be studied from the rectal-neck pressure profile include: maximum rectal-neck pressure, maximal closing rectal-neck pressure, as well as functional and anatomical rectal-neck lengths. Mean rectal-neck pressure and the pressure index could also be calculated. Normal profilogram was bell shaped (Fig. VII.62). The ascending limb showed a two-step rise, the first rise of which was gradual and affected by internal anal sphincter tone while the second was steep and evoked by external and internal anal sphincter tone. A formula was introduced to calculate separately the pressure induced by each of the external and internal sphincters. In constipated subjects, two patterns of rectal-neck pressure profile could be recognized: inertia and obstructed. Each pattern had its characteristic parameters and curve configuration. In addition, the rectal-neck pressure profile was able to define whether obstructive constipation was caused by external or internal sphincter spasm and whether fecal incontinence was partial or complete. The rectal-neck pressure profile is useful in evaluating sphincter activity at various levels along the rectal-neck length. It also measures the individual sphincter activity. Furthermore, it can help to identify some types of constipation and fecal incontinence.

Water Enema Test

Anorectal investigations can also be performed by a recently introduced, simple office test – the water enema test [36]. Water (1.5 l) contained in a gradu-

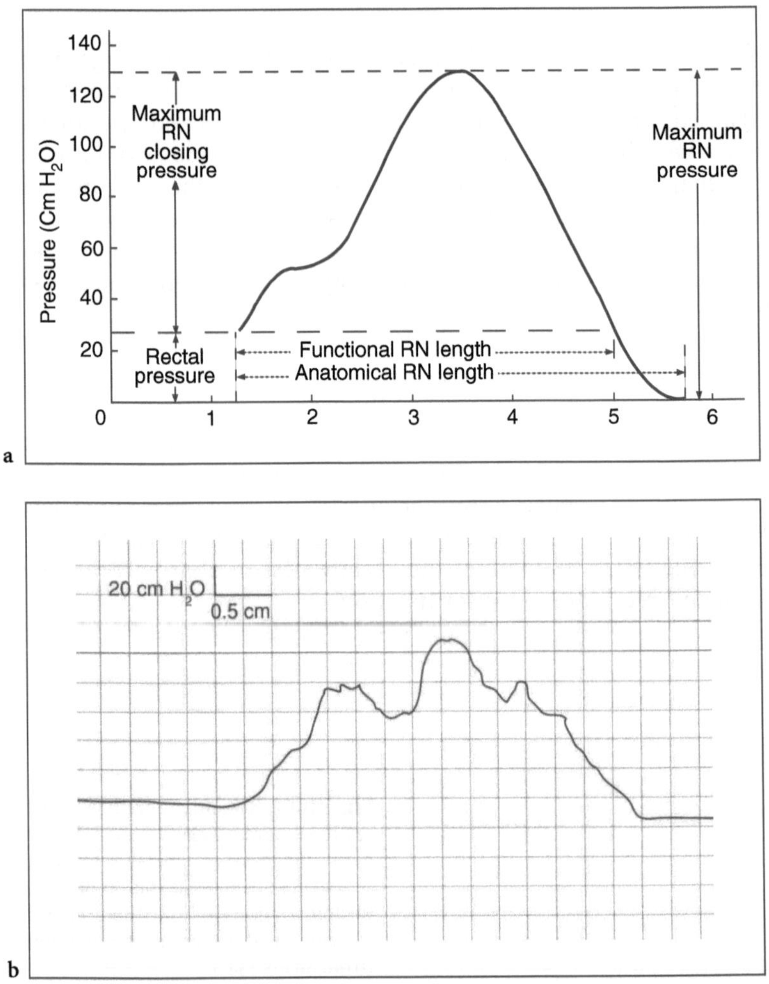

Fig. VII.62. Anal pressure profilometry. Normal rectal-neck pressure profile (**a**). Rectal-neck pressure profile in constipated subject (**b**) (from Shafik [35])

ated vessel and incubated at 37°C is instilled under gravity into the rectum through a 16F Nelaton catheter at a rate of 150 ml/min. The subject is asked to report on the first rectal sensation as well as on the desire and urge to evacuate. The volume of water infused at the time of these occurrences is determined and compared with standard levels in controls. Defecation disorders may be identified with this easy and noninvasive test.

Fecal-Leak Test

To assess results of repair and the degree of fecal incontinence, another simple office test was performed in 24 patients with complete incontinence who had undergone direct suture operation [37]. Rectal pressure and infusion volume were recorded during rectal filling with saline at a rate of 50 cc/min. Two rectal-leak pressures were determined: resting and coughing. Before incontinence repair, coughing rectal-leak pressure was significantly higher than the resting one whereas the infused saline volume at the two pressure levels showed an insignificant difference. After operative repair, 16 patients who became totally continent had no leakage. Six patients who improved following partial incontinence exhibited a significant increase in resting and coughing rectal-leak pressures compared with preoperative values. Infused saline volume at the two leak pressures also increased significantly. The two patients who remained incontinent after repair showed an insignificant difference in resting and coughing rectal-leak pressure or infused saline volume against prerepair levels. The degree of continence increased with the increase in resting and coughing rectal pressure. Resting rectal-leak pressure determines outlet resistance under normal conditions while coughing rectal-leak pressure determines outlet resistance under stress conditions. The rectal-leak pressure test is a simple, reproducible, and cost-effective test to assess incontinence and the results of treatment.

Transcutaneous Electrorectography

A transcutaneous recording of rectal electric activity, or an electrorectography, was obtained from 24 healthy volunteers with a mean age of 39.6 years [38]. A silver-silver chloride electrode was applied laterally to each of the two sacroiliac joints, and a third one was placed midway between the left greater trochanter and ischial tuberosity. The reference electrode was applied to the right lower limb. At least two 20-min recording sessions were performed for each of the 24 subjects. In addition, an intrarectal electrorectographic recording was done in ten of the 24 subjects using silver-silver chloride electrodes attached to the rectal mucosa by suction. Pacesetter potentials (PPs) were recorded transcutaneously. The wave was triphasic, with a small positive, a large negative, and another small positive deflection (Fig. VII.63). PPs had a regular rhythm and were reproducible. The mean frequency was 3.1 cycles/min. Transcutaneously recorded PPs could be confirmed by the intrarectal route. Both routes had similar electrorectographic recordings

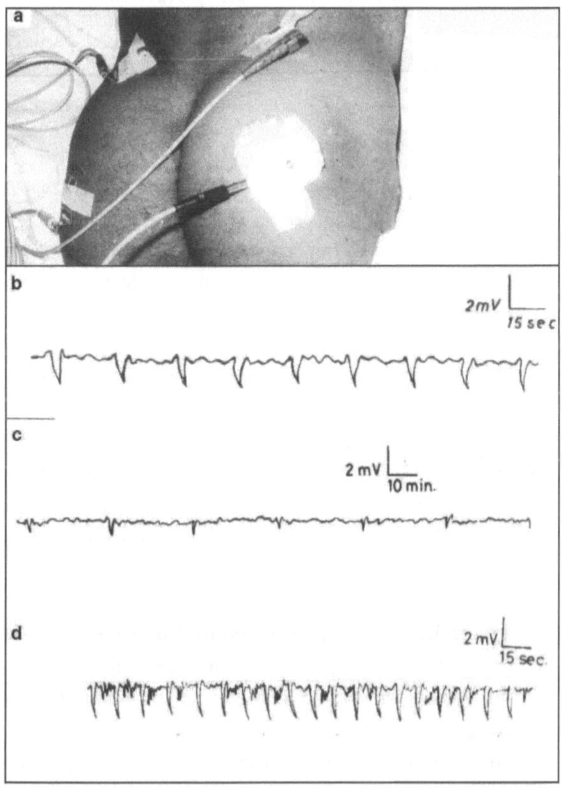

Fig. VII.63. Transcutaneous electrorectogram. Electrodes applied to skin (**a**); electrorectogram in normal subject (**b**); electrorectogram in constipation due to rectal inertia, pacesetter potentials show low frequency, amplitude, and velocity of conduction, a condition we call "bradyrectia" (**c**); electrorectogram of obstructive constipation showing abnormally high frequency, a condition we call "tachyrectia" (**d**) (from Shafik [38])

except for the action potentials, which did not show in the transcutaneous electrorectogram.

Reflexometry

Additional investigative tools to obtain reliable, objective, and substantial information on the physiologic state of pelvic floor muscles and the nerves supplying them are the reflexes described above [4, 19–24, 29, 39, 40]. Evaluation of reflex actions of the pertinent musculature contributes to establishing the diagnosis in anorectal disorders with even greater accuracy, in a more comprehensive manner, and in less time because the approach is direct. The technique follows an easy principle: a balloon-tipped catheter is introduced into the rectum and a needle electrode, inserted into the muscle to be tested, records the response of the muscle to distension of the rectal balloon. Detectable changes in latency or amplitude of motor unit action potentials or the evoked response may indicate a defect in the reflex pathway that could be due to muscle or nerve damage.

Andrological Investigations

Recent studies have shown that anorectal pathological conditions, in particular, acute and chronic anal fissures, and external anal sphincter injuries, were found to be associated in some cases with erectile dysfunction [41, 42]. These findings seem to be related to the close relationship of the external anal sphincter to the bulbocavernosus muscle which is a muscle of erecttion. The bulbocavernosus muscle, was found to be an extension of the external anal sphincter and pathologic conditions in volving the external sphincter may affect the erectile process [42]. For these reasons, while investigating patients with anorectal condition, it seem indicated to inquire about, and investigate form erectile dysfunction.

References

1. Shafik A (1975) A new concept of the anatomy of the anal sphincter mechanism and the physiology of defecation. I. The external anal sphincter: a triple loop system. Invest Urol 12:412–419
2. Shafik A, El-Sherif MYoussef A, El-Sibai O (1995) Surgical anatomy of the pudendal nerve and its clinical implications. Clin Anat 8:110–115
3. Shafik A, Doss S (1999) Study of the surgical anatomy of the somatic terminal innervation to the anal and urethral sphincters: Role in anal and urethral surgery. J Urol 161:85–89
4. Shafik A (1980) A new concept of the anatomy of the anal sphincter mechanism and the physiology of defecation. IX. The single loop continence. A new theory of the mechanism of anal continence. Dis Colon Rectum 23:37–43
5. Shafik A (1981) A new concept of the anatomy of the anal sphincter mechanism and the physiology of defecation. XI. Anal incontinence: a technique for repair: Am J Proct Gastroenterol Col Rect Surg 32:18–23
6. Shafik A (1999) The physioanatomic entirety of the external anal sphincter with the bulbocavernosus muscle: A new concept. Arch Androl 42:45–54
7. Shafik A (1976) A new concept of the anatomy of the anal sphincter mechanism and the physiology of defecation. III. The longitudinal anal muscle; anatomy and role in anal sphincter mechanism. Invest Urol 13:271–277
8. Shafik A (1981) A new concept of the anatomy of the anal sphincter mechanism and the physiology of defecation. XIII. Rectal prolapse: a concept of pathogenesis. Am J Proct Gastroent Col Rect Surg 32: 6–13
9. Shafik A (1975) A new concept of the anatomy of the anal sphincter mechanism and the physiology of defecation. II. Anatomy of the levator ani muscle with special reference to puborectalis. Invest Urol 13:175–182
10. Shafik A (1979) A new concept of the anatomy of the anal sphincter mechanism and the physiology of defecation. VIII. Levator hiatus and tunnel: anatomy and function. Dis Colon Rectum 22:539–549
11. Shafik A (1983) A new concept of the anatomy of the anal sphincter mechanism and the physiology of defecation. XVIII. The levator dysfunction syndrome. A new syndrome with report of 7 cases. Coloproctology 5:158–165
12. Shafik A (1985) A new concept of the anatomy of the anal sphincter mechanism and the physiology of defecation. XXV. Anorectal mobilization in the treatment of rectal lesions. Further study. Coloproctology 7:107–112
13. Shafik A (1986) A new concept of the anatomy of the

anal sphincter mechanism and the physiology of defecation. XXIX. Reversion to normal defecation after combined excision operation and end colostomy for rectal cancer. Am J Surg 151:278–284
14. Shafik A (1987) A new concept of the anatomy of the anal sphincter mechanism and the physiology of defecation. XXVIII. Complete rectal prolapse: a technique of repair: Coloproctology 9:345–352
15. Shafik A (1984) A new concept of the anatomy of the anal sphincter mechanism and the physiology of defecation. XX. The pelvic double-sphincter control complex. Theory of pelvic organ continence with clinical application. Urology 23:611–618
16. Shafik A (1997) Study on the origin of the external anal, urethral, vaginal and prostatic sphincters. Int Urogynecol J Pelvic Floor Dysfunct 8:126–129
17. Shafik A (1998) A new concept of the anatomy of the anal sphincter mechanism and the physiology of defecation. Mass contraction of the pelvic floor muscles. Int Urogynecol J Pelvic Floor Dysfunct 9:28–32
18. Shafik A (1982) A new concept of the anatomy of the anal sphincter mechanism and the physiology of defecation. XVII. Mechanism of defecation. Coloproctology 4:49–54
19. Shafik A (1991) Constipation. Some provocative thoughts. J Clin Gastroenterol 13:259–267
20. Shafik A (1991) Straining-levator reflex. The description of a new reflex and its clinical significance. Coloproctology 13:314–319
21. Denny-Brown D, Robertson EG (1935) An investigation of the nervous control of defecation. Brain 58:256–310
22. Shafik A (1990) A new concept of the anatomy of the anal sphincter mechanism and the physiology of defecation. XLII. Recto-puborectalis reflex. Coloproctology 12:170–172
23. Shafik A (1993) The recto-levator reflex. The description of a new reflex and its clinical application. Preliminary report. Clin Physiol Biochem 10:13–17
24. Shafik A (1991) Levator-puborectalis reflex: Its role in elimination. Pract Gastroenterol 15:28–35
25. Mahieu P, Pringot J, Bodart P (1984) Defecography 1. Description of a new procedure and results in normal patients. Gastrointest Radiol 9:247–251
26. Mahieu P, Pringot J, Bodart P (1984) Defecography 2. Contribution to the diagnosis of defecation disorders. Gastrointest Radiol 9:253–261
27. Barnes PR, Lennard-Jones JE (1984) Patients with constipation of different types have difficulty in expelling a balloon from the rectum. Gut 25:562–563
28. Lestar B, Penninckx FM, Kerremans RP (1989) Defecometry. A new method for determining the parameters of rectal evacuation. Dis Colon Rectum 32:197–201
29. Shafik A (1991) Straining puborectalis reflex: Description and significance of a "new" reflex. Anat Record 229:281–284
30. Shafik A, Khalid AM (1992) Fecoflowmetry in fecal incontinence. Eur Surg Res 24:61–68
31. Shafik A, Khalid A (1993) Fecoflowmetry: A new parameter assessing rectal function in normal and constipated subjects. Dis Colon Rectum 36:32–42
32. Shafik A, Abdel-Moneim K (1992) Fecoflowmetry: A new parameter assessing rectal function. Int Surg 77:190–194
33. Shafik A, El-Sibai O, El-Gohary H et al (1999) Residual rectal fluids in normal, constipated and incontinent subjects. Techn Coloproctol 3:19–21
34. Shafik A, Khaled AM (1991) Rectometry. A new method assessing rectal function. Coloproctology 13:237–243
35. Shafik A (1992) Rectal neck pressure measurement. Technique and role in assessment of rectal neck disorders. Coloproctology 14:42–49
36. Shafik A (1992) Water enema test. A parameter for assessing rectal function. Pract Gastroenterol 16: 24J–24P
37. Shafik A (1992) Fecal leak test. Simple test for assessing degree of fecal incontinence. Gut [Suppl 2] 37: A25, 302
38. Shafik A, Nour A, Abdel-Fattah A (1995) Transcutaneous electrorectography. Human electrorectogram from surface electrodes. Digestion 56:479–482
39. Shafik A (1997) Deflation reflex. Description and clinical significance. Anat Rec 249:405–408
40. Shafik A, El-Sibai O (2001) Rectal inhibition by inferior rectal nerve stimulation in dogs: Recognition of a new reflex: The 'voluntary anorectal inhibition reflex. Eur J Gastroent Hepatol 13:413–418
41. Shafik A, El-Sibai O (2000) The anocavernosal erectile dysfunction syndrome. II. Anal fissure and erectile dysfunction. Int J Import Rcs 12:279-283
42. Shafik A (2001) Injured external anal sphincter in erectilo dysfunction. Andrologia 33:35-41

Section VIII

Treatment Options for Fecal Incontinence

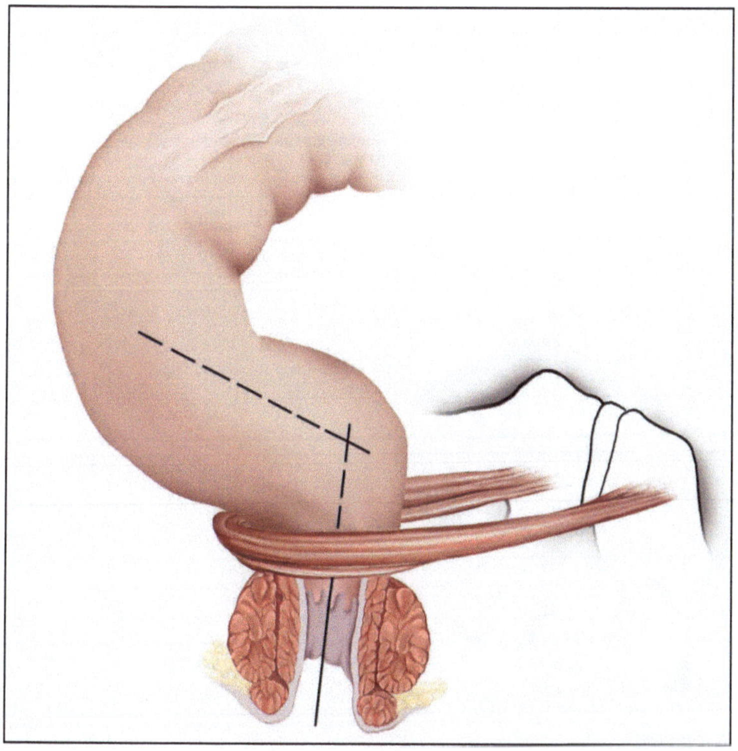

VIII.1. Introduction

G.A. Santoro, G. Di Falco

The treatment of incontinence remains somewhat empirical although considerable advances have been made in understanding the pathophysiology of the condition in recent years [1]. The purpose of this section is to characterize this disorder and to put into perspective the numerous procedures that have been described for the treatment of this condition [2–6].

Normal continence depends on cognitive function, stool volume and consistency, colonic transit, rectal compliance, anorectal sensation, anorectal reflexes, and sphincter control (Fig. VIII.1). Anal incontinence is the inability to control the release of bowel contents, and it can be partial (liquid and gas) or complete (solid). It is important to differentiate between minor levels of functional loss and the clinical state in which there is a serious disruption of normal life. Minor degrees of anal incontinence are defined as the occasional fecal staining of underwear (fecal leakage or soiling or seepage),

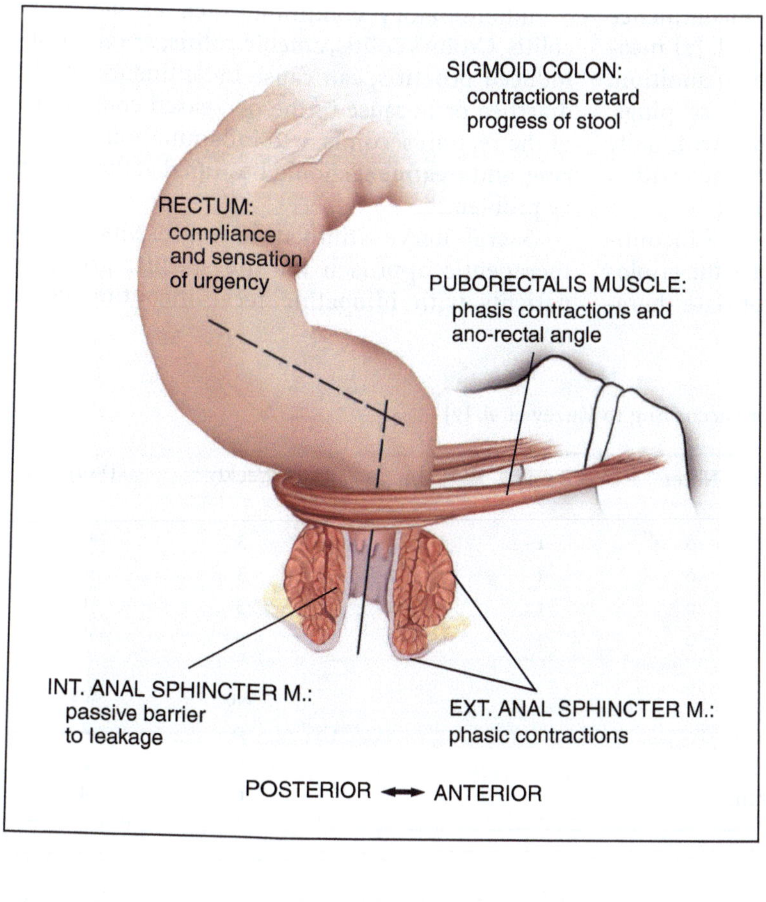

Fig. VIII.1. Pelvic floor components involved in the mechanisms for preserving continence

Table VIII.1. Grading of fecal incontinence according to Parks [4]

Grade	
Parks I	Fully continent
Parks II	Soiling or incontinence to gas
Parks III	Incontinence to liquid stool
Parks IV	Incontinence to solid stool

incontinence of flatus, incontinence in the presence of loose stool only, or rectal urgency. These symptoms are relatively common, especially with increasing age, and most patients can be satisfactorily managed by nonoperative therapy (diet, drugs, bowel training, sphincter exercises, improved hygiene). Major incontinence is defined as the frequent and inadvertent voiding per anum of formed stool and represents the most severe form of fecal incontinence. Several incontinence severity scales have been described in the last 10 years [4–9]. Parks [4] was one of the first to describe such a system (Table VIII.1). This system is very simple, and it is one of the most frequently utilized. However, it does not take into account the frequency of symptoms. St. Mark's incontinence scoring system proposed by Vaizey et al. [7] measures frequency and consistency and, in addition, includes questions on the use of pads or plugs, antidiarrheal medications, interference with daily activities, and association of incontinence with a strong urge to defecate (Table VIII.2) [7].

There are many and varied causes of incontinence, and it is important to categorize the etiology of incontinence so that an appropriate therapeutic approach can be selected (Table VIII.3) [10]. Diagnosing the cause and assessing the severity of the condition precede any treatment [10–12]. Anorectal physiology investigations, such as endoanal ultrasound [12–18], anal manometry [19, 20], pudendal nerve terminal motor latency [21], mucosal electrosensitivity [22], electromyography [23–25], and magnetic resonance [26–27] help the clinician in determining the nature of the incontinence. Most patients have acquired anal incontinence secondary to obstetric laceration [28–36], previous anorectal surgery (such as fistulotomy or hemorrhoidectomy) [37–40], or trauma (such as impalement). These injuries are the most amenable to surgical management, specifically the anal sphincteroplasty [31–44]. Other causes of incontinence, such as long-standing prolapse or third- to fourth-degree hemorrhoids, often respond to treatment of the primary disorder alone. More difficult to treat are the neurogenic injuries, such as those resulting from massive neuromuscular trauma, myelomeningocele or demyelinating diseases of the spinal cord, and diabetic neuropathy. A procedure suited to injuries of this type is to create a neosphincter with the gracilis muscle transposition [45–49] or the artificial bowel sphincter [50].

Inflammatory condition, such as ulcerative colitis, Crohn's colitis, amebic colitis, or radiation-induced proctitis, can cause incontinence by the diarrhea or because of the decreased compliance of the rectum secondary to inflammation or scarring, and treatment should be aimed at the primary problem.

Sacral nerve stimulation represents a new therapeutic approach for the specific group of patients with idiopathic fecal incontinence in

Table VIII.2. St. Mark's incontinence score according to Vaizey et al. [7]

Clinical condition	Never	Rarely	Sometimes	Weekly	Daily
Incontinence to solid stool	0	1	2	3	4
Incontinence to liquid stool	0	1	2	3	4
Incontinence to gas	0	1	2	3	4
Alteration in lifestyle	0	1	2	3	4
				No	Yes
Need to wear a pad or plug				0	2
Taking constipating medicines				0	2
Lack of ability to defer defecation for 15 min				0	4

Table VIII.3. Etiology of fecal incontinence

Category	Mechanism	Common causes
Functional	Rapid transit	Irritable bowel syndrome, inflammatory bowel disease, tumors
	Pelvic floor dyssynergia	Idiopathic, spinal cord injury
	Psychological	Dementia, psychosis, behavioral
Sphincter weakness	Sphincter muscle injury	Obstetrical trauma, accidental trauma, surgical trauma
	Pudendal nerve injury	Obstetrical trauma, idiopathic, peripheral neuropathy
	Central nervous system injury	Spina bifida, spinal cord injury, cerebrovascular accident
Sensory loss	Afferent nerve injury	Diabetic neuropathy, spinal cord injury

which traditional pelvic repair would not be effective [51–53]. An innovative treatment is radiofrequency energy delivered to the anal sphincter, creating precise submucosal thermal lesions. Over time, these lesions are resorbed, and the tissue contracts [54–55]. In patients in whom there is no functioning sphincter muscle at all and in whom it is impractical to create a neosphincter, a defunctioning stoma is often the best option.

There now follows a critical appraisal of the different procedures available for the treatment of fecal incontinence.

References

1. Henry MM, Swash M, Phillips RKS (1992) Faecal incontinence. In: Henry MM, Swash M (eds) Coloproctology and the pelvic floor. Butterworth-Heinemann, Oxford, pp 257–304
2. Santoro GA, Bartolo DCC (2000) Incontinence surgery. In: Beynon J, Carr ND (eds) Recent advances in coloproctology. Springer, London, pp 123–134
3. Rudolph W, Galandiuk S (2002) A practical guide to the diagnosis and management of fecal incontinence. Mayo Clin Proc 77:271–275
4. Parks AG (1975) Anorectal incontinence. J R Soc Med 68:21–30
5. Pescatori M, Anastasio G, Bottini C, Mentasti A (1992) New grading and scoring for anal incontinence. Evaluation of 335 patients. Dis Colon Rectum 35:482–487
6. Jorge JM, Wexner SD (1993) Aetiology and management of faecal incontinence. Dis Colon Rectum 36:77–97
7. Vaizey CJ, Carapeti E, Cahill JA, Kamm MA (1999) Prospective comparison of fecal incontinence grading systems. Gut 44:77–80
8. Rockwood TH, Church JM, Fleshman JW (1999) Patient and surgeon ranking of the severity of symptoms associated with fecal incontinence. Dis Colon Rectum 42:1525–1532
9. Rockwood TH, Church JM, Fleshman JW (2000) Fecal incontinence quality of life scale: quality of life instrument for patients with fecal incontinence. Dis Colon Rectum 43:9–17
10. Whitehead WE, Wald A, Norton NJ (2001) Treatment options for fecal incontinence. Dis Colon Rectum 44:131–144
11. Keighley MRB, Fielding JWL (1983) Management of faecal incontinence and results of surgical treatment. Br J Surg 70:463–468
12. Liberman H, Faria J, Ternent CA et al (2001) A prospective evaluation of the value of anorectal physiology in the management of fecal incontinence. Dis Colon Rectum 44:1567–1574
13. Stoker J, Halligan S, Bartram CI (2001) Pelvic floor imaging. Radiology 218:621–641
14. Bartram CI (2003) Ultrasound. In: Bartram CI, DeLancy JOL (eds) Imaging Pelvic Floor Disorders. Springer, Berlin Heidelberg New York, pp 69–79
15. Thakar R, Sultan A (2004) Anal endosonography and its role in assessing the incontinent patient. Best Pract Res Clinic Obstet Gynaec 18:157–173
16. Sultan AH, Kamm MA, Talbot IC et al (1994) Anal endosonography for identifying external sphincter defects confirmed histologically. Br J Surg 81: 463–465
17. Gold DM, Bartram CI, Halligan S et al (1999) Three-

dimensional endoanal sonography in assessing anal canal injury. Br J Surg 86:365–370
18. Christensen AF, Nyhuus B, Nielsen MB, Christensen H (2005). Three-dimensional anal endosonography may improve diagnostic confidence of detecting damage to the anal sphincter complex. Br J Radiol 78:308–311
19. Sentovich SM, Blatchford GJ, Rivela LJ et al (1997) Diagnosing anal sphincter injury with transanal ultrasound and manometry. Dis Colon Rectum 40:1430–1434
20. Perry RE, Blatchford GJ, Christensen MA et al (1990) Manometric diagnosis of anal sphincter injuries. Am J Surg 159:112–117
21. Fleshman JW (1995) Determination of pudendal nerve terminal motor latency. In: Smith LE (ed) Practical guide to anorectal testing. Igaku-Shoin, New-York, pp 221–226
22. Hoffmann BA, Timmcke AE, Gathright JB Jr et al (1995) Fecal seepage and soiling: a problem of rectal sensation. Dis Colon Rectum 38:746–748
23. Law PJ, Kamm MA, Bartram CI (1990) A comparison between electromyography and anal endosonography in mapping external anal sphincter defects. Dis Colon Rectum 33:370–373
24. Tjandra JJ, Milsom JW, Schroeder T, Fazio VW (1993) Endoluminal ultrasound is preferable to electromyography in mapping anal sphincter defects. Dis Colon Rectum 36:689–692
25. Gantke B, Schafer A, Enck P, Lubke H (1993) Sonographic, manometric and myographic evaluation of the anal sphincters morphology and function. Dis Colon Rectum 36:1037–1041
26. Williams AB, Malouf AJ, Bartram CI et al (2001) Assessment of external anal sphincter morphology in idiopathic fecal incontinence with endocoil magnetic resonance imaging. Dig Dis Sci 46:1466–1471
27. Rociu E, Stoker J, Eijkemans MJC et al (1999) Fecal incontinence: endoanal US versus endoanal MR imaging. Radiology 212:453–458
28. Oberwalder M, Dinnewitzer A, Baig K et al (2004) The association between late-onset fecal incontinence and obstetric anal sphincter defects. Arch Surg 139:429–432
29. Varma A, Gunn J, Gardiner A et al (1999) Obstetric anal sphincter injury: a prospective evaluation of incidence. Dis Colon Rectum 42:1253–1260
30. Zetterstrom JP, Mellgren A, Jensen LL et al (1999) Effect of delivery on anal sphincter morphology and function. Dis Colon Rectum 42:1253–1260
31. Nichols CM, Gill EJ, Nguyen T (2004) Anal sphincter injury in women with pelvic floor disorders. Obstet Gynecol 104:690–696
32. Snooks SJ, Setchell M, Swash M, Henry MM (1984) Injury to innervation of pelvic floor sphincter musculature in childbirth. Lancet 2:546–550
33. Sultan AH, Kamm MA, Hudson CN et al (1993) Anal sphincter disruption during vaginal delivery. N Engl J Med 329:1905–1911
34. Donnelly V, Fynes M, Campbell D et al (1998) Obstetric events leading to anal sphincter damage. Obstet Gynecol 92:955–961
35. Handa VL, Danielsen BH, Gilbert WM (2001) Obstetric anal sphincter lacerations. Obstet Gynecol 98:225–230
36. Lee SJ, Park JW (2000) Follow-up evaluation of the effect of vaginal delivery on the pelvic floor. Dis Colon Rectum 43:1550–1555
37. Bennett RC, Friedman MHW, Goligher JC (1963) Late results of haemorrhoidectomy by ligature and excision. BMJ 2:216–219
38. Speakman CT, Burnett SJ, Kamm MA, Bartram CI (1991) Sphincter injury after anal dilatation demonstrated by anal endosonography. Br J Surg 78:1429–1430
39. Khubchandani IT, Reed JF (1989) Sequelae of internal sphincterotomy for chronic fissure in ano. Br J Surg 76:431–434
40. Kennedy HL, Zegarra JP (1990) Fistulotomy without external sphincter division for high anal fistula. Br J Surg 77:898–901
41. Fang DT, Nivatvongs S, Vermeulen FD et al (1984) Overlapping sphincteroplasty for acquired anal incontinence. Dis Colon Rectum 27:720–722
42. Ctercteko GH, Fazio VW, Jagelman DG et al (1988) Anal sphincter repair: a report of 60 cases and review of the literature. Aust NZJ Surg 58:703–710
43. Miller R, Orrom WJ, Cornes H et al (1989) Anterior sphincter plication and levatorplasty in the treatment of faecal incontinence. Br J Surg 76:1058–1060
44. Zorcolo L, Covotta L, Bartolo DCC (2005) Outcome of anterior sphincter repair for obstetric injury: comparison of early and late results. Dis Colon Rectum 48:524–531
45. Faucheron JL, Hannoun L, Thome C, Parc R (1994) Is fecal continence improved by nonstimulated gracilis muscle transposition? Dis Colon Rectum 37:979–983
46. Konsten J, Baeten CGMI, Havenith MG, Soeters PB (1993) Morphology of dynamic graciloplasty compared with the anal sphincter. Dis Colon Rectum 35:559–563
47. Seccia M, Menconi C, Balestri R, Cavina E (1994) Study protocols and functional results in 86 electrostimulated graciloplasties. Dis Colon Rectum 37:897–904
48. Baeten CGMI, Geerdes BP, Adang EMM et al (1995) Anal dynamic graciloplasty in the treatment of intractable faecal incontinence. N Engl J Med 332:1600–5
49. Wexner SD, Gonzalez-Padron A, Rius J et al (1996) Stimulated gracilis neosphincter operation. Dis Colon Rectum 39:957–964
50. Wong WD, Jensen LL, Bartolo DCC, Rothenberger DA

(1996) Artificial anal sphincter. Dis Colon Rectum 39:1345–1351

51. Malouf AJ, Vaizey CJ, Nicholls RJ, Kamm M (2000) Permanent sacral nerve stimulation for fecal incontinence. Ann Surg 232:143–148
52. Ganio E, Ratto C, Masin A et al (2001) Neuromodulation for fecal incontinence: outcome in 16 patients with definitive implant. The initial Italian Sacral Neurostimulation Group (GINS) experience. Dis Colon Rectum 44:965–970
53. Matzel KE, Kamm MA, Stosser M et al (2004) Sacral spinal nerve stimulation for faecal incontinence: multicentre study. Lancet 363:1270–1276
54. Takahashi T, Garcia-Osogobio S, Valdovinos MA et al (2002) Radio-frequency energy delivery to the anal canal for the treatment of fecal incontinence. Dis Colon Rectum 45:915–922
55. Efron JE, Corman ML, Fleshman J et al (2003) Safety and effectiveness of temperature-controlled radio-frequency energy delivery to the anal canal (Secca procedure) for the treatment of fecal incontinence. Dis Colon Rectum 46:1606–1618

VIII.2. Surgical Treatment of Fecal Incontinence

L. Zorcolo, D.C.C. Bartolo

Patients with major fecal incontinence often do not benefit from medical treatment or biofeedback and thus are proposed for surgery. Different surgical options are available, the choice of which depends on the type of incontinence, the severity of symptoms, and the compliance of the patient. The efficacy of surgery still remains difficult to assess, but it is quite evident that none of the operations can guarantee a return to perfect continence. Surgical treatment for fecal incontinence can be divided in two main groups:

1. Operations to reinforce the existing muscles
   - Anterior sphincter repair (ASR)
   - Postanal repair
   - Total pelvic floor repair

2. Operations to create a neosphincter
   - Muscle transposition
     - Nonstimulated graciloplasty
     - Gluteoplasty
     - Dynamic graciloplasty (DGP)
   - Artificial bowel sphincter (ABS)

Other surgical options, such as stoma creation or colonic conduit, can help improve the quality of life when nothing else can be done.

In this chapter, we will focus on indications, techniques, and outcomes of the most common procedures, which are ASR and (less commonly) postanal repair for the first group, and stimulated graciloplasty and ABS for the second group. New procedures, such as sacral nerve modulation and implantation of sphincteric bulking material, also aim to improve continence through the existing muscles. These emerging operations have a very low morbidity and no mortality and, especially the former, seem to be valid alternatives to major procedures. These will be discussed in separate chapters.

Reinforcement of the Existing Sphincter

Anterior Sphincter Repair

Obstetric trauma is considered to be the commonest cause of fecal incontinence, and current opinion based on anal endosonography is that the majority of these patients have structural sphincter damage [1]. The first-line treatment for this condition is ASR. This is a relatively simple operation with low morbidity. However, its efficacy following recent longer-term outcome analyses has been recognized to be substantially less than previously reported.

Patient Selection

This operation should be considered in all incontinent patients with a demonstrable external sphincter defect, unresponsive to conservative treatment. Some authors argue that patients with abnormally prolonged pudendal nerve terminal motor latency (PNTML), especially if bilaterally prolonged, are not good candidates for repair [2–5], but this has not been confirmed by others [6–9]. There is a general agreement that results are probably poorer in older patients, in those with associated evacuatory disorders, and in the presence of multiple defects. However, none of these are absolute contraindications to the repair.

Notes on Techniques

Preoperatively, patients receive bowel preparation with stimulants or osmotic laxatives, antibiotics, and thromboembolic prophylaxis. Covering stoma has been demonstrated to be unnecessary [6, 10, 11]. Under general anesthesia, the patient is placed in a modified lithotomy position and catheterized. The prone jack-knife position can also be used and is more popular in North America, but we find that with the buttocks protruding well beyond the flexed knees, there is good exposure (Fig. VIII.2). A curvilinear incision is made in the anterior perineum at the edge of the pigmented anal skin. The incision is parallel to the anal margin and is extended for about 180° (Fig. VIII.3). The wound can be exposed with Gelpi or Lone Starr retractors, and the external sphincter ring is identified and progressively freed up.

Dissection is initiated in the midline, where scar tissue is present, and carried out in either direction, searching for the retracted edges of the sphincter muscle. Detection of the residual muscle may be facilitated by the use of diathermy. Once identified, the two ends of the external sphincter are mobilized from surrounding fat and from the internal sphincter up to the level of the levator muscles (Fig. VIII.4). Care must be taken

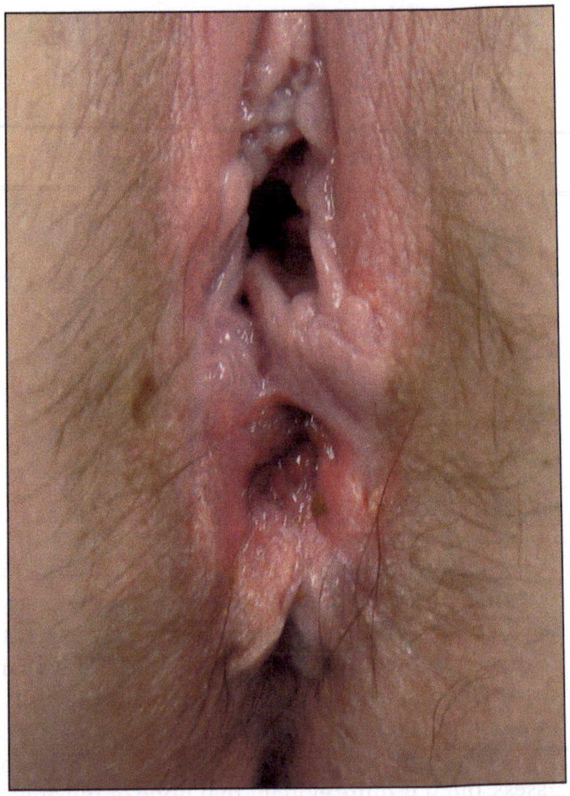

Fig. VIII.2. Exposure of the operative field in Lloyd-Davies position. This lady had an extensive EAS scar with disruption of the perineal body

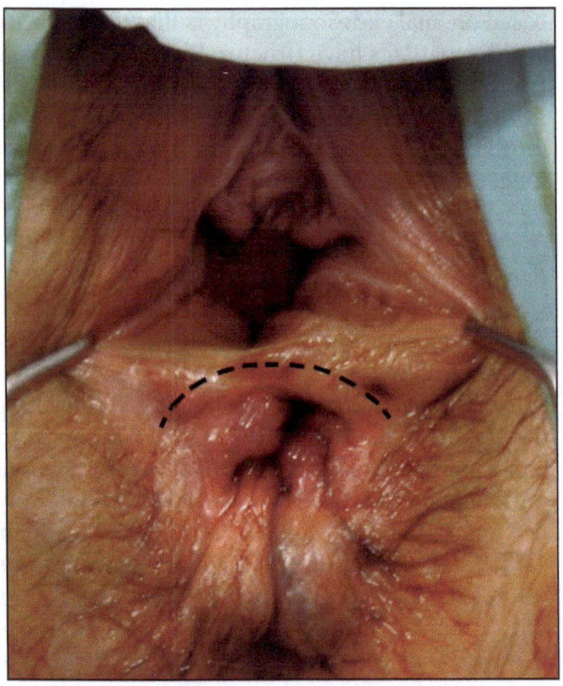

Fig. VIII.3. A curvilinear incision is made ad the edge of pigmentated skin (dotted line)

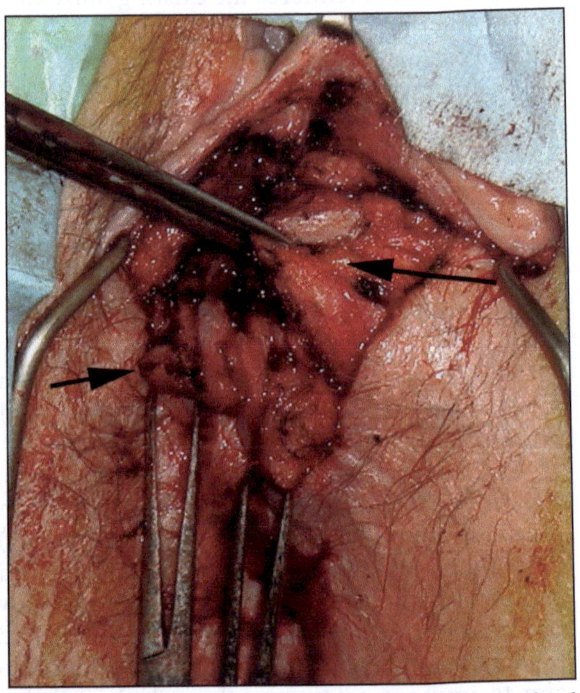

Fig. VIII.4. The two ends of the external sphincter are freed up (black arrows)

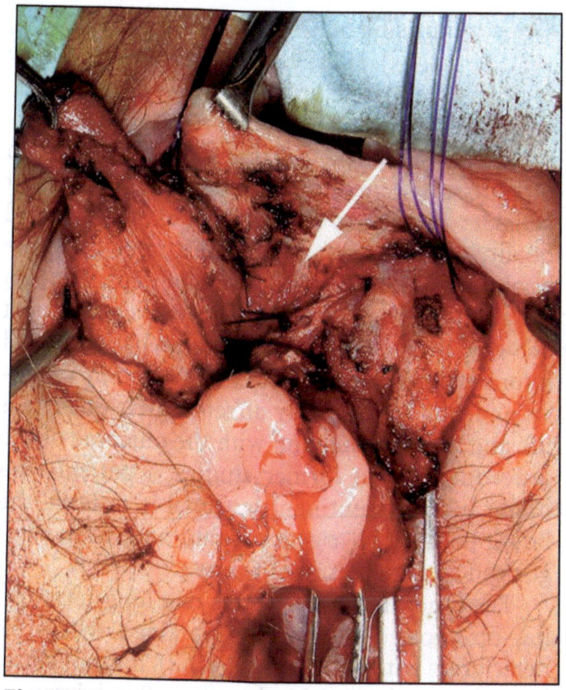

Fig. VIII.5. Levatoroplasty with interrupted stitches (white arrow)

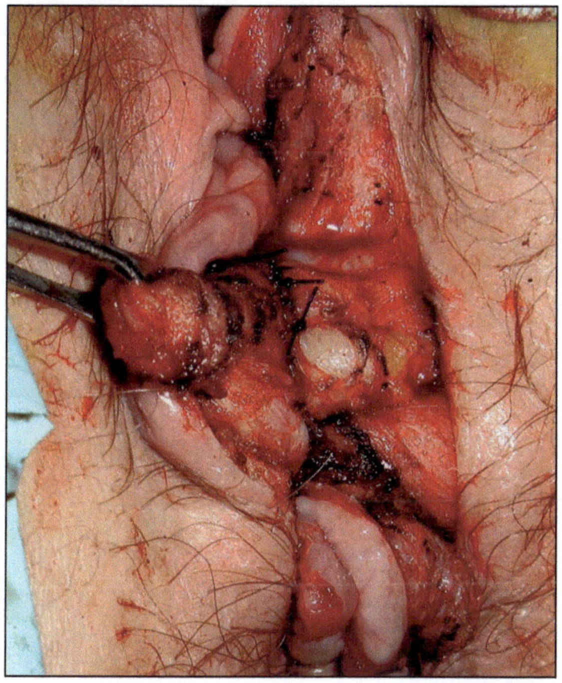

Fig. VIII.6. Overlapping of the two ends of the external sphincter

posterolaterally, where the branches of the pudendal nerve enter the muscle. The scar tissue found anteriorly must not be excised because it will be used for the repair. However, it can be divided in the midline to facilitate mobilization of the two ends of the sphincter. If the internal anal sphincter is clearly identified, this can be imbricated separately from the external one, but this procedure did not appear to offer any benefit [9, 12]. At this stage, a levatorplasty can be added to tighten the anterior pelvic floor and reconstruct the perineal body (Fig. VIII.5). In this case, the levator muscles on each side are approximated together with interrupted stitches of a slow absorbable suture [i.e., 2/0 polydioxanone (PDS)]. The finding that levatorplasty improved outcome has been supported by some series [13–15] but not by others [4].

Finally, the two ends of the external sphincter are overlapped by suturing the scar tissue from one end to the middle part of the opposite sphincter muscle. Usually, 3–5 interrupted mattress stitches of 2/0 PDS on each side are placed, and they are tied snugly but not too tightly in order to avoid muscular ischemia (Fig. VIII.6). When scar tissue is not clearly evident, the sphincter ring can be plicated rather than divided and overlapped. Hemostasis must be meticulous. At the end of the procedure, the wound, which was originally transverse, can be usually closed in an inverted "Y" fashion, thus increasing the distance between anus and vagina (Fig. VIII.7). We often leave a small opening if there is any tension in order to minimize the risk of infection. Occasionally, it may be necessary to create an advancement or an island flap to cover the repair. Postoperatively, the urinary catheter is kept in situ for 24–36 h, and a normal diet is reintroduced the day after operation, supplemented with bulking laxatives to optimize stool consistency and avoid straining and impaction. Bowel confinement and the use of antidiarrheal drugs have been demonstrated to be unnecessary and are associated with more complications [16]. Daily wound cleansing is practiced.

Complications

ASR can be considered a relatively simple procedure with low morbidity and no mortality. The most common complication is wound infection. In the authors' experience, this occurred in 24 patients (26%). Five required an examination under anesthesia while one developed perineal

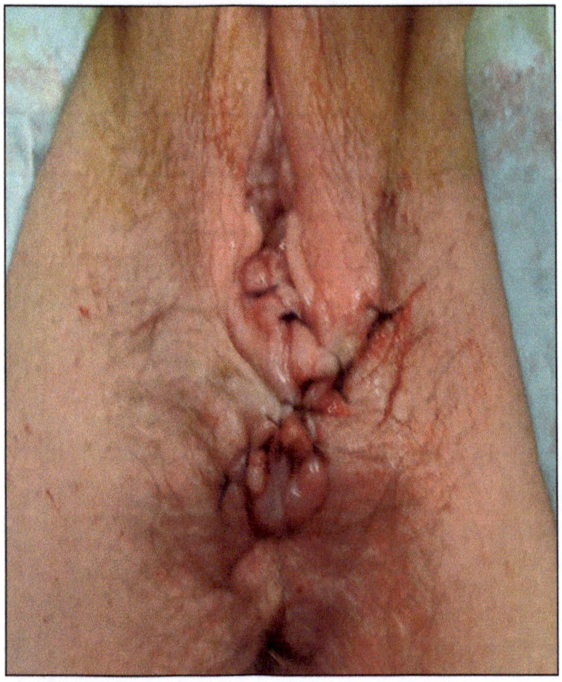

Fig. VIII.7. Wound closure. The perineal body has been reconstructed

sepsis and required a colostomy that was closed 2 months later. Other complications were prolonged anal pain (8%) and dyspareunia (6%) [9]. These figures were consistent with the reported literature [2, 6, 17, 18]. Wound infection did not, in fact, appear to be significantly associated with failure; the literature is not clear on this point, with some authors reporting an increased risk for breakdown of the repair [2] while others found no deleterious effect [17, 18]. However, it significantly prolongs healing time. Recently, it has been reported that closing the wound with an island flap lowers the incidence of dehiscence to 15% [19]. Our current practice is often to leave part of the wound open. Some authors have reported a higher incidence of dyspareunia when the sphincter repair was augmented with a levatorplasty [8]. Our series and those of others have not confirmed this correlation. Sphincter repair can also cause evacuation difficulties, such as the need to strain and incomplete evacuation. This occurred in about 16% of the patients in our series [9].

Outcome

Anterior anal sphincter repair has been reported to achieve good results in 69–97% of patients in series comprising between 12 and 88 patients [2, 6, 10, 11, 17, 20–25]. However, these figures are likely to be overestimated. In fact, early reports attributed success to even minor improvements in control, and most of them based their evaluation on inappropriate incontinence scores that did not consider important factors such as urgency and quality of life. As recently demonstrated by Byrne et al. [26], quality of life is highly dependent on the ability to be able to leave the home. Our report showed that even though many patients had improved, they were severely restricted by urgency, and this significantly affected their quality of life and their satisfaction with the outcome of the procedure [9]. In former studies, a patient who might be fully continent but unable to leave the house because of urgency would have been categorized as a successful outcome.

The other important fact is that long-term follow-up showed that results obtained with ASR deteriorate with time (Table VIII.4). It is not clearly understood why this happens. Breakdown of the repair can occur, but this usually happens in the early period after surgery and therefore is an unlikely explanation. Some opine that dissection of the muscles for overlapping may impair innervation [7], but the most probable explanation is that there is a progressive weakening of the overlapped muscle due to normal aging or to the nature itself of the obstetric trauma [28], which may involve other perineal muscle and may include nerve damage.

Postanal Repair

This operation was developed by Parks [30] in an attempt to treat patients with idiopathic or neurogenic incontinence with an intact anal sphincter. At the time, ultrasonography was not available, and the only way to identify defects with certainty was serial electromyographic needle puncture of the perineum to document sphincter defects or integrity. Technically, with the patient in prone jack-knife or lithotomy positions, the intersphincteric plane is entered through a posterior V-shaped incision, and the opposite limbs of the ischiococcygeus, ileococcygeus, and puborectalis muscles are approximated together in order to strengthen the pelvic floor and restore the acute angulation at the anorectal junction. Further studies have shown that the success of this procedure, which only benefits, at most, 30–40% of patients

Table VIII.4. Long-term results of anterior sphincter repair

Author	Year	Patients (*n*)	Median FU (months)		Excellent/good		Fair/poor		Patients fully continent[a]	
			S-T	L-T	S-T	L-T	S-T	L-T	S-T	L-T
Londono-Shimmer et al [2]	1994	94		58		50%		50%		n.r.
Karoui et al [8]	2000	74	3	40	81%	51%	19%	49%	49%	28%
Malouf et al [7]	2000	46	15	77	79%	59%	21%	41%	n.r	n.r.
Morren et al [27]	2001	55		40		56%		44%		n.r.
Halverson et al [28]	2002	49		62		45%		55%		12%
Gutierrez et al [29]	2004	130	36	120	64%	41%	36%	59%	18%	6%
Zorcolo et al [9]	2005	73	10	70	68%	54%	32%	46%	36%	16%

[a] Patients fully continent or incontinent to flatus

FU follow-up, *S-T* short-term follow-up, *L-T* long-term follow-up, *n.r.* data not reported

treated [31–33], does not depend on the modification of the anorectal angle but is dependent on the recreation of a high pressure zone in the anal canal [34, 35]. Because of the low success rate, and since it has been demonstrated that the same results are achieved with an anterior sphincteroplasty [36], this procedure has become less frequently performed. The combination of postanal repair with anterior levatorplasty is called total pelvic floor repair, but there is no evidence supporting the use of this combined procedure [37].

Creation of a Neosphincter

For patients with severe idiopathic or neurogenic incontinence or those with congenital anomalies or a destroyed sphincter, neosphincter creation is an alternative to a definitive stoma. This can be achieved either with transposition of healthy skeletal muscle or with insertion of prosthetic material. The muscles that can be used are basically gluteus maximus and gracilis because their vascular supplies allow transposition to the pelvic floor. Gracilis muscle has been demonstrated to be the most suitable for this purpose while gluteoplasty is burdened by higher functional deficit [38] and thus is only rarely performed.

Patient Selection

Patients selected for graciloplasty or artificial sphincter are those with severe fecal incontinence who fail to respond to conservative treatment or first-line surgery. Although there are no limits to age, it seems reasonable not to perform these operations in old patients with very limited activities and a short life expectancy. Furthermore, nonmotivated patients, those with psychological instability, low mental capacity, significant comorbidity, poor functional status, severe arthritis, or other disabilities limiting the use of the hands, or patients with Crohn's disease or other chronic diarrheal state, should not be considered for sphincter replacement [39].

Dynamic Graciloplasty

Pickrell et al. first described gracilis muscle transposition [40] in 1952, but results were disappointing due to the inability of the muscle to maintain sustained contraction. More recently, the demonstration that chronic low-frequency (10–12 Hz) electrical stimulation transforms fatigue-prone type II skeletal muscle into fatigue-resistant type I muscle allowed the transposed gracilis to work as a sphincter [41, 42]. For these reasons, DGP has become the most common procedure to create a neosphincter.

Notes on Techniques

Initially, this operation was performed in three or two steps. In the three-stage procedure, the first stage consisted of devascularization of the distal part of the gracilis and creation of a loop colostomy, the second stage consisted of transposition of the muscle around the anus, and the third stage consisted of colostomy closure. In the two-stage procedure, devascularization was avoided. However it has been clarified that neither preliminary vascular delay nor fecal diversion have a role in reducing postoperative complications and outcome of DGP [43, 44], and thus it is now common practice to perform this operation in a single stage. Bowel preparation and antibiotic and thromboembolic prophylaxis is recommended. Under general anesthesia, the patient is placed in the modified Lloyd-Davies position, and catheterization is delayed until the end of the procedure. This avoids a potential risk of infection from the exposed catheter. Through a 10- to 15-cm incision in the medial aspect of the upper thigh, the left gracilis is mobilized (Fig. VIII.8), taking care to preserve its main neurovascular bundle located on the anterolateral side about one quarter of the way from the groin to the knee. This pedicle is the fulcrum about which the gracilis is rotated to reach the perineum. Blunt dissection is continued in the adductor canal. Another little medial incision at the distal thigh allows complete muscular dissection and the identification of a second blood vessel arising from the superficial femoral system. Finally, a 2-cm incision at the knee allows division of the tendon at its insertion to the tibia. When the muscle is fully mobilized and ready for the transposition, an electrode is positioned either epineurally or intramuscularly. The epineural electrode is placed over the main nerve trunk and sutured to the underlying adductor muscle with nonabsorbable sutures while intramuscular electrodes are usually fixed near the entry point of the nerve into the muscle. In both cases, the best area is chosen with a stimulation test.

Theoretically, with epineural stimulation, the whole muscle fibers are recruited and the necessary voltage is reduced, with a consequently longer battery life, but a direct comparison between the two techniques showed a significantly higher rate of lead displacement and failure for epineural stimulation [45–47]. However, new generation bipolar electrode paddles (i.e., model 3961 Medtronic) have lowered the risk of displacement [45]. Once the electrode has been positioned, the lead is tunneled to the homolateral iliac fossa where a subfascial pocket is made to accommodate the stimulator. Initially, the device was placed subcutaneously, but this resulted in a high rate of displacement [48]. Two lateral perineal incisions are made, and a circumanal tunnel is created in the extrasphincteric plane (Fig. VIII.9). This can be particularly difficult anteriorly, especially in patients with extensive scarring of the perineum. In these cases, an incision of the posterior vagina wall can help in creating the tunnel thereby avoiding inadvertent perforation of the anal canal [48].

With a further subcutaneous tunnel, the thigh incision is reached and the muscle is delivered to the perineum to be wrapped around the anus. Wrapping can be performed in various ways (Fig. VIII.10), but usually the choice is for the gamma (γ) configuration in which the muscle passes anterior to the anus and after a 360° loop its tendon is attached to the periosteum of the contralateral ischiatic tuberosity with a nonabsorbable suture (Fig. VIII.11). If the muscle is not long enough to reach the contralateral ischium, its tendon can be

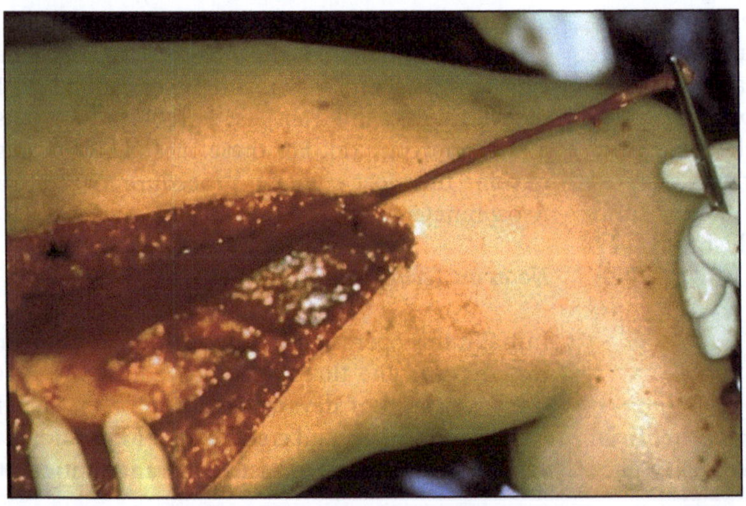

Fig. VIII.8. Gracilis muscle is detached from its distal insertion and fully mobilised

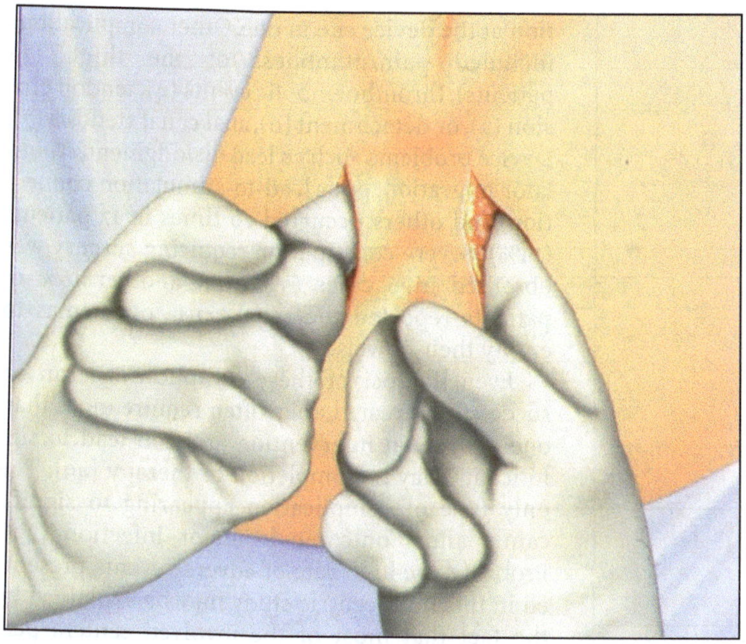

Fig. VIII.9. The anal canal is completely surrounded trough two lateral incisions

attached to the homolateral ischial tuberosity after a 270° loop in what is called an alpha (α) configuration. Epsilon configuration is when the muscle is initially passed posteriorly to the anus and then wrapped for 360° and attached to the contralateral ischiatic tuberosity. This is only possible with a long muscle. Fixing the tendon has to be done after moving the thigh back in a neutral position. The neosphincter should be snug but not too tight on the surgeon's finger. Frequent pitfalls, especially in inexpert hands, are inadequate fixation of the tendon, with subsequent tendon detachment, and a tendency to make the wrap too tight, which can lead to erosion and anal canal perforation. Thigh, abdominal, and perineal wounds are washed out with gentamicin solution and closed with interrupted stitches. Redivac drains can be left in situ for 24–48 h. Postoperatively, wounds are cleaned regularly, and the patient is kept on stool softeners.

Early stimulation (after 2 weeks) is recommended to avoid muscular atrophy. The surgeon can adjust all stimulation parameters via a computer that communicates with the stimulator by a radiofrequency coil. Initially, the stimulation is set to be intermittent, and the length of activation time is progressively increased over 6–8 weeks

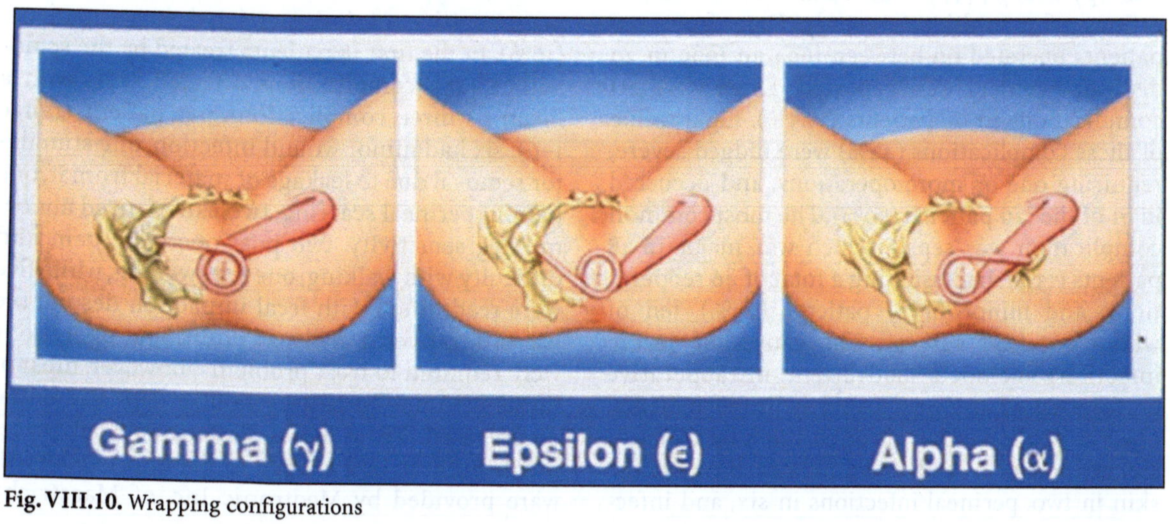

Fig. VIII.10. Wrapping configurations

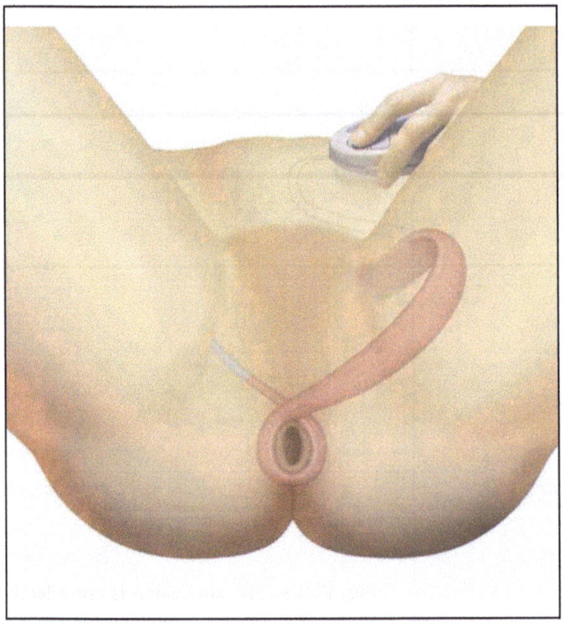

Fig. VIII.11. Final position of gracilis and stimulator

until the muscle develops fatigue resistance. After this period, continuous activation may be commenced. The patient is given a remote control to turn off the stimulator prior defecation. Latest controllers also allow the patient to increase or decrease the stimulation voltage within a preset range.

Complications

The rate of complications is high, but fortunately, most of them can be managed without affecting the outcome. In 2001, the Dynamic Graciloplasty Therapy Group [49] published the overall complications of a multicenter study. Data from 120 patients operated on between 1994 an 1999 in 20 dedicated centers were reported. There were 211 complications in 93 patients (77.5%). Eighty-nine of these complications (42%) were judged severe, requiring one or more operations, and occurred in 61 of the 120 patients (50%). The most common complication was sepsis, which was major in 18 patients (15%), necessitating a total of 46 reoperations, and minor in 29 patients (24%), ten of whom required surgery. The causes of severe infections included inadvertent intraoperative perforation of the anal canal in three patients, erosion of the tendon through the anal canal in six, erosion of a lead or stimulator through the skin in two, perineal infections in six, and infection at the device site in one. Other complications included pain/numbness of the thigh (38 patients), thromboembolic events (4), tendon erosion (2), or detachment (6), anal canal stenosis (7). Device problems such as lead dislodgment, stimulator migration, poor lead-to-stimulation connection, and others occurred 20 times in 17 patients (14%). Severe constipation requiring surgery was observed in 6 cases (5%), but another 16% of patients reported the regular use of enemas to empty their bowels.

Even if most of these complications can be successfully treated, they often require more than one additional intervention and can lead to significant delay in completion of therapy [49]. The only type of complication appearing to significantly affect outcome is major infection [49]. Probably, the high rate of adverse events presented in this multicentric study may be explained by the fact that most of the involved centers performed less than ten graciloplasty procedures. Other studies demonstrated that morbidity is lower in larger, single-center series [50, 51], but the figures are still quite disappointing (Table VIII.5). Rongen et al. [48] reported 138 complications in 200 patients, most of them occurring in the early years of their experience. Infections leading to explantation of the stimulator occurred eight times in the first 20 patients (40%) and only 16 times in the remaining 180 (9%). This significant reduction was related to a proper antibiotic prophylaxis and to the use of topical antibiotics such as gentamicin sponge-release. Other complications, such as anal perforation, tendon erosion, or stimulator or lead displacement, were also lowered with increasing experience. Evacuation disorders, which are not uncommon in the early postoperative period, persisted in 32 patients (16%). In the first 18 patients treated by the senior author [43], complications affected 50%, with a mean of three complications per patient (range 1–6): six had minor wound infection, one stimulator removal due to leakage of material from it, one painful perineal scarring, two experienced abnormal leg sensitivity, two post-operative pain and difficulty with walking, one leg swelling, while five were readmitted with fecal impaction despite the use of laxatives. Finally, 23 additional operations were required to treat problems; however, most of these were due to battery failure with the initial device used. These necessitated new lead placements because of a change to the improved hardware provided by Medtronic Inc. of Maastricht.

Table VIII.5. Complications and results of dynamic graciloplasty

Author	Year	Patients (n)	Patients with complications	Median FU (months)	Success
Christiansen et al [52]	1998	13	10 (77%)	7–27	11 (85%)
Cavina et al [53]	1998	31	23 (74%)		26 (84%)
Sielezneff et al [43]	1999	18	9 (50%)	20	14 (81.2%)
Dynamic Graciloplasty Therapy Study Group [49, 54]	2000	120	93 (77,5%)	12	89 (74%)
Konsten et al [45]	2001	81	n.r.	n.r.	46 (57%)
French multicenter [55]	2002	24	12 (50%)	21 (3–72)	19 (79%)
Wexner et al [44]	2002	88	n.r.	24	49 (56%)
Seccia et al [56]	2003	36	n.r	n.r.	27 (75%)
Rongen et al [48]	2003	200	138 (69%)	60	145 (72%)
Belgium multicenter [47]	2004	60	44 (73%)	48 (13–117)	33 (55%)
Thornton et al [57]	2004	38	26 (68%)	60 (1–112)	6/33 (18%)
Bartolo (unpublished data)	2005	25			17 (68%)

There were no erosion complications. Moreover, none of the complications caused failure and did not affect the outcome of the procedure.

Outcome

Functional results of DGP are often good, with improved or normal continence achieved in a majority of patients. Percentages varied from 55 to 85% [41, 43, 47, 48, 52–56, 58]. Less favorable results are obtained in patients treated for congenital incontinence (Table VIII.6); no other variables have been correlated with success or failure [44, 54]. The largest single-center study, conducted by Rongen et al. [48] regards 200 patients with a minimum follow-up of 2 years and a median follow-up of 5 years. They reported that 145 patients (72.5%) were either fully continent or incontinent to flatus. The number of failures was significantly higher among the first 20 cases treated, demonstrating that this is not a simple procedure and a learning curve is necessary. That study also showed that, differently form anterior sphincter repair, continence achieved with DGP does not deteriorate with time. However, this fact was not been confirmed by Thornton et al. [57]: about one third of their patients followed up for a median of 60 months deteriorated and received an end colostomy, and only 18% of the total maintained a good continence status. Results from other centers are reported in Table VIII.5.

Table VIII.6. Success categorized by cause of fecal incontinence (adapted from Rongen et al. [48])

Cause	Patients (n)	Success rate
Congenital	28	52%
Trauma	98	82%
Idiopathic	58	72%
Neurologic	16	80%
Total	200	72%

Artificial Sphincter

After being successfully used in urinary incontinence [59], artificial sphincter has also been implanted to treat severe fecal incontinence [60]. This is an alternative to skeletal muscle transposition, especially in patients with neurological diseases affecting the lower body, such as myasthenia gravis or diabetic neuropathy [60, 61]. The artificial bowel sphincter (ABS) (American Medical System, Minnetonka, MN, USA), which is currently the most widely used system, maintains continence through a fluid-filled cuff that surrounds the anal canal. The cuff is connected to a little pump, usually placed subcutaneously in the scrotum or labia majora, and to a reservoir balloon implanted in the prevesical space (Figs. VIII.12-VIII.13). Squeezing the pump forces the fluid from

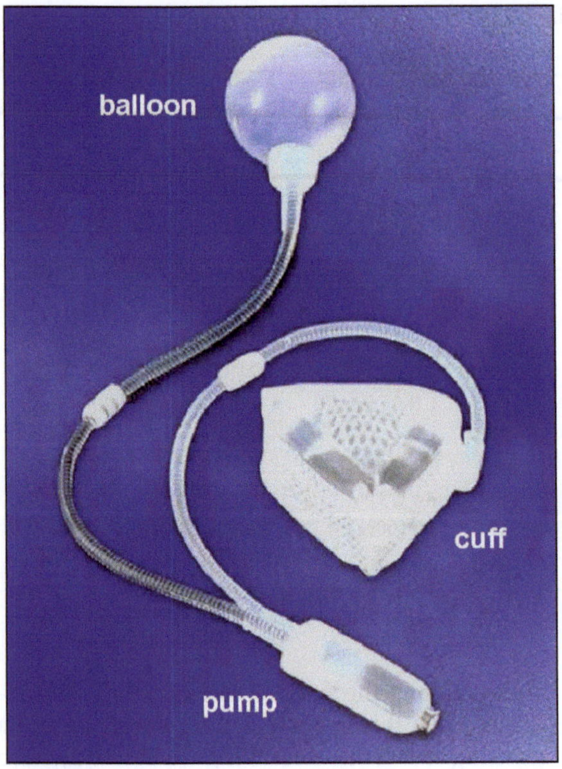

Fig. VIII.12. The artificial bowel sphincter

the cuff into the reservoir and allows defecation. Positive abdominal pressure then makes the fluid gradually return to the cuff, thus keeping the anal canal closed.

Note on Techniques

Implant is performed under general or spinal anesthesia with the patient in the modified lithotomic position. Preoperative bowel preparation and antibiotic prophylaxis are strongly recommended. A tunnel is created around the anus in the extrasphincteric space to accommodate the cuff. This can be done either through two lateral curvilinear incisions or through a single anterior incision. This second approach is preferred in women because it allows entry to the rectovaginal septum, usually thinned and scarred, avoiding damage to the two organs. The tunnel should be created as proximal as possible (at least 5 cm from the skin [62]) to minimize the risk of skin erosion. At this point, the cuff can be placed.

The cuff is available in two widths: 2 and 2.9 cm, each with lengths varying from 9 to 14 cm. The appropriate size is chosen with a cuff sizer present in the kit. Prior the positioning, the cuff is filled with a radiopaque solution, emptied again to remove all the air bubbles, then passed circumferentially around the anus, taking care to end with the tube anteriorly at the site chosen for pump placement (left side for right-handed patients and vice versa). A suprapubic transverse incision is made, and the prevesical space is reached after dividing the rectal fascia and separating the linea alba. Before accommodating the balloon, a plane is bluntly dissected below Scarpa's fascia into the scrotum or labia where the pump will be positioned. The tubing from the cuff is also passed subcutaneously to the abdominal wound. At this point, the pump device can be placed into the labia or scrotum with the deactivation button facing medially. The balloon is filled with a specific amount of fluid (usually 40 ml) to reach a pressure of 80–90 cm H_2O and placed in the retropubic space; the tubing from the cuff and the balloon are cut to the appropriate length and connected to the pump. The perineal incisions are closed in multiple absorbable layers in order to separate the device from the skin as much as possible and to prevent its dislocation. The suprapubic incision is also closed in layers, with the tubing remaining above the fascia. During the operation, careful aseptic techniques and wound irrigation

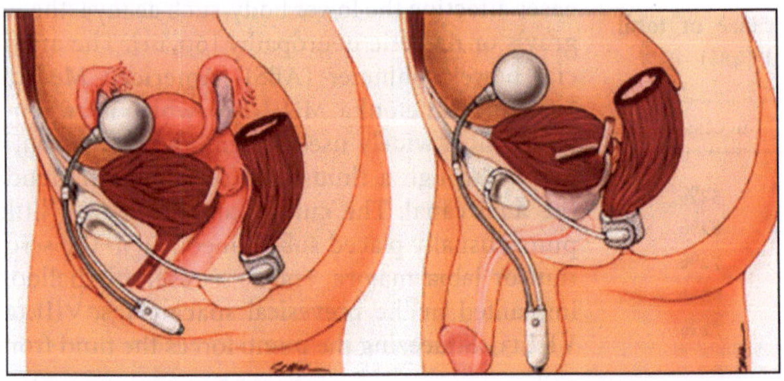

Fig. VIII.13. ABS positioning in woman and in man

Table VIII.7. Complication rates and definitive explantation of artificial bowel sphincter

Author	Year	Patients (n)	FU (months)	Reoperations (n)	Explants (n)	Reimplant	Definitive explant
Vaizey et al [64]	1998	6	10 (5–13)	1 (17%)	1	0	1 (17%)
Christiansen et al [65]	1999	17	60 (60–120)	6 (35%)	7	0	7 (41%)
O'Brien et al [66]	2000	13	n.r.	4 (31%)	3	0	3 (23%)
Altomare et al [67]	2001	28	19 (7–41)	7 (25%)	7	0	7 (25%)
Altomare et al. [68][a]	2004	28	50		11		11 (39%)
Devesa et al [62]	2002	53	26 (7–55)	16 (30%)	10	2	10 (19%)
Ortiz et al [69]	2002	22	28 (6–48)	6 (27%)	9	2	7 (32%)
Lehur et al [70]	2002	16	25 (7–49)	2 (12%)	5	1	4 (25%)
Wong et al [71]	2002	112	12	73 (65%)	41	7	34 (30%)
Michot et al [72]	2003	25	34 (7–60)	8 (32%)	5		5 (20%)
Parker et al [73]	2003	45	91-39[b]	29 (64%)	20	2	18 (40%)

[a] Same patients at long-term

[b] Two groups of patients: I group (10 patients): mean follow-up 91 months; II group (35 patients): mean follow-up 39 month

with antibiotic solution are recommended in order to minimize the risk of infection. Postoperatively, intravenous antibiotics are continued for 48 h, wounds are cleaned regularly, and the urinary catheter in female patients is left in place for 2–3 days. The device is activated after 4–6 weeks, provided that all the wounds are healed.

Complications

As recently published in a review about safety and effectiveness of ABS [63], no mortality has been associated with this operation, but almost all series reported a high reoperation rate (12-65%) and a significant proportion of definitive explantation of the device, with percentages varying from 17 to 41% (Table VIII.7). Moreover, these figures may increase in the long term, as noticed by Altomare et al. [68] and by Ortiz et al. [69], who calculated a 44% cumulative probability of device explantation at 48 months. The most common reason for removal is infection. Other causes, which usually develop during follow-up, are erosion of the skin or of the anal canal, and mechanical problems such as cuff rupture or loss of device function. Tables VIII.8 and 9 show the type and frequency of early and late complications, as noted in the wider single-center series presented in the literature [62]. Among 53 patients in this series, there were 33 early and 29 late complications requiring 16 reoperations (30%) and a definitive explant in ten patients (19%).

Outcome

When the device is not explanted, it is usually able to improve the continence, with all studies reporting a significant reduction in mean incontinence score. However, early success rates of 70-80% with a high proportion of patients fully continent [60, 74, 75] have not been subsequently confirmed in larger series and over the long term

Table VIII.8. Early complications after artificial bowel sphincter (adapted from Devesa et al. [62])

Early complications	Patients (n=53)	Percent
Wound separation	8	15%
Infection	7	13%
Hematoma	7	13%
Fever of unknown origin	1	2%
Urethral fistula	1/18	5.5%
Impaction	5	9%
Diarrhea	4	8%
Total	**33**	**62%**

Table VIII.9. Late complications after artificial bowel sphincter (adapted from Devesa et al. [62])

Late Complications	Patients (n=50)[a]	Percent
Cuff erosion	5	10
Pump erosion	4	8
Primary infection	3	6
Impaction	11	22
Pain	4	8
Pump malfunction	1	2
System leaks	1	2
Total	**29**	**58**

[a] Two patients were explanted in the early postoperative period, and one was missing after discharge from the hospital

(Table VIII.10). Results from a multicentercohort study involving the majority of centers dedicated to this procedure [71] indicate that only 53% of patients enrolled in the study were considered clinical successes at 1 year from implantation. In the series of Ortiz et al. [69], almost all patients with a functioning device (68% of the total) were able to control solid stools, but only four (27%) were fully continent. Long-term results from the Italian multicenter trial [68] are also disappointing: of 21 patients with a functional device, 14 (66%) were fully continent after a mean follow-up of 19 months, but only eight of them (28% of the entire series) remained continent after 50 months.

Good results and patient satisfaction may also be jeopardized by the occurrence of defecation difficulties. This event is quite common with ABS (see Table VIII.10) and not rarely, it needs to be corrected surgically. Fecal impaction requiring regular enemas ranges from 6 to 83% [63]. In the series by Parker et al. [73], surgery to correct defecation problems was necessary in 11% of patients. In the Italian multicenter trial [68], 50% of patients with functioning ABS no longer activated the pump because of obstructed defecation. The cause of this problem is unclear. Sometimes it may be from technical problems, such as closing the cuff to tightly around the anus [73, 76]. For this reason, Parker et al. [73] recommended a cuff not 1 cm but 2 cm larger than the measured size. Another possible explanation is that the quick refill of the cuff after being emptied would favor the persistency of feces in the rectum, which may become impacted [77]. Altomare et al. [68] suggest that in the long term, the artificial sphincter, because of the surrounding fibrosis, acts mainly as a passive obstacle to the passage of feces (like a Thiersch's sling) rather than as a dynamic sphincter.

Table VIII.10. Complication rate and definitive explantation of artificial bowel sphincter

Author	Year	Patient (n)	Mean FU	Patients with functioning device	Improved continence[a]	Overall success	Patients with defecation difficulties
Vaizey et al [64]	1998	6	9 (4–12)	5	5 (100%)	83%	80%
Christiansen et al [65]	1999	17	60 (60–120)	8	8 (100%)	47%	n.r.
O'Brien et al [66]	2000	13	n.r.	10	9 (90%)	69%	20%
Devesa et al [62]	2002	53	26 (7–55)	43	29 (65%)	55%	22%
Ortiz et al [69]	2002	22	28 (6–48)	15	14 (93%)	64%	13%
Lehur et al [70]	2002	16	25 (7–49)	12	11 (92%)	69%	42%
Wong et al [71]	2002	112	12	78[b]	51 (84%)	53%	37%
Michot et al [72]	2003	25	34 (7–60)	20[c]	15 (79%)	60%	37%
Parker et al [73]	2003	45	91-39[d]	27	19 (70%)	42%	11%
Altomare et al [68]	2004	28	50	17	8 (47%)	28%	50%

[a] Percentages refer to patients with functioning device
[b] Outcome available for 61 patients
[c] Outcome available for 19 patients
[d] Two groups of patients: I group (10 patients): mean follow-up 91 months; II group (35 patients): mean follow-up 39 months

Other Surgical Options

Colostomy and Colonic Conduit

Fecal diversion does not confer continence, but it gives patients back the possibility of controlling their bowel movements and an acceptable personal and social life [78]. The creation of a colostomy should not be considered a treatment failure but an option for those patients with severe incontinence not suitable for major operations. Usually, an end sigmoid colostomy with preservation of the rectum is chosen. Sometimes, in presence of persistent rectal symptoms such as leakage of mucus or blood, a subsequent proctectomy can be associated [79].

Another alternative is antegrade colonic irrigation, either through an appendicostomy or a cecostomy (Malone procedure [80]) or through the creation of a colonic conduit. The possibility of irrigating and empty the colon can improve defecation disorders and promote fecal continence. This is particularly useful in those forms of incontinence secondary to sensory and motor disorders that also result in rectal evacuatory difficulties [81]. However, this wash-out procedure can cause abdominal discomfort, resulting in unpleasantness for many patients. Appendicostomy is technically easier but has a higher rate of complications, such as stenosis or reflux of colonic contents; moreover, the appendix is often absent in adults or is too narrow to allow the passage of a catheter. A colonic conduit is typically created after mobilizing and dividing the hepatic flexure. The proximal transverse colon is intussuscepted to form an antireflux valve and then tunneled to the skin while the bowel continuity is restored by an end-to-side anastomosis between the ascending colon and the distal transverse colon. This procedure can also be useful in patients with DGP or artificial sphincter who developed severe evacuatory problems [82].

Conclusions

Many options are available to treat fecal incontinence, but surgeons and patients should have a clear understanding that none of the proposed operations can guaranty a complete return to normal status and that there are no preoperative variables at the moment that can predict whether a treatment will be successful or not. A correct assessment of the causes and severity of symptoms with diary data and validated incontinence [83] and quality of life scores [26] is important to orientate the choice of the treatment. Yet conservative therapies and minor procedures should always be offered first, limiting major operations, such as creation of a new sphincter, to very select cases. Anterior sphincter repair, because of its simplicity and very low morbidity rate, could be the initial procedure when a defect is clearly demonstrated. However, a realistic appraisal of the short and long-term relatively poor outcome may encourage more patients to accept a nonoperative approach.

DGP and ABS should be reserved for cases of severe incontinence in which easier procedures are not feasible or have failed. In both options, case selection is a critical aspect for success: ABS is clearly more indicated in fecal incontinence due to neurological disease that affects the muscles of the lower extremity while patients with a very thin or scarred perineum caused by obstetric trauma, perianal infection, previous surgery, or radiation might be best treated with a DGP. It is difficult to assert if one procedure is better than the other because no direct comparisons have been done. A randomized controlled trial would be useful, but it would be difficult to accomplish because of the limited number of patients and the limited number of surgeons with sufficient experience in both methods [39].

Although continence is improved in a large number of patients, DGP is a difficult operation with a high morbidity rate. Fortunately, most problems can be successfully managed and, at the end of the day, they do not affect the outcome, but patients (and surgeons) need to be really motivated and agree to the possibility of many admissions and reoperations to achieve a good result. Another problem with this procedure is that it is expensive, also considering that the impulse generator does has a median life of 7–8 years [48], after which it needs to be substituted. Nevertheless, Adang et al. [84] produced data showing that overall costs of DGP are lower than those of long-term stoma care. ABS is technically easier and also cheaper than DGP. Besides, it requires less training and gives the patient immediate continence. However, this procedure suffers from a high explantation rate and more technical problems than DGP. Furthermore, results seem to be not as good as thought early on, and difficult defecation is a frequent problem [63]. Our opinion is that in expert hands, DGP can satisfy a higher number of patients. However, both DGP and ABS should remain limited to a small number of centers in which adequate patient volume and surgical experience help to assure low morbidity and satisfactory outcome. For those patients with untreatable incontinence or in whom major operations are contraindicated, end colostomy remains an option that affords an acceptable quality of life.

There is a relatively new treatment called sacral neuromodulation (SNM), which seems to be able to significantly improve symptoms in most patients with severe incontinence, irrespective of the nature of the incontinence. This procedure, which is the topic of next chapter, is easy to perform and almost without complications. Moreover, this is the only operation in which outcome can be predicted with a preliminary test – peripheral nerve evaluation (PNE) – which selects with an accuracy close to 100% patients who are good candidates for definitive implantation of the stimulator. For all these reasons this new procedure may become the treatment of choice when surgery is required.

References

1. Burnett SJ, Bartram CI (1991) Unsuspected sphincter damage following childbirth revealed by anal endosonography. Br J Radiol 64:225–227
2. Londono-Shimmer EE, Garcia-Duperly R, Nicholls RJ et al (1994) Overlapping anal sphincter repair for faecal incontinence due to sphincter trauma: five year follow-up functional results. Int J Colorectal Dis 9:110–113
3. Nikiteas N, Korsgen S, Kumar D, Keighley MR (1996). Audit of sphincter repair: factors associated with poor outcome. Dis Colon Rectum 39:1164–1170
4. Gilliland R, Altomare DF, Moreira H et al (1998) Pudendal neuropathy is predictive of failure following anterior overlapping sphincteroplasty. Dis Colon Rectum 41:1516–1522
5. Sangwan YP, Coller JA, Barrett RC et al (1996) Unilateral pudendal neuropathy: impact on outcome of anal sphincter repair. Dis Colon Rectum 39: 686–689
6. Young CJ, Mathur MN, Eyers AA, Solomon MJ et al (1998) Successful overlapping anal sphincter repair: relationship to patient age, neuropathy, and colostomy formation. Dis Colon Rectum 41:344–349
7. Malouf AJ, Norton CS, Engel AF et al (2000) Long-term results of overlapping anterior anal-sphincter repair for obstetric trauma. Lancet 355:260–265
8. Karoui S, Leroi AM, Koning E et al (2000) Results of sphincteroplasty in 86 patients with anal incontinence. Dis Colon Rectum 43:813–820
9. Zorcolo L, Covotta L, Bartolo DC (2005) Outcome of anterior sphincter repair for obstetric injury: comparison of early and late results. Dis Colon Rectum 48:524–531
10. Engel AF, Kamm MA, Sultan AH et al (1994) Anterior anal sphincter repair in patients with obstetric trauma. Br J Surg 81:1231–1234
11. Hasegawa H, Yoshioka K, Keighley MR (2000) Randomized trial of faecal diversion for sphincter repair. Dis Colon Rectum 43:961–964
12. Lam TC, Kennedy ML, Chen FC et al (1999) Prevalence of faecal incontinence: obstetric and constipation related risk factors: a population-based study. Colorectal Dis 1:197–203
13. Aitola P, Hiltunen KM, Matikainen M (2000) Functional results of anterior levatorplasty and external sphincter plication for faecal incontinence. Ann Chir Gynaecol 89:29–32
14. Miller R, Orrom WJ, Cornes H et al (1989) Anterior sphincter plication and levatoroplasty in the treatment of faecal incontinence. Br J Surg 76:1058–1060
15. Stricker JW, Schoetz DJ, Coller JA, Veidenheimer MC (1988) Surgical correction of anal incontinence. Dis Colon Rectum 31:533–540
16. Nessim A, Wexner SD, Agachan F et al (1999) Is bowel confinement necessary after anorectal surgery? Dis Colon Rectum 42:16–23
17. Ctercteko GC, Fazio VW, Jagelmann DG et al (1988) Anal sphincter repair: a report of 60 cases and review of the literature. Aust NZ J Surg 58:703–710
18. Rasmussen O, Puggaard L, Christiansen J (1999) Anal sphincter repair in patients with obstetric trauma. Dis Colon Rectum 42:193–195
19. Draganic B, Eyers AA, Solomon MJ (2001) Island flap perineoplasty decreases the incidence of wound breakdown following overlapping anterior sphincter repair. Colorectal Dis 3:387–391
20. Parks AG, McPartlin JF (1971) Late repair of injuries of the anal sphincter. Proc Roy Soc Med 64:1187–1189
21. Christiansen J, Pedersen IK (1987) Traumatic anal incontinence: results of surgical repair. Dis Colon Rectum 30:189–191
22. Oliveira L, Pfeifer J, Wexner SD (1996) Physiological

and clinical outcome of anterior sphincteroplasty. Br J Surg 83:502–505
23. Sangalli MR, Marti MC (1994) Results of sphincter repair in post-obstetric faecal incontinence. J Am Col Surg 179:583–586
24. Fleshman JW, Peters WR, Shemesh EI et al (1991) Anal sphincter reconstruction: anterior overlapping muscle repair. Dis Colon Rectum 34:739–743
25. Wexner SD, Marchetti F, Jagelman DG (1991) The role of sphincteroplasty for faecal incontinence re-evaluated: a prospective physiologic and functional review. Dis Colon Rectum 34:22–30
26. Byrne CM, Pager CK, Rex J et al (2002) Assessment of quality of life in the treatment of patients with neuropathic faecal incontinence. Dis Colon Rectum 45:1431–1436
27. Morren GL, Hallbook O, Nystrom PO et al (2001) Audit of anal sphincter repair. Colorectal Dis 3:17–22
28. Halverson AL, Hull TL (2002) Long-term outcome of overlapping anal sphincter repair. Dis Colon Rectum 45:345–348
29. Gutierrez AB, Madoff RD, Lowry AC et al (2004) Long-term results of anterior sphincteroplasty. Dis Colon Rectum 47:727–732
30. Parks AG (1975) Anorectal incontinence. Proc Roy Soc Med 68:681–690
31. Jameson JS, Speakman CT, Darzi A et al (1994) Audit of postanal repair in the treatment of faecal incontinence. Dis Colon Rectum 37:369–372
32. Setti-Carraro P, Kamm MA, Nicholls RJ (1994) Long-term results of postanal repair for neurogenic faecal incontinence. Br J Surg 81:140–144
33. Matsuoka H, Mavrantonis C, Wexner SD et al (2000) Postanal repair for faecal incontinence – is it worthwhile? Dis Colon Rectum 43:1561–1567
34. Browning GG, Parks AG (1983) Postanal repair for neuropathic fecal incontinence: correlation of clinical results and anal canal pressure. Br J Surg 70:101–104
35. Yoshioka K, Hyland G, Keighley MR (1988) Physiological changes after postanal repair and parameters predicting outcome. Br J Surg 75:1220–1224
36. Orrom WJ, Miller R, Cornes H et al (1991) Comparison of anterior sphincteroplasty and postanal repair in the treatment of idiopathic faecal incontinence. Dis Colon Rectum 34:305–310
37. Van Tets WF, Kuijpers JHC (1998) Pelvic floor procedures produce no consistent changes in anatomy or physiology. Dis Colon Rectum 41:365–369
38. Christiansen J, Hansen CR, Rasmussen O (1995) Bilateral gluteus maximus transposition for anal incontinence. Br J Surg 82:903–905
39. Madoff RD, Beaten CGMI, Christiansen J, et al (2000) Standards for anal sphincter replacement. Dis Colon Rectum 43:135–141
40. Pickrell KL, Broadbent TR, Masters FW, Metzger JT (1952) Construction of a rectal sphincter and restoration of anal continence by transplanting the gracilis muscle: a report of four cases in children. Ann Surg 135:853–862
41. Baeten CG, Konsten J, Spaans F et al (1991) Dynamic graciloplasty for treatment of faecal incontinence. Lancet 338:1163–1165
42. Williams NS, Patel J, George BD et al (1991) Development of an electrically stimulated neoanal sphincter. Lancet 338:1166–11699
43. Sielezneff I, Malouf AJ, Bartolo DC et al (1999) Dynamic graciloplasty in the treatment of patients with faecal incontinence. Br J Surg 86:61–65
44. Wexner SD, Baeten C, Bailey R et al (2002) Long-term efficacy of dynamic graciloplasty for faecal incontinence. Dis Colon Rectum 45:809–818
45. Konsten J, Rongen MJ, Ogunbiyi O et al (2001) Comparison of epineural or intramuscular Nerve electrodes for stimulated graciloplasty. Dis Colon Rectum 44:581–586
46. Mavrantonis C, Billotti VL, Wexner SD (1999) Stimulated graciloplasty for treatment of intractable faecal incontinence: critical influence of the method of stimulation. Dis Colon Rectum 42(4):497–504
47. Penninckx F (2004) Belgian section of colorectal surgery. Belgian experience with dynamic graciloplasty for faecal incontinence. Br J Surg 91:872–878
48. Rongen MGM, Uludag O, Naggar KE et al (2003) Dis Colon Rectum 46:716–721
49. Matzel KE, Madoff RD, LaFontaine LJ et al (2001) Dynamic Graciloplasty Therapy Study Group. Complications of dynamic graciloplasty: incidence, management, and impact on outcome. Dis Colon Rectum 44:1427–1435
50. Baeten CGMI, Gerdes BP, Adang EMM et al (1995) Anal dynamic graciloplasty in the treatment of intractable faecal incontinence. N Engl J Med 332:1600–1605
51. Geerdes BP, Heineman E, Konsten J et al (1996) Dynamic graciloplasty. Complication and management. Dis Colon Rectum 39:912–917
52. Christiansen J, Rasmussen OO, Lindorf-Larsen K (1998) Dynamic graciloplasty for severe anal incontinence. Br J Surg 85:88–91
53. Cavina E, Seccia M, Banti P, Zocco G (1998) Anorectal reconstruction after abdominoperineal resection. Experience with double-wrap graciloplasty supported by low-frequency electrostimulation. Dis Colon Rectum 41:1010–1016
54. Baeten CG, Bailey HR, Bakka A et al (2000) Safety and efficacy of dynamic graciloplasty for fecal inconti-

nence: report of a prospective, multicenter trial. Dynamic Graciloplasty Therapy Study Group. Dis Colon Rectum 43:743–751

56. Seccia M, Lippolis PV, Menconi C (2003) Applied electrophysiology of transposed muscle stimulation: practical considerations and surgical experience on graciloplasty for faecal incontinence. Acta Biomed Ateneo Parmense 74S2:84–88
55. Bresler L, Reibel N, Brunaud L et al (2002) Dynamic graciloplasty in the treatment of severe faecal incontinence. French multicentric retrospective study. Ann Chir 127:520–526
57. Thornton MJ, Kennedy ML, Lubowskj DZ, King DW (2004) Long-term follow-up of dynamic graciloplasty for faecal incontinence. Colorectal Dis 6:470–476
58. Mander BJ, Wexner SD, Williams NS et al (1999) Preliminary results of a multicenter trial of the electrically stimulated gracilis neoanal sphincter. Br J Surg 86:1543–1548
59. Montague DK (1992) The artificial urinary sphincter (AS 800): experience in 166 consecutive patients. J Urology 147:380–382
60. Christiansen J, Lorentzen M (1989) Implantation of artificial sphincter for anal incontinence. Report of five cases. Dis Colon Rectum 32:432–436
61. Moff RD, Baeten CG, Christiansen J et al (2000) Standards for anal sphincters replacement. Dis Colon Rectum 43:135–141
62. Devesa JM, Rey A, Hervas PL et al (2002) Artificial anal sphincter. Complications and functional results of a large personal series. Dis Colon Rectum 45:1154–1163
63. Mundy L, Merlin TL, Maddern GJ, Hiller JE (2004) Sistematic review of safety and effectiveness of an artificial bowel sphincter for faecal incontinence. Br J Surg 91:665–672
64. Vaizey CJ, Kamm MA, Gold DM et al (1998) Clinical, physiological and radiological study of a new purpose-designed artificial bowel sphincter. Lancet 352:105–109
65. Christiansen J, Rasmussen OO, Lindorff-Larsen K (1999) Long-term results of artificial anal sphincter implantation for severe anal incontinence. Ann Surg 230:45–48
66. O'Brien PE, Skinner S (2000) Restoring control: the Acticon Neosphincter artificial bowel sphincter in the treatment of anal incontinence. Dis Colon Rectum 43:1213–1216
67. Altomare DF, Dodi G, La Torre F et al (2001) Multicenter retrospective analysis of the outcome of artificial anal sphincter implantation for severe faecal incontinence. Br J Surg 88:1481–1486
68. Altomare DF, Binda GA, Dodi G et al (2004) Disappointing long-term results of the artificial anal sphincter for faecal incontinence. Br J Surg 91:1352–1353
69. Ortiz H, Armendariz P, DeMiguel M et al (2002) Complications and functional outcome following artificial anal sphincter implantation. Br J Surg 89:877–881
70. Lehur PA, Zerbib F, Neunlist M et al (2002) Comparison of quality of life and anorectal function after artificial sphincter implantation. Dis Colon Rectum 45:508–513
71. Wong WD, Congliosi SM, Spencer MP et al (2002) The safety and efficacy of the artificial bowel sphincter for faecal incontinence. Results from a multicentric cohort study. Dis Colon Rectum 45:1139–1153
72. Michot F, Costaglioli B, Leroi AM, Denis P (2003) Artificial anal sphincter in severe faecal incontinence. Outcome of prospective experience with 37 patients in one institution. Ann Surg 237:52–56
73. Parker SC, Spencer MP, Madoff RD et al (2003) Artificial bowel sphincter. Long-term experience at a single institution. Dis Colon Rectum 46:722–729
74. Lehur PA, Glemain P, Bruley des Varannes S (1998) Outcome of patients with an implanted artificial anal sphincter for severe faecal incontinence. A single institution report. Int J Colorectal Dis 13:88–92
75. Wong WD, Jensen LL, Bartolo DCC, Rothenberger DA (1996) Artificial anal sphincter. Dis Colon Rectum 39:1345–1351
76. Lehur PA, Roig JV, Duinslaeger M (2000) Artificial anal sphincter : prospective clinical and manometric evaluation. Dis Colon Rectum 43 :1100–1106
77. Savoye G, Leroi AM, Denis P, Michot F (2000) Manometric assessment of an artificial bowel sphincter. Br J Surg 87:586–589
78. Vaizey CJ, Kamm MA, Nicholls RJ (1998) Recent advances in the surgical treatment of faecal incontinence. Br J Surg 95:596–603
79. Catena F, Wilkinson K, Phillips RKS (2002) Untreatable faecal incontinence: colostomy or colostomy and proctectomy? Colorectal Disease 4:48–50
80. Malone PS, Ransley PG, Kiely EM (1990) Preliminary report: the antegrade continence enema. Lancet 336:1217–1218
81. Briel JW, Schouten WR, Vlot EA et al (1997) Clinical value of colonic irrigation in patients with continence disturbances. Dis Colon Rectum 40:802–805
82. Saunders JR, Eccersley AJP, Williams NS (2003) Use of a continent colonic conduit for treatment of refractory evacuatory disorder following construction of an electrically stimulated gracilis neoanal sphincter. Br J Surg 90:1416–1421
83. Vaizey CJ, Carapeti E, Cahill JA, Kamm MA (1999) Prospective comparison of faecal incontinence grading systems. Gut 44:77–80
84. Adang EMM, Engel GI, Rutten FFH et al (1998) Cost-effectiveness of dynamic graciloplasty in patients with faecal incontinence. Dis Colon Rectum 41:725–733

VIII.3. New Treatment Options for Fecal Incontinence: Radiofrequency Delivery and Bulking Agents

M. Trompetto, C. Pastore, A. Realis Luc

Fecal incontinence is a benign functional disorder having a negative impact on patient's lifestyle and overall quality of life. The severity of the disturbance depends on a variety of anatomical, pathophysiological, and psychological factors and, in spite of the possibility of using a great amount of anatomophysiological investigation to define its severity, its treatment is often stepwise, beginning with dietary measures, antimotility agents, different kinds of pelvic exercises, and biofeedback.

Surgical treatments may be an option for patients not responding to conservative management and are tailored to the specific cause of the incontinence. Overlapping sphincteroplasty is effective for patients with sphincter defects, but its long-term results are far from being good. Stimulated graciloplasty and artificial bowel sphincter are plagued by a high percentage of complications, and the promising short-term results of sacral nerve stimulation have yet to be confirmed.

With these unsatisfactory clinical results, the attention of coloproctologists has moved to less invasive treatments such as the injection of bulking agents and the use of radiofrequency energy.

These new options could be a good alternative, especially for the majority of cases in which the sphincter defect is minimal or absent, as in patients with keyhole deformity of the anal canal, "weakness" of the internal sphincter, or in patients in which the social impact of the disorder does not match with the results of the functional investigations.

Radiofrequency Energy Delivery (Secca Procedure)

Radiofrequency energy has been used in many different diseases, particularly in patients with benign prostatic hyperplasia, joint capsule laxity, and mostly, in cases of gastroesophageal reflux disease. The rationale for its use in selected cases of fecal incontinence is the possibility of taking advantage of the heat delivered by the radiofrequency energy that seems be able to provoke some advantageous anatomical changes in the anal canal. In fact, the effects of the treatment seem to result in an rapid contraction of the collagenous tissue followed by wound healing and a consequent new remodeling and a certain grade of tightening of the anal canal.

Technique

The procedure can be considered as an outpatient technique. An antibiotic prophylaxis with ciprofloxacin 500 mg twice daily and metronidazole 500 mg three times daily for 3 days is advisable. No bowel preparation is needed, but a small enema 1 h before the procedure allows dealing with a clean rectum. Patients are positioned in the classic jackknife position and receive intravenous benzodiazepine and a narcotic for sedation. Then a local anesthesia is administered (lidocaine or bupivacaine with or without epinephrine).

The Secca device comprises an anoscopic bar-

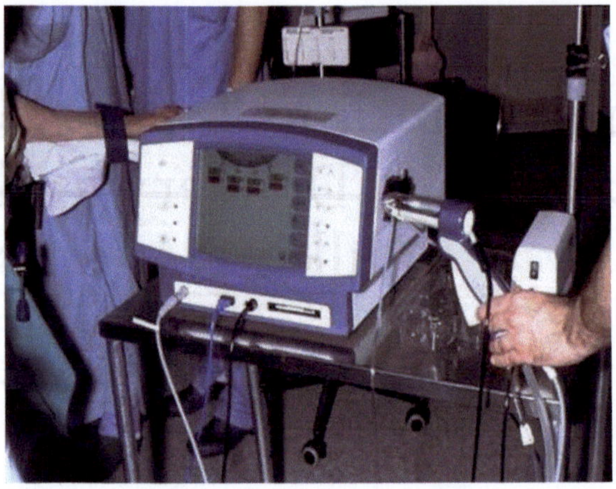

Fig. VIII.14. Secca device and anoscopic barrel

rel with four nickel-titanium curved needle electrodes (22 gauge, 6 mm in length; Curon Medical) (Figs. VIII.14 and 15). Thermocouples are present within the tip and at the base of each needle to monitor tissue and mucosal temperatures, respectively, during radiofrequency delivery. On deployment, there is a reduction in electrical impedance, indicating the proper contact of the electrode with the submucosal layer.

Digital examination and anoscopy are performed, then the device is positioned under direct visualization within the anal canal, allowing the proper penetration of the needles starting 1 cm distal to the dentate line (Fig. VIII.16). When the needles are deployed in the tissue, the generator delivers radiofrequency energy to each needle for 90 s at a preselected temperature of 85°C. The mucosa is preserved by thermal lesions, cooling it

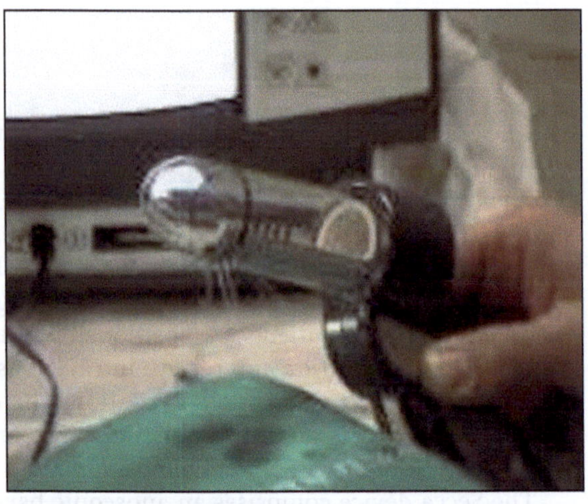

Fig. VIII.15. Anoscopic barrel

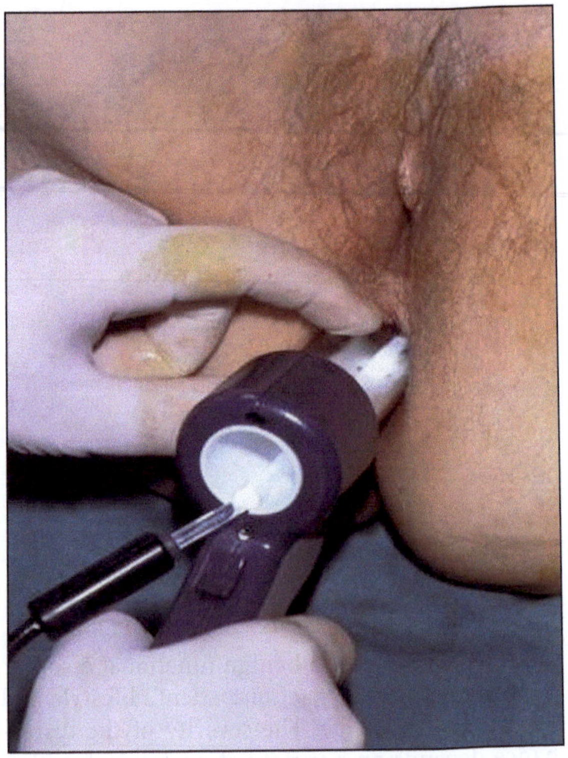

Fig. VIII.16. Positioning of the anoscopic barrel

by delivering chilled water (45°C) to the base of each needle. A series of three to four other similar procedures are performed proximally until 15 mm from the dentate line for a total of 16–20 lesion sets (Fig. VIII.17). Patients can be discharged approximately 2 h after treatment.

Results

To date, very few papers have been published on this technique, especially about its safety and feasibility [1, 2]. Short-term results seem to be satisfactory while only one article confirms their maintenance 2 years after the treatment [3]. The procedure-related complications consist of some anoderm ulcerations requiring accurate local wound care, cases of antibiotic-associated diarrhea, minor bleeding, transient anal pain, and fever without clinical signs of perianal infection. Probably, the technique does not preclude patients from undergoing more invasive procedures if the certain degree of scarring provoked within the anal canal, which may be the main reason of improvement of continence, makes subsequent treatment more difficult.

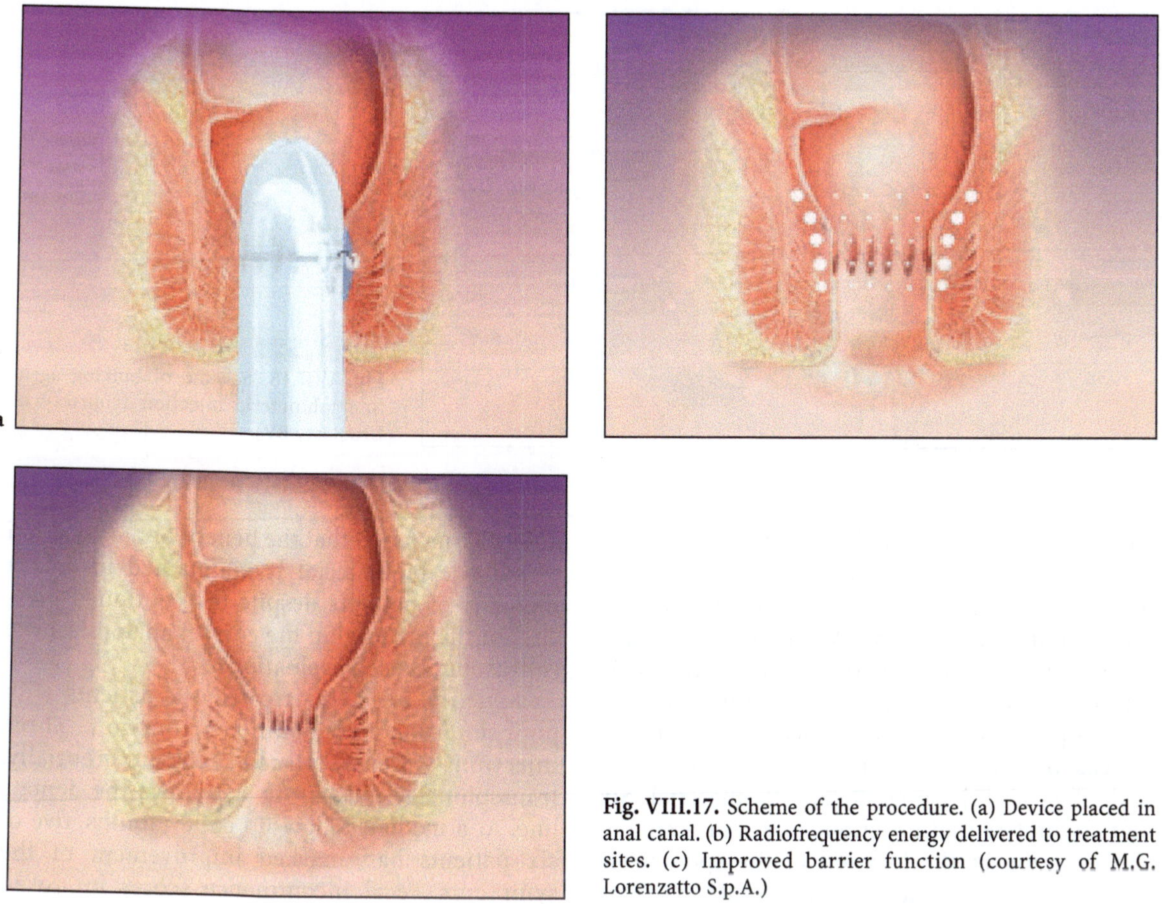

Fig. VIII.17. Scheme of the procedure. (a) Device placed in anal canal. (b) Radiofrequency energy delivered to treatment sites. (c) Improved barrier function (courtesy of M.G. Lorenzatto S.p.A.)

Bulking Agents

Looking at the good results obtained by urologists in enhancing the function of the vesical neck [4, 5], local injections of collagen, polytetrafluoroethylene, and autologous fat have been used for passive fecal incontinence with opposing results (Fig. VIII.18). The use of new types of bulking agents, such as silicone-based biomaterials, calcium hydroxyapatite, and Durasphere, have been considered only recently. The few reports in the literature to date do not allow comparison of the results of the injection with the current traditional treatments [6].

Technique

Treatment, whatever bulking agent is used, can be performed on a outpatient procedure basis, and an antibiotic prophylaxis (metronidazole 500 mg 3 times daily and ciprofloxacin 500 mg twice daily for 5 days) is mandatory. After cleansing the anoperineal area with povidone-iodine soap, local anesthesia is performed (lidocaine or bupivacaine with or without epinephrine) (Fig. VIII.19). The needle for the injection must be inserted in the skin at 2.5 cm from the anal margin and pushed forward to reach the intersphincteric space (Fig. VIII.20), controlled by a finger put in the anal canal. The bulking agent must be slowly injected, perceiving with the finger the formation of a small, elastic ball protruding in the anal canal. In the majority of cases, three or four injections are needed to tighten the anal canal, but the number of perianal injections and the volume of the biomaterial injected can vary from case to case, depending on the size and location of the sphincteric defect or on a generalized sphincteric disfunction (Fig. VIII.21 and 22).

Results

Tjandra et al. [7] treated 82 patients using an injectable silicone biomaterial (Bioplastique) to

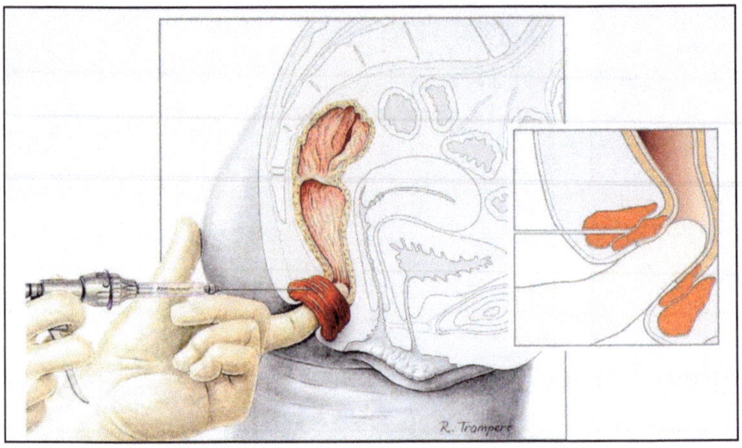

Fig. VIII.18. Scheme of bulking agent intersphincteric injection (courtesy of Uroplasty BV)

augment the internal anal sphincter. No significant complications occurred. Fecal continence improved significantly in all patients (median >50% improvement by Wexner's continence score) and 93% percent of patients had >50% improvement in the global quality of life scores.

Ten patients with passive incontinence due to a weak or disrupted sphincter were injected by Malouf et al. [8] using silicone biomaterial. Six had circumferential injections and four a single-site injection in the location of the sphincteric rupture. Five patients had moderate pain or minor ulceration at the injection site. No other complication occurred. At 6 weeks, six patients showed a marked improvement or a complete cessation of leakage. A further patient improved after a second injection. Three patients had no improvement. At 6 months, only two of the seven improved patients maintained good results. The authors concluded that the benefit of the injection of silicone biomaterial is maintained in only a minority of patients despite the continued presence of the material in the correct anatomical site (ultrasound-based evaluation).

Kenefick et al. [9] treated six patients with poor internal anal sphincter function. Three injections were placed circumferentially, transsphincterically, at or just above the dentate line. At a median follow-up of 18 months, five of six patients had marked improvement of the symptoms. Fecal incontinence scores improved from a median of 14/24 before to 8/24 after treatment, as well as SF-36 quality of life physical and social function scores. There was also a corresponding physiological increase in maximum anal resting and squeeze pressures. There were no complications.

Davis et al. [10] treated 18 patients with persis-

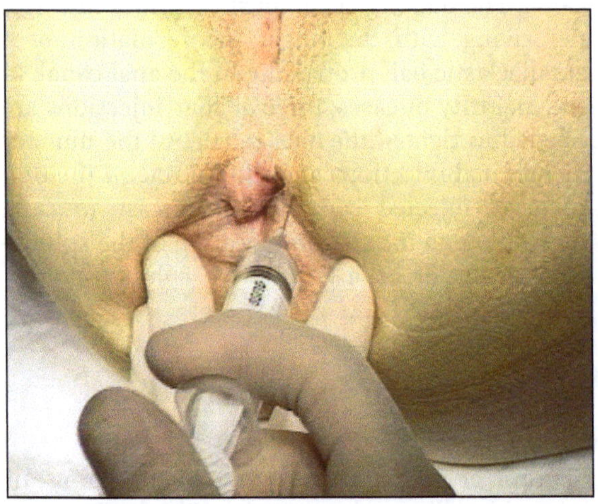

Fig. VIII.19. Perianal local anesthetic injection

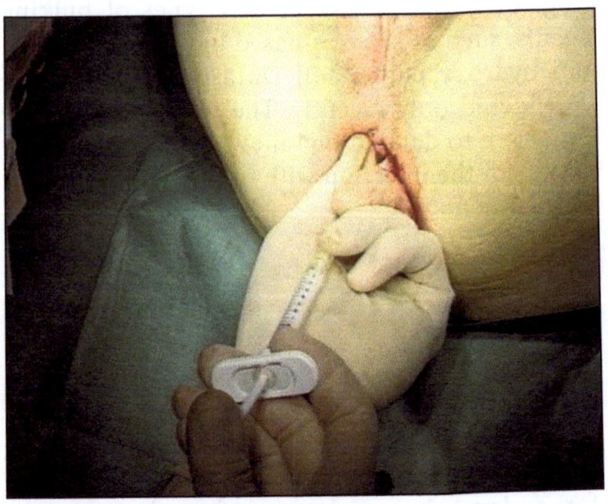

Fig. VIII.20. Intersphincteric injection

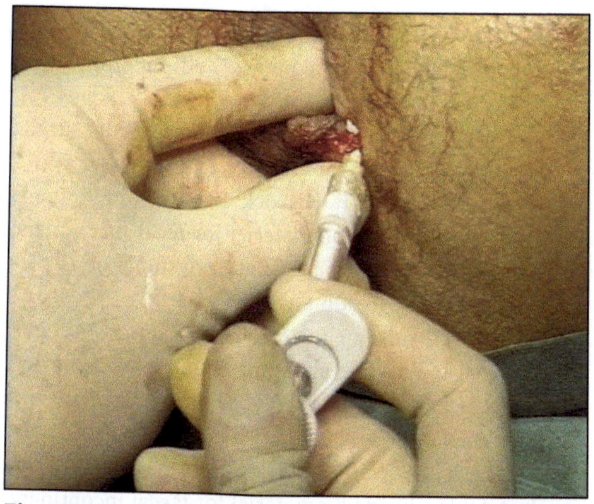

Fig. VIII.21. Checking the endoanal protrusion resulting from the intersphincteric injection

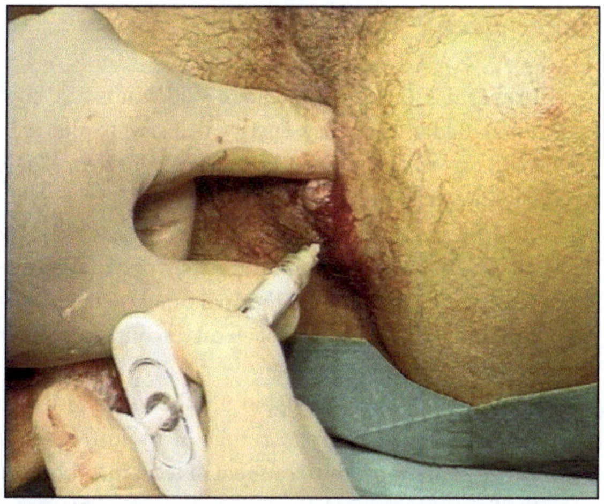

Fig. VIII.22. Further injection around the anal canal

tent fecal leakage/soiling using injections of Durasphere to restore anal canal symmetry. Anorectal physiological parameters, apart from the maximum tolerable rectal volume at 12 months, showed no significant improvement, also if patients achieved a significant improvement in continence grading, satisfaction and quality of life scores (lifestyle, coupling, depression, and embarrassment).

Personal Experience

Our experience is based on a pilot study using injections of Coaptite, a calcium hydroxyapatite suspension in a hydrosoluble gel, in 17 patients with passive fecal incontinence due to an internal anal sphincter dysfunction. Three or four injections (1 ml each) were given in ten patients and six injections in seven, regularly distributing the biomaterial all around the anal canal. Wexner's score for continence, daily diary, endoanal ultrasound (Figs. VIII.23), and monitoring of the safety parameters were used for evaluation of results, with a median follow-up of 10 months. Thirteen patients had a marked improvement, with a reduction in the incontinence score from 8.3 to 2.6. Patients who had three injections improved more than patients receiving six injections. No major or minor complications occurred.

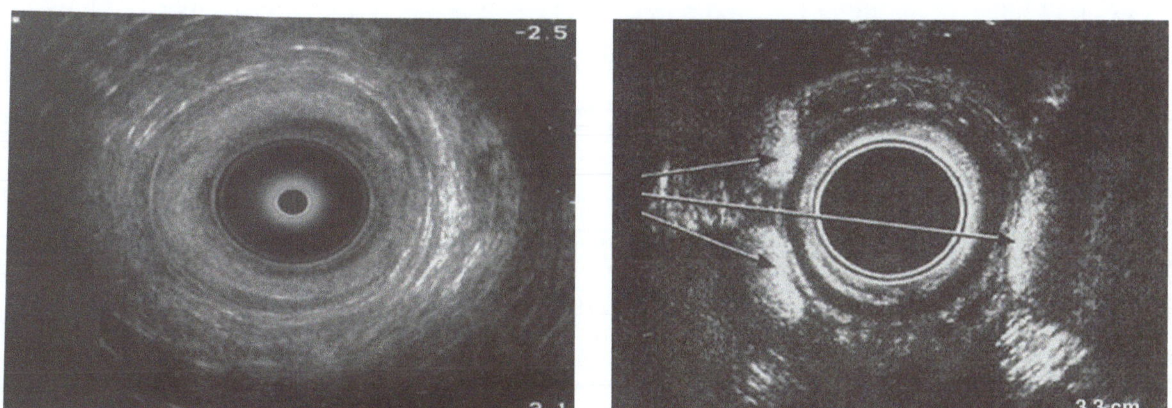

a b

Fig. VIII.23. Preoperative ultrasound showing a multiple rupture of a thin internal anal sphincter (**a**). Postinjection ultrasound showing correct positioning of the bulking agent (*arrows*) (**b**)

References

1. Takahashi T, Garcia-Osogobio S, Valdovinos MA et al (2002) Radio-frequency energy delivery to the anal canal for the treatment of fecal incontinence. Dis Colon Rectum 45:915–922
2. Efron JE, Corman ML, Fleshman J et al (2003) Safety and effectiveness of temperature-controlled radio-frequency energy delivery to the anal canal (Secca procedure) for the treatment of fecal incontinence. Dis Colon Rectum 46:1606–1618
3. Takahashi T, Garcia-Osogobio S, Valdovinos MA et al (2003) Extended two-year results of radio-frequency energy delivery for the treatment of fecal incontinence (the Secca procedure). Dis Colon Rectum 46:711–715
4. Mayer R, Lightfood M, Jung I (2001) Preliminary evaluation of calcium hydroxyapatite as a transurethral bulking agent for stress urinary incontinence. Urology 57:434–438
5. Dmochowski R, Appell RA (2003) Advancements in minimally invasive treatment for female stress urinary incontinence: radiofrequency and bulking agents. Curr Urol Rep 4:350
6. Person B, Wexner SD (2005) Advances in the surgical treatment of fecal incontinence. Surg Innov 12:7–21
7. Tjandra JJ, Lim JF, Hiscock R, Rajendra P (2004) Injectable silicone biomaterial for fecal incontinence caused by internal anal sphincter dysfunction is effective. Dis Colon Rectum 47:2138–2146
8. Malouf AJ, Vaizey CJ, Norton CS, Kamm MA (2001) Internal anal sphincter augmentation for fecal incontinence using injectable silicone biomaterial. Dis Colon Rectum 44:595–600
9. Kenefick NJ, Vaizey CJ, Malouf AJ et al (2002) Injectable silicone biomaterial for faecal incontinence due to anal sphincter dysfunction. Gut 51: 225–228
10. Davis K, Kumar D, Poloniecki J (2003) Preliminary evaluation of an injectable anal sphincter bulking agent (Durasphere) in the management of fecal incontinence. Aliment Pharmacol Ther 18: 237–243

Invited Commentary

S.D. Wexner

I very much enjoyed reading the section on "Treatment Options for Fecal Incontinence" in the textbook *Benign Anorectal Diseases*. The introduction by Santoro and Di Falco was very enlightening. I would emphasize within the section that the evaluating physician or surgeon must determine which treatment the patient will tolerate. For example, an elderly patient confined to a nursing home may not be a suitable candidate for one of the more advanced procedures, such as sacral nerve stimulation, stimulated graciloplasty, or artificial bowel sphincter. Conversely, a young, active patient with significant incontinence would most likely be willing to try any viable alternative. The reason for the importance of determining candidates for potential treatment at this early stage is to avoid subjecting patients to more evaluation than is required for the potentially proposed treatment. Specifically, in the case of the elderly patient who might be reasonably managed with only medical therapy, perhaps with additional biofeedback therapy and a rectoanal cleansing regimen, I would recommend a limited physiological investigation. Conversely, in the patient who would potentially require a more advanced surgical procedure, a complete physiologic evaluation would be routinely undertaken. It is also important to differentiate the degree of incontinence, and for this reason, the authors prefer the Vaizey classification. However, we still rely on its predecessor, the Cleveland Clinic Florida/Wexner incontinence score [1]. In addition, to assess the impact on quality of life, we also employ the Rockwood American Society of Colon and Rectal Surgeons (ASCRS) fecal incontinence score [2]. With some combination of a fecal incontinence score and a fecal incontinence quality-of-life scale, we can usually appropriately ascertain potential therapy and therefore suggest the best evaluation for each patient.

The section by Zorcolo and Bartolo is certainly a comprehensively written and extensively referenced section. In addition to reading the description of the techniques, I found the tables quite useful. To address these various techniques individually, we still utilize an overlapping sphincter repair. Although our initial success rate was in the range of 75%, like many more recently published reports, we have noted that the success rate has significantly declined to probably 35% with a 10-year follow-up [3–6]. At this point, I counsel all patients prior to overlapping sphincter repair that the operation will represent the first stage in an effort to correct the problem. I further explain that they may go on to require either a repeat sphincter repair, an artificial bowel sphincter, sacral nerve stimulation, graciloplasty, the use of injectables, radiofrequency, or some combination of these alternatives at a later time. Therefore, I feel that it is important to set the expectations appropriately low and not to rely upon the initial 75–95% success rates. If the expectations are set appropriately meagre, patients are not surprised if they experience deterioration, and patients who have no initial improvement are also not surprised.

Certainly, the results in Table VIII.4 showing long-term success rates ranging from 6% to 28% are within the realm of expectations. In one recent study, we showed the importance of overlapping scar rather than muscle in obtaining optimal results. Therefore, we continue to employ the overlapping technique.

Like Laurberg et al. [7], Londono-Schimmer et al. [8], and Sangwan et al. [9], we found a significant impact of pudendal nerve status upon the outcome of anterior sphincter repair. Gilliland et al. [4] specifically assessed 77 patients in whom we noted a 66% success rate of anterior sphincter repair or lateral sphincter repair in those without pudendal neuropathy compared with 17% in those with pudendal neuropathy. Accordingly, we might even consider deferring sphincter repair and not inducing additional scarring, knowing the poor long-term outcome of sphincter repair and being cognizant of additional, newer treatment options. While this approach may seem heretical, it may also offer the best outcome of success. In addition, based upon a prospective randomized trial, we no longer utilize bowel confinement [10].

One change in our recommendations for local surgical procedures has been the discontinued use of postanal repair [11]. As the authors note, our success rate of 33% is certainly less than stellar. Prior to the advent of injectables and radiofrequency, we did occasionally offer postanal repair for the patient with "neurogenic" fecal incontinence. We justified offering a postanal repair when there was no discrete readily remediable anterior defect. The study by Matsuoka et al. [11] evaluated 21 patients, ten of whom had prior sphincter repairs, and reported a mean of 6.8 (range 0.5–22) years of fecal incontinence. There was no mortality, 5% morbidity, and although the success rate was only 35%, the specific rate decrease of preoperative fecal incontinence was 16.7 to a postoperative 2.6. Nevertheless, at the present time, it seems that both injectables and radiofrequency are potentially less morbid with similar success rates. Therefore, postanal repair is no longer utilized at our institution.

I very much enjoyed reading the section on neosphincter. Basically, based upon our extensive experience with the graciloplasty, we found a high morbidity but reasonable expectations of success in patients in whom the stimulated graciloplasty continued to work [12–15]. In publication of the multicenter experience of 129 patients after stimulated graciloplasty, we reported a fairly consistent improvement of 62% of patients 12 months following the procedure to 66% at 24 months. The most important determinant of success was the use of intramuscular rather than direct nerve stimulation, with success rates of 93% and 10%, respectively [12]. Sadly, the Medtronics Corporation (who manufactures the stimulator) did not pursue Food and Drug Administration (FDA) approval in the United States, and therefore, we can no longer offer this often much needed therapy. Although this therapy required significant determination by both the surgeon and the patient because of the myriad of potential complications, technical difficulties, and cost, it did offer significant benefit to appropriately selected patients in many instances. In point of fact, patients with significant tissue loss may not be candidates for artificial bowel sphincter and certainly cannot undergo sacral nerve stimulation. Because we no longer offer stimulated graciloplasty in the United States, these patients are often condemned to a permanent stoma. One option that we have occasionally taken is the use of the nonstimulated graciloplasty technique followed by an artificial bowel sphincter. However, it will certainly be simpler to perform a single operation rather than multiple ones.

When an appropriate amount of tissue exists, the artificial bowel sphincter may be an option [16]. We use the same technique as described by the authors and have certainly demonstrated similar results. The main problem with this operation remains extrusion of the device even at a late stage. We have had some patients with excellent success who many years later have had extrusion and required explantation of the sphincter. Nonetheless, given the absence of availability of stimulated graciloplasty in the United States, the artificial bowel sphincter is often the procedure of choice. We have even successfully implanted a sphincter in patients with concomitant artificial urinary sphincter and perineal implants.

Despite the excellent work by Williams and others [17], we have not employed the Malone procedure and instead relied upon a standard colostomy or enemas in patients who do not wish a stoma. When the patient does require or request a stoma, our preference is for a laparoscopically constructed end colostomy to which irrigation can be performed. Such irrigation can obviate the need for routine wearing of an appliance.

The most exciting new treatment that we employ is the sacral nerve stimulation procedure [18, 19]. We have performed almost 20 procedures to date and have been very impressed with both the ease of the electrode implantation as well as the durability of the device and functionality of the methodology. While the data have not yet been published, we are certainly optimistic. Particularly given our experience with high morbidity with the stimulated graciloplasty and the high rate of extrusion of the artificial bowel sphincter, sacral nerve stimulation is certainly a welcome alternative.

Jost [18] reported 30 patients who underwent electrical nerve stimulation for fecal incontinence. He reported not only improvement in pudendal nerve amplitude from 0.5 ms to 0.8 ms but also improvement in incontinence from a score of 7.3–7.1. Osterberg et al. [19] also reported the use of electrical nerval stimulation with a double-plugged pulse generator. With follow-up at 3 and 12 months, improvement was noted in 46% and 38% of patients, respectively.

I also very much enjoyed the section by Trompetto, Pastore, and Realis Luc. Injectables and radiofrequency both have a significant role in the treatment of fecal incontinence. Our experience with injectables has thus far been limited to carbon-coated beads. Weiss et al. [20] noted an excellent initial response with a diminished although still modest long-term success rate. Specifically, we performed an open-label study of ten patients in whom carbon-coated beads were injected. The 80% initial improvement waned to 23% at 2 months and remained at 30% at 6 months, with improvement reported in all four scales of the fecal incontinence quality-of-life scores at 3 months. The procedure is simple with minimal complications.

The success rate of radiofrequency has been perhaps somewhat more impressive [21–23]. Takahashi et al. [21] initially reported on ten women of a mean age of 55.9 years who underwent radiofrequency treatment. There were a few minor complications, and at 1-year follow-up, there was significant improvement in incontinence with reduction in the incontinence score from 13.5 to 5 and improvement in all major scales of fecal incontinence quality of life (lifestyle, depression, coping, embarrassment). A subsequent 2-year follow-up [22] showed that incontinence scores persistent, with good improvement from 13.8 preoperatively to 7.3 at 2 years, persistent improvement of all four fecal incontinence quality-of-life scales and social functioning SF-36 scores, as well as elimination of the use of pads in four of patients.

In the largest investigator multicenter study, Efron et al. [23] reported 50 patients with a mean length of fecal incontinence of 15 years. Fecal incontinence scores improved from 14.5 prior to the procedure to 11.7 at 6 months. Improvements were noted in all four major components of the fecal incontinence quality-of-life scale, in the SF-36 social functioning scale, and in the mental health scores. There were few adverse events and manometrically objective documentation of improvement in maximum tolerable volume from 245 cc to 210 cc at 6 months. Similarly, the threshold volume improved from 23 cc preprocedure to 15 cc at 6 months.

The last potential option is the Procon incontinence device [24]. In our initial pilot investigation, seven patients completed a 14-day trial and significant improvement was noted from a baseline incontinence score of 12.7 to a posttreatment incontinence score of 5.2. Quality of life was also noted to improve from 95.3 preprocedure to 135.5 postprocedure. Five of the seven patients reported complete satisfaction although two of the seven reported difficulty in handling the device.

In conclusion, there are many new exciting alternatives for the treatment of fecal incontinence. Twenty years ago, anterior sphincter repair and postanal repair were the only two options other than a colostomy. However, now patients can be offered any number of revisionary, reconstructive, augmentative, or replacement therapies as well as alternative types of stomas. The difficulty now is not a dearth of therapy but rather a plethora of therapies, potentially making appropriate selection rather difficult. The following algorithm (Fig. VIII.24) will hopefully help guide the reader into one potential schema for decision making.

Specifically, patients are basically divided into two large groups. One group of patients has isolated and potentially surgically correctable anterior sphincter defects while the second group has either no defect or multifocal defects. In the absence of pudendal neuropathy, the first group will generally be treated by anterior overlapping sphincter repair. Patients with pudendal neuropathy despite a single anterior-based defect and patients with multifocal defects or no defect will be considered for some of the alternative therapies.

I wish to thank the editors for inviting me to author this commentary and wish to congratulate them on an excellent textbook.

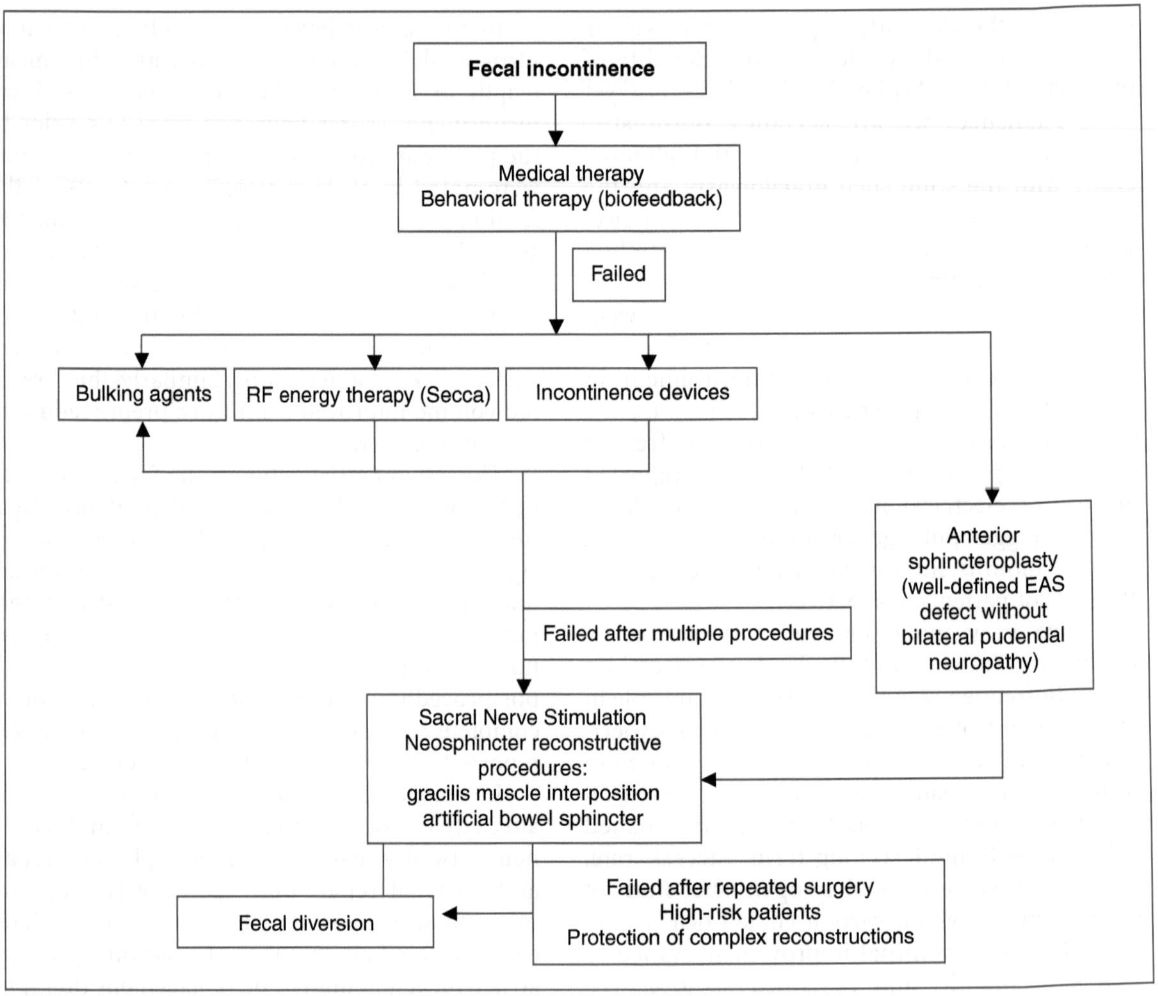

Fig. VIII.24. Algorithm for choosing appropriate therapy for fecal incontinence. *RF* radiofrequency, *SNS* sacral nerve stimulation, *EAS* external anal sphincter

References

1. Jorge JMN, Wexner SD (1993) Etiology and management of fecal incontinence. Dis Colon Rectum 36:77–97
2. Rockwood TH, Church JM, Fleshman JW et al (2000) Fecal incontinence quality of life scale: quality of life instrument for patients with fecal incontinence. Dis Colon Rectum 43:9–16
3. Oliveira L, Pfeifer J, Wexner SD (1996) Physiological and clinical outcome of anterior sphincteroplasty. Br J Surg 83:502–505
4. Gilliland R, Altomare DF, Moreira H Jr et al (1998) Pudendal neuropathy is predictive of failure following anterior overlapping sphincteroplasty. Dis Colon Rectum 41:1516–1522
5. Wexner SD, Marchetti F, Jagelman DG (1991) The role of sphincteroplasty for fecal incontinence reevaluated: a prospective physiologic and functional review. Dis Colon Rectum 34:22–30
6. Giordano P, Renzi A, Efron J et al (2002) Previous sphincter repair does not affect the outcome of repeat repair. Dis Colon Rectum 45:635–640
7. Laurberg S, Swash M, Snooks SJ, Henry MM (1988) Neurologic cause of idiopathic incontinence. Arch Neurol 45:1250–1253
8. Londono-Schimmer EE, Gracia-Duperly R, Nichols RJ et al (1994) Overlapping anal sphincter repair for faecal incontinence due to sphincter trauma: five year follow up functional results. Int J Colorectal Dis 9:110–113
9. Sangwan YP, Coller JA, Barrett RC et al (1996) Unilateral pudendal neuropathy. Impact on outcome of anal sphincter repair. Dis Colon Rectum 39:686–689
10. Nessim A, Wexner SD, Agachan F et al (1999) Is bowel confinement necessary after anorectal reconstructive

surgery? A prospective, randomized, surgeon blinded trial. Dis Colon Rectum 42:16–23

11. Matsuoka H, Mavrantonis C, Wexner SD et al (2000) Postanal repair for fecal incontinence: is it worthwhile? Dis Colon Rectum 43:1561–1567
12. Mavrantonis C, Billotti VL, Wexner SD (1999) Stimulated graciloplasty for treatment of intractable fecal incontinence: critical influence of method of stimulation. Dis Colon Rectum 42:497–504
13. Wexner SD, Baeten C, Bailey R et al (2002) Long term efficacy of dynamic graciloplasty for fecal incontinence. Dis Colon Rectum 45:809–818
14. Baeten C, Bailey R, Bakka A (2000) Safety and efficacy of dynamic graciloplasty for fecal incontinence: report of a prospective, multicenter trial. Dynamic Graciloplasty Therapy Study Group. Dis Colon Rectum 43:743–751
15. Matzel KE, Madoff RD, LaFontaine LJ et al (2001) Dynamic Graciloplasty Therapy Study Group. Complications of dynamic graciloplasty: incidence, management, and impact on outcome. Dis Colon Rectum 44:1427–1435
16. Wong WD, Congolisi S, Spencer M et al (2002) The safety and efficacy of the artificial bowel sphincter for fecal incontinence: results for a multicenter cohort study. Dis Colon Rectum 45:1139–1153
17. Malone PS, Ransley PG, Kiely EM (1990) Preliminary report: the antegrade continence enema. Lancet 336:1217–1218
18. Jost WH (1998) Electrostimulation in fecal incontinence: relevance of the sphincteric compound muscle action potential. Dis Colon Rectum 41:590–592
19. Osterberg A, Graf W, Eeg-Olofsson K et al (1999) Is electrostimulation of the pelvic floor an effective treatment for neurogenic fecal incontinence? Scand J Gastroenterol 34:319–324
20. Weiss EG, Wexner SD, Efron J, Nogueras JJ (2002) Submucosal injection of carbon coated beads is a successful and safe office-based treatment of fecal incontinence. Colorectal Dis 4:34
21. Takahashi T, Garcia-Osobogio S, Valdovinos MA et al (2002) Radiofrequency energy delivery to the anal canal for the treatment of fecal incontinence. Dis Colon Rectum 45:915–922
22. Takahashi T, Garcia-Osogobio S, Valdovinos MA et al (2003) Extended 2-year results of radiofrequency energy delivery for the treatment of fecal incontinence (the Secca procedure). Dis Colon Rectum 46:711–715
23. Efron JE, Corman ML, Fleshman J et al (2003) Safety and effectiveness of temperature-controlled radiofrequency energy delivery to the anal canal (Secca procedure) for the treatment of fecal incontinence. Dis Colon Rectum 46:1606–1612
24. Giamundo P, Welber A, Weiss EG et al (2002) The Procon incontinence device: a new nonsurgical approach to preventing episodes of fecal incontinence. Am J Gastroenterol 97:2328–2332

VIII.4. Neuromodulation for Fecal Incontinence

C. Ratto, D. F. Altomare

Fecal incontinence (FI) is the lack of control in evacuation of feces (liquid or solid) from the bowel. Estimated prevalence of this functional disorder ranges from 3.5% for women to 2.3% for men [1], with a rising percentage with age. However, the true incidence is likely to be higher due to the individual embarrassment to confess this problem and social stigma related to it [2]. FI is considered as distressing and socially incapacitating, with an enormous economic cost for patients and society.

Traumatic sphincter lesions, or idiopathic degeneration of the sphincter muscles, spinal injury or other neurological causes have been considered the most frequent causes of FI in adults. Obstetric injuries are the most frequent cause of FI in women; 4–6% of women having a vaginal delivery will suffer from FI [3]. Traditionally, treatment has been primarily conservative (diet, antidiarrheal drugs, rehabilitation, and biofeedback) [4–6]. Many patients have been recommended to use absorbent pads and anal plugs only. In the past but also recently, different types of biomaterials have been injected in patients with internal anal sphincter dysfunction and secondary passive incontinence. Recent application of these bulking agents is under evaluation to determine long-term results [7, 8]. Overlapping sphincteroplasty is performed for external anal sphincter defects. Although early results have shown improvement in 70–80% of patients [9, 10], long-term efficacy seems to be significantly decreased with time [11]. In cases with wide or multiple sphincter lesions, dynamic graciloplasty or artificial bowel sphincter implantation may be performed [12, 13]. The first option seems have a lesser incidence of long term complications and a significantly higher therapeutic efficacy than the second. Permanent stoma placement is another surgical option in extremely poor, intractable conditions or in patients who cannot be treated with the above-mentioned surgical procedures.

A large number of patients present with FI due to idiopathic pelvic neuropathy or lesions of pelvic nerves, iatrogenic or secondary to other pelvic diseases or dysfunctions. These clinical conditions could involve the neural supply of the anorectal region, including both somatic and autonomic (sympathetic and parasympathetic) nervous systems. Sacral nerves are the common site of these dual nerve supplies [14].

Electrical stimulation of sacral nerves has been thought to excite both nervous systems and thus "modulate" specific functions due to this complex nerve supply. Expected results of such stimulation should be to give additional impulses not only to an inadequate pelvic floor musculature and pelvic organs [15] but also to the sensitive pelvic fibers [16]. This therapeutic approach is called sacral neuromodulation (SNM) or sacral nerve stimulation (SNS).

The first application of SNM was in 1906 [17] for patients with micturition alterations. The first SNM implant in humans was performed in 1981 [18] in patients with urinary urge incontinence and nonobstructive urinary retention. Over time, a concomitant improvement in bowel symptoms was noted in some patients treated for urinary disorders [19]. An increased anorectal junction angle and an increased anal canal resting pressure were documented and suggested to improve FI [14]. As a result, SNM has been used to treat FI since 1995. Today, patient selection criteria from the available reports [6, 20–26] remain widely heterogeneous. Primarily, inclusion criteria were poor FI (at least one episode of either solid or liquid stool leakage per week) and failure of conservative treatment. Thereafter, functional defects of the striated pelvic musculature (without sphincter lesion) were the main criteria used in the early studies [20]. Enrolled patients had decreased manometric squeeze pressure but normal pudendal nerve terminal motor latency (PNTML).

More recently, other, more precise, indications have been investigated, including FI due to idiopathic sphincter degeneration [6, 27], iatrogenic internal sphincter damage [28], partial spinal cord injury [6, 29, 30], scleroderma [31], limited lesions of internal or external anal sphincters [20, 22, 25, 32], rectal prolapse repair [28, 33], and low anterior resection of the rectum [34–38]. Actually, patient selection should take into consideration results of preliminary conservative treatment and features from physiology examinations (anorectal manometry, endoanal ultrasonography, and anorectal electrophysiology). Incontinent patients without sphincters lesions with residual, even if reduced, sphincteric or reflex function should be candidates for the percutaneous nerve evaluation (PNE) test to evaluate response to therapy. This is an optimal approach for patient selection to a permanent SNM implant.

Main contraindications to SNM are: sacral bony abnormalities, poor skin alterations in the site of electrode placement, wide anal sphincter lesions, pregnancy, coagulation disorders, mental or psychological disturbances, presence of cardiac pacemaker or implantable defibrillator, patients with high risk of infection, patients with intractable inflammatory bowel disease or presently with colorectal cancer, future needs of magnetic resonance imaging (MRI). Some physician considers previous pelvic irradiation as a contraindication to SNM; however, in patients with previous radiotherapy to the pelvis, FI could develop, being a secondary effect of both irradiation and surgery. SNM application in these conditions seems to be effective [37].

Technique of Sacral Neuromodulation

SNM presents peculiar characteristics if compared with other surgical options for FI treatment. The first step, the PNE test, is both a diagnostic procedure and a test of therapeutic efficacy. The second step is permanent implant of the SNM system. Only if the PNE test produced good results in improving FI can a permanent implant be considered.

Peripheral Nerve Evaluation

The PNE test must be considered a fundamental phase of SNM therapy. It permits the implantation of an electrode adjacent to the sacral nerves in order to both evaluate their response to stimulation during the implantation procedure and following period and assess the clinical efficacy on defecation disturbances. Indeed, the PNE test, when affecting significant improvement, allows a 100% positive predictive value [6, 26, 31, 32, 39] of response to permanent chronic stimulation.

Traditionally, the electrode implanted for the PNE test is monopolar and used temporarily, limited to the test period. However, progress in the implantation technique has opened wider opportunities for performing the PNE test. Because electrostimulation of the sacral nerves elicits contractions of the striated pelvic floor muscles and a possible variety of sensations in the pelvis, the PNE test procedure is preferably performed under local anesthesia. With the patient in the prone position (Fig. VIII.25) and under sterile conditions, a few skin landmarks are identified bilaterally (Fig. VIII.26) in order to facilitate the insertion of sheathed needles into S2, S3, or S4 foramina. S3 is the most preferred because sacral nerves

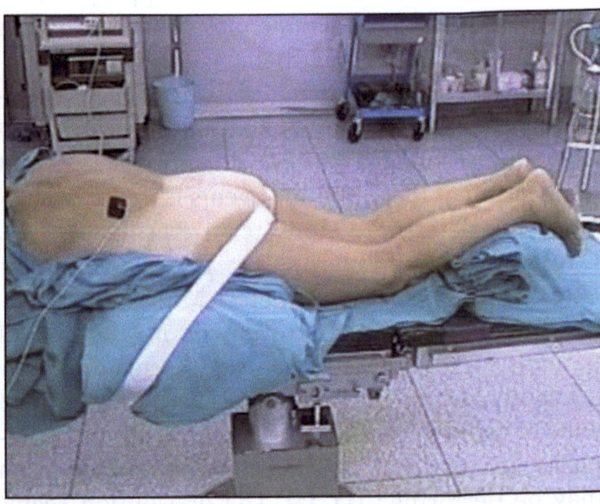

Fig. VIII.25. Prone position required during application of sacral neuromodulation device

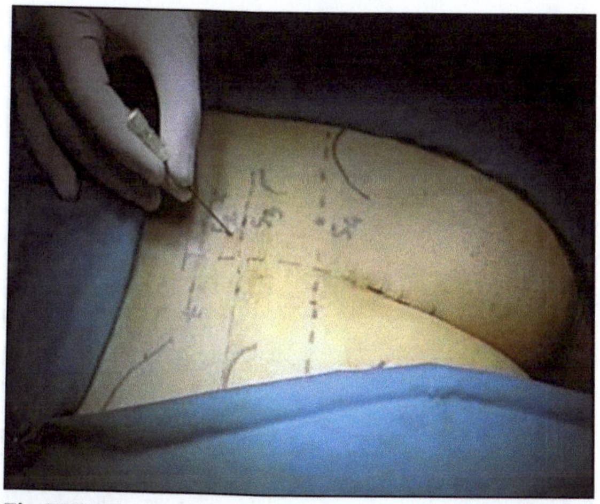

Fig. VIII.26. Skin landmarks identified addressing the introduction of a needle during a sacral neuromodulation implant

are very close to the ventral side of this foramen. It is medial to the upper edge of the greater sciatic notch and a finger's breath from the sacral spine. Correct insertion into S3 foramen is confirmed by needle electrostimulation via a portable stimulator, which determines a "bellows response" (contraction and relaxation of the external anal sphincter and levator ani), and plantar flexion of the ipsilateral big toe; moreover, a sensory response is produced in the vagina/scrotum, perineum, and perianal region. On the other hand, with stimulation through S2 foramen, a contraction of the perineal muscles and external rotation of the leg can be seen while pulses through S4 foramen gives a circular contraction of the external anal sphincter but no toe flexion. Position of the needle is checked by anteroposterior and/or lateral fluoroscopy views of the sacral area. When a good response is observed, an electrode is inserted and the needle gently removed. Electrode position is checked again by both electrostimulation and fluoroscopy. Thereafter, the electrode is secured on the skin by adhesive dressing and connected to the stimulator, which is programmed (pulse width, 210 μs; frequency, 25 Hz; amplitude, from 1 to 10 V) for a minimum 14-day test period. During this time, the patient collects a diary of normal bowel movements and micturition episodes, as well as episodes of fecal and urinary incontinence. Also, a quality of life questionnaire can be completed and anorectal manometry performed. At the end of the test period, the temporary electrode is removed, and results are evaluated. If the clinical improvement concerns at least 50% of FI episodes, a permanent implant of the electrostimulator is planned. If the PNE test results are not clearly positive, a new PNE test could be programmed. If negative, a different approach should be investigated. The most frequent complication during the PNE test performed with a monopolar temporary electrode is lead dislodgement, causing possibly a false negative result of the test in patients in whom SNM could really be effective. Moreover, in a relevant number of patients showing good results during the PNE test, implantation of a definitive electrode provokes a different response, possibly due to a different position of the electrode and its relationship with sacral nerves. Then, it could be reasonable to use the new model of a definitive quadripolar electrode for the PNE test. As described below, the electrode can be implanted by a percutaneous technique under local anesthesia and connected to the external stimulator. With this lead, the PNE test period can be longer for a more precise assessment of the response, eventually changing more frequently the electrical field (trying different electrode combinations) and stimulation parameters. The electrode can be removed under local anesthesia in case of negative results, but, if positive, implantation of the definitive stimulator only is necessary. In some cases, more than one temporary electrode can be placed for a wider stimulation involving sacral nerves bilaterally. Consequently, a bilateral implant of definitive electrodes could be indicated [6, 24, 34].

Permanent Implant

Patients showing significant improvement following the PNE test are candidates for a permanent implant. The implant technique has been modified over the time. The first implant procedure needed to be performed under general anesthesia given without curare in order to avoid striated muscle blockage during stimulation. Sacral foramen chosen for the PNE test had to be found again by needle, repeating both electrostimulation and fluoroscopy in order to reproduce a response similar to the PNE test. Then, a long median incision (from 10 cm to 12 cm) of the presacral skin was required for insertion of the definitive electrode, which was directly inserted into the foramen and secured to the sacral periosteum. Changes in implant technique have been

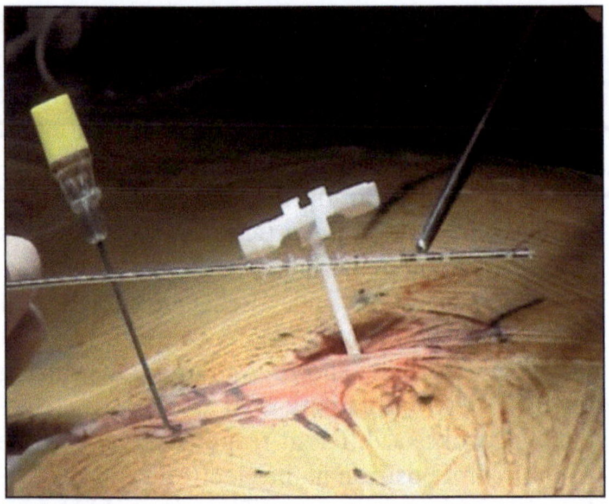

Fig. VIII.27. The quadripolar tined lead used for percutaneous implant

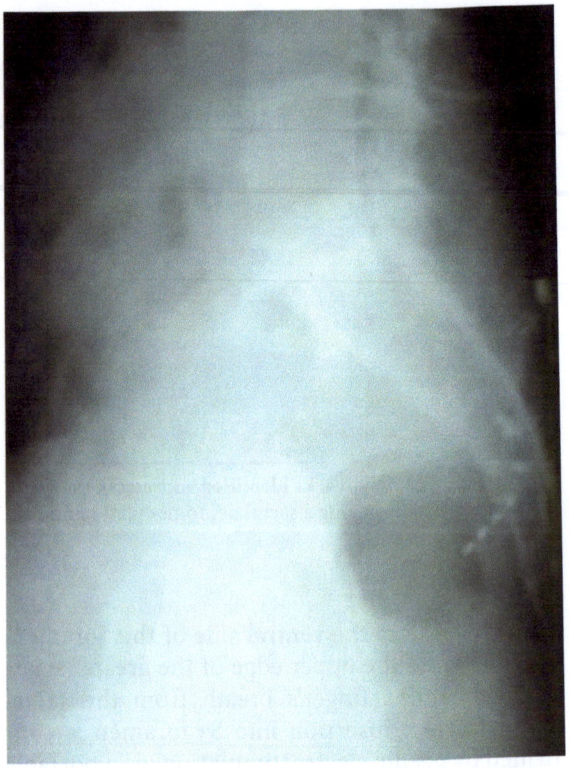

Fig. VIII.29. Radiographic image of an implanted quadripolar electrode

tried in order to simplify electrode introduction, first with minimal skin incision [40], then by a percutaneous insertion of a tined lead [41, 42]. Both these procedures do not need general anesthesia but are suitable of local anesthesia. This makes the procedure simpler and allows the surgeon to obtain the patient's cooperation in identifying appropriate responses. The ultimate model of electrode, the tined lead (Fig. VIII.27), is inserted using a Seldinger method and spontaneously fixed within the sacral foramen after removal of the introducer (Fig. VIII.28). Electrostimulation and fluoroscopy are necessary to confirm correct electrode position (Fig. VIII.29). The electrode must be tunnelized subcutaneously and connected to an extension directed to the external stimulator when a two-stage implant has been planned or to the definitive stimulator in case of a single-stage implant. Also, the procedure for the stimulator insertion has been modified over time. Initially, it was implanted in a subcutaneous pocket into the anterior abdominal quadrant: it required a prolonged operative time, including changing the patient's position. Successively, its placement in a pocket located in the gluteal area (Fig. VIII.30) was suggested as a more time-reducing method and as being more comfortable for the patient [43, 44].

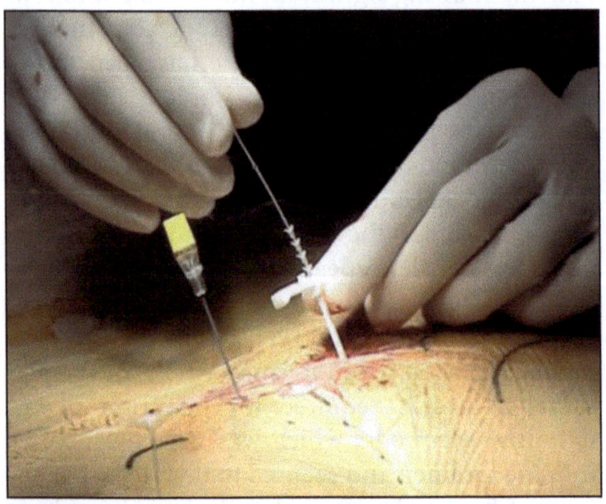

Fig. VIII.28. Introduction of the tined lead

Similar parameters used during the PNE test are selected for permanent stimulation, even though they may be changed in order to obtain the best response. Modification of the parameters is made using a telemetric programmer. The surgeon can use a programmer to modify all parameters of electrostimulation while the patient can use another model of programmer for modification of pulse amplitude (within a programmed range under physician control) or to switch off the stimulator when required. Battery life is related to the settings, with an estimated life ranging from 6 to 8 years.

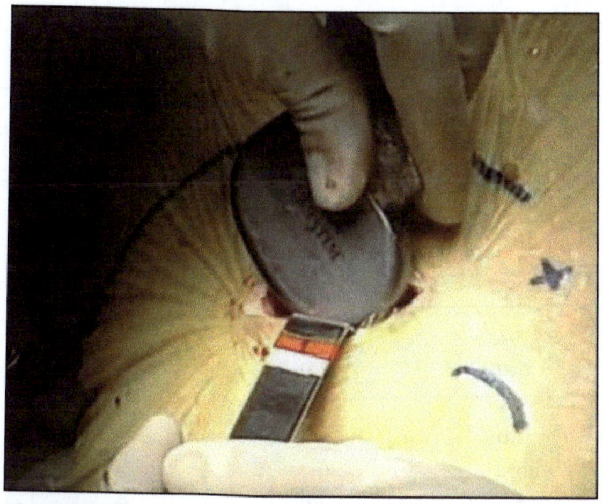

Fig. VIII.30. Implant of the sacral neuromodulation electrostimulator into a subcutaneous pocket in the gluteal area

Settings

Usually, the external stimulator is set at a frequency ranging between 10 and 25 Hz, with a pulse width of 210 µs and an amplitude a little below or above the referred threshold sensation. The most common sensations felt by the patient are a tingling or tapping in the buttock, anus, down the leg, or in the vagina. The sensations could be different in location, type, and intensity, depending on which of the four electrodes is activated as anode or cathode. Preferred electrode polarity is determined by considering the lowest amplitude required to elicit patient sensations. The stimulator could be used as an anode, but with this configuration, pain at the stimulator implantation site is frequently noted by the patient. No significant adverse event has been reported following the stimulator implant. All complications were curable. In case of an infection at the implant site, it is possible to remove the device and reimplant a new one after the infection has resolved.

Complications and Adverse Events

Complications from SNM are an uncommon event, ranging from 5% to 26% [6, 26, 43, 45]. Only minor wound infection has been reported during the PNE test [26]. Rarely, the permanent SNM device needs to be explanted due to a complication (<5%). Pain at the electrostimulator site could be quite common in thinner patients. Wound infection is usually superficial, rarely being a cause of electrode removal (a later reimplantation could be planned). Electrode dislodgement after temporary implant is quite frequent and has significant impact on clinical interpretation of SNM efficacy. On the other hand, migration after permanent implant is rarer. In a review by Jarrett et al. [46], adverse events were documented in ten out of 266 (3.8%) patients receiving the PNE test (nine electrode dislodgements, one superficial skin infection). Adverse events were seen in 19 of 149 (12.8%) patients permanently implanted: three implant infections (requiring implant removal, one reimplanted), eight lead dislodgements (in seven patients, five reimplanted), six implant-related pain (treated with drug therapy), and one superficial wound dehiscence (spontaneous healing).

Results of SNM Clinical Application

Evaluation of clinical results of SNM is of interest not only to assess, at the present, the therapeutic impact of this approach on FI but also to interpret its potential mechanisms of actions. In the early reports, the patient diary about the number of FI episodes was the main indicator of therapy effectiveness. Manometric measures have been used to evaluate SNM effects on anorectal physiology. Moreover, a few score systems are also actually used to measure severity of incontinence, for example, the Cleveland Clinic Incontinence Score [47] and patient quality of life, for example, the SF-36 [48] or the Fecal Incontinence Quality of Life (FIQL) Index [49]. Most reports concern patient series from single centers, but multicenter studies and reviews are available.

Effects on Patient Symptoms

As showed in Table VIII.11, all literature reports have documented a significant reduction of FI episodes in patients treated with SNM. In an European multicenter study [52] evaluating results following permanent implant in 34 incontinent patients (median follow up 23.9 months), frequency of incontinence episodes fell from 16.4±19.3 to 3.1±5.5 at 12 months and 2.0±3.3 at 24 months (p<0.0001), with a statistically significant reduction of days passed with incontinence, with stain, or with pads. Incontinence disappeared completely in 37% of patients. A significant recov-

Table VIII.11. Pre- and postsacral neuromodulation definitive implant results: episodes of incontinence

Authors	Year of publication	Patients (*n*)	Episodes of incontinence (n/week)		
			Preimplant	Postimplant	Pre- vs. postvariation
Vaizey [23]	1999	9	13.7	1.9	⇓
Malouf [25]	2000	5	18.2	1.4	⇓
Ganio [50]	2001	5	4.8	0	⇓
Leroi [32]	2001	6	3.2	0.5	⇓
Rosen [6]	2001	16	6.0	2.0	⇓
Ganio [21]	2001	16	5.5	0.3	⇓
Kenefick [26]	2002	15	11.0	0	⇓
Matzel [36]	2003	16	40.0	0	⇓
Jarrett [28]	2004	46	7.5	1.0	⇓
Altomare [45]	2004	14	14	0.5	⇓
Uludag [51]	2004	75	7.5	0.7	⇓

⇓ Decrease of postimplant vs. preimplant value

ery of ability to postpone defecation and completely empty the bowel was also obtained under SNM. In our recent analysis concerning rectal sensation in 16 patients permanently implanted, in all cases with constant or inconstant alteration before treatment, rectal discrimination was completely recovered following SNM. Feeling of complete evacuation was also recovered in almost all patients [53].

Consequently, measurement of FI scores significantly improved in all series, as reported in Table VIII.12. In 88 patients definitively implanted with an SNM system and registered by the Italian Sacral Neuromodulation Group (GINS), the mean Cleveland Clinic Incontinence Score fell from 15.2 to 6.6 ($p<0.0001$) [55]. Jarrett et al. [46] recently reported data from a literature review on SNM. Starting from 106 relevant reports published, they selected only six patient series [6, 27, 28, 32, 35, 36] and a double-blind crossover study [56, 57] according to very strict criteria. In patient series, a total of 266 patients included in the selected studies had a PNE test; 149 (56%) went on to permanent implantation, ranging from 26.7% to 80% in the single patient series. Complete continence to solid and liquid feces was reported in 41% to 75% of untreated patients. After permanent implantation, 75–100% of patients experienced at least 50% improvement in the number of incontinence episodes. Also, significant improvement in the ability to defer defecation and in Cleveland Clinic Incontinence Scores was reported.

Table VIII.12. Pre- and postsacral neuromodulation definitive implant results: incontinence score

Authors	Year of publication	Patients (*n*)	Incontinence score[a]		
			Preimplant	Postimplant	Pre- vs. postvariation
Malouf [25]	2000	5	18.2	1.4	⇓
Matzel [36]	2003	16	40.0	0	⇓
Rasmussen [54]	2004	37	16	6.0	⇓
Altomare [45]	2004	14	15	5.5	⇓
Ratto [55]	2005	88	15.2	6.6	⇓

[a] Cleveland Clinic Fecal Incontinence Score [47]

⇓ Decrease of postimplant vs. preimplant value

Recently, Leroi et al. [57] reported results of the first double-blind multicenter study performed in France in a significant number of cases (27 patients) with definitive SNM implantation for FI. The authors randomized blinded patients in a crossover protocol to stimulation ON or OFF for 1-month periods. The patients chose the preferred period of stimulation, which was continued for a final 3 months. Frequency of FI episodes was significantly lower during the ON than OFF period during both the crossover phase and final stage of the study and was associated with a significant improvement of ability to postpone defecation, incontinence score, and anal sphincter function. These features indicate that the observed effectiveness of SNM is not due to a placebo effect.

Effects on Patient Quality of Life

SNM seems able to improve patient state of health and quality of life, as reported by all studies (Table VIII.13), even if not always with statistical significance. In the European multicenter study [52] assessing patient state of health with the SF-36 questionnaire, all domains (except for bodily pain) resulted in improved long-term follow-up when compared with baseline state. In particular, social functioning and mental health were constantly and significantly better 12 months after SNM implantation. In that study, all quality of life variables improved from baseline to 12 months postimplant score. In the GINS report [55], all SF-36 parameters were significantly improved at 12-months median follow-up after permanent SNM implant. Moreover, a statistical improvement was observed in physical, psychic, and social functions evaluated with the Rockwood Quality of Life Questionnaire [49]. From a review by Jarrett et al. [46], patients' quality of life improved in the six series evaluated.

Effects on Physiological Parameters

Most studies report findings from anorectal manometry considered useful in an attempt to interpret mechanisms of SNM action. They are summarized in Tables VIII.14, 15, and 16. However, the effects of SNM on physiological parameters are not consistent and are often contrasting. Resting pressure increased after SNM in most series (Table VIII.14), even if the reported increase was slight in comparison with preoperative data that it very rarely reached statistical significance [6, 21, 23, 25, 26, 58]. Also, squeeze pressure showed increased values (Table VIII.15) when measured after SNM implantation but rarely reached statistical significance when compared with pretreatment data [6, 20- 23, 26, 28, 36, 50]. In other series [25, 32, 51], no change or even decreased values were reported. Even more confusing data have been reported concerning rectal sensation (Table VIII.16). Vaizey et al. [23] reported results in nine treated patients. Mean postimplant rectal sensation levels increased in comparison with baseline values. However, Malouf et al. [25] found a decreased threshold level, no change in the urgency value, and an increased maximum tolerated volume in five patients after SNM compared

Table VIII.13. Pre- and postsacral neuromodulation definitive implant results: impact on quality of life

Authors	Year of publication	Patients (*n*)	Scale	Results
Malouf [25]	2000	5	SF-36	Improvement of all parameters
Ganio [21]	2001	16	SF-36	Improvement of all parameters
Kenefick [26]	2002	15	SF-36	Improvement of social activities and physic health
Jarrett [28]	2004	46	SF-36	Improvement of general health, mental health, emotional role, social function, vitality
Altomare [45]	2004	14	FIQL	Improvement of all parameters
Ratto [55]	2005	88	SF-36	Improvement of all parameters except bodily pain

FIQL Fecal incontinence quality of life

Table VIII.14. Pre- and postsacral neuromodulation definitive implant results: manometric maximum resting pressure

Authors	Year of publication	Patients (n)	Maximum resting pressure (mmHg; mean)		
			Preimplant	Postimplant	Pre- vs. postvariation
Vaizey [23]	1999	9	40[a]	57[a]	⇑
Malouf [25]	2000	5	40[a]	49[a]	⇑
Matzel [22]	2001	6	63	65	≅
Ganio [50]	2001	5	42	65	⇑
Leroi [32]	2001	6	77	61	⇓
Rosen [6]	2001	16	28	50	⇑
Ganio [21]	2001	16	38	49	⇑
Kenefick [26]	2002	15	35[a]	49[a]	⇑
Matzel [36]	2003	16	63	59	≅
Jarrett [28]	2004	46	46[a]	49[a]	≅
Altomare [45]	2004	14	36.5	32	≅
Uludag [51]	2004	75	50	48	≅
Ratto [55]	2005	88	60.5	71.9	≅

[a] Values measured in cmH_2O
⇓ Decrease of postimplant vs. preimplant value
⇑ Increase of postimplant vs. preimplant value
≅ Similar postimplant vs. preimplant values

Table VIII.15. Pre- and postsacral neuromodulation definitive implant results: manometric maximum squeeze pressure

Authors	Year of publication	Patients (n)	Maximum squeeze pressure (mmHg; mean)		
			Preimplant	Postimplant	Pre- vs. postvariation
Matzel [20]	1995	3	68	111	⇑
Vaizey [23]	1999	9	33[a]	75[a]	⇑
Malouf [25]	2000	5	80[a]	81[a]	⇑
Matzel [22]	2001	6	38	93	⇑
Ganio [50]	2001	5	67	82	⇑
Leroi [32]	2001	6	57	40	⇓
Rosen [6]	2001	16	59	120	⇑
Ganio [21]	2001	16	67	83	⇑
Kenefick [26]	2002	15	43[a]	69[a]	⇑
Matzel [36]	2003	16	69	97	≅
Jarrett [28]	2004	46	63[a]	93[a]	⇑
Altomare [45]	2004	14	72	62	≅
Uludag [51]	2004	75	83	82	≅
Ratto [55]	2005	88	84.5	99.3	≅

[a] Values measured in cmH_2O
⇓ Decrease of postimplant vs. preimplant value
⇑ Increase of postimplant vs. preimplant value
≅ Similar postimplant vs. preimplant values

Table VIII.16. Pre- and postsacral neuromodulation definitive implant results: assessment of rectal sensation

Authors	Year of publication	Patients (*n*)	Rectal sensation (ml; mean)			
			Parameters	Preimplant	Postimplant	Pre- vs. postvariation
Vaizey [23]	1999	9	Threshold	45	145	⇑
			Urgency	73	173	⇑
			Max. tol. vol.	95	175	⇑
Malouf [25]	2000	5	Threshold	45	30	≈
			Urgency	70	80	≈
			Max tol. vol.	95	130	≈
Leroi [32]	2001	6	Urgency	175	124	⇓
			Max tol. vol.	203	200	≈
Ganio [21]	2001	16	Threshold	58.5	37	≈
			Urgency	118.0	87.7	⇓
Kenefick [25]	2002	15	Threshold	47	34	⇓
Matzel [36]	2003	16	Threshold	40	25	≈
			Urgency	60	70	≈
			Max tol. vol.	150	200	⇑
Jarrett [28]	2004	46	Threshold	41	27	⇓
			Urgency	92	71	⇓
			Max tol. vol.	129	107	⇓
Altomare [45]	2004	14	Threshold	64	70	≈
			Urgency	145	120	≈
			Max tol. vol.	250	250	≈
Ratto [55]	2005	88	Threshold	54.3	46.5	≈
			Urgency	119.9	97.9	≈

Max tol. vol. Maximum tolerated volume
⇓ decrease of post-implant vs. pre-implant value
⇑ increase of post-implant vs. pre-implant value
≈ similar post-implant vs. pre-implant values

with pretreatment data. Leroi et al. [32], in six implanted patients, detected a decreased urgency and comparable mean values of maximum tolerated volume following SNM. Ganio et al. [50] reported a decrease in rectal sensation parameters after definitive SNM implant in five patients. In the multicenter GINS study [21], 16 patients were studied after definitive SNM implant. Both mean threshold and urgency values decreased when compared with pretreatment data (but only the difference in urgency was statistically significant). Kenefick et al. [26] reported a decreased mean threshold level after SNM in 15 patients. In a series of 16 patients, Matzel et al. [36] found a decreased mean threshold level, a similar mean urgency value, and an increased mean maximum tolerated volume. Jarrett et al. [28] reported in a large series of 46 patients implanted at St. Mark's Hospital a significant improvement of sensory function measured as threshold sensation, urgency sensation, and maximum tolerated volume. In a study on 15 patients, Uludag et al. [16] specifically investigated the effects of SNM on the rectum. Patients were submitted to barostat measurements of rectal sensation and compliance before and after a 3-week PNE test. In 14 of those patients, threshold sensation, urge sensation, and maximum tolerated volume decreased significantly during stimulation. Median rectal wall tension decreased significantly related to all filling sensations while rectal compliance was similar before and during stimulation.

These contrasting data are of no help in better understanding whether rectal sensation has a primary role in the development of FI in patients treated with SNM, and, on the other hand, what the real effect of this therapy is on impaired rectal sensation. In a recent evaluation [59], we assumed that the conflicting results reported in other series reflected the obvious differences in pathogenesis causing FI in the patients treated. Indeed, there are incontinent patients with either a hyposensitive or hypersensitive rectum while others present normal rectal sensation. Reevaluation after definitive SNM implant led to apparently incomprehensible results. However, it is conceivable that SNM acts primarily by "modulating" the effects produced by the electrostimulation on the nerves. Thus, it has been postulated that there is a difference in the effect elicited on the initially hypersensitive or normosensitive rectum (expected to increase sensation levels) and that elicited on the primitive hyposensitive rectum (expected to decrease sensation levels). When evaluated in this light, the results of definitive SNM showed that the majority of patients reflected this hypothetical response mechanism, particularly as far as urgency and maximum tolerated volume are concerned (80% of patients). These patients had the best clinical improvement in FI as opposed to patients who showed different effects of SNM on rectal sensation.

Conclusion

SNM can be considered as an effective therapeutic approach to treat patients suffering from FI associated with some kind of neuropathy as the primary or secondary cause. A large number of reports demonstrate the effectiveness of this therapy in improving the FI and patients' quality of life. In all series, episodes of FI are reported to be significantly decreased and FI scores are improved. Urgency is frequently reduced, and altered rectal sensations, compared with those reported by patients preoperatively, are significantly ameliorated in most cases. Also, improvement of almost all variables measuring quality of life represents one of the most important results obtained by SNM application in this group of patients with severe psychological, social, and behavioral problems due to FI.

However, the mechanisms of action of SNM are still not well understood. SNM seems to play a multiple role, combining a variety of effects on anal sphincters and rectal sensation and motility via a modulated stimulation of the different nerve pathways involved in defecation physiology, including afferent and efferent connections with the central nervous system. A better understanding of action mechanisms will allow assessment of which clinical conditions are appropriate candidates for SNM. However, the actual evaluation with clinical and instrumental assessment of FI, together with the PNE test, gives the best approach to selecting patients for definitive implantation of an SNM device. In most cases, clinical results observed during the PNE test are reproducible, long-term durable, and not susceptible to the placebo effect.

References

1. MacLennan AH, Wilson DH, Wilson D (2000) The prevalence of pelvic floor disorders and their relationship to gender, age, parity and mode of delivery. Br J Obstet Gynaecol 107:1460–1470
2. Johanson JF, Lafferty J (1996) Epidemiology of faecal incontinence: the silent affliction. Am J Gastroenteol 91:33–36
3. MacArthur C, Bick D, Keighley MR (1997) Faecal incontinence after childbirth. Br J Obstet Gynaecol 104:46–50
4. Cheetham MJ, Kenefick NJ, Kamm MA (2001) Non-surgical treatment of faecal incontinence. Hosp Med 62:538–541
5. Norton C, Kamm MA (2001) Anal sphincter biofeedback and pelvic floor exercises for faecal incontinence in adults – a systematic review. Aliment Pharmacol Ther 15:1147–1154
6. Rosen HR, Urbarz C, Holzer B et al (2001) Sacral nerve stimulation as a treatment for fecal incontinence. Gastroenterology 121:536–541
7. Kenefick NJ, Vaizey CJ, Malouf AJ et al (2002) Injectable silicone biomaterial for faecal incontinence due to internal anal sphincter dysfunction. Gut 51:225–228
8. Vaizey CJ, Kamm MA (2005) Injectable bulking agents for treating faecal incontinence. Br J Surg 92:521–527
9. Barisic G, Krivokapic Z, Markovic V et al (2000) The role of overlapping sphincteroplasty in traumatic fecal incontinence. Acta Chir Iugosl 47(Suppl 1):37–41
10. Engel AF, Kamm MA, Sultan AH et al (1994) Anterior anal sphincter repair in patients with obstetric trauma. Br J Surg 81:1231–1234

11. Malouf AJ, Norton CS, Engel AF et al (2000) Long-term results of overlapping anterior anal-sphincter repair for obstetric trauma. Lancet 355:260–265
12. Baeten CG, Bailey HR, Bakka A et al (2000) Safety and efficacy of dynamic graciloplasty for fecal incontinence: report of a prospective, multicenter trial. Dynamic Graciloplasty Therapy Study Group. Dis Colon Rectum 43:743–751
13. Lehur PA, Glemain P, Bruley des Varannes S et al (1998) Outcome of patients with an implanted artificial anal sphincter for severe faecal incontinence. A single institution report. Int J Colorectal Dis 13:88–92
14. Matzel K, Schmidt RA, Tanagho EA (1990) Neuroanatomy of the striated anal continence mechanism: implications for the use of neurostimulation. Dis Colon Rectum 33:666–673
15. Tanagho EA (1993) Concepts of neuromodulation. Neurourol Urodyn 12:487–488
16. Uludag O, Morren GL, Dejong CH, Baeten CG (2005) Effect of sacral neuromodulation on the rectum. Br J Surg 92:1017–1023
17. Frankl-Hochwart LV, Zuckerkandl O (1906) Die nervösen Erkrankungen der Harnblase. In: Nothnagel HA, Hölder A (eds) Spezielle Pathologie und Therapie, vol 109, Wien, p 109
18. Tanagho EA, Schmidt RA (1982) Bladder pacemaker; scientific basis and clinical future. J Urol 20:614–619
19. Pettit PD, Thompson JR, Chen AH (2002) Sacral neuromodulation: new applications in the treatment of female pelvic floor dysfunction. Curr Opin Obstet Gynecol 14:521–525
20. Matzel K, Stadelmaier M, Hohenfellner FP (1995) Electrical stimulation of sacral spinal nerves for treatment of faecal incontinence. Lancet 346:1124–1127
21. Ganio E, Ratto C, Masin A, Realis Luc A et al (2001) Neuromodulation for fecal incontinence: outcome in 16 patients with definitive implant. The initial Italian Sacral Neurostimulation Group (GINS) experience. Dis Colon Rectum 44:965–970.
22. Matzel K, Stadelmaier U, Hohenfellner M, Hohenberger W (2001) Chronic sacral spinal nerve stimulation for faecal incontinence: long-term results with foramen and cuff electrodes. Dis Colon Rectum 44:59–66
23. Vaizey CJ, Kamm MA, Turner IC et al (1999) Effects of short-term sacral nerve stimulation on anal and rectal function in patients with anal incontinence. Gut 44:407–412
24. Stadelmaier U, Dahms S, Bittorf B et al (2001) Efferent innervation patterns during sacral nerve stimulation. Dis Colon Rectum 44:A2
25. Malouf AJ, Vaizey CJ, Nicholls RJ, Kamm MA (2000) Permanent sacral nerve stimulation for faecal incontinence. Ann. Surg 232:143–148
26. Kenefick NJ, Vaizey CJ, Cohen RC et al (2002) Medium-term results of permanent sacral nerve stimulation for faecal incontinence. Br J Surg 89:896–901
27. Ganio E, Realis Luc A, Ratto C et al (2003) Sacral nerve modulation for fecal incontinence: functional results and assessment of the quality of life. http://www.colorep.it/Rivista%20CEC/sacral_nerve_modulation_for_feca.htm. Cited 28 Nov 2005
28. Jarrett ME, Varma JS, Duthie GS et al (2004) Sacral nerve stimulation for faecal incontinence in the UK. Br J Surg 91:755–761
29. Bernstein AJ, Peters KM (2005) Expanding indications for neuromodulation. Urol Clin North Am 32:59–63
30. Jarrett ME, Matzel KE, Christiansen J et al (2005) Sacral nerve stimulation for faecal incontinence in patients with previous partial spinal injury including disc prolapse. Br J Surg 92:734–739
31. Kenefick NJ, Vaizey CJ, Nicholls RJ et al (2002) Sacral nerve stimulation for faecal incontinence due to systemic sclerosis. Gut 51:881–883
32. Leroi AM, Michot F, Grise P, Denis P (2001) Effect of sacral nerve stimulation in patients with faecal and urinary incontinence. Dis Colon Rectum 44:779–789
33. Jarrett ME, Matzel KE, Stosser M et al (2005) Sacral nerve stimulation for fecal incontinence following surgery for rectal prolapse repair: a multicenter study. Dis Colon Rectum 48:1243–1248
34. Matzel KE, Stadelmaier U, Bittorf B et al (2002) Bilateral sacral spinal nerve stimulation for fecal incontinence after low anterior rectum resection. Int J Colorectal Dis 17:430–434
35. Uludag O, Dejong HC (2002) Sacral neuromodulation for faecal incontinence. Dis Colon Rectum 45:34–36
36. Matzel KE, Bittorf B, Stadelmaier U, Hohenberger W (2003) Sacral nerve stimulation in the treatment of faecal incontinence. Chirurg 74:26–32
37. Ratto C, Grillo E, Parello A et al (2005) Sacral neuromodulation in treatment of fecal incontinence following anterior resection and chemoradiation for rectal cancer. Dis Colon Rectum 48:1027–1036.
38. Jarrett ME, Matzel KE, Stosser M et al (2005) Sacral nerve stimulation for faecal incontinence following a rectosigmoid resection for colorectal cancer. Int J Colorectal Dis 20:446–451
39. Ganio E, Masin A, Ratto C et al (2001) Short-term sacral nerve stimulation for functional anorectal and urinary disturbances: results in 40 patients: evaluation of a new option for anorectal functional disorders. Dis. Colon Rectum 44:1261–1267
40. Ratto C, Morelli U, Paparo S et al (2003) Minimally invasive sacral neuromodulation implant technique: modifications to the conventional procedure. Dis Colon Rectum 46:414–417

41. Spinelli M, Malaguti S, Giardiello G et al (2005) A new minimally invasive procedure for pudendal nerve stimulation to treat neurogenic bladder: description of the method and preliminary data. Neurourol Urodyn 24:305–309
42. Spinelli M, Weil E, Ostardo E et al (2005) New tined lead electrode in sacral neuromodulation: experience from a multicentre European study. World J Urol 23:225–229
43. Hohenfellner M, Matzel KE, Schultz-Lampel D et al (1997) Sacral neuromodulation for treatment of micturition disorders and faecal incontinence. In: Hohenfellner R, Fichtner J, Novick A (eds) Innovations in Urologic Surgery, 2nd edn. ISIS Medical Media, Oxford, pp 129–138
44. Scheepens W, Weil EH, van Koeveringe GA et al (2001) Buttock placement of the implantable pulse generator: a new implantation technique for sacral neuromodulation – a multicenter study. Eur Urol 40: 434–438
45. Altomare D, Rinaldi M, Petrolio et al (2004) Permanent sacral nerve modulation for faecal incontinence and associated urinary disturbances. Int J Colorectal Dis 19: 203–209
46. Jarrett ME, Mowatt G, Glazener CM et al (2004) Systematic review of sacral nerve stimulation for faecal incontinence and constipation. Br J Surg 91:1559–1569
47. Jorge JMN, Wexner SD (1993) Aetiology and management of faecal incontinence. Dis Colon Rectum 36:77–79
48. Ware JE (1993) SF-36 Health Survey, manual and interpretation. Health Institute, New England Medical Center, Boston
49. Rockwood TH, Church JM, Fleshman JW et al (2000) Faecal Incontinence Quality of Life Scale: quality of life instrument for patients with faecal incontinence. Dis Colon Rectum 43:9–16
50. Ganio E, Realis Luc A, Clerico G, Trompetto M (2001) Sacral nerve stimulation for treatment of fecal incontinence: a novel approach for intractable fecal incontinence. Dis Colon Rectum 44:619–629
51. Uludag O, Koch SM, van Gemert WG et al (2004) Sacral neuromodulation in patients with fecal incontinence: a single-center study. Dis Colon Rectum 47:1350–1357
52. Matzel KE, Kamm MA, Stosser M et al (2004) Sacral spinal nerve stimulation for faecal incontinence: multicentre study. Lancet 363:1270–1276
53. Ratto C, Parello A, Doglietto GB (2005) Sacral neuromodulation could interfere on rectal sensation in fecal incontinence patients recovering rectal discrimination and emptying. Dis Colon Rectum 48:650
54. Rasmussen OO, Buntzen S, Sorensen M et al (2004) Sacral nerve stimulation in fecal incontinence. Dis Colon Rectum 47:1158–1162
55. Ratto C, Altomare (Corridge)DF, Ganio E et al (2005) A Significant improvement of quality of life and health status following sacral neuromodulation in faecal incontinence patients. Proceedings of Second Joint Meeting of European Council of Coloproctology and European Association of Coloproctology, Bologna, Italy, 15–17 September 2005, p 163
56. Vaizey CJ, Kamm MA, Roy AJ, Nicholls RJ (2000) Double-blind crossover study of sacral nerve stimulation for fecal incontinence. Dis Colon Rectum 43:298–302
57. Leroi AM, Parc Y, Lehur PA et al (2005) Efficacy of sacral nerve stimulation for fecal incontinence: results of a multicenter double-blind crossover study. Ann Surg 242:662–669
58. Rao SS (2004) Pathophysiology of adult fecal incontinence. Gastroenterology 126:S14–22
59. Ratto C, Petrolino M, Altomare DF et al (2004) The effects of sacral neuromodulation on rectal sensation can predict improvement of fecal incontinence. Dis Colon Rectum 47:611

Invited Commentary

K.E. Matzel

The authors have provided a thorough overview of sacral nerve stimulation (SNS) for anorectal dysfunction, with special focus on the multicenter experience of the Italian Sacral Neuromodulation Group (GINS). Since its first application for the treatment of fecal incontinence [1], SNS has constantly evolved. Conceptual considerations, patient selection, outcome measures, technique, and knowledge of its mechanism of action have all changed. Today, SNS is a valuable addition to our armamentarium.

After its initial application based on a physiologic concept, the technique of SNS began to be applied through a pragmatic approach. The initial use was confined to patients with deficient striated anal sphincter and levator ani function, but with no morphologic defect [1, 2], in whom electrical stimulation would recruit residual function of the continence organ. The common denominator of the heterogeneous etiologies addressed was reduced function and intact morphology. Initial indications and positive clinical outcomes were confirmed by single-center reports [3, 4] and recently in a prospective multicenter study [5–8].

Recording of anorectal activity during temporary testing suggested that the effect of SNS was not limited to the striated sphincter muscle [9]. Subsequently, indications for permanent SNS were successfully expanded to deficiencies of the smooth-muscle internal anal sphincter, limited structural defects, and functional deficits of the external and internal sphincter [10].

During the initial work, it became apparent that the two-step selection of patients with both acute and temporary phases of diagnostic stimulation was highly predictive of therapeutic effect. Consequently, as stated above, patient selection was no longer based on the conceptual consideration of the potential mechanism of action but became a more pragmatic, trial-and-error approach. The short- and long-term effects of SNS based on this pragmatic patient selection process are favorable and confirm its appropriateness [11, 12].

Studies vary with regard to design, number of patients, and manner of reporting clinical outcome. Most studies comprise patients with greatly varying pathophysiologic conditions, thus outlining the spectrum of patients who might benefit from SNS. This aggregation of various underlying pathophysiologic conditions prevents firm conclusions regarding the mechanism of action of SNS. Only recently, case reports or small series have begun to focus on well-defined clinical and/or physiologic conditions [6–8, 13–15].

The manner in which outcome is reported has been modified. Most commonly, it is demonstrated as an improvement in symptoms, such as decreased episodes of incontinence or days with incontinence during the observation period. However, because surgical restoration of function also aims to improve quality of life, various quality-of-life instruments – some unspecific, others disease specific – have been introduced [11, 12]. Not surprisingly, quality of life is significantly improved if clinical symptoms are ameliorated [11, 12].

The technique has undergone continuous development. Test stimulation for patient selection carries little risk and has limited invasiveness; thus, it is being used more liberally to explore potential indications. Acute and temporary test stimulation can be performed on one or many nerves. Two technical options are available: wire leads that need to be removed after the screening phase; and so-called two-staged implants with tined leads, which can remain for use as a permanent electrode if screening proves successful. This tined-lead placement through a trocar system is also most commonly used for permanent electrode positioning. Although the superiority of this approach has not yet been proved, it is broadly accepted and is today the preferred technique owing to its limited invasiveness. Because the percutaneous acute phase and the temporary stimulation phase are of pivotal importance in patient selection, the two technical options deserve to be compared regarding ease, predictive value, and cost effectiveness.

Despite the very positive clinical outcome of SNS, its increased use, and broadened acceptance, our knowledge of its mechanism of action remains limited. Multiple efforts have been made to correlate clinical outcome with results of anorectal physiology testing [11, 12], but the observations of the effect of chronic SNS vary greatly among published reports. Results can be contradictory; some are inconclusive and unconvincing. In most studies, patients represent widely varying pathophysiology, thus preventing firm conclusions on mechanism of action. The clinical effect of SNS is likely multifactorial, based on multiple physiologic functions. Understanding the relative importance of each of these functions and their dependence on pathophysiologic preconditions is unclear. It may simply be that SNS works differently in different patients.

For the future, interrelated clinical, physiological, and technical issues should be addressed to increase our knowledge of the appropriate uses of SNS and its mechanism of action. To correlate clinical and physiologic findings better, some case reports and small case series have investigated the effect of SNS in well-defined anorectal physiology and distinct conditions: e.g., patients with muscular dystrophy [13]; patients who have undergone rectal resection and neoadjuvant chemoradiation [14]; patients with a sphincteric gap before surgical repair [15]; patients with neurologic dysfunction [6]; after rectal prolapse [7]; and after rectal resection for cancer [8]. Initial results are promising but require confirmation in large prospective trials. It is hoped that this approach will reliably predict responders – both clinically and physiologically – and thus potentially omit the need for test stimulation.

By applying SNS to patients with sphincteric disruption [15] in whom surgical repair is planned, and thus potentially avoiding the need for repair, the current treatment algorithm for fecal incontinence is challenged. This is of special interest, as we have learned in recent years that the short-term benefit of sphincteric repair deteriorates over time; indeed, after 5 years, it has been shown to be less favorable [16, 17]. However, data of the long-term efficacy and durability of SNS are themselves diffuse. A multinational registry could be helpful for both long-term follow-up and subgroup analysis.

In patients in whom electrode placement at the level of the sacral spinal nerve is not possible, new techniques may be helpful for peripheral stimulation: e.g., tibial [18] or pudendal [19]. Again, the effectiveness and reliability of this latest technical evolution must be confirmed.

To increase its efficacy, SNS has been applied bilaterally in only a few patients [20]. However, whether bilateral stimulation per se improves the clinical response is still unclear; depending on the individual innervation pattern, unilateral stimulation of more than one nerve may also be beneficial [21]. Validity, accuracy, and reproducibility of electrophysiologic testing – whether during treatment to monitor functional changes or during the initial operation to optimize electrode placement – must continue to be investigated.

Indications of SNS have been expanded beyond fecal incontinence to slow-transit constipation and outlet obstruction. Preliminary data indicate that SNS may work in both conditions [22] and that its clinical benefit is not likely to be a placebo effect [23]. Based on these findings, a prospective multicenter trial is ongoing.

Since the introduction of SNS to colorectal surgery, some of our traditional thinking has been challenged by unexpected findings. Still, as this is a dynamic process dealing with a relatively new concept, we constantly need to reconsider our current understanding of neurostimulation in the treatment of anorectal functional disorders. Future research should focus on patient selection based on defined morphologic and physiologic conditions, on novel indications with the diagnostic approach of acute and temporary test stimulation and new techniques, on long-term outcome, on increasing efficacy either by technical modifications or by an individualized approach based on physiologic findings, and on the role and value of SNS in the treatment algorithm.

References

1. Matzel KE, Stadelmaier U, Hohenfellner M, Gall FP (1995) Electrical stimulation for the treatment of faecal incontinence. Lancet 346:1124–1127
2. Matzel KE, Stadelmaier U, Hohenfellner M, Gall FP (1995) Permanent electrostimulation of sacral spinal nerves with an implantable neurostimulator in treatment of fecal incontinence. Chirurg 66:813–817
3. Leroi AM, Michot F, Grise P, Denis P (2001) Effect of sacral nerve stimulation in patients with fecal and urinary incontinence. Dis Colon Rectum 44:779–789
4. Ganio E, Masin A, Ratto C et al (2001) Neuromodulation for fecal incontinence: outcome in 16 patients with definitive implant. The initial Italian Sacral Neurostimulation Group (GINS) experience. Dis Colon Rectum 44:965–970
5. Matzel KE, Kamm MA, Stösser M et al (2004) MDT 301 Study Group. Sacral nerve stimulation for fecal incontinence: a multicenter study. Lancet 363:1270–1276
6. Jarrett ME, Matzel KE, Christiansem J et al (2005) Sacral nerve stimulation for faecal incontinence in patients with previous partial spinal injury including disc prolapse. Br J Surg 92:734–739
7. Jarrett ME, Matzel KE, Stosser M et al (2005) Sacral nerve stimulation for fecal incontinence following surgery for rectal prolapse repair: a multicenter study. Dis Colon Rectum 48:1243–1248
8. Jarrett ME, Matzel KE, Stosser M et al (2005) Sacral nerve stimulation for faecal incontinence following a rectosigmoid resection for colorectal cancer. Int J Colorectal Dis 20:446–451
9. Vaizey CJ, Kamm MA, Turner IC et al (1999) Effects of short term sacral nerve stimulation on anal and rectal function in patients with anal incontinence. Gut 44:407–412
10. Malouf AJ, Vaizey CJ, Nicholls RJ, Kamm M (2000) Permanent sacral nerve stimulation for fecal incontinence. Ann Surg 232:143–148
11. Matzel KE, Stadelmaier U, Hohenberger W (2004) Innovations in fecal incontinence: Sacral nerve stimulation. Dis Colon Rectum 47:1720–1728
12. Tjandra JJ, Lim JF, Matzel KE (2004) Sacral nerve stimulation – an emerging treatment for faecal incontinence. ANZ J Surg 74:1098–1106
13. Buntzen S, Rasmussen OO, Ryhammer AM et al (2004) Sacral nerve stimulation for treatment of fecal incontinence in a patient with muscular dystrophy: report of a case. Dis Colon Rectum 47:1409–1411
14. Ratto C, Grillo E, Parello A et al (2005) Sacral neuromodulation in treatment of fecal incontinence following anterior resection and chemoradiation for rectal cancer. Dis Colon Rectum 48:1027–1036
15. Conaghan P, Farouk R (2005) Sacral nerve stimulation can be successful in patients with ultrasound evidence of external anal sphincter disruption. Dis Colon Rectum 48:1610–1614
16. Halverson AL, Hull TL (2002) Long-term outcome of overlapping anal sphincter repair. Dis Colon Rectum 45:345–348
17. Malouf AF, Norton CS, Engel AF et al (2000) Long-term results of overlapping anterior anal sphincter repair for obstetric trauma. Lancet 366, 260–265
18. Queralto M, Portier G, Cabarrot PH et al (2005) Preliminary results of peripheral transcutaneous neuromodulation in the treatment of idiopathic fecal incontinence. Int J Colorect Dis (*E-pub*)
19. Matzel KE, Stadelmaier U, Besendörfer M, Hohenberger W (2005) Pudendal stimulation for anorectal dysfunction – the first application of a fully implantable microstimulator. Colorect Dis 7(1):45–143
20. Matzel KE, Stadelmaier U, Bittorf B et al (2002) Bilateral sacral spinal nerve stimulation for fecal incontinence after low anterior resection. Int J Colorect Disease 17:430–434
21. Matzel KE, Stadelmaier U, Hohenfellner M et al (1999) Asymmetry of pudendal motor function assessed during intraoperative monitoring. Gastroenterology 116:4508
22. Jarrett MED , Mowatt G, Glazener CMA et al (2004) Systematic review of sacral nerve stimulation for faecal incontinence and constipation. Br J Surg 91:1559–1569
23. Kenefick NJ, Vaizey CJ, Cohen CR et al (2002) Double-blind placebo-controlled crossover study of sacral nerve stimulation for idiopathic constipation. Br J Surg 89:1570–1571

VIII.5. Incontinence: Biofeedback and Other Nonoperative Modalities

G. Bazzocchi, B. Salvioli

Introduction

Fecal incontinence is a potentially devastating symptom that is more common than usually accepted and which increases in prevalence with age. The involuntary loss of stool is a distressing, disabling, and underreported condition with prevalence in the overall population of 0.1–1.5% [1, 2]. As many as 5–15% of healthy subjects have been reported to loose bowel control at least occasionally. Prevalence increases with age [3], and the condition is estimated to afflict at least three million US citizens. After vaginal delivery, at least 10–15% of women experience temporary fecal incontinence [4]. However, the exact incidence of fecal incontinence is unknown, and wide variations in reported data are probably due to disparity in the definition of incontinence as well as the methods of data collection.

There is no single mechanism responsible for fecal incontinence. Theoretically, any factor that interrupts the balance between central control and the muscular and neural structures of the pelvic floor could lead to fecal incontinence. The pathophysiological mechanisms can be subdivided into: (1) Structural and functional defects of the anal sphincters following surgical, obstetric, or traumatic injury; (2) Neurogenic incontinence, in which primary or secondary neuropathic processes impair motor and/or sensory components of the continence mechanisms; (3) Urgency incontinence, in which unrestrained expulsionary forces (rectal and/or colonic) threaten to overcome a sphincteric mechanism that is essentially normal.

Depending on the severity of symptoms, fecal incontinence should be classified as being of minor or major degree (Table VIII.17) [5]. Minor incontinence consists of partial soiling or loss of control of flatus or liquid stool. Major incontinence has been defined as "deficient control of stool of normal consistency" [6] and includes most cases of traumatic and gross neurologic defects. Based on anorectal physiology testing, five types of deficits can be identified as being associated with fecal incontinence (Table VIII.18).

Nonoperative Strategies

The first approach in the management of fecal incontinence rests with nonoperative modalities, which can avoid, at least in a select group of patients, surgical intervention. Indications for nonoperative options are: initial approach to treatment; pudendal neuropathy; before reconstructive surgery; neuropathic incontinence; surgical failure.

Recognizing the underlying causes is crucial for consequent management of patients with fecal incontinence. Supportive treatment includes dietary modification, a scheduled bowel program, drug therapy, local disposables, and biofeedback. Nonoperative treatment options for fecal incontinence are described in Table VIII.19.

Bowel Habit and Dietary Modification

Institutionalized patients with fecal incontinence need to be followed carefully by qualified personnel who provide hygienic measures by cleaning

Table VIII.17. Causes of fecal incontinence

Minor incontinence	
Normal sphincters and pelvic floor	Diarrheal states: irritable bowel syndrome, inflammatory bowel disease, infectious, malabsorption syndrome, short-gut syndrome, radiation enteritis
	Surgery: fistula, colostomy
Abnormal sphincter or pelvic floor function	Fecal impaction, perianal surgery, prolapse (rectal, mucosal)
Major incontinence	
Traumatic	Accidental, obstetrical, operative
Drugs	Antibiotics, laxatives, intoxication
Complete rectal prolapse	
Colorectal malignancy	
Congenital	Muscular/anatomic
	Neurologic (Hirschsprung's disease)
	Lumbar meningomyelocele
Neurological	Idiopathic
	Central: cerebral, multiple strokes, dementia/degenerative disorders, trauma
	Spinal: multiple sclerosis, tumors/metastases, degenerative diseases (e.g., B12 deficiency), tabes dorsalis
	Peripheral: cauda equina (tumor/trauma), peripheral neuropathy (diabetes, multiple sclerosis)
Musculoskeletal	Myotonic dystrophy
	Polymyositis
Collagen vascular disease	Scleroderma
	Amyloidosis

Modified from Swash [5]

the perianal skin following soiling episodes and avoiding skin excoriation by means of moist tissue paper and zinc oxide cream or calamine lotion [7]. Disposable bodyworns are preferred to underpads in protecting skin by preventing soiling of linen [8]. In these patients, supportive measures such as habit training and education have been shown to improve general well-being [9].

In patients with fecal impaction and overflow incontinence, especially when motility is reduced, a regular program of emptying the rectum with bisacodyl/glycerol suppositories or enemas may

Table VIII.18. Types of deficits associated with fecal incontinence

Hyposensitive rectum	Sensory nerve damage
	Rectal dilatation from chronic constipation
External anal sphincter weakness	Prolonged second stage labor
	Surgery
	Radiation
	Episiotomy
Internal anal sphincter weakness	Surgery
	Rectal dilatation from chronic constipation
Noncompliant rectum	
Dyssynergic defecation	

Table VIII.19. Nonoperative modalities in fecal incontinence

Treatment of underlying condition	
Educational	Habit training/counseling
Hygienic measures/skin care/toilet scheduling	Suppositories/enemas
Dietary	Fiber, food intolerance
Pharmacological (*per os*)	Antidiarrheal opiate agents, anticholinergic, bile-acid-binding resin
	Tricyclic antidepressant
	5-HT_3 antagonist
Pharmacological (*in situ*)	Phenylephrine gel
Local disposables	Anal plugs, Procon device
Local injection	Bulking agents
Biofeedback therapy	Sphincter strengthening
	Rectal sensory conditioning
	Sensory-motor coordination training

be useful. Short-term follow-up studies report a success rate of 60–80% [10]. Daily osmotic laxative (lactulose 10 ml twice daily) plus weekly enema is curative in aged patients with dementia [11].

Dietary manipulations are necessary in patients with diarrhea and incontinence due to underlying lactose or fructose intolerance [12]. Fibers can increase fecal mass by absorbing water or, otherwise, increase colonic fermentation, worsening diarrhea. Psyllium and gum agar has been proved to be effective in reducing incontinence episodes by promoting more formed stools than placebo [13]. Fiber intake is contraindicated in patients with fecal impaction [14]. Limiting coffee could be helpful since coffee enhances the gastrocolonic reflex and increases colonic motility [15]. Enemas are useful to induce bowel movements and leave the rectum empty between evacuations.

Medical Strategy

For minor degrees of incontinence, dietary management with bran and fiber supplement with antidiarrheals, to produce firmer stools, may be all that is needed. The key to these simple approaches is making the stools more solid. In this regard, primary treatment of any medical conditions predisposing to diarrhea must be undertaken. These may include the diagnosis and treatment of malabsorptive states, the correction of dietary indiscretions, the best possible control of diabetes mellitus, and the treatment of bacterial overgrowth (systemic sclerosis and other pseudo-obstructions). Antidiarrheals must be used in adequate doses and in an effective way if firmer stools are to be achieved. For patients with severe urgency, prophylactic use of antidiarrheals prior to periods of stress, with reduced access to toilet facilities, may be especially helpful. Loperamide 4 mg, diphenoxylate 5 mg, or codeine sulfate 60 mg may need to be used regularly – up to four times daily in severe examples. Loperamide increases internal sphincter tone [16], reduces stool weight [17], increases colonic transit time [18], and improves passive incontinence following proctocolectomy [19]. Diphenoxylate/atropine may represent an alternative option [20]. Codeine phosphate may achieve the same benefit but may cause drowsiness.

The tricyclic antidepressant amitriptyline has been proved to be efficacious in fecal incontinence [21] since it allows formation of firmer stool by decreasing the amplitude and frequency of rectal motor complex and increasing colonic transit [22]. The 5-HT_3 antagonist alosetron slows colonic transit, increases colonic compliance to distention, and decreases visceral hypersensitivity [23]. This drug is indicated, under severe restricted conditions, for women with diarrhea-predominant irritable bowel syndrome [24], but there are no data showing that it improves continence.

Patients with weakness of the internal anal sphincter may benefit by application of topical phenylephrine gel. This α_1 agonist agent has a dose-dependent effect in increasing resting pressure in healthy subjects and in patients with fecal incontinence [25] although randomized controlled trials are disappointing [26]. Phenylephrine gel has also been valuable in patients with ileoanal pouches without pouchitis [27].

Local Disposables

Polyurethane or cotton anal plugs are available [28] and, if tolerated, restore barrier function and serve as an absorbent [29]. They may be useful in cases with impaired rectal sensation, in institutionalized patients, or in patients with neurological diseases [30]. The Procon incontinence device consists of a disposable, pliable, rubber catheter with an infrared photointerrupter sensor and flatus vent holes, which acts as a temporary mechanical barrier to stool leakage. Stool entering the rectum is sensed by the photointerrupter sensor, which alerts the patient to an imminent bowel movement [31].

Bulking agents, [e.g., autologous fat [32], glutaraldehyde cross-linked (GAX) collagen [33], Durasphere [34], Bioplastique [35], thoroughly described in a recent review [36], have been used to attempt to seal the anal canal [37]. Although the main indication for these agents has always been urinary incontinence, they can be used as an alternative treatment for passive fecal incontinence. Inadequate experience and lack of randomized controlled trials limit their use in patients with fecal incontinence [36].

Biofeedback Training

Biofeedback is a strategy based on operating condition derived from the psychological learning theory and is an effective therapy in patients with fecal incontinence associated with impaired functioning of the puborectalis muscle and external anal sphincter muscles [38, 39]. Continence is a complex mechanism in which different anatomical and functional parts interplay, and any condition that alters this equilibrium can theoretically cause defecation disorders [40]. The puborectalis muscle and external anal sphincter complex are striated muscles under conscious control that can be voluntary taught to strengthen and relax [40].

Biofeedback training in fecal incontinence is aimed at instructing patients how to recognize and achieve control of their striated muscle sphincter apparatus by means of techniques that are directed to modification of rectal perception and increased external anal sphincter responsiveness [38]. Modes of therapeutical action imply that a patient is able to comprehend and is willing to cooperate with therapist. Different devices can be utilized and vary from visual, verbal, or auditory feedback. Patients with fecal incontinence are taught to squeeze anal muscles without increasing intra-abdominal pressure or inappropriately contracting thigh or gluteal muscles [41]. Essentially, three modalities of treatment are employed to teach the patients to exercise anal muscles.

The first modality consists of anal manometric catheter, intra-anal electromyography (EMG) electrodes, or perianal external EMG electrodes. Ultrasound has been used as well to monitor sphincter contraction [42]. Pressures or EMG signals are displayed on a monitor or chart recorder [43] (Fig. VIII.31) to illustrate to the patient how the sphincter functions and to teach how to isolate anal sphincter contraction from buttocks and abdominal effort. Portable devices are available to customize home treatment and to monitor progress.

The second mode consists of a three-balloon system to facilitate sensor-motor coordination by correctly identifying rectal distention and responding by immediate contraction to compensate for inhibition of the internal anal sphincter [39].

The third approach implies sensory impairment retraining, and the patient is taught to discriminate smaller volumes of balloon distention by gradually reducing rectal volume inflation [41].

The goals of biofeedback therapy in fecal incontinence are basically targeted at improving sphincter strength and endurance, improving rectal sensation, and yielding sensory-motor coordination. Muscle strength [44] and duration of squeeze are important in preserving continence [45], and some authors have focused biofeedback treatment on improving force and endurance [45, 46]. Patients are taught to isolate pelvic muscles and to perform maximal voluntary contraction, concentrating on both the amplitude and duration of the squeeze. Moreover, repeated contractions and relaxations are recommended at the beginning and end of home exercises. These quick contract and relax exercises improve strength and function of fast-twitch muscle fibers in order to prevent accidents caused by increased intra-abdominal pressure exacerbated during coughing, pulling, and lifting. To build up endurance, in

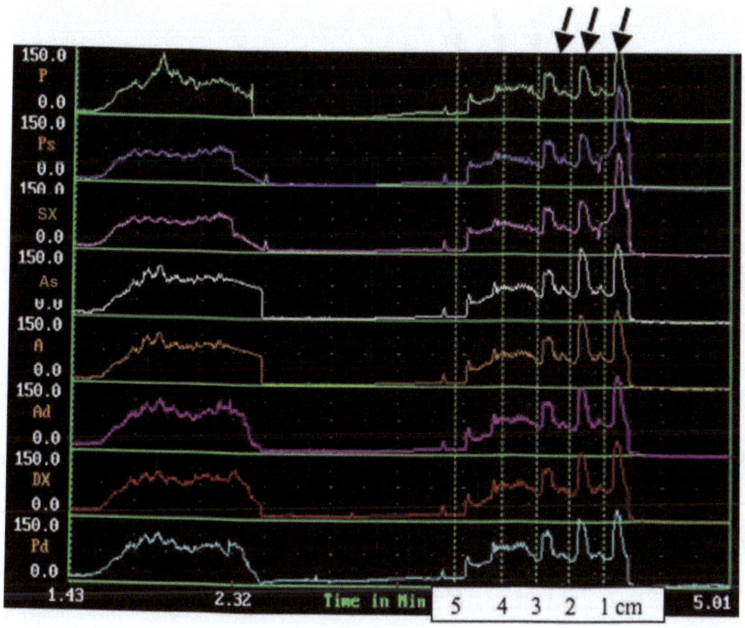

Fig. VIII.31. Anorectal manometry recording in a normal subject with an 8-radial-channel probe in anticlockwise direction, from *P* to *Pd*. On the *left* part of the panel, during longitudinal resting pullout at constant speed of 1 mm/s, pressure profiles show symmetric length and tone of the anal canal. Maximum tone recorded is around 80 mmHg. On the *right*, during 1-cm stationary pullout, squeeze pressures are recorded. Note (*arrows*) voluntary contraction induces a progressive increase of resting sphincter tone from 3 cm to 1 cm from anal verge, which is symmetric in each channel. *P* posterior, *PS* left posterior, *Sx* left, *As* left anterior, *A* anterior, *Ad* right anterior, *Dx* right, *Pd* right posterior

patients with an adequate maximal contraction, submaximal squeezc is requested. Figures VIII.32 and VIII.33 show a manometric tracing of a patient with fecal incontineuce. Other authors have focused on increase of responsiveness of the external sphincter to rectal distention [41] while others have tried to modify both [47, 48].

External anal sphincter defect following obstetric trauma does not always lead to incontinence, and this could be explained by counterbalanced strengthening of the puborectalis muscle. In fact, levator ani contraction has been demonstrated to be an independent variable with the strongest correlation to severity of incontinence and with the strongest predictive value of response to treatment [49]. The unresponsiveness of the external sphincter to retraining [41, 50] could be due to perineal muscular damage or to

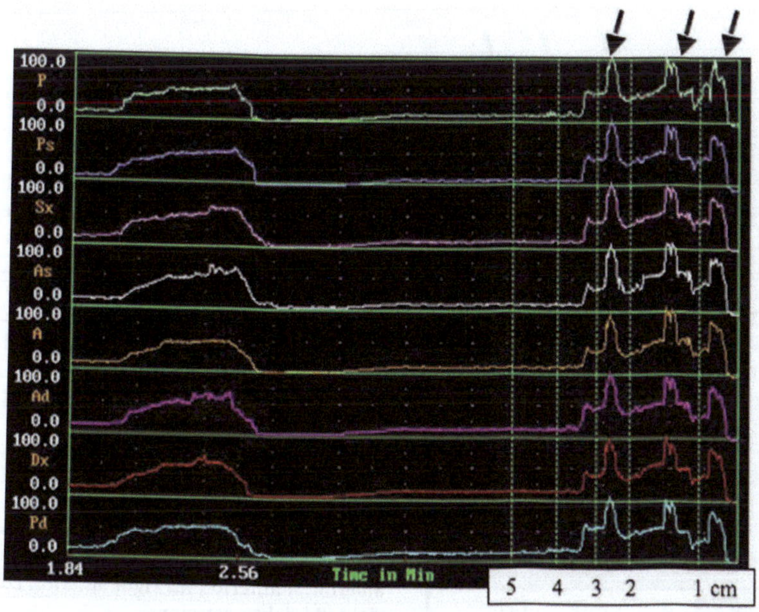

Fig. VIII.32. Anorectal manometry recording in a patient with fecal incontinence. Symmetry and pressure values of anal resting tone (*left*) are within normal ranges. Voluntary squeeze pressures (*arrows*) are reduced, as maximum values are constantly <100 mmHg at each level, with symmetric decrease. These manometric patterns suggest a weakness of striated perineal muscles not related with a structural defect of the external anal sphincter. In this case, retraining treatment is indicated. *P* posterior, *PS* left posterior, *Sx* left, *As* left anterior, *A* anterior, *Ad* right anterior, *Dx* right, *Pd* right posterior

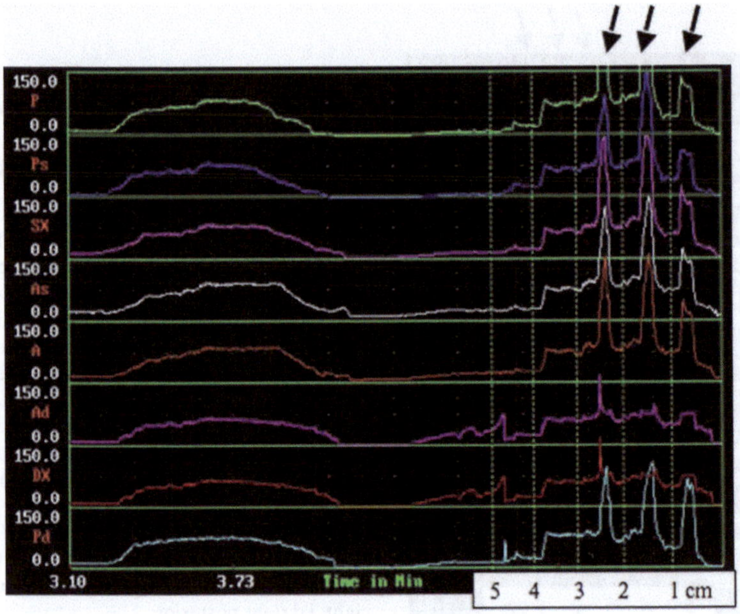

Fig. VIII.33. Anorectal manometry in a patient with fecal incontinence. Anal resting tone is reduced but not symmetrically. Note lower (<50 mmHg) pressure profiles in posterior quadrants (*P*, *Pd*) than in left and anterior quadrants (*SX*, *As*, *Ad*), where pressures reach 80–90 mmHg. These patterns suggest limited damage of the internal anal sphincter structure. Also, voluntary squeeze shows an asymmetric pattern (*arrows*). In this case, biofeedback training may be useful for improving stool continence, in particular to enhance the ability to postpone defecation. *P* posterior, *PS* left posterior, *Sx* left, *As* left anterior, *A* anterior, *Ad* right anterior, *Dx* right, *Pd* right posterior

short, instead of more prolonged, treatment [51] (Fig. VIII.34).

Amelioration of rectal sensitivity and sensory-motor coordination are believed to be important factors related to improvement [52, 53]. The enhanced ability to contract anal sphincters with biofeedback training is likely to modify urgency by reducing large-bowel peristalsis and to induce retrograde peristalsis. Patients with a hypersensitive rectum (e.g., urge incontinence) are trained to encourage relaxation and suppression of urgency in response to increasing volume of rectal balloon distention. The mechanisms by which training augments rectal perception are probably based on recruitment of sensory neurons adjacent to damaged afferent pathways. In those who are insensitive to distention, the aim is to lower the threshold for first sensation, using progres-

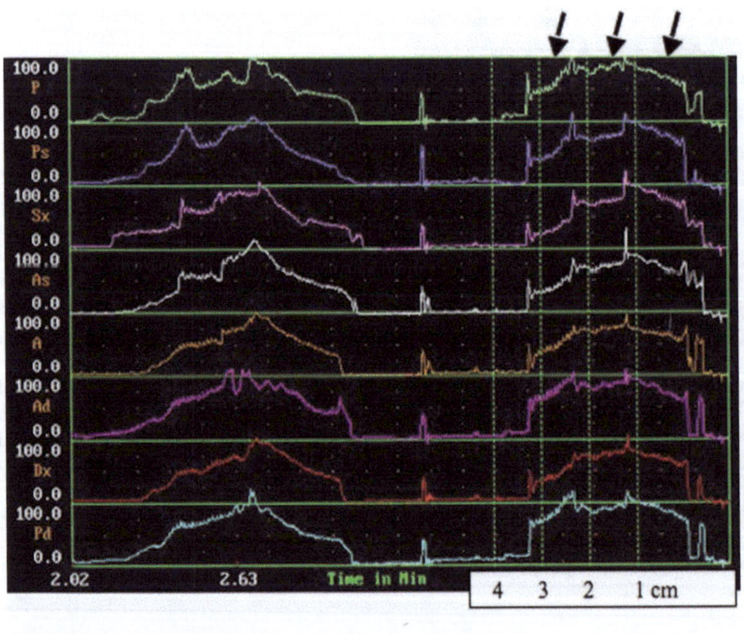

Fig. VIII.34. Anorectal manometry in a patient with fecal incontinence. Symmetry and pressure values of anal resting tone (*left*) are within normal ranges. In this patient, pressures are even increased. Conversely from the previous cases, voluntary contractions induce no changes in the anal tone: at 3, 2 and 1 cm from anal verge, there is no increase in squeeze pressures (*arrows*) along the anal canal. These manometric patterns suggest a total deficit of striated muscles, as it occurs when there is a complete interruption of the neural pathway. In this case, retraining treatment is not indicated since there is no possibility to improve the efficacy of muscle contraction. *P* posterior, *PS* left posterior, *Sx* left, *As* left anterior, *A* anterior, *Ad* right anterior, *Dx* right, *Pd* right posterior

Table VIII.20. Indications and selection criteria for biofeedback therapy in fecal incontinence

Potential indications	Sphincter dysfunction secondary to obstetric or surgical trauma
	Idiopathic fecal incontinence
	Fecal or anal seepage
	Fecal incontinence in neuropathy
Selection Criteria	
Manometric criteria	Weak resting or squeeze sphincter pressure
	Impaired rectal sensation
	Impaired rectal compliance
	Mild or moderate pudendal neuropathy
Subjective criteria	Age (no age preclusion, as long as cognitive function is intact)
	Motivation
	Ability to follow suggestions and cooperate

sively reduced balloon rectal volumes. By coordination training, patients learn how to promptly contract pelvic floor muscles as balloon rectal distension is perceived without increasing intra-abdominal pressure.

In patients with fecal seepage, a small amount of stool matter may seep out during sampling reflex or spontaneously [54], and conventionally, they are grouped together with passive or urge-incontinent patients during assessment and management [55]. It has recently been found that these patients show fairly distinctive manometric and defecation patterns compared with incontinent patients, revealing that a combination of impaired rectal perception and incomplete evacuation (i.e., dyssynergic defecation) are at the basis of development of fecal seepage. Biofeedback strengthening exercises could thus be ineffective, suggesting that correction of the underlying mechanism by improving sensation and rectoanal coordination facilitates a more complete evacuation [56].

General indications and selection criteria for biofeedback therapy in fecal incontinence are reported in Table VIII.20. Success is highly dependent on the motivation of the patient and that of the therapeutic team – in physical medicine, behavioral medicine, dietetics, and gastroenterology. The authors believe that anorectal manometry is key in patient selection for biofeedback treatment. Multimodal biofeedback training (i.e., enhancing of strength, rectal sensory perception, sensory-motor coordination) is the approach of choice [41], but since pathophysiology of fecal incontinence is multifactorial [57], customized treatment is preferable.

There is an abundance of literature on biofeedback therapy in fecal incontinence and, overall, success is reported to be around 70% [48, 58–60] that is sustained even at long-term follow-up [61]. It has been suggested that biofeedback therapy efficacy diminishes with time [62], but a recent study showed that therapy produces persistent clinical and anorectal function improvement at 12 months of follow-up [63]. A Cochrane review identified only five out of 109 studies which met criteria included in their analysis and concluded that there is not enough evidence suggesting the utility of biofeedback as treatment in fecal incontinence, which aspects are the most helpful, or which patients are most likely to be helped [47]. Lack of uniformity in methodologies, lack of randomized controlled study, heterogeneous patient population, small sample size, short follow-up periods, and lack of validated outcome measures are all variables that limit evaluation of success rate of this technique [64].

The mechanism of improvement of biofeedback is far from being elucidated. Progress in patients with intact sphincters may be related to enhanced ability of contracting the external sphincter that reduces large-bowel movements and induces retrograde peristalsis [65]. In patients with sphincteric damage, biofeedback could increase the residual functional capacity [66] (Fig. VIII.35, VIII.36). Its effect on the internal anal sphincter is debatable and could be the result of modification of autonomic function, as demonstrated in patients with constipation using laser Doppler rectal mucosal blood flow [67] (Fig. VIII.37).

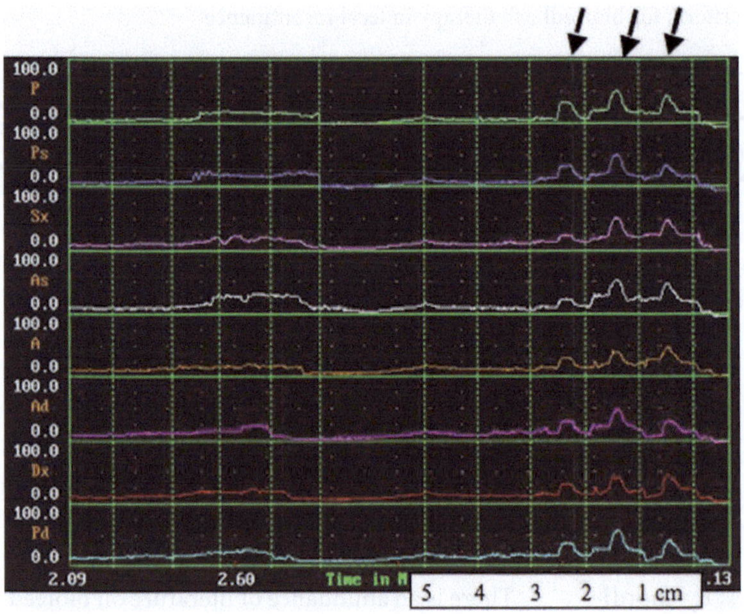

Fig. VIII.35. Anorectal manometry in a patient with fecal incontinence. Symmetry and pressure values of anal resting tone (*left*) are within normal ranges. Conversely, voluntary squeeze pressures (*arrows*) are reduced, with asymmetric decrease. Note there is a complete contractile deficiency of *Ad* and *DX* quadrants where no peaks during squeeze (*asterisks*) are recorded. Moreover, different from the normal pattern, squeeze pressure at 1 cm from the anal verge is lower than values at 3 and 2 cm in the left wall (*P, Ps, SX, As, A*). In this case, asymmetries of voluntary contraction are indicative of limited damage of the external anal sphincter ring. In this case biofeedback could increase the residual functional capacity. *P* posterior, *PS* left posterior, *Sx* left, *As* left anterior, *A* anterior, *Ad* right anterior, *Dx* right, *Pd* right posterior

It is questionable whether biofeedback has a specific effect above and beyond an interactive educational intervention alone [58, 59, 65], and a study conducted to compare education/verbal instruction plus biofeedback versus education/verbal instruction alone concluded that incontinent patients had a good response to both [68]. Patients receiving biofeedback, unlike the control group, showed an increase of manometric parameters (resting and squeeze pressures), and complete response to treatment was present, respectively, in 86% versus 46% of patients, hence questioning whether the author's conclusion about lack of differences was due to a type II error. However, the results of this study are confirmed by a large, randomized study comparing different modalities of treatment (i.e., standard medical/nurse advice, advice plus verbal

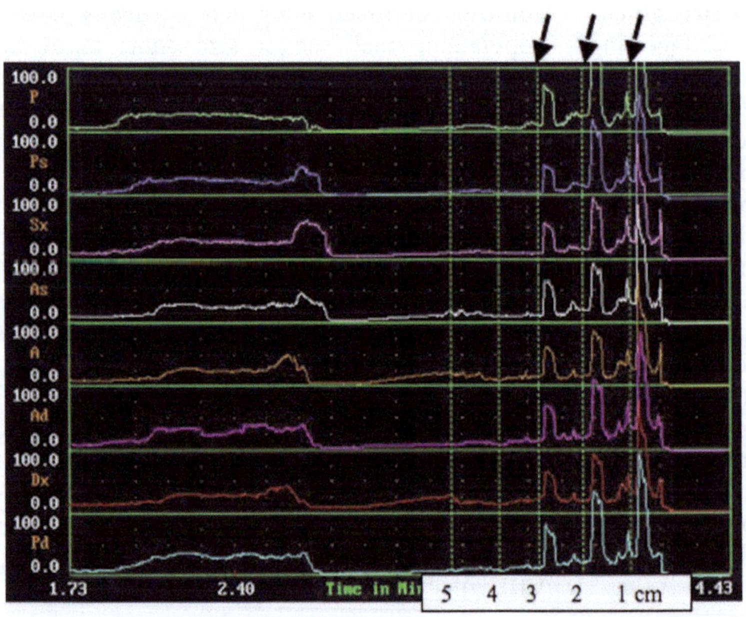

Fig. VIII.36. Anorectal manometry in a patient with fecal incontinence. Note the symmetric decrease in resting tone related to an internal anal sphincter deficiency. In contrast, squeeze pressures (*arrows*) are within normal ranges, with values reaching up to 200 mmHg at 1 cm from anal verge. In this case, biofeedback training is debatable. *P* posterior, *PS* left posterior, *Sx* left, *As* left anterior, *A* anterior, *Ad* right anterior, *Dx* right, *Pd* right posterior

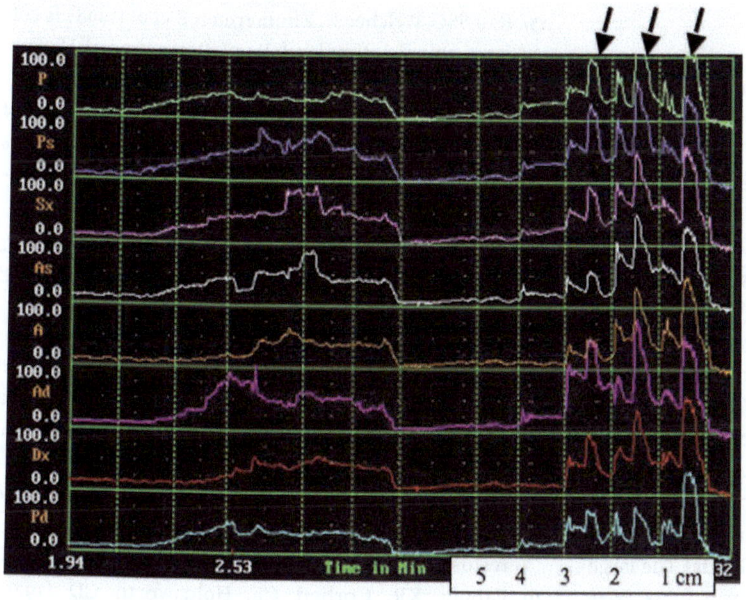

Fig. VIII.37. Anorectal manometry in a patient with fecal incontinence. Longitudinal resting pullout shows an important and symmetric decrease in tone along the entire anal canal. This pattern indicates a deficit of the internal anal sphincter involving likewise the entire sphincter ring. On the other hand, voluntary squeeze (*arrows*) induces a symmetric increase in pressure, albeit reduced (<60 mmHg), that is indicative of an intact external sphincter structure and preserved neural control. In this case, retraining treatment is indicated since striated muscle activity may be improved by biofeedback. *P* posterior, *PS* left posterior, *Sx* left, *As* left anterior, *A* anterior, *Ad* right anterior, *Dx* right, *Pd* right posterior

instruction on sphincter exercise, hospital-based computer-assisted sphincter pressure biofeedback, hospital biofeedback plus home EMG device) showing an overall improvement in 50% patients, sustained at 1 year of follow-up, in all four groups [69]. These conclusions suggest that patient coping strategies and interaction with therapists seem to play a key role in improvement of continence.

Predictors of outcome are not well established. Biofeedback can increase both rectal sensation and external anal sphincter contraction [70], but this improvement is not always associated with significant changes in any of the objective indices of sphincter function, nor to symptom improvement [71]. Success has been correlated to structural intact sphincters [65] while other studies did not find such correlation [72, 73]. Sphincter squeeze duration may be more important than strength [45, 74]. Success seems to correlate more with improvement in rectal sensation than with sphincteric strengthening [41, 75] and also with an increase of feeling of control and self-confidence.

Poor prognostic factors for biofeedback outcome are dementia, cognitive impairment, anus deformity, megarectum [76], and total absence of rectal sensitivity [77]. Pudendal neuropathy seems to be a negative factor for biofeedback success [71, 78] even though in another study, symptomatic improvement was not precluded by neurology damage [71]. More recently, evidence demonstrated that impaired defecatory maneuvers and younger age [79] are poor predictive factors of biofeedback outcome. The paradoxical coexistence of defecatory difficulties in incontinent patients is one worsening factor that has to be taken in account. Preexistent dyssynergic defecation and excessive straining may lead to perineal damage [80, 81] that can eventually lead to frank fecal incontinence.

Summary

Fecal incontinence is an unvoiced and stressful symptom that recognizes multiple etiologies. Some examples need to be treated medically by measures aimed at reducing stool frequency and improving stool consistency and that can be reinforced by biofeedback directed to improving motor and/or sensory functions. Biofeedback is a safe procedure and represents the first-line conservative therapy following failure of medical or supportive aid in fecal incontinence patients. Future placebo-controlled randomized studies are needed to better evaluate pelvic floor retraining in nonresponders to advice/education only and sensory retraining in incontinent patients. Outcomes should include standardized measures, validated quality of life questionnaires, and long-term assessment of therapeutic success.

References

1. Whitehead WE, Schuster MM (1985) Fecal incontinence. In: Whitehead WE, Schuster MM (eds) Gastrointestinal disorders: behavioral and physiological basis for treatment. Academic Press, Orlando, pp 229 -275
2. Leigh RJ, Turnberg LA (1982) Fecal incontinence: The unvoiced symptom. Lancet 12:1349–1351
3. Enck P, Bielefeldt K, Rathamann W et al (1991) Epidemiology of faecal incontinence in selected patients groups. Int J Colorectal Dis 6:143–146
4. Roberts RO, Jacobsen SJ, Reilly WT et al (1999) Prevalence of combined fecal and urinary incontinence: a community-based study. J Am Geriatr Soc 47:837–841
5. Swash M (1991) Pathophysiology of incontinence. In: Phillips SF, Pemberton JH, Shorter RG (eds) The large intestine: Physiology and disease. Raven Press, New York, pp 697–708
6. Mandelstam DA, Henry MM, Swash M (1985) Faecal incontinence. In: Henry MM, Swash M, (eds) Coloproctology and the pelvic floor: pathophysiology and management. Butterworths, Boston, pp 217–281
7. Leung F, Rao SSC (2001) Treatment of fecal incontinence in the elderly. In: Mezey MD, Callahan CM et al (eds) The encyclopedia of elder care: The comprehensive resource on geriatric and social care. Springer, Berlin Heidelberg New York, pp 261-264
8. Shirran E, Brazzelli M (2000) Absorbent products for containing urinary and/or faecal incontinence in adults. (Systematic Review). Cochrane Database of Systematic Reviews 2:CD001406
9. Chassagne P, Landrin I, Neveu C et al (1999) Fecal incontinence in the institutionalized elderly: incidence, risk factors, and prognosis. Am J Med 106:185–190
10. Lowery SP, Srour JW, Whitehead WE et al (1985) Habit training as treatment of encopresis secondary to chronic constipation. J Pediatr Gastroenterol Nutr 4:397–401
11. Tobin GW, Brocklehurst JC (1986) Fecal incontinence in residential homes for the elderly: prevalence, aetiology and management. Age Ageing 15:41–46
12. Choi YK, Johlin FC Jr, Summers RW et al (2003) Fructose intolerance: an under-recognized problem. Am J Gastroenterol 98:1348–1353
13. Bliss DZ, Jung HJ, Savik K et al (2001) Supplementation with dietary fiber improves fecal incontinence. Nurs Res 50:203–213
14. Voderholzer WA, Schatke W, Muhldorfer BE et al (1997) Clinical response to dietary fiber treatment of chronic constipation. Am J Gastroenterol 92:95–98
15. Rao SSC, Welcher K, Zimmerman B et al (1998) Is coffee a colonic stimulant? Eur J Gastroenterol Hepatol 10:113–118
16. Read M, Read NW, Barber DC et al (1982) Effects of loperamide on anal sphincter function in patients complaining of chronic diarrhea with fecal incontinence and urgency. Dig Dis Sci 27:807–814
17. Herbst F, Kamm MA, Nicholls RJ (1998) Effects of loperamide on ileoanal pouch function. Br J Surg 85:1428–1432
18. Sun WM, Read NW, Verlinden M (1997) Effects of loperamide oxide on gastrointestinal transit time and anorectal function in patients with chronic diarrhea and faecal incontinence. Scand J Gastroenterol 32:34–38
19. Hallgren T, Fasth S, Delbro DS et al (1994) Loperamide improves anal sphincter function and continence after restorative proctocolectomy. Dig Dis Sci 39:2612–2618
20. Palmer KR, Corbett CL, Holdsworth CD (1980) Double-blind cross-over study comparing loperamide, codeine and diphenoxylate in the treatment of chronic diarrhea. Gastroenterology 79:1272–1275
21. Farrar JT (1982) The effects of drugs on intestinal motility. Clin Gastroenterol 11:673–681
22. Santoro GA, Eitan BZ, Pryde A et al (2000) Open study of low-dose amitriptyline in the treatment of patients with idiopathic fecal incontinence. Dis Colon Rectum 43:1676–1682
23. Mayer EA, Berman S, Derbyshire SW et al (2002) The effect of the 5-HT3 receptor antagonist, alosetron, on brain responses to visceral stimulation in irritable bowel syndrome patients. Aliment Pharmacol Ther 16:1357–1366
24. Andresen V, Hollerbach S (2004) Reassessing the benefits and risks of alosetron: what is its place in the treatment of irritable bowel syndrome? Drug Saf 27:283–292
25. Cheetham MJ, Kamm MA, Phillips RK (2001) Topical phenylephrine increases anal canal resting pressure in patients with faecal incontinence. Gut 48:356–369
26. Carapeti EA, Kamm MA, Phillips RK (2000) Randomized controlled trial of topical phenylephrine in the treatment of faecal incontinence. Br J Surg 87:38–42
27. Carapeti EA, Kamm MA, Nicholls RJ et al (2000) Randomized controlled trial of topical phenylephrine for fecal incontinence in patients after ileoanal pouch construction. Dis Colon Rectum 43:1059–1063
28. Mortensen N, Humphreys MS (1991) The anal continence plug: a disposable device for patients with anorectal incontinence. Lancet 338:295–297
29. Norton C, Kamm MA (2001) Anal plug for faecal incontinence. Colorectal Dis 32–37

30. Tuteja AK, Rao SSC (2004) Recent trends in diagnosis and treatment of faecal incontinence. Aliment Pharmacol Ther 19:829–840
31. Giamundo P, Welber A, Weiss EG et al (2002) The procon incontinence device: a new nonsurgical approach to preventing episodes of fecal incontinence. Am J Gastroenterol 97:2328–2332
32. Shafik A (1995) Perianal injection of autologous fat for treatment of sphincteric incontinence. Dis Colon Rectum 38:583–587
33. Kumar D, Benson MJ, Bland JE (1998) Glutaraldehyde cross-linked collagen in the treatment of faecal incontinence. Br J Surg 85:978–979
34. Davis K, Kumar D, Poloniecki J (2003) Preliminary evaluation of an injectable anal sphincter bulking agent (Durasphere) in the management of faecal incontinence. Aliment Pharmacol Ther 18:237–243
35. Kenefick NJ, Vaizey CJ, Malouf AJ et al (2002) Injectable silicone biomaterial for faecal incontinence due to internal anal sphincter dysfunction. Gut 51:225–228
36. Vaizey CJ, Kamm MA (2005) Injectable bulking agents for treating faecal incontinence. Br J Surg 92:521–527
37. Shafik A (1993) Polytetrafluoroethylene injection for the treatment of partial fecal incontinence. Int Surg 78:159–161
38. Engel BT, Nikoomanesh P, Schuster MM (1974) Operant conditioning of rectosphincteric responses in the treatment of fecal incontinence. N Engl J Med 290:646–649
39. Buser WD, Miner PB (1986) Delayed rectal sensation with fecal incontinence. Successful treatment using anorectal manometry. Gastroenterology 91:1186–1191
40. Rao SS (2004) Pathophysiology of adult fecal incontinence. Gastroenterology 126:S14–S22
41. Miner PB, Donnelly TC, Read NW (1990) Investigation of mode of action of biofeedback in treatment of fecal incontinence. Dig Dis Sci 35:1291–1298
42. Solomon MJ, Rex J, Eyers AA et al (2000). Biofeedback for fecal incontinence using transanal ultrasonography: novel approach. Dis Colon Rectum 43:788–792
43. Diamant NE, Kamm MA, Wald A et al (1999) AGA technical review on anorectal testing techniques. Gastroenterology 116:735–760
44. MacLeod JH (1987) Management of anal incontinence by biofeedback. Gastroenterology 93:291–294
45. Chiarioni G, Scattolini C, Bonfante F et al (1993) Liquid stool incontinence with severe urgency: anorectal function and effective biofeedback treatment. Gut 34:1576–1580
46. Macleod JH (1987) Management of anal incontinence by biofeedback. Gastroenterology 93:291–294
47. Norton C, Hosker G, Brazzelli M (2000) Effectiveness of biofeedback and/or sphincter exercises for the treatment of fecal incontinence in adults. Cochrane Electronic Library 2:CD 002111
48. Heymen S, Jones KR, Ringel Y et al (2001) Biofeedback treatment of fecal incontinence: a critical review. Dis Colon Rectum 44:728–736
49. Fernandez-Fraga X, Azpiroz F, Malagelada JR (2002) Significance of pelvic floor muscles in anal incontinence. Gastroenterology 123:1441–1450
50. Loening-Baucke V (1990) Efficacy of biofeedback training in improving faecal incontinence and anorectal physiologic function. Gut 31:690–695
51. Aziporz F, Fernandex-Fraga X, Merletti R et al (2005) The puborectalis muscle. Neurogastroenterol Motil 17 [Suppl 1]:68–72
52. Bharucha AE (2003) Fecal incontinence. Gastroenterology 124:1672–1685
53. Whitehead WE, Wald A, Norton NJ (2001) Treatment options for fecal incontinence. Dis Colon Rectum 44:131–144
54. Miller R, Bartolo DC, Cerbero F, Mortensen NJ (1988) Anorectal sampling: a comparison of normal and incontinent patients. Br J Surg 75:44–47
55. Hoffmann BA, Timmcke AE, Gathright JB Jr et al (1995) Fecal seepage and soiling: a problem of rectal sensation. Dis Colon Rectum 38:746–748
56. Rao SSC, Stessman M, Kempf J (1999) Is biofeedback therapy (BT) useful in patients with anal seepage? Gastroenterology 116:G4636
57. Rao SSC, Patel RS (1997) How useful are manometric tests of anorectal function in the management of defecation disorders? Am J Gastroenterol 92:469–475
58. Rao SSC, Welcher KD, Happel J (1996) Can biofeedback therapy improve anorectal function in fecal incontinence? Am J Gastroenterol 91:2360–2366
59. Enck P (1993) Biofeedback training in disordered defecation. A critical review. Dig Dis Sci 38:1953–1960
60. Rao SSC (1998) The technical aspects of biofeedback therapy for defecation disorders. Gastroenterologist 6:96–103
61. Enck P, Daublin G, Lubke HJ et al (1994) Long-term efficacy of biofeedback training for fecal incontinence. Dis Colon Rectum 37:997–1001
62. Ferrara A, De Jesus A, Gallagher JT et al (2001) Time-related decay of the benefits of biofeedback therapy. Tech Coloproctol 5:131–135
63. Ozturk R, Niazi S, Stessman M et al (2004) Long-term outcome and objective changes of anorectal function after biofeedback therapy for fecal incontinence. Aliment Pharmacol Ther 20:667–674
64. Norton C (2004) Behavioral management of fecal incontinence in adults. Gastroenterology 126:S64–S70
65. Herbst F, Kamm MA, Morris GP et al (1997)

Gastrointestinal transit and prolonged ambulatory colonic motility in health and fecal incontinence. Gut 41:381–389
66. Norton C, Kamm MA (1999) Outcome of biofeedback for fecal incontinence. Br J Surg 86:1159–1163
67. Emmanuel AV, Kamm MA (1997) Successful response to biofeedback for constipation is associated with specifically improved extrinsic autonomic innervation to the large bowel. Gastroenterology 112 [Suppl]:A729
68. Ilnyckyj A, Fachnie E, Tougas G (2005) A randomized-controlled trial comparing an educational intervention alone vs education and biofeedback in the management of faecal incontinence in women. Neurogastroenterol Motil 17:58–63
69. Norton C, Chelvanayregam S, Wilson-Barnett J et al (2003) Randomized controlled trial of biofeedback for fecal incontinence. Gastroenterology 125:1320–1329
70. Berti Riboli E, Frascio M, Pitto G et al (1988) Biofeedback conditioning for fecal incontinence. Arch Phys Med Rehabil 69:29–31
71. Bharucha AE (2004) Outcome measures for fecal incontinence: anorectal structure and function. Gastroenterology 126 [Suppl 1]:S90–S98
72. Leroi AM, Dorival MP, Lecouturier MF et al (1999) Pudendal neuropathy and severity of incontinence but not presence of an anal sphincter defect may determine the response to biofeedback therapy in fecal incontinence. Dis Colon Rectum 42:762–769
73. Rieger NA, Wattchow DA, Sarre RG et al (1997) Prospective trial of pelvic floor retraining in patients with fecal incontinence. Dis Colon Rectum 40:821–826
74. Patankar SK, Ferrara A, Levy JR et al (1997) Biofeedback in colorectal practice. Dis Colon Rectum 40:827–831
75. Wald A (1983) Biofeedback for neurogenic fecal incontinence: rectal sensation is a determinant of outcome. J Pediatr Gastroenterol Nutr 2:302–306
76. Whitehead WE, Thompson WG (1993) Motility as a therapeutic modality. In: Schuster MM (ed) Atlas of gastrointestinal motility in health and disease. Williams & Wilkins, Baltimore, pp 300–316
77. Cerulli MA, Nikoomanesh P, Schuster MM (1979) Progress in biofeedback conditioning for fecal incontinence. Gastroenterology 76:742–746
78. Van Tets WF, Kuijpers JH, Bleijenberg G (1996) Biofeedback treatment is ineffective in neurogenic fecal incontinence. Dis Colon Rectum 39:992–994
79. Fernandez-Fraga X, Azpiroz F, Aprici A et al (2003) Predictors of response to biofeedback treatment in anal incontinence. Dis Colon Rectum 46:1218–1225
80. Kiff ES, Barnes PR, Swash M (1984) Evidence of pudendal neuropathy in patients with perineal descent and chronic straining at stool. Gut 25:1279–1282
81. Snooks SJ, Barnes PR, Swash M et al (1985) Damage to the innervation of the pelvic floor musculature in chronic constipation. Gastroenterology 89:977–981

Invited Commentary

M. Camilleri

Drs. Bazzocchi and Salvioli have provided a treatise of the current state of knowledge on the non-operative and, particularly, the behavioral approach to the treatment of fecal incontinence. They identify the evidence for efficacy or lack of efficacy by means of a scholarly review of the literature and their own vast experience in practice. What to do in the foreseeable future is based on the scholarly interpretation by Bazzocchi and Salvioli. However, the significant burden of fecal incontinence, even in the general population [1–3], supports the need for synthesis of critical or systematic deficiencies in the published literature and to point to relevant clinical questions that remain largely unanswered.

1. In patients with fecal incontinence, it is essential to classify the phenotype more thoroughly to be able to appraise the efficacy of any treatment modality. Thorough appraisal of the phenotype may necessitate the measurement of resting and squeezing anal sphincter pressures, duration of voluntary sphincter contraction, rectal sensation, anatomical deficits in the internal and external anal sphincters, anatomy and function of the pelvic floor, degree of prolapse or perineal descent, colonic transit, and function of the pudendal nerve [4]. There is no study in the literature that has measured all of these functions in a large series in a therapeutic trial. Novel imaging methods have been introduced, including magnetic resonance imaging (MRI), allowing assessment and, hopefully, integration of structure, function, and symptom correlation [5–7], but their impact on the management of patients or the appraisal of therapies for incontinence is still unclear.
   Appraisal of treatment efficacy must include critical functions as covariates in the analysis. In sensation-based biofeedback, a quantitative assessment of baseline rectal sensation and possibly pudendal nerve function are clearly important covariates of response. In retraining the external anal sphincter, patient cognition, sphincter integrity or the nature and size of tears, and duration and magnitude of pretreatment squeeze sphincter contraction are likely to be important covariates in the outcome of retraining. When these matters are not rigorously controlled, the null hypothesis that treatment A is superior to treatment B cannot be adequately tested. Given the large number of potential covariates, the sample size of most studies is inadequate. In multivariate analyses, it is customary to include ten patients for every potential factor associated with outcome. The literature is replete with examples of studies in which the phenotype is inadequately characterized, the analysis excludes covariates, and per-protocol (rather than intent-to-treat) analysis is performed.
   Does the lack of accounting of anatomical and physiological factors among treatment groups or the dropout of 31 of 171 participants account for the inability to demonstrate superiority of biofeedback over simple education [8]? Are groups sufficiently matched for severity of incontinence? The severity of incontinence in clinically relevant terms must be considered for such comparisons, and several question-

naires/instruments have been developed for this purpose [9–12]. Yet it is unclear whether any have been validated adequately for responsiveness in the context of nonoperative interventions. Is this because the instruments were invalid, the outcome measures were not standardized [13], or the treatments were ineffective?

2. There is significant heterogeneity among studies of fecal incontinence and difficulty appraising efficacy of treatment. This is illustrated by the fact that when Cochrane reviews have appraised the efficacy of physical therapies [14], drug therapies [15], or physical barriers [16], they comment on the poor quality of trials and the need for further larger, well-designed controlled trials. Moreover, poor characterization or heterogeneity of patients included in medication trials do not allow a clear distinction as to whether medication actually improved diarrhea and urgency rather than fecal incontinence.
   Heterogeneity in the actual delivery of therapy includes sensation- versus electromyographic (EMG)- or contraction-based biofeedback, variation in the number and duration of sessions, different goals, and expected outcomes. All of these factors contribute to the lack of understanding of the true efficacy of these therapies. Poor data quality and the significant concerns about heterogeneity and type II errors have not prevented policy makers from making rash judgments on the reimbursement by third-party payers for these types of treatments. Review bodies are often insufficiently savvy to appraise the clinical significance or pitfalls of these negative studies.
   The academic community and journal editors have a duty to protect deserving patients from being denied the chance to potentially benefit from nonoperative treatments. Health care professionals in the field of fecal incontinence should study the approach and diligent and tenacious work of a group of nurses called the Society of Urologic Nurses and Associates/ Wound Ostomy & Continence Nurses Society (SUNA/WOCN) Continence Coalition who have expertise in the management of urinary incontinence. This group joined forces with professional organizations and prominent individuals to approach, with one message and one voice, the Centers for Medicare & Medicaid Services (CMS) (formerly the Health Care Financing Administration). The outcome was a national coverage decision in the United States for the use of biofeedback and pelvic floor electrical stimulation in the treatment of urinary incontinence [17].
3. Studies need to characterize predictors of poor response. Bazzocchi and Salvioli address the evidence suggesting which factors are predictive of a poor response to nonoperative intervention. Clearly, application of this information in practice may save unnecessary effort and expense, as well as triage patients toward alternative treatments.
4. The mechanism whereby retraining, education, or biofeedback results in improved continence is still largely unclear. Understanding the physiological mechanisms associated with improvement may provide opportunities to identify altered function and pharmacologically enhance it. The basis for improved function with biofeedback is unclear. Does biofeedback really result in retroperistalsis and, if so, can this be enhanced pharmacologically for additional or accelerated response to treatment?
5. For many of the other nonbiofeedback or educational therapies, such as anal plugs and medications, evidence for efficacy is also weak. The importance of formal, randomized, controlled trials is emphasized by the penchant for treatments to be effective in open-label trials that used a physiological endpoint, such as sphincter pressure [18], only to prove ineffective in the subsequent randomized, controlled trials [19]. Novel nonoperative approaches, such as the Secca procedure [20], require further studies of efficacy now that it is clear that it can be delivered safely.
6. Practical management steps. In practice, the clinician often initiates education, bowel toilet, and relief of obstruction to defecation when present and then pursues a trial of fiber or an antidiarrheal agent to identify patients with simple incontinence secondary to rapid transit. This approach excludes those with mild incontinence from further costly, or time-consuming, or aggressive treatments. The next steps are, as detailed by Bazzocchi and Salvioli, often determined by local expertise. There is still much variation in the method used for delivery of therapy and outcomes measured.

Summary

More needs to be known about the pathophysiology of incontinence, the role of the pelvic floor and anal sphincters [21, 22], the most useful tests, and the pharmacology of the anal sphincters [23]. Patients need to be carefully characterized in clinical trials and in practice, and covariates must be included in the appraisal of therapeutic efficacy. Methods to deliver non-operative treatment and to measure the outcomes of treatment need to be improved and standardized to permit meaningful, large, randomized controlled trials.

The clinician is left with few evidenced-based options. Alas, the patient is left with the frustration and embarrassment of a socially stigmatizing disorder that may, indeed, be devastating and costly in the absence of suitable reimbursement for the therapist-intensive biofeedback.

As Sir Winston Churchill stated in a speech at the height of the devastation of London in 1942:

Now this is not the end.
It is not even the beginning of the end.
But, it is, perhaps, the end of the beginning.

Acknowledgments: The author is supported by RO1-DK54681, RO1-DK67071 and K24-DK02638 grants from National Institutes of Health. The excellent secretarial support of Mrs. Cindy Stanislav is gratefully acknowledged.

References

1. Perry S, Shaw C, McGrother C et al (2002) Incontinence Study Team. Prevalence of faecal incontinence in adults aged 40 years or more living in the community. Gut 50:480–484
2. Bharucha AE, Zinsmeister AR, Locke GR et al (2005) Prevalence and burden of fecal incontinence: a population-based study in women. Gastroenterology 129:42–49
3. Goode PS, Burgio KL, Halli AD et al (2005) Prevalence and correlates of fecal incontinence in community-dwelling older adults. J Am Geriatr Soc 53:629–635
4. Person B, Wexner SD (2005) Advances in the surgical treatment of fecal incontinence. Surg Innov 12:7–21
5. Fletcher JG, Busse RF, Riederer SJ (2003) Magnetic resonance imaging of anatomic and dynamic defects of the pelvic floor in defecatory disorders. Am J Gastroenterol 98:399–411
6. Klingele CJ, Bharucha AE, Fletcher JG et al (2005) Pelvic organ prolapse in defecatory disorders. Obstet Gynecol 106:315–320
7. Bharucha AE, Fletcher JG, Harper CM et al (2005) Relationship between symptoms and disordered continence mechanisms in women with idiopathic faecal incontinence. Gut 54:546–555
8. Norton C, Chelvanayagam S, Wilson-Barnett J (2003) Randomized controlled trial of biofeedback for fecal incontinence. Gastroenterology 125:1320–1329
9. Jorge JM, Wexner SD, Morgado PJ Jr et al (1994) Optimization of sphincter function after the ileoanal reservoir procedure. A prospective, randomized trial. Dis Colon Rectum 73:419–423
10. Vaizey CJ, Carapeti E, Cahill JA, Kamm MA (1999) Prospective comparison of faecal incontinence grading systems. Gut 44:77–80
11. Rockwood TH, Church JM, Fleshman JW et al (1999) Patient and surgeon ranking of the severity of symptoms associated with fecal incontinence: the fecal incontinence severity index. Dis Colon Rectum 42:1525–1532
12. Bharucha AE, Locke GR 3rd, Seide BM, Zinsmeister AR (2004) A new questionnaire for constipation and faecal incontinence. Aliment Pharmacol Ther 20:355–364
13. Bharucha AE (2004) Outcome measures for fecal incontinence: anorectal structure and function. Gastroenterology 126 [Suppl 1]:S90–S98
14. Hay-Smith J, Herbison P, Morkved S (2002) Physical therapies for prevention of urinary and faecal incontinence in adults. Cochrane Database Syst Rev 2:CD003191
15. Cheetham M, Brazzelli M, Norton C, Glazener CM (2003) Drug treatment for faecal incontinence in adults. Cochrane Database Syst Rev 3:CD002116
16. Deutekom M, Dobben A (2005) Plugs for containing faecal incontinence. Cochrane Database Syst Rev 3:CD005086
17. Thompson DL (2002) The national coverage decision for reimbursement for biofeedback and pelvic floor electrical stimulation for treatment of urinary incontinence. J Wound Ostomy Continence Nurs 29:11–19
18. Cheetham MJ, Kamm MA, Phillips RK (2001) Topical phenylephrine increases anal canal resting pressure in patients with faecal incontinence. Gut 48:356–359
19. Carapeti EA, Kamm MA, Phillips RK (2000)

Randomized controlled trial of topical phenylephrine in the treatment of faecal incontinence. Br J Surg 87:38–42
20. Efron JE, Corman ML, Fleshman J et al (2003) Safety and effectiveness of temperature-controlled radio-frequency energy delivery to the anal canal (Secca procedure) for the treatment of fecal incontinence. Dis Colon Rectum 46:1606–1616
21. Enck P, Hinninghofen H, Merletti R, Azpiroz F (2005) The external anal sphincter and the role of surface electromyography. Neurogastroenterol Motil 17 [Suppl 1]:60–67
22. Azpiroz F, Fernandez-Fraga X, Merletti R, Enck P (2005) The puborectalis muscle. Neurogastroenterol Motil 17 [Suppl 1]:68–72
23. Rattan S (2005) The internal anal sphincter: regulation of smooth muscle tone and relaxation. Neurogastroenterol Motil 17 [Suppl 1]:50–59

SECTION IX

Treatment Options for Anal Fistulas

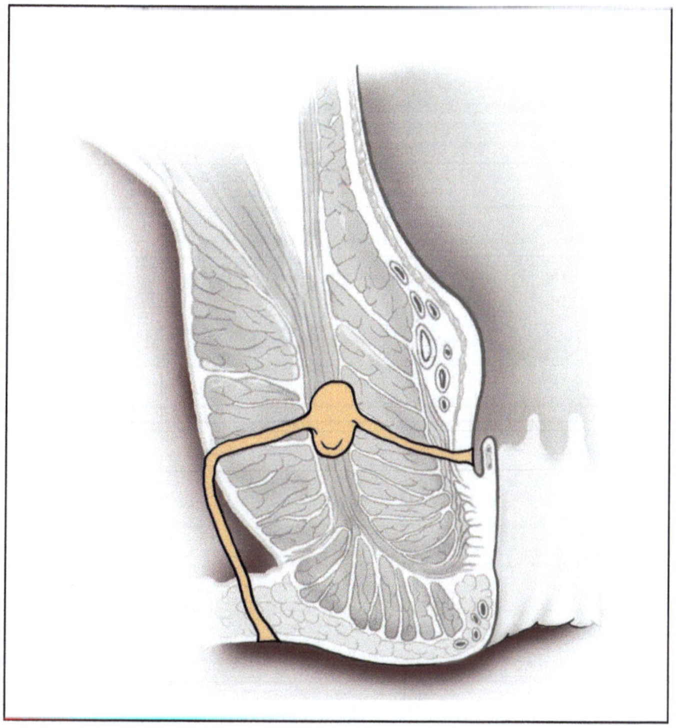

Treatment Options for Anal Fistulas

T.L. Hull

Anal fistulas result from anorectal sepsis. Common culprits that lead to sepsis and hence a fistula include cryptoglandular infections, trauma, Crohn's disease, radiation damage, malignancy, and atypical microbe infections. Multiple treatment options exist for dealing with fistulas, but treatment starts with a comprehensive history and physical exam. The history includes prior treatment, bowel habits, overall patient health and surgical history, obstetrical history, and medications. On physical exam, it is important to view the external opening and look for evidence of purulent drainage. A digital exam is done to assess inflammation, induration, and sphincter status. The course of the fistula is determined, which in turn allows approximation of the amount of muscle involved with the track. If any portion of the physical exam of the anus is compromised due to pain, consideration is given for examination being done under anesthesia so that accurate evaluation may be obtained. The entire treatment plan depends on accurate anatomical and pathological classification.

Probably the most important aspect of the initial exam is to determine if undrained sepsis exists. Antibiotics are not enough, and evidence of induration, pain, cellulites, or other septic features requires immediate intervention with drainage. Usually, drainage is accomplished by making an incision over the area of maximum flatulence while also trying to stay close to the ring of the external sphincter, avoiding injury. This allows for the shortest fistula tract if one remains after drainage. The most common drainage methods are insertion of a mushroom-headed catheter into the abscess cavity or performing a wide cruciate incision on the skin over the cavity. Both will allow for complete drainage and prevent premature closure of the skin edges. If an obvious tract exists, a seton of inert material can be loosely tied. Packing, especially tightly in the cavity, should be avoided unless the goal of the packing is to obtain hemostasis. The packing should be removed the next day, and the incision should be planned initially large enough so that no further packing is required to facilitate drainage. A primary fistulotomy is advocated by some in this setting and will be further discussed below.

After the sepsis has resolved, a fistula tract may form. At this stage, the treatment plan is formulated. The optimal goals of therapy are to eliminate the tract and sepsis while preserving fecal continence. This is influenced by the etiology of the fistula, the course of the tract, and the initial sphincter status. It is helpful to classify the fistula as intersphincteric, transsphincteric (low and high), suprasphincteric, and extrasphincteric when planning treatment options. This classification highlights the amount of sphincter involved in the tract.

Commonly accepted treatment options, each of which will be discussed later, are:

- Fistulotomy
- Advancement flap (semicircular, sleeve, transabdominal pull through, anocutaneous)
- Closure of internal opening
- Seton (cutting and loose drainage)
- Fibrin sealant
- Other

Fistulas resulting from Crohn's disease or radiation therapy as well as rectovaginal fistulas will also be mentioned separately under special situations. The use of a stoma will also be commented on under special situations.

Fistulotomy

Fistulotomy involves identifying the internal opening and unroofing the fistula tract similarly to opening a roof over a tunnel. Excision of the tract is not necessary. Since any muscle enveloped in the tract will be divided, it is important to estimate the amount of sphincter muscle that will be cut. Therefore, this therapy is appropriate for intersphincteric fistulas and low transsphincteric fistulas.

Identification of the internal opening is essential for successful treatment with a fistulotomy. If a false tract is inadvertently created, the true source of sepsis is not eradicated. Imaging studies may be helpful to guide the surgeon as to where the internal opening appears to be located. When performing the operative exam, as the anal retractor is first inserted, precise observation may demonstrate a drop of pus where the internal opening is located, so it is important to be observant when initially inserting the anal retractor. Injection of hydrogen peroxide in the external opening may demonstrate bubbles from the internal opening. Since the anal retractor may occlude the tract, when injecting the peroxide, rotation or using a retractor that only rests against half of the circumference (such as a Hill Ferguson) may prevent the occlusion. Injection of milk has also been used to see the internal opening. Methylene blue injected into the tract can be messy. It should be used if other methods fail to demonstrate the internal opening. The intention is that it will stain the tract and allow it to be followed beyond bends that prohibit probing.

Fistulotomy can also be done at the time of primary abscess drainage. This is somewhat controversial since not all abscesses will form a definite fistula tract. Three studies compared initial treatment of drainage and fistulotomy with drainage alone. Table IX.1 summarizes the results of these studies. Recurrence was higher with drainage only, and fecal incontinence rates were comparable.

Fistulotomy performed for a mature tract (not done at the initial drainage) appears to have varied results. Abcarian [4] summarized the results of fistulotomy with the thoughts that more complex fistulas have increased risk of recurrence and increased risk of incontinence. He felt that the skill of the operating surgeon is an important factor and the most likely cause of recurrence is failure to identify and adequately deal with the internal opening. Interestingly, he cited a literature review published in 1968 that found the recurrence rate varied from 0.7% to 26.5% and the rate of anal incontinence from 5–40%.[5] Abcarian further reported on his review of multiple, more recent papers and discovered a similar wide variation, [6-9] although the three studies cited in Table IX.1 [1-3], where fistulotomy was done in the face of drainage, had more promising results.

Considering anal incontinence after fistulotomy, one study looked at this problem when performed for intersphincteric anal fistulas [10]. They studied 45 patients before and greater than 6 months after surgery. They found a significant decrease in maximal resting anal pressure after operation. The squeeze pressures were similar to preoperative levels. Comparing pre- and postoperative continence scores, scores were significantly poorer for women and those who had lower preoperative resting pressures. The authors concluded that patients with low preoperative resting pressures should cautiously undergo fistulotomy. As pointed out by Nelson [11], the true answers can only be discovered by well-conducted randomized controlled trials with uniform assess-

Table IX.1. Initial treatment of anal fistula: drainage alone versus drainage and fistulotomy

Author	Number	Recurrence	Incontinence	Distinguishing features
Oliver [1]	172	29% vs 0%	0% vs 2.8%	Prospective randomized; follow-up 1 year
Ho [2]	52	25% vs 0%	0% vs 0%	Prospective randomized; perianal abscess; follow-up 15 months; manometry performed pre- and postop: no difference; operative time, healing time, hospital stay: comparable
Cox [3]	72	44% vs 21%	21% vs 21%	Retrospective; ischioanal abscess; follow-up 15 months

ment of disturbances of continence. These studies have yet to be performed and published. In the meantime, it is prudent to be cautious and fully inform patients regarding the risk of postoperative anal incontinence as well as recurrence.

Advancement Flaps

Advancement flaps have been advocated to treat fistulas that transverse significant sphincter complex or anterior fistulas in women. Generally, these are high transsphincteric or suprasphincteric. This type of complex tract may predispose the patient to fecal incontinence if a fistulotomy is performed. There are multiple variations on the technique.

Advancement Rectal Flap

The *advancement rectal flap* involves mobilization of at least mucosa and submucosa. Some include internal sphincter with the flap, and others mobilize well into the rectum to advance the rectal wall. All agree that the base of the flap must be wide enough (usually twice the width of the apex) to ensure adequate blood supply to the tip of the flap. The flap is raised and the fistula tract cored out. The fistula is then closed on the rectal side with absorbable sutures. The tip of the flap is trimmed to eliminate the area where the fistula had gone through the mobilized tissue of the flap. The flap is advanced down, while avoiding any tension, and sewn to the neodentate line with absorbable sutures. The external os is left open and may need to be enlarged to ensure adequate drainage.

Several studies have looked at results in a retrospective fashion. Zimmerman et al. [12] reported on treating 105 non-Crohn's patients who had a transsphincteric fistula. None were rectovaginal fistulas. At a median follow-up of 14 months, 69% were successful. Of all variables examined, only smoking was found to significantly influence healing (60% of smokers with a healed flap versus 79% of nonsmokers; p=0.037). Ortiz et al. [13] reported on 103 patients with high transsphincteric or suprasphincteric fistulas who were treated with endorectal advancement flaps. The etiology of all fistulas was cryptoglandular, and the recurrence rate was 7%. When examining factors affecting success, the level of the fistula did not affect outcome. The authors also stated that previous repairs did not affect outcome; however only 15% had previous repairs and they emphasized in the discussion that this was the first prospective study where few patients had previous repairs. Continence disturbance was noted in 8%, and this is one of the only studies that prospectively looked at continence before and after the surgery. A study by Schouten et al. [14] with 99 patients at a median follow-up of 12 months found a recurrence rate of 25%, with a disturbance in continence of 35%. They attributed the high degree of incontinence to the use of a Parks' retractor for exposure, which overstretches the sphincter during the operation. Two papers reported from the Cleveland Clinic in Ohio and Florida in the same journal [15, 16] examined factors affecting success of the endorectal advancement flap for non-Crohn's fistulas. One study with 48 patients reported a recurrence rate of 23%, and the other with 66 patients had a 33% recurrence rate. Factors associated with success were prior

Table IX.2. Results of advancement rectal flap

Author	Number	Success rate	Follow-up	Distinguishing features
Zimmerman [12]	105	69%	14 months	Non-Crohn's; no RVF; smoking decreases success
Ortiz [13]	103	93%	12 months	All cryptoglandular; 8% disturbed continence postop.; few had previous repair
Schouten [14]	99	75%	12 months	35% incontinence possibly from Parks' retractor
Mizrahi [15]	66	67%	40 months	Continence deterioration was more common in patients who underwent previous repairs
Sonada [16]	48	77%	17 months	Success higher if prior drainage of seton used and in those with increased body surface area

RVF rectovaginal fistula

drainage with a seton and higher body surface area (>100). Continence worsened in 9% and was associated with previous repairs. Table IX.2 summarizes the results of cited studies using advancement rectal flaps.

Advancement Sleeve Flap

In selected situations, a "sleeve" of rectum is chosen as the flap type. This includes patients with a failed flap where scarring limits the mobility of a semicircular flap. Additionally, for patients with anal stenosis from scar or Crohn's disease (provided in Crohn's disease the rectum and colon are minimally affected), this repair could be chosen. A mucosectomy is performed in the anal canal, and the rectum is fully mobilized circumferentially. The plane of mobilization is similar to the one used when performing an Altmeier procedure for rectal prolapse. If mobility cannot be obtained from the transanal route, transabdominal mobilization of the rectum and advancement of the rectum out the anus is executed. The fistula tract is cored out and closed with absorbable sutures, just as in the advancement rectal flap. The tube of rectum is trimmed and sewn to the neodentate line with absorbable sutures similar to a coloanal hand-sewn anastomosis. In instances where the anastomosis would be in close proximity to the newly closed fistula, multiple tracts exist, or where there have been failed previous repairs, a delayed closure is considered. The fistula is cored out and closed, as above, but the rectum is advanced through the anus 4–6 inches and wrapped with gauze. Then approximately 5 days later, the end is amputated and sewn in place. This delay allows the healthy rectum to adhere to the raw edges of the anal canal and closed fistula area prior to the anastomosis. Proximal diversion is strongly considered for all sleeve advancements and nearly mandatory if there will be a delayed closure. Advancement rectal sleeves done transanally for fistulas from Crohn's disease [17] resulted in 62% being healed at 1 year. Of variables studied, only simultaneous bowel resection improved success rates ($p=0.008$).

Anocutaneous Advancement Flap

This procedure is advocated by some for complex fistulas. The reduced time of stretching the anal sphincter makes this option attractive over rectal advancement flaps. Nelson et al. [reported an extensive study of their institution's 65 patients who underwent 73 flaps [18]. Island flaps were used, and 17 recurrences developed in 13 patients. Factors associated with recurrences were male gender, previous fistula treatment, large fistulas needing combined flaps (with the use of a rectal flap also), and the simultaneous fibrin glue injection. They concluded that the internal sphincter opening should be closed and fibrin glue should not be done simultaneously. Using an anocutaneous advancement flap in 23 patient with a transsphincteric fistula, Zimmerman et al. [19] reported successful closure in 46%. Success was inversely correlated with the number of prior attempts at treatment. Additionally, 30% had deterioration of continence after this type of repair. Based on these results, the authors concluded that if the patient has had less than two previous repairs, success is moderate. If they have had two or more repairs, success is poor. Based on success and possible deterioration of continence, they felt that transanal advancement rectal flaps were a better choice for transsphincteric fistulas. Other studies were more optimistic, with Amin et al. [20] reporting 83% healing with "preserved continence" at a median follow-up of 19 month in 18 patients. Hossack et al. [21] reported 94% success with this technique, and additionally, postoperative continence scores improved in 70%. Sungurtekin et al. [22] also had a 91% success rate, with no changes of continence and minimal complications.

It is unclear why there is such variation in the anocutaneous advancement flap. Review of the techniques shows they are all similar, and reports include similar complex cases. Table IX.3 summarizes the results.

Closure of the Internal Opening

In an effort to reduce fecal incontinence, closure of the internal opening is an attractive option. Athanasiadis et al. [23] reported on this technique for 90 patients with transsphincteric fistulas who underwent 106 operations. In this group, 41 underwent the procedure for recurrent fistulas. The median follow-up was 2.6 years. The technique involved first sparingly excising the internal opening along with the intersphincteric portion of the tract. The external opening was next

Table IX.3. Results of anocutaneous flap

Author	Number	Success rate	Follow-up	Characteristics
Nelson [18]	65	80%		Failure associated with male gender, previous fistula treatment, large fistula, simultaneous fibrin glue injection
Zimmerman [19]	23	46%		Success inversely correlated with number of prior repairs; 30% had deterioration of continence
Amin [20]	18	83%	19 months	No incontinence
Hossack [21]	16	94%		Incontinence improved in 70%
Sungurtekin [22]	65	91%	32 months	No continence changes and minimal complications

excised with a wide elliptical excision, including excising the entire tract up to the external sphincter complex. The internal opening was closed in layers, with the first layer being interrupted sutures through the internal sphincter. The next layer was mucosa and submucosa. The rows were placed horizontally or vertically, depending on what led to the least tension. Two or three sutures were then placed in the external sphincter. They reported suture line dehiscence in 15 patients (14%), and 12 needed reoperation. The overall total reoperation rate was 22.5%, with 18% due to fistulas and 4.5% due to sepsis. Recurrence rate was 18%, and 94% were fully continent. Koehler et al. [24], from the same institution as Athanasiadis et al., reported on 11 patients with a posterior horseshoe fistula that had fistulectomy and direct closure of the opening only. All sepsis was initially drained, and they only used this technique on soft, elastic, anal canals. No recurrences occurred. Thomson et al. [25] reported results in a similar procedure for deep anal fistulas. For 44 patients, there was a 59% healing rate. This study concluded that this procedure seemed inferior to methods with flap reinforcement. Literature studying this method overall is sparse, but it appears to be an attractive option since no muscle is divided. The true incidence of recurrence is not clear reviewing current literature.

Setons

An inert thread can be inserted through the tract and tied loosely for continued drainage or gradually tightened as a cutting seton. Several informative papers cite results of both techniques. When considering a cutting seton, the Birmingham experience [26] of 32 patients with cryptoglandular fistulas (81% transsphincteric) found that 29% of fistulas recurred. Continence disturbances occurred in 15 of 28 patients (three major, seven minor, five soiling). Interestingly, only seven reported their continence was worse after the cutting seton. Major incontinence only occurred in women who had previous vaginal deliveries. They concluded that patients should be warned regarding the high recurrence rate and the use of a cutting seton avoided in women with an anterior fistula and a history of a vaginal delivery. Isbister et al. [27] reviewed records of 47 patients with transsphincteric fistulas. A cutting seton was used if greater that 30% of the internal sphincter would be divided by fistulotomy. Setons were tightened in the operating room every 3–4 weeks. Setons were tightened once in 34%, twice in 40%, and greater than three times in 25% of cases. Mean follow-up was 1.1 years, with only one recurrence recorded. Continence was compared before and after treatment. When considering patients who were fully continent before surgery, 9.5% were significantly incontinent to gas and 21.4% were occasionally incontinent to gas after the procedure. Despite the excellent "cure" rate cited in this study, the new problem of gas incontinence is worrisome. Similarly, Mentes et al. [28] used a cutting seton (made from the elastic of a surgical glove) for 20 patients with fistulas that encompassed greater than 50% of the sphincter complex or were located anteriorly in woman. After the initial placement and tightening, no further tightening was done, and 45% had cut through at 1 month and all by 3 months. There was one recurrence of a fistula (5%) at 8 months, and 20% of patients reported worsening of anal continence although pre- and postoperative incontinence scores were similar. Other authors report no incontinence using a seton. Theerapol et al. [29] used a cutting seton for 47 patients. Seventy percent underwent placement in the clinic without anesthesia. The median healing time was 9 weeks (range 4–62), with 78% complete healing and no incontinence reported in any patients.

The idea of placing the seton and later removing it as the definitive treatment was investigated by Buchanan et al. [30]. Twenty patients who were treated with a loose seton for at least 10 years previously were contacted. At long-term follow-up, 16/20 had recurrent or persistent sepsis. Results were similar for cryptoglandular- and Crohn's-related causes. The recurrence in some occurred up to 60 months after seton removal. The authors recommend that prior to seton removal, patients should be counseled to emphasize that although some are cured, many develop recurrent sepsis, requiring further surgery. When considering Crohn's-related fistulas, a loose seton can effectively treat sepsis without deterioration in continence. However, two studies [31, 32] showed that 20–30% of patients with indwelling setons can develop further sepsis, requiring additional procedures for drainage.

In summary, setons are valuable to drain sepsis and may be used as definitive treatment for some. Loose indwelling setons, which are later removed, may be all that is needed, and certainly, loose setons can preserve the anus in selected individuals with significant Crohn's disease. Cutting setons can also be effective, but like other treatments described above, alterations in continence can occur. Careful counseling is required before its use regarding possible disturbances of continence.

Fibrin Sealant

During the last 13 years, considerable enthusiasm has been generated for using fibrin sealant as an alternative to cutting setons and advancement flaps in the treatment of complex anal fistulas. Initially, autologous fibrin glue was made by the surgeon, but today, commercially available fibrin glue can be used.

Cintron et al. [33] reported on the results of their prospectively maintained database using this treatment. At 1 year, 54% of 26 patients who had treatment with autologous fibrin tissue adhesive and 64% of 53 treated with commercial fibrin sealant were healed. It is of note that the internal opening was not closed at instillation. Most recurrences occurred by 3 months, but some continued to recur up to 11 months after treatment. Sentovich [34] also examined long-term outcome; however, he placed a draining seton for 2 month before instilling the fibrin glue. At a median follow-up of 22 months (range 6–46), 60% of 48 fistulas were closed. Retreatment with fibrin glue increased the closure rate to 69%. Of note, 6% had recurrence, which occurred greater than 6 months after treatment. One patient who failed fibrin glue treatment seemed to have a more complicated tract created after the treatment. No other complications were noted. Similarly, of 48 patients treated by Loungnarath et al. [35], durable healing was found only in 31%. These authors noted that initial healing was common, but recrudescence was frequent with most occurring within 3 months. The success rate did not change if patients had failed previous treatment. Considering ways to improve success, Zmora et al. [36] instilled fibrin glue in conjunction with an endorectal advancement flap in 13 patients and compared the results to 24 patients treated with instillation in the tract alone. The success rate at a mean follow-up of 12 months was 54% in the flap group and 33% in the instillation only group. Noncryptoglandular fistulas tended to have a higher rate of success. There was no morbidity associated with the fibrin glue.

With the thought that failure may be caused by persistent infection in the tract or early expulsion of the fibrin clot, Singer et al. [37] randomized patients to three groups prospectively. Group one had cefoxitin added to the sealant ($n=24$), group two had surgical closure of the internal opening ($n=25$), and group three had both ($n=26$). At a mean follow-up of 27 months, initial healing was 21%, 40%, and 31%, respectively ($p=0.38$). Therefore, neither of these two changes in technique improved the success rate. Table IX.4 summarizes these studies using fibrin sealants.

Predicting clinically who will recur after treatment was assessed by Buchanan et al. [38] prospectively. Of 22 patients, 77% had skin healing at 14 days. However, only 14% remained healed at 16 months. At 3 months, patients had magnetic resonance imaging (MRI) and clinical assessment to predict healing. MRI with short tau inversion recovery sequence combined with dynamic contrast-enhanced MRI predicted outcome in 100% versus short tau inversion recovery sequence

Table IX.4. Results using fibrin glue

Author	Type	Number	Success rate	Follow-up	Characteristics
Cintron [33]	Autologous fibrin tissue adhesive	26	54%	12 months	Most failures within first 3 months but some as late as 11 months; internal opening not closed
	Commercial fibrin sealant	53	64%	12 months	
Sentovich [34]	Fibrin glue	48	60%	22 months	Initially 2 months with seton in place before instillation of glue
Loungnarath [35]	Commercial fibrin sealant	48	31%		
Zmora [36]	Fibrin glue	24	33%	12 months	Fistulas of noncryptoglandular origin had higher success
	Fibrin glue under advancement flap	13	54%	12 months	
Singer [37]	Cefoxitin with commercial sealant	24	21%	27 months	
	Closure of internal opening with commercial sealant	25	40%	27 months	
	Both cefoxitin and closure of internal opening with commercial sealant	26	31%	27 months	

alone (94%) or clinical assessment (71%) (p=0.02). The authors concluded that there was poor healing using this treatment for complex fistulas and that MRI predicted outcome before clinical assessment.

In summary, successful treatment with fibrin sealant is possible, but differences in the type of fistula, etiology, protocol for treatment, and follow-up make comparisons of studies and recommendations for its use impossible. However, as Person and Wexner [39] concluded after a review of its use in the literature, this treatment is simple and carries a low risk of morbidity and can be repeated. Many of these fistulas will otherwise require surgery, which also may have a success rate less than desired (such as advancement flaps) and be associated with greater morbidity. Therefore, this procedure should still be considered in the treatment algorithm, but patients need to be aware that success rates are not high.

Other Treatments

Surgeons are continually looking for ways to improve treating anal fistulas, especially those felt to be complex. Autologous stem cell transplantation for a rectovaginal fistulas from perianal Crohn's disease was reported in 2003 [40]. The stem cells were obtained from liposuction of abdominal fat and underwent a complex preparation. The prepared inoculum was injected into the rectal mucosa after the internal opening had been closed from the vaginal side. The rectal mucosa was deemed too friable to approach the closure transanally. At 3 months, despite continued anal canal disease, the rectovaginal fistula remained closed.

Insertion of a biocompatible mesh made from porcine small intestinal submucosa (Surgisis) has successfully been used to separate the rectovaginal septum in a patient being treated with a recurrent rectovaginal fistula. The mesh was felt to be instrumental in the successful closure of the tract [41]. Similarly, in two patients with insufficient native tissue to allow adequate closure of a large rectovaginal fistula, porcine dermal graft was placed in the rectovaginal septum to separate the vagina and rectum. Successful outcome was reported over 6 months after the repair in both patients.[42].

Both these treatments require further study but may show promise in treating all types of fistulas.

Special Situations

Anorectovaginal fistulas present special challenges. Normally, thin tissue between the anorectal region and the vagina may be a culprit leading to reduced success with closure techniques. Fistulotomy anteriorly in women is to be avoided due to the risk of fecal incontinence from loss of muscle continuity or a key-hole deformity. The anterior muscle should be assessed in women, especially if a vaginal delivery has occurred previously. If there is no sphincter defect, an advancement flap is considered. Results vary, but success rates appear to be 40–60% [15, 16]. If there is an anterior muscle defect, the success of an advancement flap with loss of underlying muscle is compromised. In those situations, recreating a fourth-degree tear by doing a fistulotomy and then fully repairing the rectal mucosa and overlapping the muscle should be considered. Interposition of healthy tissue, such as a gracilis interposition, is done when other treatment failures result in significant loss of healthy tissue in the rectovaginal septum but an intact sphincter complex exists. However, porcine grafts may be another alternative, as previously discussed.

For radiation-induced anorectovaginal fistulas, the tissue must be soft and supple. This may require a stoma for proximal diversion, but for some women, the tissue damage from the radiation precludes ever having acceptable tissue. Interposition with gracilis muscle is an option, but many patients are elderly, and a permanent stoma is the best choice to improve their quality of life.

Crohn's-related anal fistulas present a special challenge. Fistulotomy can be performed for superficial fistulas in patients with quiescent anal and rectal disease; however, sometimes a loose indwelling seton, as described above, is a better choice if healing may be compromised. Successful advancement flaps can be done if the tissue has minimal to no evidence of active Crohn's disease in the anus and the rectum. The two Cleveland Clinic papers cited above (under flaps) found that fistulas from Crohn's disease were predictive of failure [15, 16], with success in about 50%. With new agents such as Remicade, which may alleviate the inflammation and active disease, success with flaps may improve. It is also logical to have proximal disease under control prior to performing the anorectal closure surgery for fistulas. The study cited above concerning sleeve advancement [17] did find that simultaneous bowel resection was associated significantly with successful outcome. However, definitive statements cannot be universally made.

Finally, what about the use of a stoma when doing a complicated repair? A stoma does not guarantee success [15], and no study has definitely found it to offer an advantage. However, a stoma should be considered if there is a complex redo operation, such as a complex flap, or other adverse features exit, such as a patient with diarrhea from various causes.

Conclusion

The most appropriate management of an anal fistula is based upon the cause of the fistula and its relationship to the sphincters. The goal of eradicating the fistula while preserving continence must always be considered when planning treatment. Since 70% of fistulas are intersphincteric, fistulotomy will be the treatment choice for most anal fistulas. However, the complex fistula, which includes transsphincteric, suprasphincteric, extrasphincteric, anorectovaginal, and radiation-induced, deserve special consideration. Multiple methods have been used to close these fistulas, including various types of flaps, primary internal opening closure, and instillation of fibrin sealant. No treatment provides results that approach consistently greater than 90% success rate, so patients must be apprised of the possibility of failure and treatment tailored to the overall fistula conditions. Figure IX.1 outlines the ideas for treatment.

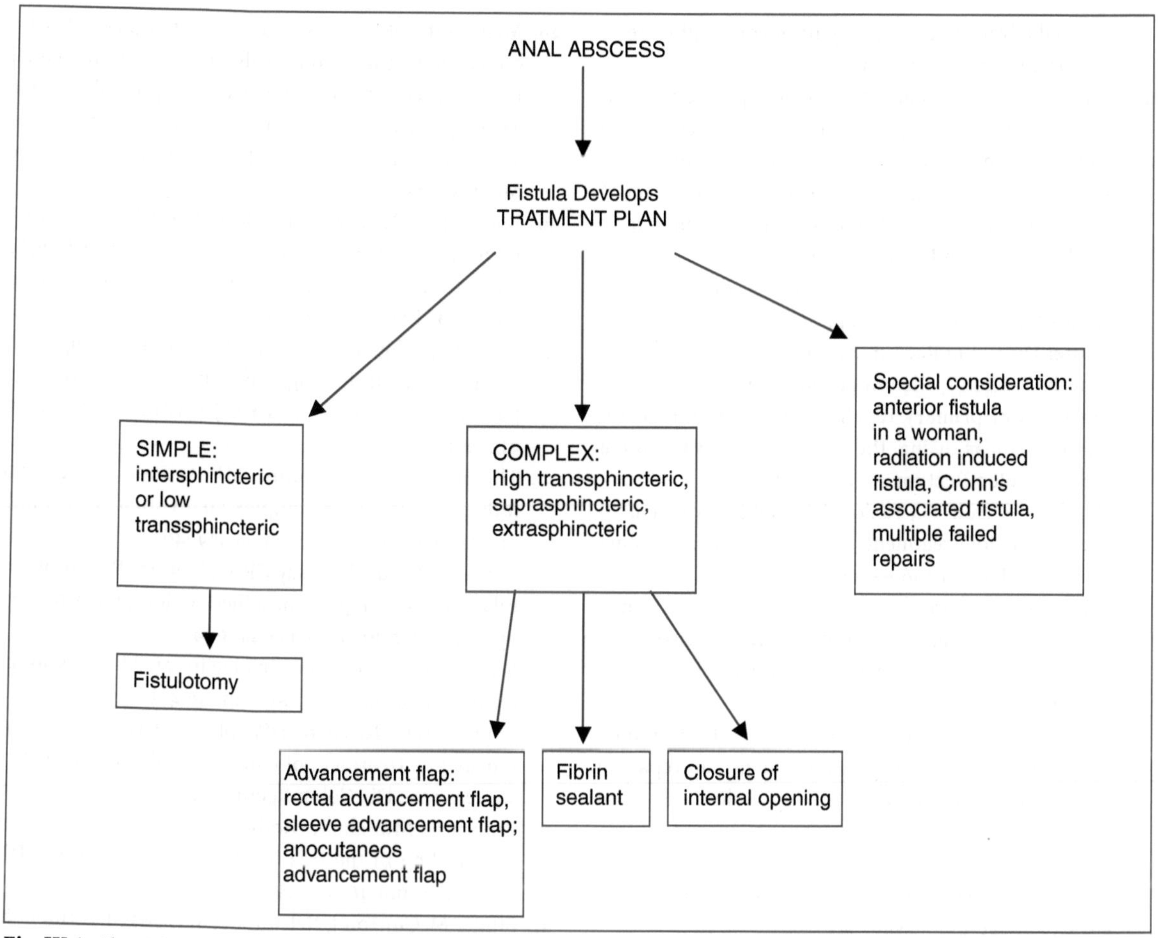

Fig. IX.1. Algorithm for treatment of anal fistulas

References

1. Oliver I, Lacueva FJ, Vicente FP et al (2003) Randomized clinical trial comparing simple drainage of anorectal abscess with and without fistula track treatment. Int J Colorectal Dis 18:107–110
2. Ho YH, Tan M, Chui CH et al (1997) Randomized controlled trial of primary fistulotomy with drainage alone for perianal abscesses. Dis Colon Rectum 40:1435–1438
3. Cox SW, Senagore AJ, Luchtefeld MA, Mazier WP (1997) Outcome after incision and drainage with fistulotomy for ischiorectal abscess. Am Surg 63:686–689
4. Abcarian H (1996) The "lay open" technique. In: Phillips RKS, Lunniss PJ (eds) Anal fistula surgical evaluation and management. Chapman and Hall Medical, London, pp 73–80
5. Lilius HG (1968) Investigation of human fetal anal ducts and intermuscular glands and a clinical study of 150 patients. Acta Chir Scand 383[Suppl]:3–88
6. Parks AG, Stitz RW (1976) The treatment of high fistula-in-ano. Dis Colon Rectum 19:487–499
7. Kuijpers JHC (1982) Diagnosis and treatment of fistula-in-ano. Neth J Surg 34:147–152
8. Ramanujan PS, Prasad ML, Abcarian H, Tan A (1984) Perianal abscess and fistula: a study of 1023 patients. Dis Colon Rectum 27:593–597
9. Mazier WP (1971) The treatment and care of anal fistulas. A study of 1000 patients. Dis Colon Rectum 14:134–144
10. Chang SC, Lin JK (2003) Change in anal continence after surgery for intersphincteral anal fistula: a functional and manometric study. Int J Colorectal Dis 18:111–115
11. Nelson R (2002) Anorectal abscess fistula: what do we know? In: Beart RW (ed) The Surgical Clinics of North America, vol 82. WB Saunders, Philadelphia, pp 1139–1151
12. Zimmerman DDE, Delemarre JBVM, Gosselink MP et al (2003) Smoking affects the outcome of transanal

mucosal advancement flap repair of trans-sphincteric fistulas. Br J Surg 90:351–354
13. Ortiz H, Marzo J (2000) Endorectal flap advancement repair and fistulectomy for high trans-sphincteric and suprasphincteric fistulas. Br J Surg 87:1680–1683
14. Schouten WR, Zimmerman DDE, Briel JW (1999) Transanal advancement flap repair of transsphincteric fistulas. Dis Colon Rectum 42:1419–1423
15. Mizrahi N, Wexner SD, Zmora O et al (2002) Endorectal advancement flap: are there predictors of failure? Dis Colon Rectum 45:1616–1621
16. Sonoda T, Hull T, Piedmonte MR, Fazio VW (2002) Outcomes of primary repair of anorectal and recto-vaginal fistulas using the endorectal advancement flap. Dis Colon Rectum 45:1622–1628
17. Marchesa P, Hull TL, Fazio VW (1998) Advancement sleeve flaps for treatment of severe perianal Crohn's disease. Br J Surg 85:1695–1698
18. Nelson RL, Cintron J, Abcarian H (2000) Dermal island-flap anoplasty for transsphincteric fistula-in-ano: assessment of treatment failures. Dis Colon Rectum 43:681–684
19. Zimmerman DD, Briel JW, Gosselink MP, Schouten WR (2001) Anocutaneous advancement flap repair of transsphincteric fistulas. Dis Colon Rectum 44:1474–1480
20. Amin SN, Tierney GM, Lund JN, Armitage NC (2003) V-Y advancement flap for treatment of fistula-in-ano. Dis Colon Rectum 46:540–543
21. Hossack T, Solomon MJ, Young JM (2005) Ano-cutaneous flap repair for complex and recurrent supra-sphincteric anal fistula. Colorectal Dis 7:187–192
22. Sungurtekin U, Sungurtekin H, Kabay B et al (2004) Anocutaneous V-Y advancement flap for the treatment of complex perianal fistula. Dis Colon Rectum 47:2178–2183
23. Athanasiadis S, Helmes C, Yazigi R, Kohler A (2004) The direct closure of the internal fistula opening without advancement flap for transsphincteric fistulas-in-ano. Dis Colon Rectum 47:1174–1180
24. Koehler A, Risse-Schaaf A, Athanasiadis S (2004) Treatment for horseshoe fistulas-in-ano with primary closure of the internal fistula opening: a clinical and manometric study. Dis Colon Rectum 47:1874–1882
25. Thomson WH, Fowler AL (2004) Direct appositional (no flap) closure of deep anal fistula. Colorectal Dis 6:32–36
26. Hasegawa H, Radley S, Keighley MR (2000) Long-term results of cutting seton fistulotomy. Acta Chir Iugoslavica 47:19–21
27. Isbister WH, Sanea N (2001) The cutting seton: an experience at King Faisal Specialist Hospital. Dis Colon Rectum 44:722–727
28. Mentes BB, Oktemer S, Tezcaner T et al (2004) Elastic one-stage cutting seton for the treatment of high anal fistulas: preliminary results. Tech Coloproctol 8:159 162
29. Theerapol A, So BY, Ngoi SS (2002) Routine use of setons for the treatment of anal fistulae. Singapore Medical J 43:305–307
30. Buchanan GN, Owen HA, Torkington J et al (2004) Long-term outcome following loose-seton technique for external sphincter preservation in complex anal fistula. Br J Surg 91:476–480
31. Takesue Y, Ohge H, Yokoyama T et al (2002) Long-term results of seton drainage on complex anal fistulae in patients with Crohn's disease. J Gastroenterology 37: 912–915
32. Thornton M, Solomon MJ (2005) Long-term indwelling seton for complex anal fistulas in Crohn's disease. Dis Colon Rectum 48:459–463
33. Cintron JR, Park JJ, Orsay CP et al (2000) Repair of fistulas-in-ano using fibrin adhesive: long-term follow-up. Dis Colon Rectum 43:944–949
34. Sentovich SM (2003) Fibrin glue for anal fistulas: long-term results. Dis Colon Rectum 46:498–502
35. Loungnarath R, Dietz DW, Mutch MG et al (2004) Fibrin glue treatment of complex anal fistulas has low success rate. Dis Colon Rectum 47:432–436
36. Zmora O, Mizrahi N, Rotholtz N et al (2003) Fibrin glue sealing in the treatment of perineal fistulas. Dis Colon Rectum 46:584–589
37. Singer M, Cintron J, Nelson R et al (2005) Treatment of fistulas-in-ano with fibrin sealant in combination with intra-adhesive antibiotics and/or surgical closure of the internal fistula opening. Dis Colon Rectum 48:799–808
38. Buchanan GN, Bartram CI, Phillips RK et al (2003) Efficacy of fibrin sealant in the management of complex anal fistula: a prospective trial. Dis Colon Rectum 46:1167–1174
39. Person B, Wexner SD (2004) Novel technology and innovations in colorectal surgery: the circular stapler for treatment of hemorrhoids and fibrin glue for treatment of perianal fistulae. Surgical Innovation 11:241–252
40. Garcia-Olmo D, Garcia-Arranz, Garcia LG et al (2003) Autologous stem cell transplantation for treatment of rectovaginal fistula in perianal Crohn's disease: a new cell-based therapy. Int J Colorectal Dis 18:451–454
41. Pye PK, Dada T, Duthie G, Phillips K (2004) Surgisistrade mark mesh: a novel approach to repair of a recurrent rectovaginal fistula. Dis Colon Rectum 47:1554–1556
42. Moore RD, Miklos JR, Kohli N (2004) Rectovaginal fistula repair using a porcine dermal graft. Obstet Gynecol 104:1165–1167

Invited Commentary

S.D. Wexner

Not unexpectedly, Dr. Hull has authored a well-researched, readily comprehensible, appropriately comprehensive, and authoritatively referenced chapter. She has achievied these goals in a well-written chapter wich is both logically constructed and clinically useful. She has emphasized all of the important points relative to anal fistulas.

Firstly, she has reviewed the etiology and pathophysiology of fistulas and secondly emphasized how the various treatments relate to their etiology and pathogenesis. She has very capably pointed out that no panacea exists as a treatment for fistulous disease. Although Dr. Hull notes 70% that of fistulas are intersphincteric and fistulotomy will undoubtedly be the best choice in these instances, the complex fistulas, including transsphincteric, suprasphincteric, extrasphincteric, anovaginal, rectovaginal, and radiation-induced all deserve special consideration. The problem, as Dr. Hull notes in her review, is that flaps, primary closure, and fibrin glue all were initially touted as having almost universal success rates. However, with the passage of time, the success rates of any of these treatments are at best in the vicinity of 70%. In addition Dr. Hull mentions the associations of compromise in bowel continence after fistula treatment and cautions the reader about which treatments may predispose more than others to such problems. I am particularly impressed by the algorithm in which she points out that drainage or possible fistulotomy is the first step. I agree with her algorithm in which intersphincteric or low transsphincteric fistula is treated with fistulotomy whereas complex fistulae may be treated by a variety of advancement flaps, fibrin sealant, or closure of the internal opening. Again, the algorithm highlights the special consideration in certain situations. I might have added the role of cutting setons and drainage setons to this algorithm, as I personally favor the use of setons in many situations. When possible, the seton can allow better eradication of active sepsis prior to definitive treatment. In other cases, the seton can allow for the slow and controlled performance of a fistulotomy without compromise of continence.

I readily admit to my patients with complex anal fistulas that their problem is more difficult to treat than is virtually any other problem that confronts the colorectal surgeon. The myriad of available treatments attests to the lack of universal success of any single treatment or any combination of treatments. The surgeon who approaches fistulous disease must have an honest and lengthy discussion with the patient at each visit, but especially at the first visit, explaining the difficulties in obtaining success. This discussion usually centers around obtaining whatever preoperative assessments may be beneficial. Such assessment can range from the simplicity of an office evaluation to anal ultrasonography with hydrogen peroxide instillation, intra-anal coil or external surface magnetic resonance imaging (MRI), or an examination under anesthesia. I have not found fistulography to be of significant value and prefer anal ultrasonography with hydrogen peroxide [1] or MRI to delineate the relation of fistula tracks to the anal musculature. Examination under anesthesia allows several possibilities, including injection of hydrogen peroxide, milk, or methylene blue. I favor hydrogen peroxide as it does not discolor the track, and when it "bubbles through," it helps readily delineate the area for probing. One other possible method that I occasionally employ is cutting down on the fistula track, gradually opening it and following the granulation tissue to its origin. Certainly, one of the most important parts of treating complex fistulas is not to be overly aggressive. If the internal opening cannot be readily delineated through all of these various means, then curettage and drainage of the track with placement of a mushroom-tipped catheter is something that I employ. Contingent upon the progress of the patient, the drain might either be removed or injected with hydrogen peroxide during anal ultrasonography to try to delineate the track and the internal opening.

Complex anovaginal, pouch-vaginal, and radiation-induced rectourethral fistulas are special circumstances. In each of these situations, my preference is for a gracilis interposition. As we have noted in several prior publications, our success rate is quite favorable with this methodology, transposing healthy tissue into the previously infected space [2, 3]. Occasionally, an endorectal advancement flap is a useful adjunct if a gracilis transposition heals parts but not all of the fistula [4].

Regardless of the treatment employed, the surgeon should be cognizant of the multiple therapeutic options and should discuss them with the patient. Failure of an initial treatment, such as a cutting seton, should not deter further treatment, but again, one must be cognizant of any potential damage of that treatment. For example, if a cutting seton has divided muscle, then prior to any consideration of additional muscle division, it may be beneficial to obtain anal manometry and/or anal ultrasonography. Alternatively, if an advancement flap has retracted, one must consider why and perhaps employ alternative therapy. The surgeon should at all times be flexible given the multiple approaches and should be willing to individualize them based upon the individual circumstance.

Once again, I wish to commend Dr. Hull upon this excellent chapter and thank the editors for having solicited my comments.

References

1. Cheong DM, Nogueras JJ, Wexner SD, Jagelaman DG (1993) Anal endosonography for recurrent anal fistulas: image enhancement with hydrogen peroxide. Dis Colon Rectum 36:1158–1160
2. Zmora O, Potenti FM, Wexner SD et al (2003) Gracilis muscle transposition for iatrogenic rectourethral fistula. Ann Surg 237:483–487
3. Cera SM, Wexner SD (2005) Muscle transposition: Does it still have a role? Clinics in colon and rectal surgery 18:46–54
4. Mizrahi N, Wexner SD, Zmora O et al (2002) Endorectal advancement flap: are there predictors of failure? Dis Colon Rectum 45:1616–1621

Section X

Current Concepts in Management of Outlet Obstruction

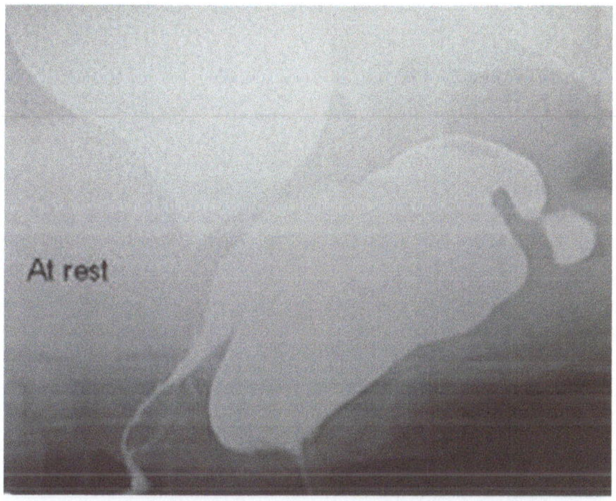

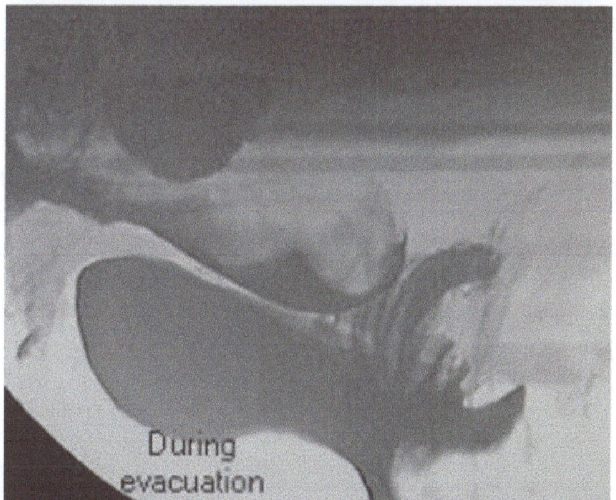

Current Concepts in Management of Outlet Obstruction

A. Infantino, R. Bellomo, F. Galanti, L. Pisegna Cerone

Outlet constipation is often characterized by disabling symptoms consisting of the strenuous effort to expel stools, a feeling of incomplete evacuation, rectal tenesmus and a repeated call to toilet, digitations, and the necessity of enemas and/or suppositories [1]. It is related to multiple alterations, variously associated and in different degrees, of the organs of the pelvis and perineum: rectocele, rectal occult-mucosal or full-thickness prolapse, and enterocele. Synchronous anatomic alterations in the urogynecological sector can also be found: uterine, vaginal, and bladder prolapses [2]. A unique pathophysiologic theory has been suggested but not yet demonstrated [3]. As a consequence of the variability of the affected organs, great difficulty in reaching a diagnosis exists, and the management and treatment of outlet constipation is, to date, far from being standardized.

Clinical Conditions

Rectocele

Rectocele is the most common anatomical alteration that can be evidentiated through inspection at straining and combined digital rectal and vaginal examinations. The presence of a rectocele, however, often does not represent by itself the cause of the symptoms of obstructed defecation. In fact, only when it is larger than 3 cm, when barium is entrapped after defecographic evacuation, in the absence of anismus, can it be considered a cause of outlet obstruction. The association between rectocele and other anatomical defects should always be considered. Incidences of 33% of occult rectal prolapse, 1.7% of sigmoidocele, and 10% of anismus have been defecographically demonstrated after a clinical diagnosis of rectocele and obstructed defecation [4]. This is very important because of the subsequent different approaches: conservative for anismus or surgical intervention for other conditions.

Rectal Intussusception

Rectal intussusception is often difficult to diagnose. Radiological findings that can be indicative of rectal intussusception can be found also in healthy people [5, 6]. Even the interpretation of radiological images is still a controversial issue [4, 7–10]. There is open discussion as to whether magnetic resonance imaging (MRI) can add more information than cystocolpodefecography [9, 10], which remains the most useful and simplest test.

Enterocele

Enterocele has been found by Mellgren et al. [11] in 19% of 2,816 defecographies, but it can be visualized at a high rate at straining [12, 13]. By itself, it does not necessarily impair defecation [14]; however, the presence of the sigma in the dislocated Douglas pouch can be a cause of compression of the rectum at straining [15]. In any case, when a surgical approach for obstructed defecation has been chosen, enterocele must be treated.

Solitary Rectal Ulcer

In patients with obstructed defecation, a solitary rectal ulcer can be diagnosed at a rate ranging from 6% to 39%. The symptoms improve significantly after behavioral therapy consisting of biofeedback and attempts to discourage the use of laxatives, enemas, and suppositories. The success rate correlates to an increase of rectal mucosal blood flow as a consequence of improved activity of extrinsic innervations of the rectum [16].

Growing attention has been paid to the psychological aspect [17]. Fifty patients (eight with slow-transit constipation, 36 with obstructed defecation, and six with mixed symptoms) were given biofeedback training: 70% found biofeedback helpful, and 62% improved, irrespective of the type of constipation. The results were related to psychological state rather than anorectal tests [17]. It has been demonstrated that in patients with functional intestinal disorders, modification of mucosal blood flow depends on the psychological state and autonomic innervations [18]. Improvement of mucosal blood flow could be secondary to both a better psychological equilibrium and better autonomic nerve stimulation.

Management of Obstructed Defecation

Treatment of outlet obstruction is often disappointing, and many authors reported no encouraging results after surgery [19, 20]. As a consequence, an initial conservative approach has been encouraged: high-fiber diet, biofeedback, and rehabilitation of the pelvic floor muscles can help to reduce symptoms of outlet obstruction [19, 20].

Rectocele

When it has been demonstrated that the predominant alteration is the rectocele, repair of the anterior rectal wall through the different approaches described (transvaginal, perineal, or transanal) should be performed. We believe that transanal techniques are to be chosen for simultaneous repair of exuberant mucosal or full-thickness rectal wall [21]. The simplest operation is the transanal suture of the anterior rectal wall [22], with satisfactory results in more than 80% of patients [23]. Depending on the size and in absence of a large rectal intussusception, Sarles operation may be carried out and combined with an anterior levatorplasty in case of contextual presence of fecal incontinence [24].

Taking into consideration new technologies, rectocele and rectal occult mucosal prolapse may be also resected with a GIA stapled with satisfactory short-term results [25]. Transanal stapled prolapsectomy and anterior levatorplasty have been successfully carried out in a small series with short follow-up [26]. The stapled transanal rectal resection (STARR) for the treatment of symptomatic rectocele was presented in 2002 [27]. After 3 months, 30% of patients had no complaints, 40% had only one to two episodes per month of

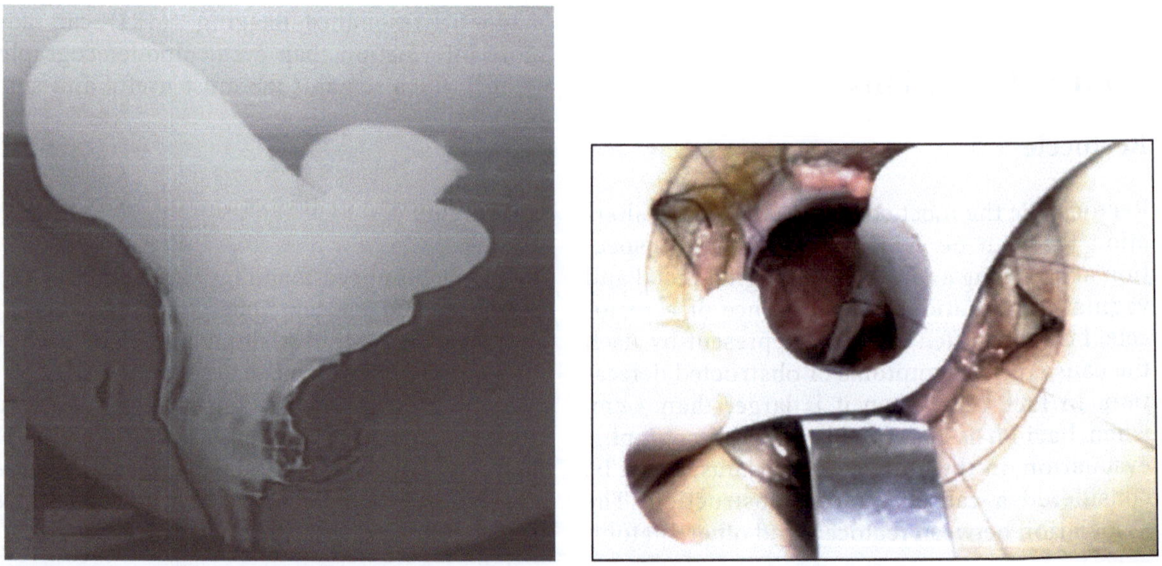

a b

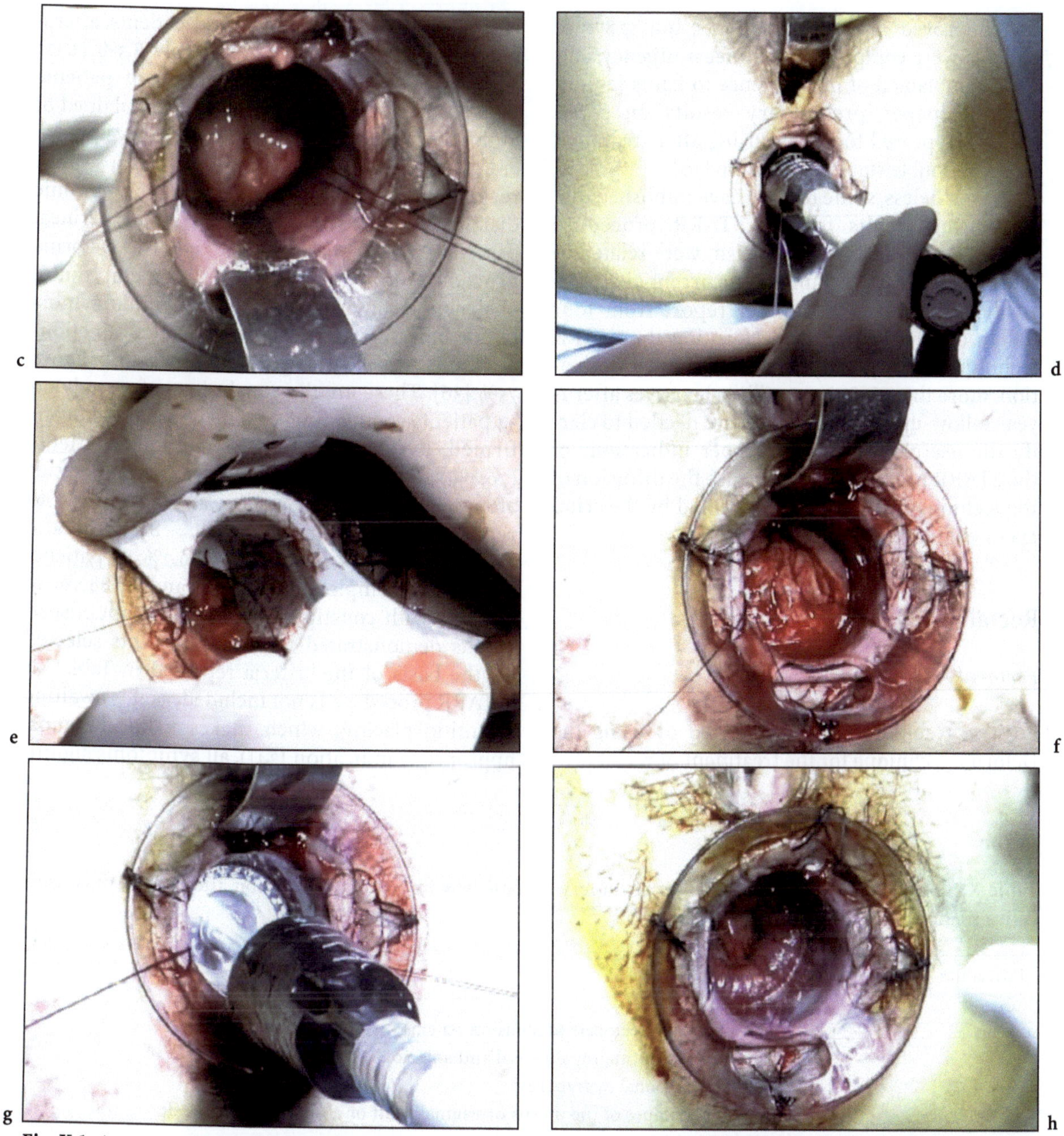

Fig. X.1. A 43-year-old woman with obstructed defecation and digital evacuation. Defecography confirmed the presence of a large rectocele associated to a posterior mucosal rectal prolapse (**a**). Stapler transanal rectal resection (STARR) procedure was performed. Three series of suture were passed through the anterior rectal wall at a distance of 5 cm from the dentate line (**b**). Anterior rectal bulging (**c**). The 33-mm circular stapler (PPH-01, Ethicon EndoSurgery) was then introduced for the anterior rectal resection (**d**). Similarly, two series of sutures were passed through the posterior rectal wall (**e**). Posterior rectal mucosal prolapse (**f**). The stapler was introduced for the second time for the posterior rectal resection (**g**). At the end of the operation, the rectum appeared unobstructed (**h**)

obstructed defecation, 13.3% had evacuation only using laxatives, and 16.6% were unchanged [27]. Afterward, a double stapler technique (Fig. X.1) was proposed and compared with STARR plus levatorplasty: the results were encouraging on outlet obstruction; however. 4/25 (16%) patients were complicated by the urge to defecate [28]. In a multicenter study, 90 patients with rectocele and rectal intussusception were treated by performing the same technique. Symptoms of obstructed defecation improved in 90% of patients, but 17.8% of patients were complicated with fecal urgency, and 8.9% complained of incontinence to flatus [29]. In a recent paper, preliminary results on seven patients appeared to be promising after treatment with the double stapler procedure [30].

Nevertheless, some reports have published disappointing results for the STARR procedure [31–34]. Anismus and neuroticism were related to severe postoperative pain and recurrent obstructed defecation [31]. In another report from four Italian centers [32], after performing the STARR technique in 65 patients with obstructed defecation, more than 60% were still on laxatives after 1-year follow-up. Further studies are needed to clarify the usefulness and the proper indications of the STARR procedure [33] because the diffusion of the technique is, to date, not justified by the criteria of evidence-based medicine [34].

Rectal Prolapse

Perineal Approach

Positive results have been reported by using the Delorme technique for the treatment of rectal prolapse [35, 36]. Among 20 operated patients, after a follow-up of at least 6 months, only 8.3% (1/12) reported fecal incontinence, and 5% of patients with preoperative constipation still complained of outlet obstruction. The negative predictive preoperative data were proximal internal prolapse with rectosacral separation at defecography, chronic diarrhea, fecal incontinence, and major perineal descent (>9 cm on straining) [35]. The Delorme procedure for the treatment of rectal outlet obstruction can be carried out with minimal morbidity and short hospital stay, with good functional results and overall patient satisfaction above 75% [36]. These are the conclusions of a study on 34 patients complaining of outlet obstruction confirmed by defecography. Twenty-six patients (76.4%) reported good to excellent overall result after the Delorme procedure, and eight (23.6%) reported fair to poor results. Symptomatic improvement was observed in 89.7% of patients who had incomplete evacuation and in 88.5% of patients with constipation [37]. Our unpublished results demonstrated that in 27 patients selected on the basis of the criteria reported in Table X.1 (STARR procedure is not included, as it is awaiting scientific placing, which makes valid the most appropriate indication [34]), all symptoms signifi-

Table X.1. Selection criteria for the choice of surgery in patients with outlet constipation after failure of conservative treatment (Modified from [38])

Procedure	Selection criteria
Sarles	• Predominance of rectocele (distension >2 cm) • Prolapse 1–10 mm (mainly mucosal and anterior) • Absence of rectoanal dyssynergy • Absence of prolapse of the uterus or vaginal vault or absence of enterocele
Delorme	• Predominance of rectal intussusception (>10 mm) • High surgical risk • Absence of prolapse of the uterus or vaginal vault or absence of enterocele • Male
Orr	• Ample rectosacral space • Enterocele • Descending perineum >9 cm during straining (at defecography) • Genital prolapse
Frykman-Goldberg	• Colonic diverticular disease • Colonic associated constipation (prevalently left at transit-times study)

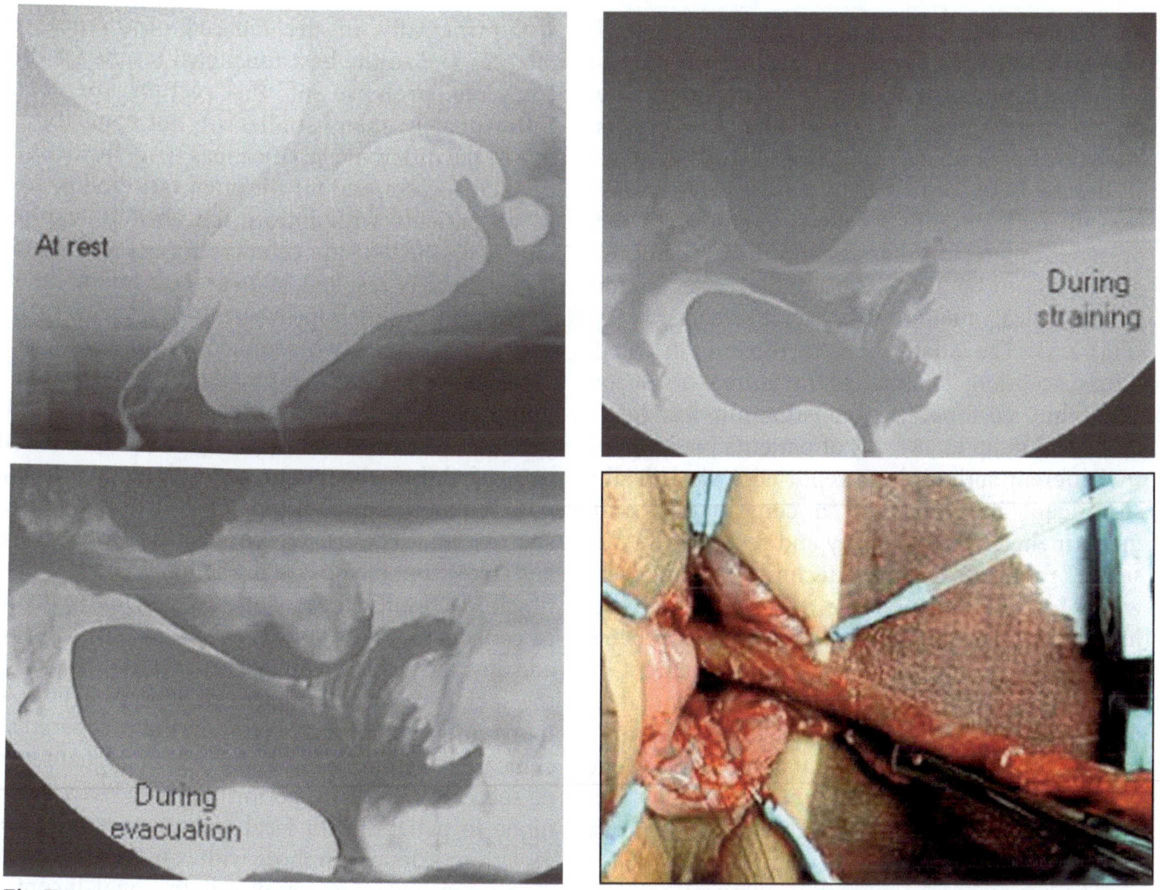

Fig. X.2. Patient complaining of outlet constipation. Cystocolpodefecography at rest (**a**), during straining (**b**), and during evacuation (**c**). The isolated mucosa of the rectum during the Delorme procedure in this patient was 18 cm (**d**)

cantly disappeared or dramatically improved, with a high rate (89%) of patient' satisfaction and no relapse evident after a medium follow-up of 30 months. We believe that these results can be justified because we included only rectal intussusception and not overt prolapse for the stringent criteria of indication for treatment according to Sielzneff et al. [38] and for the long, isolated cylinder of rectal mucosa excised (from 11 cm to 21 cm) (Fig. X.2). Indeed, one possible causes of relapse could be the incomplete dissection of the rectal and, in some cases, sigmoid wall. The good functional results on outlet obstruction are in contrast to the reduced rectal compliance after the Delorme procedure for full-thickness rectal prolapse [39]. In our study, no patients complained of postoperative fecal incontinence or urgency, and the symptoms of rectal tenesmus, false call to toilet, or inappropriate call for a very little amount of rectal content, was reduced from 21% to 4% postoperatively ($p<0.003$). In the literature, the incidence of minor complications after the Delorme procedure for rectal intussusception is reported to be between 37% and 38.2 % [37, 38]. In our experience, the complication rate was 29.6% and consisted of anastomotic substenosis (six patients), acute urinary retention (two patients), hemorrhagia (one patient), and pelvic abscess (one patient). Only this latter complication required reoperation.

Abdominal Approach

It is generally asserted that the abdominal approach is considered to be the choice for patients in health conditions while the perineal approach is reserved for older patients or patients with compromising health conditions [40]. Ripstein rectopexy, however, can be performed with low mortality and recurrence rate. Increased constipation is a problem with this procedure, especially in patients with internal rectal intussusception. In a recent study, the number of bowel movements per week significantly decreased postoperatively ($p<0.001$) [41]. The section of rectal lateral ligaments has been advocated as a cause of prolonged intestinal transit time that occurs after this operation [42, 43], even if this hypothesis has not been confirmed by a more recent paper [44]. In patients with a solitary rectal ulcer, the presence of a rectal intussusception at proctography seems to be a positive predictive factor for good surgical outcome after sacral rectopexy [45] (Fig. X.3). The anatomical correction of rectal intussusception is obtained in almost 100% of cases, but postoperative constipation has been described in up to 38–47% of patients [46–48].

Different authors have reported a statistically significant improvement in constipation and incontinence after rectopexy and resection of the sigma (Frykman-Goldberg technique) associated with a low complication rate [49–51]. An increase in anal resting and squeezing pressure has been shown and directly correlated to improvement of continence [51], which was more evident at 6 months' follow-up [52]. The incidence of postoperative constipation in patients who underwent rectopexy with resection of the sigma was reduced when compared with rectopexy without resection [50, 53, 54].

The laparoscopic approach in comparison with the laparotomic approach has shown the following advantages: reduction of postoperative pain and minor use of analgesics, reduction of surgical morbidity, minor aesthetic damage, minor recovery time, and earlier return to work [50]. Similar, however, are the results regarding the cure of a complete rectal prolapse. Access via laparoscopy seems to have a minor postoperative morbidity of between 4% and 9% but presents a more prolonged operative time, especially during the learning curve [55, 56]. Recent studies have confirmed that the retrospective [51, 57–59] or prospective comparison between the "open" technique and laparoscopy is in favor of the latter. In addition, a study on economic impact demonstrated that laparoscopic rectopexy in comparison with the open procedure, other than giving better clinical results, cost less [60].

The role of the laparoscopic approach for the treatment of rectal prolapse has been studied extensively since the end of the 1980's but only recently comparative studies with laparotomy considering the different procedures (direct suture, use of a mesh, and resection rectopexy) have been conducted. Most of the literature seems to assert that the benefits of the abdominal approach consist, principally, in the reduced occurrence of relapses and in the best functional results for the complete prolapse of the rectum [61, 62]. Unfortunately, many studies are not comparable due to the different classifications used, the definitions of success, and for the often short follow-up. In 72 patients with intestinal transit time prolonged on the left side, direct rectopexy and resection rectopexy resulted, at an average follow-up of 30 months, in an improvement or a recovery in 76% of cases and a worsening in 9% of cases [63].

Constipation and symptoms of difficult evacuation have been solved or alleviated in 70% of patients who underwent sacral rectopexy and in 64% of those who underwent colonic resection, both with a laparoscopic approach [64]. In a retrospective study comparing use of mesh, direct suture, and resection rectopexy, the latter offered better functional results, in particular for the improvement of constipation. The use of mesh did not seem to add any particular advantage [65], even considering the incidence of recurrences of prolapse [66]. A more empiric approach, based on the preoperative clinical evaluation, seems to give a greater guarantee of success; in fact, by performing the Wells technique in patients with fecal incontinence and the resection rectopexy in those with constipation, after an average follow-up of 18 months, anal incontinence and constipation improved in 80% and 91% of cases, respectively [67].

To avoid the posterior dissection of the rectum, a possible cause of postoperative constipation due to lesion of the autonomic nerves, an alternative technique has recently been proposed consisting of a ventral rectopexy performed by a laparoscopic approach [68]. After a medium follow-up of 61 months, 16/19 patients with obstructed defecation resulted asymptomatic and 28/31 incontinent patients improved significantly their continence. However, two patients developed symptoms of constipation in the postoperative period [68]. Age had no influence on the functional results obtained. The results did not differ in patients who were older or younger than 70 years [69].

Combined Repair

As already underlined, the combined repair of anterior and posterior perineum is mandatory in order to avoid multiple operations with higher risk of complications [70]. Eighty-nine patients underwent combined surgery, and 60 of these patients had a concurrent vaginal repair.

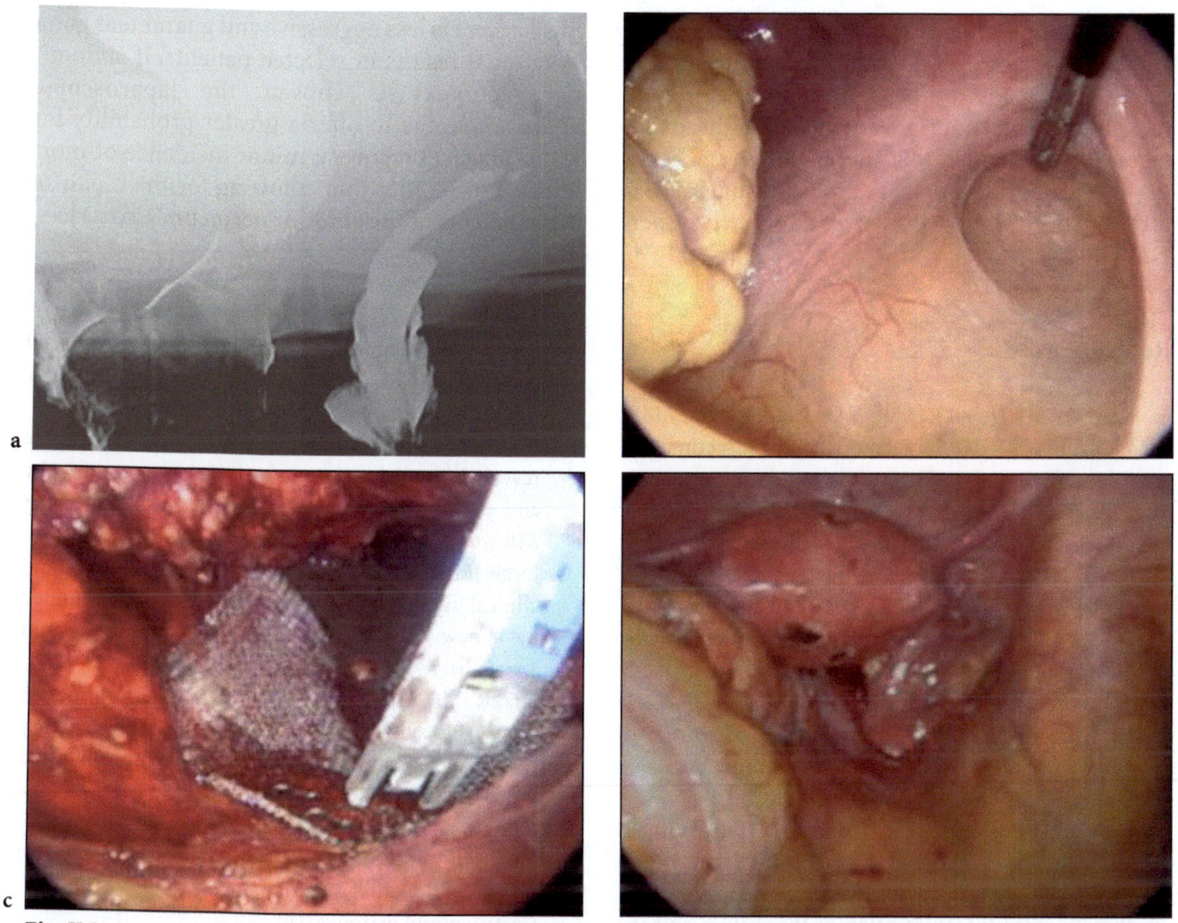

Fig. X.3. A 62-year-old woman afflicted by obstructed defecation. Cystocolpodefecography confirms suspicion of rectoanal intussusception and a large enterocele (**a**). Videolaparoscopic view of the very deep pouch of Douglas (**b**). After isolation of the rectum, sparing the hypogastric nerves, the lateral ligaments, and the uterosacral ligaments, the polypropylene mesh is fixed below the sacral promontorium and distally to the lateral wall of the rectum and the posterior vaginal fornix (**c**). End of the operation after obliteration of the pouch of Douglas by two purse-string sutures (**d**)

Improvement occurred in all major symptoms, and for all patients, this operation provided considerable relief of symptoms, with no evidence of recurrence of rectal or vaginal-vault prolapse at follow-up [71]. In case of vaginal-vault prolapse or enterocele, the associated abdominal colposacropexy with mesh has a cure rate of 90 % and a risk of mesh erosion of 3.3% [72–74].

Final Considerations

The not always encouraging results of surgery for outlet obstruction are probably not linked only to problems of technique. The centrality of the problem is not exclusively mechanic but is also, if not mostly, biological. This is confirmed by the involvement of the psyche [17, 18] and also by the global alteration of intestinal motility, not only limited to the function of the large bowel [75]. Motility alterations can be, at times, identified by anorectal manometry. Rectal hyposensitivity and sensory threshold volumes elevated beyond the normal range have been found in 33% of patients with rectocele, in 40% of rectal intussusception, and in 53% of patients with no mechanical obstruction evident on defecography [76]. This suggests that damage to the rectal wall can be associated with, and not only consequential to, rectal intussusception.

In conclusion, medical treatment must be absolutely considered at the beginning: correction of diet, implementation of fiber and water, and biofeedback, along with great attention to the patients' psychological aspects. Only after the failure of this phase should a workup for the static and dynamic evaluation of organs of the pelvis and perineum be carried out. If necessary, surgery should be proposed after a clear discussion with the patient regarding advantages and disadvantages. If it confirmed that there is no overwhelming clinical evidence that tends to suggest one form of surgical procedure over another [77], perineal access is less aggressive and guarantees good functional results in selected patients. If abdominal rectopexy is chosen, the laparoscopic approach seems to offer a greater probability for faster physical recovery, minor incidence of morbidity and – other than allowing for the repair of some defects of the anterior perineum – costs less.

References

1. Keighley MR (1993) Rectal prolapse. In: Keighley MR, Williams NS (eds) Surgery of the anus, rectum and colon. WB Saunders, London, pp 675–719
2. Thakar R, Stanton S (2002) Management of genital prolapse. BMJ 324:1258–1262
3. Petros P (2003) Changes in bladder neck geometry and closure pressure after midurethral anchoring suggest a musculoelastic mechanism activates closure. Neurourol Urodyn 22:191–197
4. Thompson JR, Chen AH, Pettit PD, Bridges MD (2002) Incidence of occult rectal prolapse in patients with clinical rectoceles and defecatory dysfunction. Am J Obstet Gynecol 187:1494–1499
5. Shorvon PJ, McHugh S, Diamant NE et al (1989) Defecography in normal volunteers: results and implications. Gut 30:1737–1749
6. Ihre T (1990) Intussusception of the rectum and the solitary rectal ulcer syndrome. Ann Med 22:419–423
7. Pomerri F, Zuliani M, Mazza C et al (2001) Defecographic measurements of rectal intussusception and prolapse in patients and in asymptomatic subjects. AJR Am J Roentgenol 176:641–645
8. Muller-Lissner SA, Bartolo DCC, Christiansen J et al (1998) Interobserver agreement in defecography – an international study. Zeit Gastroenterol 36:273–279
9. Kelvin FM, Maglinte DD, Hale DS, Benson JT (2000) Female pelvic organ prolapse: a comparison of triphasic dynamic MR imaging and triphasic fluoroscopic cystocolpoproctography. AJR Am J Roentgenol 174:81–88
10. Rentsch M, Paetzel C, Lenhart M et al (2001) Dynamic magnetic resonance imaging defecography: a diagnostic alternative in the assessment of pelvic floor disorders in proctology. Dis Colon Rectum 44:999–1007
11. Mellgren A, Bremmer S, Johansson C et al (1994) Defecography. Results of investigations in 2816 patients. Dis Colon Rectum 37:1133–1141
12. Bremmer S, Mellgren A, Holmstrom B, Uden R (1998) Peritoneocele and enterocele. Formation and transformation during rectal evacuation as studied by means of defaeco-peritoneography. Acta Radiol 39:167–175
13. Peters WA 3rd, Smith MR, Drescher CW (2001) Rectal prolapse in women with other defects of pelvic floor support. Am J Obstet Gynecol 184:1488–1494
14. Halligan S, Bartram C, Hall C (1996) Enterocele revealed by simultaneous evacuation proctography and peritoneography: does "defecation block" exist? AJR Am J Roentgenol 167:461–466
15. Jorge JM, Yang YK, Wexner SD (1994) Incidence and clinical significance of sigmoidoceles as determined by a new classification system. Dis Colon Rectum 37:1112–1117
16. Jarrett ME, Emmanuel AV, Vaizey CJ, Kamm MA (2004). Behavioural therapy (biofeedback) for solitary rectal ulcer syndrome improves symptoms and mucosal blood flow. Gut 53:368–370
17. Wang J, Luo MH, Qi QH, Dong ZL (2003) Prospective study of biofeedback retraining in patients with chronic idiopathic functional constipation. World J Gastroenterol 9:2109–2113
18. Emmanuel AV, Mason HJ, Kamm MA (2001) Relationship between psychological state and level of activity of extrinsic gut innervation in patients with a functional gut disorder. Gut 49:209–213
19. Felt-Bersma RJ, Cuesta MA (2001) Rectal prolapse, rectal intussusception, rectocele, and solitary rectal ulcer syndrome. Gastroenterol Clin North Am 30:199–222
20. Malouf AJ, Vaizey CJ, Kamm MA (2001) Results of behavioral treatment (biofeedback) for solitary rectal ulcer syndrome. Dis Colon Rectum 44:72–76
21. Tjandra JJ, Ooi B-S, Tang C-L et al (1999) Transanal repair of rectocele corrects obstructed defecation if it is not associated with anismus. Dis Colon Rectum 42:1544–1550
22. Block IR (1986) Transrectal repair of rectocele using obliterative suture. Dis Colon Rectum 29:707–711
23. Infantino A, Masin A, Melega E et al (1995) Does surgery resolve outlet obstruction from rectocele? Int J Colorectal Dis 10:97–100
24. Ayabaca SM, Zbar AP, Pescatori M (2002) Anal continence after rectocele repair. Dis Colon Rectum 45:63–69
25. D'Avolio M, Ferrara A, Chimenti C (2005) Transanal rectocele repair using EndoGIA: short-term results of a prospective study. Tech Coloproctol 9:108–114

26. Altomare DF, Rinaldi M, Veglia A et al (2002) Combined perineal and endorectal repair of rectocele by circular stapler: a novel surgical technique. Dis Colon Rectum 45:1549–1552
27. Boccasanta P, Venturi M, Cioffi U et al (2002) Selection criteria and long-term results of surgery in symptomatic rectocele. Minerva Chir 57:157–163
28. Boccasanta P, Venturi M, Salamina G et al (2004) New trends in the surgical treatment of outlet obstruction: clinical and functional results of two novel transanal stapled techniques from a randomised controlled trial. Int J Colorectal Dis 19:359–369
29. Boccasanta P, Venturi M, Stuto A et al (2004) Stapled transanal rectal resection for outlet obstruction: a prospective, multicenter trial. Dis Colon Rectum 47:1285–1296
30. Mathur P, Ng KH, Seow-Choen F (2004) Stapled mucosectomy for rectocele repair: a preliminary report. Dis Colon Rectum 47:1978–1980
31. Dodi G, Pietroletti R, Milito G et al (2003) Bleeding, incontinence, pain and constipation after STARR transanal double stapling rectotomy for obstructed defecation. Tech Coloproctol 7:148–153
32. Binda GA, Pescatori M, Romano G (2005) The dark side of double-stapled transanal rectal resection. Dis Colon Rectum 48:1830–1831
33. Pescatori M, Seow-Choen F (2003) Use and abuse of new technologies in colorectal surgery. Tech Coloproctol 7:1–2
34. Jayne DG, Finan PJ (2005) Stapled transanal rectal resection for obstructed defaecation and evidence-based practice. Br J Surg 92:793–794
35. Lechaux JP, Lechaux D, Perez M (1995) Results of Delorme's procedure for rectal prolapse. Advantages of a modified technique. Dis Colon Rectum 38:301–307
36. Berman IR, Harris MS, Rabeler MB (1990) Delorme's transrectal excision for internal rectal prolapse: patient selection, technique, and three-year follow-up. Dis Colon Rectum 33:573–580
37. Liberman H, Hughes C, Dippolito A (2000) Evaluation and outcome of the Delorme procedure in the treatment of rectal outlet obstruction. Dis Colon Rectum 43:188–192
38. Sielzneff I, Malouf A, Cesari J et al (1999) Selection criteria for rectal prolapse repair by Delorme's transrectal excision. Dis Colon Rectum 42:367–373
39. Plusa SM, Charing LA, Balaji V et al (1995) Physiologic changes after Delorme's procedure for full-thickness rectal prolapse. Br J Surg 82:1475–1478
40. Madiba TE, Baig MK, Wexner SD (2005) Surgical management of rectal prolapse. Arch Surg 140:63–73
41. Schultz I, Mellgren A, Dolk A et al (2000) Long-term results and functional outcome after Ripstein rectopexy. Dis Colon Rectum 43:35–43
42. Speakman CTM, Madden MV, Nicholls RJ, Kamm MA (1991) Lateral ligament division during rectopexy causes constipation but prevents recurrence: results of a prospective randomized study. Br J Surg 78:1431–1433
43. Scaglia M, Fasth S, Hallgren T et al (1994) Abdominal rectopexy for rectal prolapse. Influence of surgical technique on functional outcome. Dis Colon Rectum 37:805–813
44. Mollen RM, Kuijpers JH, van Hoek F (2000) Effects of rectal mobilization and lateral ligaments division on colonic and anorectal function. Dis Colon Rectum 43:1283–1287
45. Nicholls RJ (1991) Internal intussusception: the solitary rectal ulcer syndrome. In: Goldberg SM, Madoff RD (eds) Semin Colon Rect Surg 2:227–232
46. Himpens J, Cadière GB, Bruyns J, Vertruyen M (1999) Laparoscopic rectopexy according to Wells. Surg End 13:139–141
47. Broden G, Dolk A, Holmstrom B (1988) Recovery of the internal anal sphincter following rectopexy: a possible explanation for continence improvement. Int J Colorectal Dis 3:23–28
48. Mann CV, Hoffman C (1988) Complete rectal prolapse: anatomical and functional results of treatment with extended abdominal rectopexy. Br J Surg 75:34–37
49. Briel JW, Schouten WR, Boerma MO (1997) Long-term results of suture rectopexy in patients with fecal incontinence associated with incomplete rectal prolapse. Dis Colon Rectum 40:1228–1232
50. McKee RF, Lauder JC, Poon FW et al (1992) A prospective randomized study of abdominal rectopexy with and without sigmoidectomy in rectal prolapse. Surg Gynec Obstet 174:145–148
51. Huber FT, Stein H, Siewert JR (1995) Functional results after treatment of rectal prolapse with rectopexy and sigmoid resection. World J Surg 19:138–143
52. Schultz I, Mellgren A, Dolk A et al (1996) Continence is improved after the Ripstein rectopexy. Different mechanism in rectal prolapse and rectal intussusception? Dis Colon Rectum 39:300–306
53. Luukkonen P, Mikkonen U, Jarvinen H (1992) Abdominal rectopexy with sigmoidectomy vs rectopexy alone for rectal prolapse: a prospective, randomized study. Int J Colorectal Dis 7:219–222
54. Jacobs LK, Lin YJ, Orkin BA (1997) The best operation for rectal prolapse. Surg Clin North Am 77:49–71
55. Kairaluoma MV, Viljakka MT, Kellokumpu IH (2003) Open vs. laparoscopic surgery for rectal prolapse: a case-controlled study assessing short-term outcome. Dis Colon Rectum 46:353–360
56. Ashari LH, Lumley JW, Stevenson AR, Stitz RW (2005) Laparoscopically-assisted resection rectopexy for rec-

tal prolapse: ten years' experience. Dis Colon Rectum 48:982–987
57. Demirbas S, Akin ML, Kalemoglu M et al (2005) Comparison of laparoscopic and open surgery for total rectal prolapse. Surg Today 35:446–452
58. Lechaux D, Trebuchet G, Siproudhis L, Campion JP (2005) Laparoscopic rectopexy for full-thickness rectal prolapse: a single-institution retrospective study evaluating surgical outcome. Surg Endosc 19:514–518
59. Rose J, Schneider C, Scheidbach H et al (2002) Laparoscopic treatment of rectal prolapse: experience gained in a prospective multicenter study. Langenbecks Arch Surg 387:130–137
60. Salkeld G, Bagia M, Solomon M (2004) Economic impact of laparoscopic versus open abdominal rectopexy. Br J Surg 91:1188–1191
61. Senagore AJ (2003) Management of rectal prolapse: the role of laparoscopic approaches. Semin Laparosc Surg 10:197–202
62. Solomon MJ, Young CJ, Eyers AA, Roberts RA (2002) Randomized clinical trial of laparoscopic versus open abdominal rectopexy for rectal prolapse. Br J Surg 89:35–39
63. Bruch HP, Herold A, Schiedeck T, Schwandner O (1999) Laparoscopic surgery for rectal prolapse and outlet obstruction. Dis Colon Rectum 42:1189–1194
64. Kellokumpu IH, Vironen J, Scheinin T (2000) Laparoscopic repair of rectal prolapse: a prospective study evaluating surgical outcome and changes in symptoms and bowel function. Surg Endosc 14:634–640
65. Benoist S, Taffinder N, Gould S et al (2001) Functional results two years after laparoscopic rectopexy. Am J Surg 182:168–173
66. Tsugawa K, Sue K, Koyanagi N et al (2002) Laparoscopic rectopexy for recurrent rectal prolapse: a safe and simple procedure without a mesh prosthesis. Hepatogastroenterology 49:1549–1551
67. Madbouly KM, Senagore AJ, Delaney CP et al (2003) Clinically based management of rectal prolapse. Surg Endosc 17:99–103
68. D'Hoore A, Cadoni R, Penninckx F (2004) Long-term outcome of laparoscopic ventral rectopexy for total rectal prolapse. Br J Surg 91:1500–1505
69. Kaiwa Y, Kurokawa Y, Namiki K et al (2004) Outcome of laparoscopic rectopexy for complete rectal prolapse in patients older than 70 years versus younger patients. Surg Today 34:742–746
70. Nager CW, Kumar D, Kahn MA, Stanton SL (1997) Management of pelvic floor dysfunction. Lancet 350:1751
71. Collopy BT, Barham KA (2002) Abdominal colporectopexy with pelvic cul-de-sac closure. Dis Colon Rectum 45:522–526
72. Timmons MC, Addison WA, Addison SB, Cavenar MG (1992) Abdominal sacral colpopexy in 163 women with posthysterectomy vaginal vault prolapse and enterocele. Evolution of operative techniques. J Reprod Med 37:323–327
73. Fox SD, Stanton SL (2000) Vault prolapse and rectocele: assessment of repair using sacrocolpopexy with mesh interposition. Br J Obstet Gynecol 107:1371–1375
74. Visco AG, Weidner AC, Barber MD et al (2001) Vaginal mesh erosion after abdominal sacral colpopexy. Am J Obstet Gynecol 184:297–302
75. Bassotti G, de Roberto G, Sediari L, Morelli A (2004) Colonic motility studies in severe chronic constipation: an organic approach to a functional problem. Tech Coloproctol 8:147–150
76. Gladman MA, Scott SM, Williams NS, Lunniss PJ (2003) Clinical and physiological findings, and possible aetiological factors of rectal hyposensitivity. Br J Surg 90:860–866
77. Bachoo P, Brazzelli M, Grant A (2001) Surgery for complete rectal prolapse in adults (Cochrane Review). In: The Cochrane Library, 1

Invited Commentary

U. Karlbom, L. Påhlman

The majority of constipated patients experience some or several symptoms related to obstructed defecation. A sense of incomplete rectal emptying is also a symptom coherent with irritable bowel syndrome (IBS). Both constipation and IBS are common in the general population, so symptoms of obstructed defecation will be encountered frequently.

When defining slow-transit constipation, a radiological measurement of colonic transit time is always used. The transit study may also be repeated for correct diagnosis if surgery is planned. Objective measurements of rectal evacuation are not used as frequently as transit-time studies. The evacuation capacity can be assessed by a balloon expulsion tests or by defecography. Time to expel (evacuate), completeness of evacuation, or evacuation rate are examples of parameters to measure. The correlation between subjectively obstructed defecation and objectively measured evacuation is not strong. Several factors (i.e., psychological, bowel motility, sensibility) may thus be of importance when evaluating obstructed defecation, which also has been pointed out in the text.

In the workup of obstructed defecation, some diagnoses are associated with impaired rectal evacuation. Paradoxical puborectalis contraction (anismus) can be diagnosed by sphincter electromyogram (EMG) or defecography. The importance of this diagnosis has been debated, but irrespective of the diagnostic method used, the diagnosis has been related to impaired rectal evacuation. In a similar way, a rectocele has been related to delayed and incomplete evacuation. Other findings at defecography, such as mucosal infolding, internal rectal intussusception, prolapse, and enterocele, do not seem to affect rectal emptying. One possible explanation that these conditions may be a cause of symptoms is that they are occupying space in or adjacent to the rectum, which can give a sensation of incomplete emptying.

There are numerous surgical techniques – laparoscopic or traditional – for treatment of the above-mentioned conditions. The results of surgical correction of anatomy, i.e., internal rectal intussusception, are difficult to predict although some patients are relieved of symptoms whereas others have aggravated symptoms of constipation. On the other hand, repair of a rectocele seems to be associated with a high success rate, both via the anal and the vaginal route. The best technique for rectal prolapse surgery has been debated for many years. Evaluation of results is complex because local control of prolapse, fecal incontinence, and constipation has to be assessed. At present, there are some larger ongoing, randomized trials comparing surgical techniques in the treatment of rectal prolapse. This will hopefully give us a better rationale for selecting technique. The new emerging stapled transanal rectal resection (STARR) for obstructed defecation seems promising but has finally to be evaluated in a randomized manner. Optimally, these studies should not only address symptoms but also an objective measurement of rectal evacuation and a postoperative assessment if anatomical correction is achieved.

We agree with Infantino and colleagues that primary treatment of obstructed defecation is conservative. Biofeedback may be highly successful in selected patients but still have a 40–60 % success rate when used more generally. A large, nonemptying rectocele is an indication for surgery.

Subject Index

MIX
Papier aus verantwortungsvollen Quellen
Paper from responsible sources
FSC® C105338

If you have any concerns about our products,
you can contact us on
ProductSafety@springernature.com

In case Publisher is established outside the EU,
the EU authorized representative is:
Springer Nature Customer Service Center GmbH
Europaplatz 3, 69115 Heidelberg, Germany

Printed by Libri Plureos GmbH
in Hamburg, Germany